STOICHIOMETRY AND RESEARCH – THE IMPORTANCE OF QUANTITY IN BIOMEDICINE

Edited by **Alessio Innocenti**

Stoichiometry and Research – The Importance of Quantity in Biomedicine
Edited by Alessio Innocenti

Published by InTech

Janeza Trdine 9, 51000 Rijeka, Croatia

Publishing Process Manager Bojan Rafaj

Technical Editor Teodora Smiljanic

Cover Designer InTech Design Team

Additional hard copies can be obtained from orders@intechopen.com

Stoichiometry and Research – The Importance of Quantity in Biomedicine,
Edited by Alessio Innocenti
p. cm.
ISBN 978-953-51-0198-7

For EU product safety concerns:
IN TECH d.o.o., Prolaz Marije Krucifikse Kozulić 3, 51000 Rijeka, Croatia,
info@intechopen.com or visit our website at intechopen.com.

Meet the editor

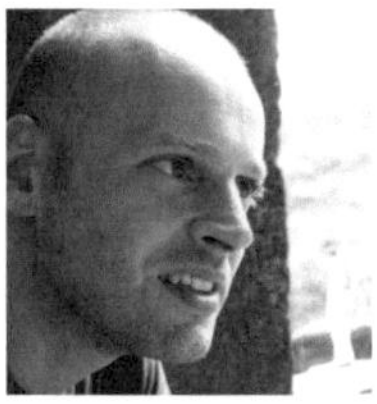

Alessio Innocenti was born in 1974. He graduated in Chemistry, with a specialization in Pharmacology, from University of Florence, Italy, in 2002. He received a PhD in Chemical Sciences from the University of Florence in 2006 and, since then, has been working as a postdoctoral Research Associate at the Department of Chemistry, University of Florence. He is responsible for the experimental assays of the research group, working on enzymatic kinetics and inhibition studies and focusing in particular on the carbonic anhydrase family. Since 2004 he has been included in four European collaborative projects involving a network of several universities and research institutes all over the European Union. His passion and enthusiasm for research has led to the publication of 133 scientific papers in peer-reviewed international journals so far. Since 2003 he has been a General Chemistry Instructor at the Department of Pharmacy at the University of Florence, trying to transmit his love for Chemistry to his students.

Contents

Preface

Science seeks to understand and explain our world, be that its physical composition (geology), chemical composition (chemistry), the way its composite matter interacts (physics), or the organisms that inhabit it (biology). We can only get an idea of what life is all about by piecing together information from each discipline to give us the big picture.

We don't have to look very far to realize that it is difficult, if not impossible, to separate biology from chemistry. After all, our body is a bag of chemicals. The proteins that form our hair, nails and muscle fibers are chemicals; the minerals that are the basis of our own bones and teeth are chemicals; even the food and drinks we consume are chemicals.

Chemistry explores life at the level of atoms and molecules. It is really all about understanding how atoms interact to form larger, more complicated substances. Biology then looks at their behavior when they are combined on a larger scale (cells, tissues, organisms, populations). Chemistry is encapsulated by a handful of essential concepts that are epitomized by the world around us. Just grasping these concepts is sufficient to get to grips with many of the key chemical principles that underpin biology.

Life is the result of thousands of different biochemical reactions occurring in every cell of our body. At first glance many of these reactions seem very complicated. Beneath the façade of complexity, however, lie simple principles and tools that give support to all chemical reactions. Some of them undergo the general concept of stoichiometry.

The word stoichiometry may sound mysterious, but it is simply based on Greek words meaning 'element measure'. It is a branch of chemistry that deals with the relative quantities of reactants and products in chemical reactions. At first blush one could think of stoichiometry as something confined to a general chemistry course or a student laboratory, but a deeper consideration of the term itself reveals a surprisingly wide range of applications. We are surrounded every day by tens of thousands of different chemical compounds with contrasting characteristics. Sometimes, the presence of a compound is essential for our existence, like O_2 in the air or glucose in the food. By contrast, the presence of a compound may be detrimental, like pollutants in the water of alcohol in our blood stream. This is the reason why we need ways of determining what is in our chemical environment, of knowing what is there and, more importantly, how much. Evaluating the amount of a compound we have in a system is often vital: too much of a compound may be toxic to the point of being lethal, too little may be equally harmful.

The aim of this book is to provide an overview of the importance of stoichiometry in the biomedical field. It contains a collection of selected research articles and reviews all providing adequate and up-to-date information related to stoichiometry from different point of views. The first section deals with host-guest chemistry, focusing on selected calixarenes, cyclodextrins and crown ethers derivatives. In the second and third sections the book presents some issues concerning stoichiometry of metal complexes and lipids and polymers architecture. The fourth section aims to to clarify the role of stoichiometry in the determination of protein interactions, while in the fifth section some selected experimental techniques applied to specific systems are introduced. The last section of the book is an attempt at showing some interesting connections between biomedicine and the environment, introducing the concept of biological stoichiometry and presenting some data that prove how the two disciplines entwine. On this basis, the present volume would definitely be an ideal source of scientific information to advanced students, junior researchers, faculties and scientists involved in biomedicine, biochemistry and other areas involving stoichiometry evaluation.

A special word of appreciation is due to Mr Bojan Rafaj, the Publishing Process Manager who oversaw and coordinated the publishing of all materials and assisted me and the authors in completing our work easily and in a timely manner. My profound thanks also to the technical editor who prepared these manuscripts for publication by InTech - Open Access Publisher.

Dr. Alessio Innocenti
Department of Chemistry,
University of Florence,
Italy

Part 1

The Importance of Stoichiometry in Host-Guest Chemistry

1

Stoichiometric Ratio in Calixarene Complexes

Flor de María Ramírez and Irma García-Sosa
Instituto Nacional de Investigaciones Nucleares
México

1. Introduction

Stoichiometry is a fundamental concept in chemistry that refers to the ratios of products and reactants in any chemical reaction. It is an important concept in both chemical reactions and biochemical processes. A stoichiometric ratio represents the relationship among the elements or molecules present in an equation. Using the correct stoichiometric amount of reactant will yield the maximum amount of product under the proper thermodynamic and kinetic conditions.

This chapter will be focused on the latest research, from our and other labs, on the determination of stoichiometric ratios for complexed species formed between substrates and calixarene receptors, the influence of size, conformation and functionalization site of calixarenes on the stoichiometry, as well as solvent effects and the stability of the complexes in the liquid and solid states. No formation (stability) constants will be discussed, although in some cases these could be mentioned.

Particular attention will be paid to the experimental methods used for stoichiometry determination. Furthermore, complexed calixarene molecules in 1:1, 1:2 and 2:1 (Substrate:Calixarene) stoichiometries calculated by Augmented MM3 and CONFLEX semiempirical procedures, and other computational calculations will be included.

The enormous number of sophisticated functionalized calixarenes published so far, forced us to be selective. Therefore, our attention will be devoted to the stoichiometry of complexes formed with parent calixarenes (Gutsche, 1989, 1998, Mandolini & Ungaro 2000) functionalized at the lower and upper rims, with linear arms, that were first reported between 1999 and 2011.

2. A brief overview of calixarenes

Calixarenes are an important group of macrocycles, considered the third best host (receptors) molecules after cyclodextrins and crown ethers (Shinkai, 1993). They are prepared by condensation reactions between para-substituted phenols and formaldehyde (Gutsche, 1989). Here, we focus on conventional *endo*-calixarenes, which have a lipophilic cavity and two rims: the polar lower rim and the apolar upper rim that provides an unusual flexibility to the calixarene that can be modulated by adjusting cavity size and the rim substituents size. Its basket-like structure, with a lipophilic cavity made up of aromatic nuclei and easily modified rims, has attracted the attention of many theoretical and experimental researchers.

With exceptions, macrocycle flexibility, i.e. conformational movement, increases with size. Calix[*n*]arenes (where *n* stands for the number of aryl groups in the macrocycle) with $n = 4$ to 20 have been synthesized (Gutsche, 1998), but only the smaller cycles ($n = 4$, 6 and 8) have been thoroughly studied. Calixarenes are versatile macrocycles with almost unlimited properties (Böhmer, 1995); they are excellent scaffolds since their conformation can be adapted to potential guests, and they can be selectively functionalized at three sites (Asfari et al., 2001; Mandolini & Ungaro, 2000). Most commonly, specific groups or substituents called pendant arms are added to the rims to impart a specific function.

Calixarenes are very attractive to researchers from numerous science and technology fields (Fig. 1). A vast array of functionalized calixarenes have been reported over the last decade (Alexandratos and Natesan, 2000; Gutsche, 1998; Lumetta et al., 2000; Mandolini and Ungaro, 2000; Mokhtari et al., 2011a, 2011b; Sliwa, 2002; Sliwa & Girck, 2010; Talanova, 2000). The challenge is to quickly synthesize suitable calixarenes on a large scale with minimal workup.

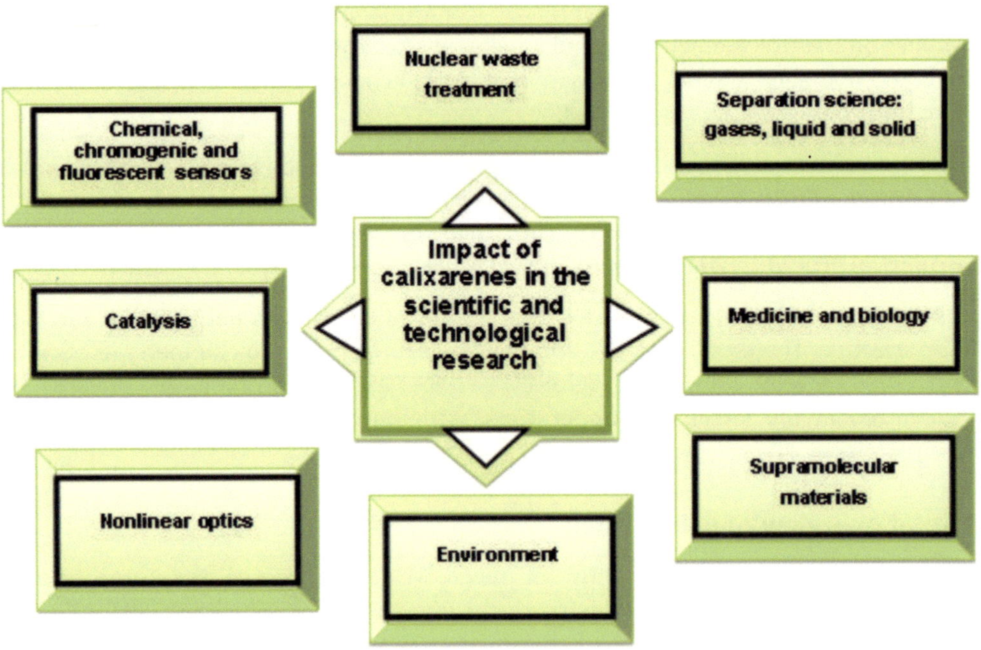

Fig. 1. Applications for calixarenes in science and technology.

In Fig. 2, a selection of recently reported calixarenes are presented.

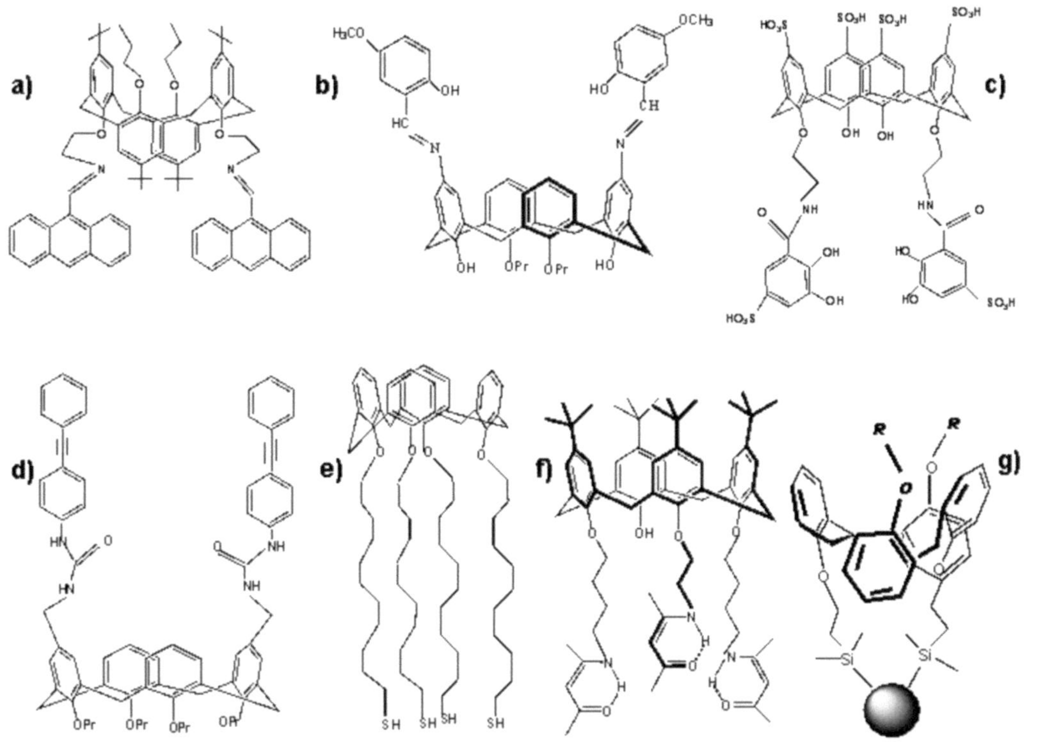

Fig. 2. Some interesting calixarene molecules built with ChemDraw Ultra 10.0 software. a) Zheng et al. (2010), b) Liang et al. (2007), c) Leydier et al. (2008), d) Bew et al. (2010), e) Snejdarkova et al. (2010), f) Sliwa& Deska, (2008), g) Sliwka-Kaszynska et al. (2009), articles cited by Mokhtari et al., 2011b.

3. Finding the stoichiometric ratio

The method of continuous variation involves a series of isomolar solutions of two reactants. It is one commonly used experimental mixing technique for determining formula and formation constants of complexes. The method is also known as Job's method, for his general development of spectrophotometric measurement techniques (Gil & Oliveira, 1990). However, it was Ostromisslensky in 1911 who (Hill & MacCarthy, 1986; Likussar & Boltz, 1971) first employed the method to establish the 1:1 stoichiometry of the adduct formed between nitrobenzene and aniline. Other methods, such as molar ratios and titration in a single flask, are also currently used to investigate the stoichiometry of complexes.

3.1 Job's method

Job's method is carried out in a batch mode (series of solutions) by mixing aliquots of two equimolecular stock solutions of two components (metal and ligand, or organic substrate and organic receptor) and diluting to a constant volume to get solutions with identical total molar concentrations but different mole fractions. The sum of the two components analytical concentration is constant while the Component 1:Component 2 ratio varies from flask to flask. Job's method is based on plotting measured absorbance (corrected for reactants absorbance) against the mole fraction of one single component. For stable complexes, the plot is a triangle, with the apex indicating the complex composition. For a moderately stable complex, the stoichiometry can be obtained from the intersection point of the curve tangents, this approximation being valid only for symmetrical plots (e.g. 1:1; 2:2). Weak complexes generally show a very curved plot.

This method works well for reactions where a single equilibrium, or simple equilibriums exist uninfluenced by ionic strength; no more than three species (two reactants and the product) can be present in solution and their complexes have to be very stable. Job's method may be applied to stoichiometric determination in two ways. The Standard Method was described above. The modified Limiting Reagent Method uses a series of solutions with a fixed "moles A" and a varying "moles B," such that the ratio moles B:moles A, goes from 0 to a value known to be larger than x (x equal to moles of B at intersection/(total moles of A plus B minus moles of B at intersection). The amount of product in each solution is then measured. Once the amount of B exceeds the stoichiometrically required amount, A becomes the limiting reagent and the amount of the formed product remains constant.

According to stoichiometric theory, the limiting reagent controls the yield, and the greatest yield is always produced at the stoichiometric equivalence point. The maximum amount of product should occur at the stoichiometric ratio that can be justified both intuitively and mathematically. For both methods, 8-15 experimental data points are required to determine the stoichiometry. The method can be applied to parameters obtained from techniques other than typical spectrophotometry, e.g. luminescence, nuclear magnetic resonance, calorimetry, conductometry.

Job's method has serious limitations for complex reactions systems where the number of species is larger than three. In these cases, two or more complexed species with different stoichiometries are formed, and/or the stability of the complexes is moderate. Moreover, the method fails when the formed complexes are only weakly stable. A simulation program (Gil & Oliveira, 1990) for reaction equilibriums has improved application of Job's method to more complicated systems.

3.2 Spectrophotometric titration

There are several experimental methods to determine stoichiometries for systems with multiple complex species in solution. Spectrophotometric titration monitored by UV/Vis is largely used because UV/Vis spectrophotometers are widely available and inexpensive. The radiant energy absorption of a solution is measured spectrophotometrically after each increment of titrant, but the evaluation is somewhat limited by the solubility of the reactants (but not the products) in water and/or organic solvent.

In macrocyclic coordination chemistry equimolar solutions of the reactants in the same solvent with the same ionic strength are prepared, and two titrations are carried out, titrating the receptor with the substrate and the substrate with the receptor, respectively. In the former, a fixed volume of the receptor solution is titrated by adding varying volumes of the substrate solution. After each addition the UV/Vis spectrum is recorded. The titrant is added until the absorbance at the analyzed wavelength does not change, or until a new band appears. Approximately 30 spectra are required, or enough data collected until a molar ratio [S]/[R]≥ 4 is reached. Specfit or Hyperquad software is used for stoichiometry evaluation.

Spectra, solution concentrations, initial volume, aliquot number and volumes, and the total final volume are fed into the Specfit software. Factor analysis reveals the number of absorbing species, and the data are fitted to models to obtain the stoichiometry of the species and their stability constants. The same steps are followed if a fixed volume of the substrate solution is titrated with a variable volume of the receptor solution.

In the case of calixarene complexes, the titration can be followed by analyzing changes in the physicochemical properties of the receptor or the substrate as the complex is formed (e.g. absorbance, luminescence, NMR chemical shifts, calorimetric changes).

4. Spectroscopic techniques

UV/Vis, ^{1}H'NMR, MS (mass spectrometry) and luminescence are the spectroscopic techniques that are most used for the elucidation of stoichiometry in calixarene complexes with organic or metallic substrates. In general, spectroscopic techniques are complementary, but if the solution contains only one complex species data from a single technique analyzed by Job or/and molar ratio methods may be sufficient. In these cases sometimes only 8 experimental points are required for a Job plot. However, if the solution contains more than two complex species, at least two different techniques and software packages are needed; in some cases the evaluation of stability constants is required to confirm the existence of a complex species in the determined stoichiometry.

The stoichiometry of isolated calixarene complexes in the solid state can be elucidated by microelemental analysis or, if possible, by its X-ray structure. If the complexes dissolve without decomposition, NMR and MS measurements are extremely useful for confirming stoichiometry.

5. Calixarene complexation

Calixarenes can interact with neutral, cationic and anionic organic substrates as well as metal ions; they are sometimes called "molecular baskets" because of this diverse capacity. Calixarenes are neutral but can act as cationic and anionic receptors if adequately functionalized (Asfari et al., 2001; Lumetta et al., 2000; Mandolini & Ungaro, 2000; Mokhtari et al., 2011a, 2011b; Sliwa & Girck, 2010). The calixarene-substrate interaction is illustrated in Fig. 3. Molecular recognition, the strength of the interaction between calixarenes and their substrates and thermodynamic and kinetic factors rule the complexes formation. It is important to keep in mind that the donating ability of solvents plays an import role (Asfari et al., 2001; Mandolini & Ungaro, 2000) in complex stability.

In organic-calixarene complexes (Fig. 3, top right), noncovalent interactions such as hydrogen bonds, π- hydrogen bonds, hydrophobic interactions, and cation-π and CH-π interactions are the main driving forces that allow stable complexes to form in the liquid and solid states (Asfari et al., 2001; García-Sosa & Ramírez, 2010; Mandolini & Ungaro, 2000).

In metal-calixarene complexes (Fig. 3, bottom right), the coordination ability of the calixarene toward the metal ion determines complex formation. Ionic and covalent interactions dominate complex formation and define calixarene complex properties including stoichiometry.

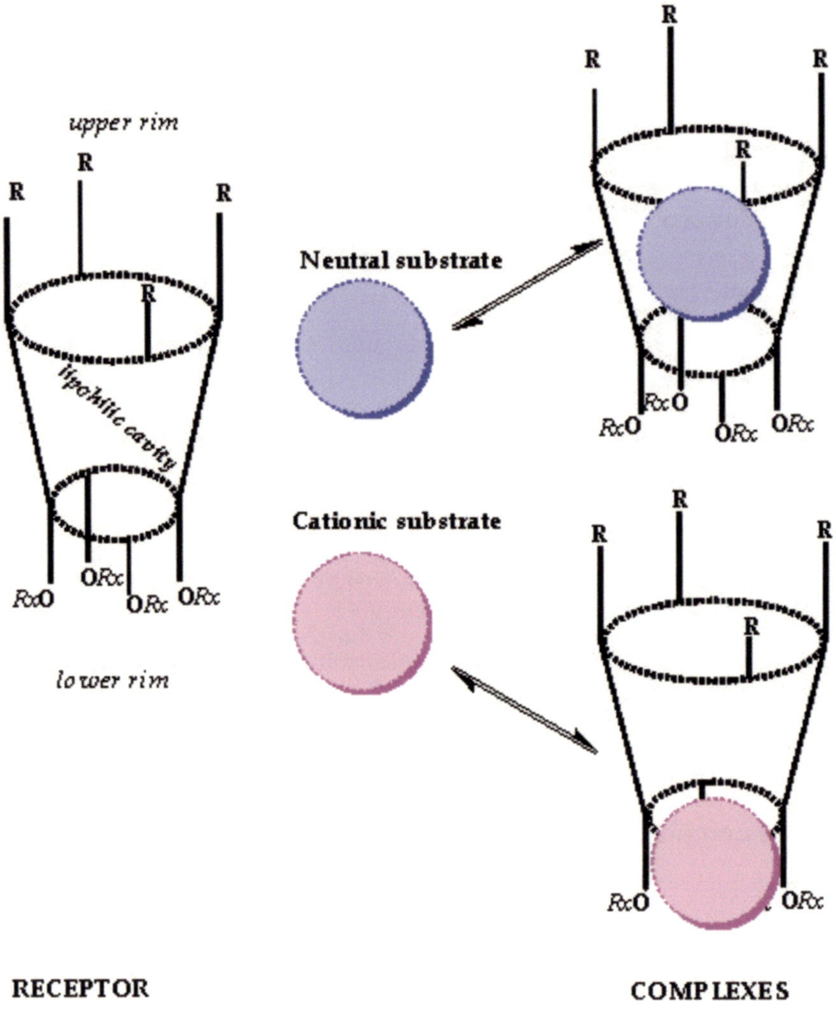

Fig. 3. Schematic representation of calixarene complexation with neutral and cationic substrates.

5.1 Stoichiometry in calixarene complexes with organic substrates in solution

There are a great number of calixarene complexes that are formed from functionalized calixarenes and organic substrates. Investigations into receptor-substrate recognition in solution afford fundamental knowledge and describe environmental, biological and medical applications. However, to the best of our knowledge, little work has been done related to stoichiometric studies of calixarene complexes for biomedical applications.

Here, we discuss some illustrative investigations.

5.1.1 Stoichiometric ratio with neutral calixarenes

Mohammed-Ziegler et al. (2003) investigated complex formation between chromogenic capped calix[4]arene derivatives comprising indophenol indicator group(s) and aliphatic amines in ethanol using UV/Vis spectroscopy. Job's method was applied to quantify the spectral changes using various molar amine/calixarene ligand ratios by maintaining a constant ligand concentration (λmax = 520–534 nm) and varying the amine concentration. A new band emerged at 652–667 nm indicating complexation and adducts with a 1:1 stoichiometry were determined. The study indicated the formation of strong polar supramolecular complexes of calix[4]arenes capped by diamide bridges with the amines, stabilized by various types of host–guest interactions and by steric effects.

Zielenkiewicz et al. (2005) have thoroughly studied the complexation of isoleucine by phosphorylated calix[4]arene in methanol. Calorimetry, NMR and UV/Vis (Job's method) spectroscopy, as well as molecular modeling methods, were used. In methanol, amino acids occur primarily in the form of zwitterions [$H_3N^+CH(R)CO_2^-$], with a protonated amino acid and a dissociated carboxylic group. The association constants determined by spectroscopy agree with data obtained by calorimetry: 25,000 for a 1:1 complex and 1700 for 1:2 isoleucine:calixarene complexes, respectively. The formation of the former is driven by favorable changes both in enthalpy and entropy during complexation while the 1:2 complex is of entropic origin.

The 1:2 complex is the result of inclusion of the amino acid's alkyl chain into the cavity of one calixarene molecule and interaction of the amino acid amino group with the phosphoryl group of a second calixarene. The more stable 1:1 complex points to electrostatic interactions between the positively charged ammonium cations of the amino acid and the phosphoryl groups of the calixarene. The phosphoryl groups appear to serve as the anchoring points for the positively charged ammonium cations of the amino acid, thus leading to a more stable inclusion complex. Complexation of isoleucine also takes place through insertion of the aliphatic moiety of the substrate molecule into the calixarene cavity. Electrostatic interactions are the dominant forces in the complexation process. Molecular modeling results fit extraordinary well with experimental values, corroborating the 1:1 and 1:2: isoleucine:calixarene(s) stoichiometries.

Halder et al. (2010) investigated the effective and selective noncovalent interactions between fullerenes (C_{60} and C_{70}) and para-tert-butylcalix[6]arene in toluene by UV/Vis and NMR methods. Both C_{60} and C_{70} form ground state noncovalent complexes with the calixarene; according to UV/Vis measurements, the complexation process is initiated by charge transfer transition. From Job's method, it was observed that both C_{60} and C_{70} form stable complexes with the calixarene ligand in a 1:1 stoichiometry. According to the binding constants, the calixarene bound strongly and selectively to C_{70}, compared with C_{60}, K = 110,000 and 32,400 $dm^3\ mol^{-1}$, respectively. Proton NMR measurements support a strong complexation between C_{70} and the calixarene ligand.

5.1.2 Stoichiometric ratio with charged calixarenes

Kunsági-Máté et al. (2004) investigated complex formation between C_{60} fullerene (dissolved in toluene) and water-soluble hexasulfonated calix[6]arenes functionalized with sulfonates in the upper rim. Photoluminescence (PL) measurements and Job's method were used for this investigation. The stoichiometry of the complex was 1:1, and related quantum chemical calculations demonstrated that the C_{60} fullerene is located deep within the cavity of the calixarene. This observation makes this calixarene a promising candidate for overcoming the natural water-repulsive character of C_{60} fullerene and could improve the application of fullerenes to biochemical processes.

Zhou et al. (2008) used spectrofluorometric titrations to investigate the inclusion behavior of *p*-(*p*-carboxyl benzeneazo) calix[4]arene with norfloxacin (fungicide) in sodium acetate-acetic acid buffer solution. The fluorescence results indicated a 1:1 complex stoichiometry. Stoichiometry was also evaluated by applying Job's method to fluorescence measurements to verify the 1:1 inclusion complex. Hydrogen bonding and structural matching effects were proposed to play important roles in the formation of the calixarene–norfloxacin complex in water. Furthermore, various factors affecting the inclusion process, such as pH value, ionic strength and surfactants, were examined in detail; the results corroborated the formation of this inclusion complex. The nature of the fungicide-calixarene interaction was mainly electrostatic. This investigation is crucial, since norfloxacin is a third-generation synthetic antibacterial fluoroquinolone agent that is used in the treatment of urinary and respiratory tract infections and gastro-intestinal and sexually transmitted diseases. Therefore, azocalix[*n*]arenes and its inclusion compounds may have potential biological and medical applications.

The effect of adding a macrocycle such as para-sulfonatocalix[6]arene on the fluorescence of benzoimidazolic fungicides such as Benomyl (BY) and Carbendazim (CZ) has been studied by Pacioni et al. (2008) using spectrofluorimetric titrations. Benomyl (BY) and Carbendazim (CZ) interact with para-sulfonatocalix[6]arene to form complexes. Calixarene enhanced the fluorescence of BY in water at pH 1.000 and 25° C. An inclusion complex with 1:1 stoichiometry was formed with the pesticide. The nature of the interactions was mainly electrostatic, i.e. cation–π and ion–ion interactions between the cationic BY and sulfonate groups. The use of macrocyclic nanocavities, compared with other methods, is a very good alternative to determine BY residues in water and fruit samples at low levels, with better or in the same order. The complexation of the neutral CZ occurs at pH 6.994. Two complexes with 1:1 and 1:2 stoichiometries were formed; the latter complex was less fluorescent than the free CZ. π-π stacking and hydrogen bonding are the main driving forces for the 1:1 and 1:2 complexes.

Organic quaternary ammonium ions have been of great interest in molecular recognition studies; paraquat (1,1′-dimethyl-4,4′-bipyridinium dichloride) is an example. Pierro et al. (2009) investigated the conformation fitting of tetramethoxy-para-carboxylatocalix[4]arene and tetrapropiloxi-para-carboxylatocalix[4]arene to paraquat in a $CDCl_3/CD_3OD$ mixture using NMR measurements. This study demonstrated that tetrapropiloxi-para-carboxylatocalix[4]arene and paraquat formed a stable complex with a 1:1 stoichiometry, as estimated by a Job plot. NMR measurements indicated that upon complexation the C_{2v}

structure of the free calixarene switches to an opposite C_{2v} pinched-cone conformation, with the two carboxylato-bearing rings pointing inward the calixarene cavity to maximize electrostatic and van der Waals interactions with the cationic paraquat. These adaptive conformational changes were fully confirmed by molecular modeling. The complexation of paraquat with tetrametoxi- para-carboxylatocalix[4]arene was also monitored with Diffusion-Ordered Spectroscopy (DOSY) NMR. DOSY has been particularly used in the characterization of host–guest systems in solution. The results indicated the formation of a complex in a 1:1 stoichiometry; in this complex, the calixarene was in the cone conformation while the free calixarene was predominantly in the partial-cone conformation.

Methiocarb [3,5-dimethyl-4-(methylthio) phenyl methylcarbamate] is one of the mostly important N-methylcarbamate pesticides, used worldwide in agriculture and health programs. Ding et al. (2011) investigated the complexation between tetrabutyl ether derivatives of p-sulfonatocalix[4]arene (SC4Bu) and methiocarb by fluorescence spectrometry in a mixture of water and DMSO. It was observed that upon the addition of methiocarb, the fluorescence intensity of SC4Bu was quenched and a slight red shift was observed for the maximum emission peak, which is indicative of a calixarene-methiocarb interaction. The results indicated that the SC4Bu-methiocarb complex was formed in a 1:1 mole ratio and that the electrostatic effect is not the main driving force. Using a modeling package it was proposed that complexation was an "external" inclusion process and that the hydrogen bonding between the methyl H atom of methiocarb and the sulfonate of SC4Bu facilitates the formation of this SC4Bu–methiocarb complex in a 1:1 stoichiometry. This study provides useful information for applying calixarenes to pesticide detection.

5.2 Stoichiometry in calixarene complexes formed with organic substrates in solid state

For years, organic frameworks have been suggested as promising gas storage substrates, but purely organic molecular crystals have received little attention. Atwood et al. (2005) studied the absorption of methane in p-tert-butylcalix[4]arene at room temperature and pressures of one atmosphere and lower. The results, supported by purely size–shape considerations, suggest that it is possible to accommodate at least two CH_4 molecules within each dimeric capsule (i.e., calixarene:substrate = 1:1). On the basis of this assumption, preliminary results indicate that on average, at 0.54 atm, 14% of capsules are occupied by two molecules of methane. The results demonstrate that low-density organic systems do indeed deserve consideration as potential sorbants for volatile gases, and that such sorption processes can occur under desirable conditions close to standard temperature and pressure.

Ferreira et al. (2010) studied the inclusion of biacetyl within p-tert-butylcalix[n=4,6]arenes in powdered solid samples using luminescence and diffuse reflectance. Lifetime distribution analysis of the phosphorescence of both complexes suggested *endo*-inclusion calixarene complexes with p-tert-butylcalix[n=4]arene, and *exo*-inclusion calixarene complexes with p-tert-butylcalix[n=6]arene. Although it is not explicit, the stoichiometry of the inclusion complexes seems to be 1:1.

Table 1 summarizes the stoichiometric ratio of some of the discussed organic complexes in solution and in the solid state.

Organic Substrate/calixarene	Technique	Method/ stoichiometry (M:L)	References
Aliphatic amines /chromogenic capped calix[4]arene derivatives	UV/Vis titration in ethanol	Job's Method/(1:1)	Mohammed-Ziegler, et al. (2003)
Isoleucine(peptide)/ phosporylated calix[4]arene.	Insight II package	Molecular Modeling /(1:1)	Zielenkiewicz et al. (2005)
	Calorimetry; NMR titration Methanol	Job's Method/ (1:1, 1:2 2:1; 1:1) /Modeling	
Norfloxacin/*p*-(*p*-carboxyl benzene-azo) calix[4]arene	Fluorescence titration	Job's Method /(1:1)	Zhou et al. (2008).
C_{60} fullerene / sulfonated calixarene	Fluorescence titration	Job's Method /(1:1)	Kunsági-Máté et al. (2004)
Adenine, guanine, cytosine, thymine /calixarene-D2EHPA	Liquid-liquid extraction	Job's Method/(1:1)	Shimojo & Goto (2005).
fullerenes (C_{60} and C_{70}) /para-tert-butylcalix[6]arene	UV/Vis titration toluene	Job's Method (1:1)	Halder et al. (2010)
Benomyl (BY) and Carbendazim (CZ)/ para-sulfonatocalix[6]arene.	fluorescence titration	Job's Method / BY(1:1), CZ(1:1, 1:2)	Pacioni, et al. (2008).
Methane/calixarene	X-ray diffraction	1:1 also modeled	Atwood et al. (2005)
paraquat / tetraalquiloxi-para-carboxylatocalix[4]arene	NMR titration/ $CDCl_3$/CD_3OD	Job's Method(1:1)	Pierro et al. (2009)
N-methylcarbamate/para-sulfonatocalix[4]arene	Fluorescence titration/ H_2O-DMSO	Molecular Modeling (1:1)	Ding et al. (2011)

Table 1. Stoichiometry of organic calixarene species, in solution and in the solid state, and the used techniques for their identification and determination.

Garcia-Sosa & Ramírez (2010) found that para-tert-butylcalix[6]arene and para-tert-butylcalix[8]arene form stable 1:1 complexes with paraquat dichloride (PQ) in the solid state (the complexes were studied in liquid and solid states). The biexponential decay of luminescence and lifetimes proved that the quaternary ammoniums (quats) of the paraquat were not in the same environment for both complexes. This fact correlated with molecular models, since two de-excitation pathways were present with very different lifetimes; the longer lifetime was associated with one methyl-pyridinium head closer to the aryl rings, and the shorter lifetime was associated with the methyl-pyridinium head far from the aryl ring. The former ring is more shielded than the latter. Solution studies (UV/Vis, luminescence) and molecular modeling suggested that the calixarenes interact with the herbicide through cation-π interactions. Paraquat is included in the para-tert-butylcalix[8]arene cavity, but only partially included in the para-tert-butylcalix[6]arene cavity. The theoretical results, in particular using MOPAC procedures, were in good agreement with experimental findings.

The preliminary test in water suggests that the stability of the PQ-para-tert-butylcalix[8]arene complex does not depend on the pH while that of PQ-para-tert-butylcalix[6]arene does. Being the former complex much more stable than the latter in aqueous media, we envision that para-tert-butylcalix[8]arene could be useful in stabilizing paraquat dichloride in solid, organic or water solutions to deposit/de-activate it as waste.

5.3 Stoichiometry of extracted species formed with organic substrates and calixarenes

Calixarenes have been used to separate organic pesticides, pharmaceuticals and dyes that pollute water. However, little attention has been dedicated to the stoichiometric ratio of the extracted species. Here, two examples are presented.

Shimojo & Goto (2005) studied the synergistic extraction of nucleobases by a combination of calixarene and D2EHPA ligands. Liquid-liquid extraction of various nucleobases with a para-tert-octylcalix[6]arene carboxylic acid derivative was carried out to elucidate its molecular recognition properties. Bis-(2-ethylhexyl)phosphoric acid (D2EHPA) was tested as a synergistic reagent to improve the extraction capability of the calixarene toward nucleobases (in buffered water). The efficiency of adenine and cytosine extraction increased drastically in the presence of both extractant ligands dissolved in isooctane. Neither calix[6]arene nor D2EHPA were very effective at nucleobase extraction. According to Job's method, the stoichiometry of the extracted stable species in the case of the better-extracted adenine was 1 adenine:1 calix[6]arene:2 D2EHPA. The authors proposed that D2EHPA is involved in the secondary coordination sphere of the calixarene-adenine complex and that its highly hydrophobic nature enhances the distribution of the complex into isooctane. Recovery of adenine from the organic phase to the aqueous receiving phase is readily achieved under acidic conditions. These results highlight the great potential of macrocyclic ligand calixarenes as extractants for bioproducts.

As seen above, calixarenes are relevant to the removal of biological or pharmaceutical compounds from wastewater. Elsellami et al. (2009) implemented a coupling process between solid–liquid extraction and photocatalytic degradation for the selective separation of amino acids from water by calix[*n*]arene carboxylic acid derivatives and degradation by activation of a photocatalyst (TiO_2) under UV light. The advantage of this liquid-solid extraction is that it selectively preconcentrates pollutants (tryptophan, phenyalanine and histidine). Apparently, the extracted complex was stabilized in a stoichiometric ratio of 1 calixarene:1 amino acid. The photodegradation followed a first-order kinetic, and the rate constant increased with amino acid concentration. Clearly, solid–liquid extraction is a simple, useful method, and the reagents are recyclable. Although these results are only preliminary, they suggest further possibilities for optimal extraction of amino acids and other pharmaceuticals.

5.4 Stoichiometry in calixarene complexes formed with metallic substrates in solution

Several books and reviews on calixarenes have been dedicated to the coordination chemistry of calixarenes with most of the metal elements of the periodic table (Alexandratos & Natesan, 2000; Lumetta et al., 2000; Mandolini and Ungaro, 2000; Mokhtari et al., 2011a, 2011b; Sliwa, 2002; Sliwa & Girck, 2010; Talanova, 2000). The most important feature of functionalized calixarenes for coordination with metal ions is that metal complexation properties depend not only on the nature of the binding groups grafted to the calixarene platform but also on their stereochemical arrangement, determined by the calixarene conformation and regulated by its size. The coordination ability of the calixarene can be completely changed, when functionalized by the same groups, by simply changing the rim these groups are attached to; the stability, selectivity and stoichiometric ratio of the metal calixarene complexes will be consequently altered. Metal ions can be highly toxic pollutants, pesticides, radionuclides, materials, nanomaterials, oligoelements, and motivate the current interest in synthesizing calixarenes with enhanced selectivity in the liquid and solid states.

5.4.1 Stoichiometric ratio with alkali and earth alkaline and metal transition ions

Joseph et al. (2009) synthesized an amide-linked lower rim 1,3-bis(2-picolyl)amine calix[4]arene derivative. Binding properties of this ligand toward ten different biologically relevant metal ions (Mn^{2+}, Fe^{2+}, Co^{2+}, Ni^{2+}, Zn^{2+}, Cu^{2+}, Na^{+}, K^{+}, Ca^{2+}, and Mg^{2+}) have been studied by fluorescence and absorption spectroscopy in methanol and aqueous methanol. This ligand is a highly discriminating fluorescence sensor that selectively detects Cu^{2+} down to a concentration of 196 and 341 ppb in methanol and 1:1 aqueous methanol, respectively, even if other metal ions are present. Based on competitive metal ion titration studies, Cu^{2+} can be sensed even in the presence of other biologically relevant ions in aqueous solution. Both the calix[4]arene platform and the pyridyl binding core are required for selective recognition of Cu^{2+}, as established by comparison of results obtained with the relevant control molecules e.g. the upper-rim-based quinoline derivative. The stoichiometry of the complex was 1:1, as calculated by a Job plot and confirmed by ESI MS. The computationally obtained structure for the Cu^{2+} complex exhibited a tetracoordinate geometry that is also seen in the blue copper protein, i.e. plastocyanin.

Dendrimers and hyperbranched molecules special properties come from their very peculiar molecular structures. Their structures have been accurately defined, and are prepared by established reactions and chosen pathways. In preliminary work, Mahouachi et al. (2006) investigated the extraction of solid zinc(2+) picrate hydrate into $CDCl_3$ solutions (10^{-3} M) by a linear dendrimer composed of six para-tertbutylcalix[4]arene linked together by amide-ethylene-amine and amide-ethylene chains. ^1H NMR spectra of the resulting solutions remained unchanged after 24 hours, indicating a stable complex. The integration ratio between the singlet of the picrate at 8.52 ppm and the aromatic protons of the linear dendrimer indicates that the stoichiometry of the complex is 2:1 (metal:ligand). However, the spectrum of the complex was broad, and the signal patterns could not be interpreted. The authors proposed that this broadening was due to metal coordination site exchange, since the ligand has three potential Zn(2+)-coordination sites, delineated by the amide functions and/or from a mixture of different arrangements of trinuclear complexes.

Sahin & Yilmaz (2011) synthesized a new fluorogenic calixarene bearing two pyrene amine groups; the ligand shows selectivity for Cu^{2+} and Pb^{2+} due to a conformational change upon chelation of the ions. Absorption ($1x10^{-4}$ M) and fluorescence ($1x10^{-6}$ M) spectra of ligands in CH_3CN/CH_2Cl_2 solutions containing 10 mol equivalents of the appropriate metal perchlorate salt were recorded. The Job method was applied to determine the stoichiometry of the complexes, and the stability constants and quenching constants were determined by fluorimetric titration. When $Cu^{2+}$and Pb^{2+} are bound to the calixarene, the pyrene monomer and excimer decreased in a ratiometric manner. This ratiometric change is attributable to a combination of heavy metal ion effects, reverse-PET (photoinduced electron transfer) and conformational changes of the pyrene during the chelation of $Cu^{2+}$and Pb^{2+} to form the 1:1 complex. The authors conclude that this calixarene acts as a selective sensor of Cu^{2+} and Pb^{2+} ions. Cu^{2+} is both a pollutant and an essential trace element, while elevated levels of Pb^{2+} in the environment cause anemia, kidney damage, blood disorders, memory loss, muscle paralysis and mental retardation by lead poisoning.

Arena et al. (2003) functionalized the 1- and 3- positions of a calix[4]arene with two dipyridyl pendants to create a ligand that complexes Cu(2+) and Co(2+). The new ligand, fixed in its 1,3-alternate conformation, forms stable complexes with both Co(2+) and Cu(2+), as shown by UV/Vis titrations carried out in acetonitrile. The stoichiometry of the main Co and Cu -calixarene species was determined by molar ratio and Job plot methods. Both methods indicated a single complex species with a 1:1 stoichiometry for Co^{2+}, and two complex species for Cu^{2+} in 1:1 and 2:1 (metal:ligand) stoichiometry. In the case of Cu^{2+}, speciation was confirmed by the multivariate and multiwavelength treatment of the data (60-70 points) using two different software packages (Specfit and Hyperquad). The existence of two complexes with the above-mentioned stoichiometry was confirmed. The authors conclude that the new ligand efficiently targets ions, and proposed that the cobalt complex is a good candidate as di-oxygen carrier, while the two copper complexes are good low molecular weight model systems for the study of copper enzyme catalytic activity in nonaqueous environments. The extracted complex species with 1:1 stoichiometry is a good candidate for nanoswitches; cyclic voltammetry studies showed reversible oxidation/reduction behavior.

Kumar et al. (2010) reported fluorescent sensors based on (N-(pyrenyl-1-methylimine)-derivatized calix[4]arenes and investigated their metal-ion binding (Li^{+}, Na^{+}, K^{+}, Pb^{2+}, Zn^{2+}, Hg^{2+} and Ag^{+}) by UV and fluorescence spectroscopy in CH_2Cl_2/CH_3CN. Two of these receptors in a cone conformation showed ratiometric sensing while the third receptor in a 1,3 alternate conformation showed 'On–Off' signaling for Pb^{2+}. The stoichiometry of Pb^{2+} with the three ligands was 1:1 as established by a Job's plot of fluorescence titrations. The cation binding properties of the ligands were examined by $^{1}H'$ NMR for Pb^{2+} in $CDCl_3$ $/CD_3CN$ (1:9 v/v). The significant downfield shift of the imino protons (>1.5 ppm) indicated strong complexation between imino nitrogen atoms and Pb^{2+} ions. Fitting the changes to the ligands fluorescence spectra with other metal ions using the nonlinear regression analysis program SPECFIT gave good fit with a 1:1 (metal:ligand) stoichiometry. The stability constant data indicated that these ligands bind strongly to Pb^{2+} ions. Ag^{+} is bound to ligands more weakly than Pb^{2+}, but more strongly than Li^{+}.

Bayrakcı et al. (2009) synthesized several dinitro-substituted calix[4]arene-based receptors for extracting chromate and arsenate anions. Chromate and arsenate anions are important because of their high toxicity and presence in soil and water. Humans are sensitive to arsenic carcinogenesis; prolonged exposure to arsenic damages the central nervous system and results in liver, lung, bladder, and skin cancers.

Chromium(6+) can be toxic, as it can diffuse as $Cr_2O_7^{2-}$ or $HCr_2O_7^{-}$ through cell membranes to oxidize biological molecules. Therefore, the treatment of waste water containing Cr(6+) prior to discharge is essential. The upper and lower rims of para-tert-butylcalix[4]arene (L) were modified in order to create binding sites for the recognition of arsenate and dichromate anions. Protonated alkylammonium forms of the ionophores showed high affinity toward dichromate and arsenate anions. Both oxyanions were extracted; extraction of the dichromate ions from water into dichloromethane follows a linear relationship between log D versus log [L] at different concentrations of L, with the slope ≈ 1 at pH=1.5, suggesting that two calixarenes form 1:1 complexes with the extracted dichromate anion.

Table 2 summarizes the stoichiometric ratio of some of the discussed metal complexes in solution.

Substrate	Techniques/Solvent	Methods/ Stoichiometry(M:L)	References
Cu^{2+}/amide linked lower rim 1,3-bis(2-picolyl)amine calix[4]	Fluorescence, UV/Vis; CH_3OH; CH_3OH-H_2O	Job plot/ ESI-MS /(1:1)	Joseph et al., 2009
Cu^{2+} and Pb^{2+}/ pyrene-armed calix[4]arene derivatives	Fluorescence titration /CH_2Cl_2/CH_3CN	Job plot/ (1:1)	Sahin & Yilmaz, 2011
$Co^{2+}$and Cu^{2+}/ 1,3-calix[4]arene with two dipyridyl pendants	UV/Vis titration/ CH_3CN	Job plot/ Specfit / Hyperquad/Co_2^{+1} (1:1)Cu^{2+}(1:1, 2:1)	Arena et al., 2003
Li^{1+},Na^{1+},K^{1+},Pb^{2+},Zn^{2+}, Hg^{2+},Ag^{2+}/(N-(pyrenyl methylimine)calix[4]	Fluorescence titration /CH_2Cl_2/CH_3CN	Job plot/Specfit/ (1:1)	Kumar et al., 2010
Cromate; Arsenate anions/ dinitro - substituted calix[4]arene	UV/Vis , Atomic absorption	Liquid-liquid extraction / (1:1)	Bayrakcı et al., 2009
Ln/tetraphosphinoylated paratertbutylcalix[4]arene	UV/Vis, NMR,ES-MS titrations/CH_3CN	Specfit/ (1:1, 1:2)	Le Saulnier et al., 1999
Ln/ tetra-ether-amide-paratertbutylcalix[4]arene	NMR titration/ CH_3CN	MINEQL$^+$ program/(1:1)	Ramirez et al., 2001
Ln/ hexaphosphinoylated paratertbutylcalix[6]arene	UV/Vis titration/ CH_3CN	Specfit/ (1:1, 1:2)	Ramirez et al., 2002
Ln/octaphosphinoylated paratertbutylcalix[8]arene	MS,UV/Vis, NMR titrations/CH_3CN	Specfit/ (1:1, 2:1)	Puntus et al., 2007
An/hexaphosphinoylated paratertbutylcalix[6]arene An, Ln/ B_6bL^6	UV/Vis titration/ CH_3CN UV/Vis	Specfit/ (1:1, 1:2) Liquid-liquid extraction/(1:1)	Ramírez et al., 2008
An, Ln/ phosphorylated calixarenes (upper rim) Ln,An/ phosphorylated calixarenes (lower rim) An, Ln/ phosphorylated calixarenes (lower and upper rims)	Microcalorimetric, UV/Vis titrations/ CH_3CN, CH_3OH UV/Vis	(1:1, 1:2) (1:1, 1:2 or 2:1) Liquid-liquid extraction (1:1, 1:2)	Karavan et al., 2010

Table 2. Stoichiometry of metal calixarene species, in solution, and the used techniques for their identification and determination.

5.4.2 Stoichiometric ratio with lanthanide and actinide ions in liquid and solid states

In the last decade, many functionalized calixarenes have been used as lanthanide ion (Ln(3+)) receptors, either to improve their photophysical properties by the antenna effect of the calixarene, or as selective extractants of Ln and actinides (An).

Le Saulnier et al. (1999) investigated the coordination chemistry of a tetraphosphinoylated para-tertbutylcalix[4]arene (B_4bL^4) with lanthanides, Ln, (Ln(3+) = La, Eu and Tb) and their luminescence. The stoichiometry of the complexes, both in solution and in the solid state, was 1:1 and 1:2 (M: B_4bL^4), as demonstrated by UV/Vis, NMR and ES-MS titrations and by applying Specfit software to UV/Vis data to determine speciation and stability constants in acetonitrile. Although the isolated complexes were very stable, the calixarene did not sensitize the Eu and Tb luminescence of the complexes.

Ramírez et al. (2001) prepared a tetra-ether-amide-para-tertbutylcalix[4]arene (L= A_4bL^4) and studied its coordination ability toward Ln(3+) = Eu, Gd, Tb, and Lu. The stoichiometry of the complex species in acetonitrile solution was demonstrated to be 1:1 (M:L) by $^1H'$- ^{13}C-NMR and ES-MS titrations. The stability constants of the 1:1 species were estimated using the MINEQL$^+$ program. A_4bL^4 reacted with Ln(3+) in acetonitrile to yield a 1:1 complex. The crystal structure of the lutetium complex $[Lu(A_4bL^4)(H_2O)](CF_3SO_3)_3$ $2Et_2O$ corroborated the 1:1 stoichiometry and showed the metal ion encapsulated in the cavity formed by the four arms. Lu was 9-coordinate, bound to the four ether and four carbonyl functions and a water molecule that was itself H-bonded to the phenolic ether functions, rigidifying the cavity formed by the pendant arms. Additionally, an ether molecule is inserted into the hydrophobic cavity defined by the aromatic rings. Both NMR (La, Lu) and luminescence (Eu, Tb) data pointed to high local symmetry at the metal center while lifetime determinations were consistent with the coordination of an inner-sphere water molecule.

Although the calixarene sensitized the luminescence of the Tb ion, the quantum yield measured in acetonitrile was relatively low (Q_{abs} = 5.8%, τ_F = 1.42 ms), particularly for Eu (Q_{abs} = 2.0%, τ_F = 0.73 ms). This is most likely due to the presence of a ligand metal charge transfer (LMCT) state that severely limits such a process. This study demonstrated once more the calixarene platform potentiality to simultaneously complex inorganic and organic guests. This finding might be helpful for modeling and designing extraction processes.

A hexaphosphinoylated para-tertbutyl calix[6]arene (B_6bL^6) was synthesized by Ramírez et al. (2002). Temperature-dependent ^1H and ^{31}P NMR studies indicate a mixture of conformers with a time-averaged C_{6v} symmetry at 405 K in dmso-d_6; $\Delta G^{\neq}$ values for conformational inter conversion processes were equal to 68(1) and 75(2) kJ mol^{-1} and reveal a semi-flexible macrocycle with alternate in-out cone conformation in DMSO and $CHCl_3$ solutions, confirmed by molecular mechanics and dynamics calculations. B_6bL^6 crystallized as a dimer, where the two calixarenes are linked through hydrogen bonding and surrounded by water and toluene molecules in the lattice. UV/Vis spectrophotometric titration of B_6bL^6 with La(3+) in acetonitrile yielded stability constants of log β_1 = 9.8 and log β_2 = 19.6 for the 1 : 1 and 1 : 2 (Ln : B_6bL^6) species, respectively.

Complexes with La, Eu, Gd and Tb in 1:1 and 1:2 (M:calixarene) stoichiometries were isolated and characterized. Lifetime determinations of the Eu(3+) and Tb(3+) complexes in acetonitrile solution were consistent with no, or little, interaction of water molecules in the inner co-ordination sphere. The B_6bL^6 sensitized the luminescence of Tb(3+) (Q_{abs} = 4.8%, τ_f = 2.1 ms, 1 :

1 complex) and Eu(3+) (Q_{abs} = 2.5%, τ = 2.0 ms, 1 : 2 complex) reasonably well in comparison with B_4bL^4. Molecular modeling calculations confirmed that the structure observed in the solid state, with phosphoryl groups interacting with water molecules, is a good model for the solution structure. The stability constants for the complexes with La(3+) were either smaller (1:1 complex) or equal (1:2) to the ones found for the corresponding B_4bL^4, in view of the larger flexibility of the calix[6]arene macrocycle. Photophysical properties were enhanced with respect to the smaller calix[4]arene, which opens the way for sensitive luminescence detection of these complexes, a definite advantage for quantifying extraction processes.

The coordination ability of the B_6bL^6 calixarene toward actinides was established by Ramírez et al. (2008). Spectrophotometric titration of uranyl with B_6bL^6 in CH_3CN yielded log β_{11} = 7.1 and log β_{12} = 12.5 for the 1:1 and 1:2 (UO_2^{2+}: B_6bL^6) species, respectively. UO_2^{2+} and Th(IV) complexes with 1:1 and 1:2 (M:L) stoichiometries were isolated and characterized. Uranyl compounds only fulfilled their CN=8 with B_6bL^6, while thorium compounds required coordinated nitrates and/or water molecules. The luminescence spectra, photophysical parameters and luminescence lifetimes of the uranyl complexes permitted an understanding of the coordination chemistry of these actinide calixarene complexes.

Energy transfer from the B_6bL^6 ligand to the uranyl ion was relevant in the 1:1 complex, with Q_{abs} = 2.0%. The uranyl complex emission revealed biexponential decay for both complexes. The conclusion that we drew from this luminescence study and comparison with the emission spectra of uranyl nitrate recorded under various experimental conditions is that coordination of uranyl to the calixarene results in stabilization of its triplet state (heavy atom effect). This coordination promotes efficient energy transfer, although incomplete in the case of the 1:2 complex. Additionally, the macrocyclic molecule(s) provide(s) a protective environment, minimizing nonradiative deactivation processes.

A de-tert-butylated calix[6]arene (A_6L^6) fitted with six ether-amide pendant arms in the lower rim was synthesized and characterized in solution (Ramírez et al., 2004). NMR spectroscopic data point to the six phenoxide units adopting an average D_{6h} conformation on the NMR time scale (1,2,3-alternate conformation). According to Augmented MM3 molecular mechanics and MOPAC quantum mechanical calculations, A_6L^6 is a ditopic ligand featuring two nonadentate coordination sites, each built from three pendant arms, and extending in opposite directions, with one arm above and the other below the main ring. A_6L^6 reacted with Ln ions (Ln(3+) = La, Eu) in acetonitrile to successively form 1:1 and 2:1 complexes. The isolated Eu 2:1 complex was luminescent (Q_{abs} = 2.5% in acetonitrile, upon ligand excitation), with bi-exponential luminescent decay, pointing to the presence of two differently coordinated metal ions, one with no bound water molecules, and the other one with two molecules bound.

According to molecular mechanics calculations, the more stable isomer was indeed asymmetric, with two nine-coordinate metal ions. Both Eu ions are bound to three bidentate arms and one monodentate triflate anion, but one metal ion completes its coordination sphere with two phenoxide oxygen atoms while the other uses two water molecules, which is consistent with IR spectroscopic and luminescence data. The two metal ion sites became equivalent in acetonitrile, and the relatively long lifetime (1.35 ms) indicates a coordination environment free of water molecules. The absence of substituents on the narrower rim of H_6L^6 (calix[6]arene) allows easy interconversion between different conformers, through either the "tert-butyl through the annulus" or "narrower rim through the annulus" pathways that facilitate 2:1 complex formation. This work demonstrated that the stoichiometry of lanthanide complexes with calixarenes can be tuned by a narrow and/or wide rim substituents suitable choice.

Puntus et al. (2007) synthesized an octa-phosphinoylated para-tertbutylcalix[8]arene (B_8bL^8), and its structure was studied in solution. According to temperature-dependent ^1H and ^{31}P NMR spectroscopic data, the calix[8]arene adopts a so-called in–out cone conformation. Its coordination ability toward Ln (Ln (3+) = La, Eu, Tb, Lu) was probed by MS, UV/Vis and NMR spectroscopic titrations. Although both 1:1 (in the presence of triflate) and 2:1 (in the presence of nitrate) Ln:B_8bL^8 complexes could be isolated in the solid state, it was clear from the titration results that the major species present in methanol (solubility problems prevented the study in acetonitrile) had a 1:1 stoichiometry (irrespective of the anion), and the minor species a 2:1 stoichiometry. Observation of the 2:1 species was consistent with the bimetallic complexes usually isolated with calix[8]arenes, but only in the presence of a nitrate counterion as a result of its bidentate chelating mode.

NMR spectroscopic data indicated a common conformation for the 1:1 complexes in solution. Ln ions were coordinated by four of the eight phosphinoyl arms, with a coordination sphere completed by methanol molecules or nitrate ions, as ascertained by IR and MS spectra. B_8bL^8 displayed a weak absorption at 360 nm that can be assigned to an intraligand charge-transfer (ILCT) state that is very sensitive to coordination. Photophysical data for the Eu 2:1 complex pointed to similar chemical environments provided by the metal ion sites and no coordinated water, contrary to what is observed in the 1:1 complex. In this work, optical electronegativity predicted the energy of the charge-transfer states in the lanthanide systems with inequivalent ligands, and extensive analysis of the vibronic satellites of the Eu($^5D_0 \rightarrow {}^7F_J$) transitions allowed the authors to draw conclusions about Eu(III) coordination.

Karavan et al. (2010) investigated the binding properties of three series of phosphorylated calixarene derivatives (bearing phosphine oxide or phosphonate groups either at the wide or the narrow rims) toward some representative lanthanide and actinide ions in solution. Complexation was studied in single media (methanol and acetonitrile) followed by UV spectrophotometric and isoperibolic (micro)calorimetric titrations (ITC). Using upper rim phosphorylated calixarenes, it was found that the solvating ability of methanol and acetonitrile influences stoichiometry, number and constant stability of the europium complex species (1:1 and/or 2:1 M: L species). In a single solvent, the major influence on the stoichiometry of a complex is the length of the substituents bound to the OP groups.

No influence of calixarene size or substituent type in the upper rim was observed in the stoichiometry of uranyl calixarene species (1:1) when lower-rim-phosphorylated calixarenes were used in methanol, while in acetonitrile, a 2:1 species was found with the de-tertbutylated tetramer derivative. Similar stoichiometries were determined for europium complex species using the tertbutylated tetramer in methanol, where a 1:2 complex species formation was also observed.

Calorimetry was very useful for the determination of stoichiometries, particularly when complexation did not induce significant spectral changes. It also provided full thermodynamic characterization of the complex species in organic solution. The influence of some structural features of the ligands on the nature of the substituents as well as the condensation degree of the calixarene moiety on the complexation thermodynamic parameters were thus established. It is clear that wide rim and narrow rim phosphine oxide derivatives formed 1:1 complexes with europium and uranyl, accompanied in some cases with 2:1 complexes or 1:2 species with europium.

The stabilization origin of the complexes is quite different for the two cations and depends on the solvent. Whereas entropy terms are generally favorable in methanol for europium complexes, the entropy contributions appear to be very negative and hence unfavorable in acetonitrile. This finding indicates the importance of solvation/desolvation in the complexation process. In contrast, the stabilization of the uranyl complexes is mostly enthalpy-driven in both solvents.

5.4.3 Stoichiometric ratio in extracted species formed with lanthanide and actinides ions

Studies of metal ion separations using liquid-liquid and liquid-solid extraction systems and the evaluation of their experimental parameters—extraction percentage, distribution (coefficients) ratios, loading capacity and the stoichiometry of the extracted species among others— allow for gaining a complete physicochemical understanding of the extraction system and its applications.

Long-lived radionuclides, actinides in particular, are the most hazardous components of nuclear waste. The recovery of these elements from waste mass, alone or combined with other elements like lanthanides before disposal or reprocessing, would significantly enhance the ecological safety and efficiency of the nuclear fuel cycle. Phosphorylated calixarenes offer numerous possibilities for selective complexation of metal ions and will likely be essential in the treatment of nuclear waste.

Here, we focus on the Ln and An extracted species with phosphinoylated (phosphorylated) calixarenes from aqueous media to organic media. The usefulness of this type of calixarene for Ln/An separation with high efficiency was proved several years ago (Lumetta et al., 2000). The stoichiometry of extracted species with a certain calixarene is not necessarily in agreement with that of its complex species. Furthermore, a functionalized calixarene with the same phosphinoylated arms in the lower rim or in the upper rim does not extract a species with the same stoichiometry (Arnaud-Neu et al., 2000; Karavan et al., 2010).

Solvent can influence the conformational arrangement of the calixarene and thus the stabilization of certain complex species. It can also compete for metal ions, affecting the M:calixarene stoichiometric ratio. Experiments were conducted on the B_6bL^6 calixarene functionalized in the lower rim mentioned above (Ramírez et al., 2008) in a liquid-liquid extraction system of metal salt/1 M HNO_3/3.5 M $NaNO_3$-calixarene in chloroform. A 1:1 stoichiometry was found for the Eu(3+), UO_2^{2+} and Th(4+) extracted species while the complexation study in acetonitrile demonstrated 1:1 and 1:2 complexes in the solution and solid state.

Karavan et al. (2010) found that for liquid–liquid extraction from nitric acid to m-nitrobenzotrifluoride uranyl extracted species were in a 1:2 stoichiometry using a pentamer functionalized on the lower rim while in methanol and in acetonitrile the uranyl complex species were in 1:1 stoichiometry. However, europium extracted species kept the same stoichiometry. In contrast, upper-rim functionalized calixarenes using the same extraction system formed 1:1 uranyl extracted species and europium in 1:1 and 1:2 stoichiometries. Thus, the size, conformation, choice of rim (upper or lower), and length and isomeric nature of the aliphatic substituents, notwithstanding solvent effects, are all factors that define the stoichiometry of extracted species.

6. Molecular modeling

Jean Marie Lehn (Lehn, 1990) established that molecular recognition is key not only to biological macromolecules but also to macrocyclic complexation. Experimental results are sometimes not sufficient to elucidate how recognition occurs, which sites coordinate, how the stereochemical arrangement influences stabilization of the complex molecule, or why the substrate physicochemical properties drastically change after interaction with a certain macrocycle. Since suitable single crystals of macrocycle complexes are difficult to obtain, simulation of complexes with molecular modeling has become extremely useful. New molecular receptors can also be designed, built and optimized with the same software, although successful prediction depends on the molecule and the calculation approach used.

Molecular modeling is mostly useful when the molecule is based on experimental data. It has to be used with a great care to avoid meaningless results. The more complicated the molecule, the less likely the model is to represent the real complex. Before 1999, only empirical calculations were used for calixarene complexes, but over the last decade, ab initio and semi-empirical calculations have been successfully attempted.

Kunsági-Máté et al. (2004) used the HYPERCHEM Professional 7 and related quantum-chemical calculations to elucidate the inclusion of C_{60} fullerene in the hexasulfonated calix[6]arene functionalized at the upper rim. The calculation showed that C_{60} lies deep in the cavity of the calixarene.

Zielenkiewicz et al. (2005) used INSIGHT II to show that a phosphorylated calix[4]arene effectively bound for the amino acid isoleucine. Based on the calculation results for 1:1 and 1:2 (isoleucine: calixarene) complexes, the inclusion of the isoleucine into the calixarene cavity stabilizes the macrocyclic skeleton in the regular cone conformation. Strong electrostatic interactions between the phosphoryl group of the calixarene and the positively charged amino group of the amino acid played an important role in the complexation process.

Atwood et al. (2005) visualized purely size–shape considerations with X-SEED to determine whether two CH_4 molecules could fit within each dimeric capsule. The calculation illustrated the capsules' excellent size–shape compatibility.

To understand the structural features of the 1:1 complex formed between an amide-linked lower rim 1,3-bis(2-picolyl)amine derivative of calix[4]arene and Cu^{2+}, Joseph et al. (2009) calculated the complex using GAUSSIAN 03 and DFT calculations. The calculated structure for the Cu^{2+} complex exhibited a tetracoordinate geometry, where all four pyridyl moieties were involved in binding and the coordination of Cu^{2+} center was a highly distorted tetrahedral.

Ding et al. (2011) calculated the most stable structures of the complex (the lowest energy was 0 kcal/mol) formed between tetrabutyl ether derivatives of p-sulfonatocalix[4]arene (SC4Bu) and the methiocarb pesticide using GAUSSIAN 03. The complexation was an "external" inclusion process, and hydrogen bonding between the methyl H atom of methiocarb and the sulfonate of SC4Bu facilitated the formation of this SC4Bu–methiocarb complex.

We have used molecular modeling in our current work with calixarenes and calixarene complexes. Structures have been built, and their minimum energies calculated, using the CAChe WorkSystem Pro 5.02 for Windows®. Free calixarenes (Ramírez et al., 2004; Ramírez et al., 2008; García-Sosa & Ramírez, 2010) and calixarenes complexed with organic substrates (García-Sosa & Ramírez, 2010) have been simulated by sequential application of Augmented MM3/CONFLEX/Augmented MM3/ MOPAC/PM5 or PM3/ MOPAC/PM5 or PM3/COSMO procedures.

MOPAC/PM5 or PM3/COSMO procedures calculate the most stable molecules under aqueous solvent effects and the heat formation of the most stable molecule (given in kcal.mol^{-1}).

The calixarene complexes formed with lanthanide and actinide ions were calculated by sequential application of Augmented MM3/CONFLEX procedures (Ramírez et al., 2004; Ramírez et al., 2008). Augmented MM3 yielded the optimum structure, and CONFLEX yielded the most stable conformers (kcal.mol^{-1}).

Fig. 4 shows the modeled structure of the de-tert-butylated calix[6]arene fitted with six ether amide pendant arms, A_6L^6 (Fig. 4, left) and its europium complex in a 2:1 (metal: ligand) stoichiometry (Fig. 4, right). The modeling shows that the free calixarene is a ditopic ligand featuring two nonadentate coordination sites; each is built from three pendant arms and extends in opposite directions, one site above, and the other under the main ring. The modeled structure of the dimetallic complex is a stable asymmetric isomer with two nine-coordinate metal ions.

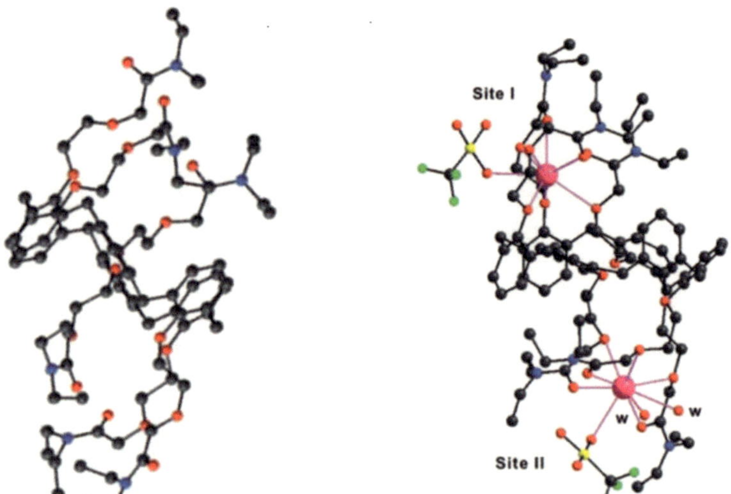

Fig. 4. Molecular modeling of A_6L^6 calixarene (left) and optimized geometry of the Eu (3+) 2:1 complex with A_6L^6 (right), as determined by MM3 Augmented and Conflex CAChe procedures (Ramírez et al., 2004).

Both Eu (3+) ions are bound to three bidentate arms and one monodentate triflate anion, but one of the metal ion completes its coordination sphere with two phenoxide oxygen atoms whereas the other uses two water molecules. These computational results are consistent with IR and luminescence data (Ramírez et al., 2004) and elucidate the luminescence behavior of the complex in solid and in solution.

7. Conclusions

The aim of this chapter was to establish the relevance of stoichiometric studies in understanding complexes formed, either in solution or in the solid state, between calixarene receptors and organic or metal substrates. Spectroscopic techniques are highly useful in investigating the stoichiometry of calixarene complexes. Nevertheless, many stoichiometric studies require more than one technique, or one that affords thermodynamic parameters. Computational calculations have gained an important place in determining the stoichiometry of calixarene complexes. Visualizing the structural arrangement of a calixarene complex with a particular stoichiometry can help elucidate how the platform of a conformational functionalized calixarene at the upper or lower rim can drastically change the physical, chemical or physicochemical properties of the complexed substrate. Great care must be taken in experimentally determining stoichiometry and in correlating these ratios with molecular modeling to avoid incorrect conclusions.

In this chapter we have focused our attention on investigations linking basic research to real problems, from pollution and water treatment, to nuclear waste treatment, fuel storage and luminescent materials. The presented examples were carefully chosen to provide sufficient knowledge of stoichiometric studies from the experimental, theoretical and applications point of view. Furthermore, these examples afford an understanding of the physical, chemical and stereochemical parameters that are responsible for the stoichiometry and structure of an organic calixarene complex or of a metal calixarene complex.

The relevancy of stoichiometry and structure of the discussed examples for their future applications is undoubted.

The increasingly interest in calixarenes resides in their versatile intrinsic properties allowing them to be functionalized and to envision their potential applications in different fields of science and technology. Particular attention has to be paid to the use of functionalized calixarenes in biomedical studies, particularly on the stoichiometry and structure of organic and/ or metal complexes with potential biomedical applications.

8. Acknowledgment

The authors thank CONACYT (México), project Nr. 36689-E and the Swiss National Science Foundation project SCOPES No 7BUPJ062293; their works cited in this chapter were developed with their support. They also thanks to Mr. Claudio Fernández from the Library of ININ for his help anytime they needed it.

9. References

Alexandratos, S. D. & Natesan, S. (2000). Coordination Chemistry of Phosphorylated Calixarenes and Their Application to Separations Science. *Industrial & Engineering Chemistry Research*, Vol. 39, No. 11, (Sept. 2000), pp.3998-4010, DOI: 10.1021 /ie000294x.

Arena, G., Contino, A., Longo, E., Sciotto, D., Sgarlata C. & Spoto G. (2003). Synthesis, Characterization of a Novel Calixarene Having Dipyridyl Pendants and Study of its Complexes with Cu(II) and Co(II). *Tetrahedron Letters*, Vol. 44, No. 29, (July 2003), pp. 5415–5418, ISSN: 0040-4039

Arnaud-Neu, F., Barboso, S., Byrne, D., Charbonnière, L. J., Schwing-Weill, M. J. &. Ulrich G. (2000). Binding of Lanthanides (III) and Thorium In: *Calixarenes for Separations* (2000) Lumetta G. J., Rogers R. D, Gopalan A. S., Editor(s) pp. 150-164, ACS Symposium Series Volume 757 American Chemical Society Washington D.C., ISBN: 0-8412-3660-7, United States of America

Asfari, M.-Z., Böhmer, V., Harrowfield J. & Vicens J. (Eds.) *Calixarenes 2001*, 2001 ISBN: 0-7923-6960-2, Kluwer Academic Publishers The Netherlands

Atwood, J L., Barbour, L. J., Thallapally, P. K. & Wirsiga, T. B. (2005). A Crystalline Organic Substrate Absorbs Methane under STP Conditions. *Chemical Communications*, (Jan. 2005), pp. 51–53, DOI: 10.1039/b416752j

Bayrakcı, M., Ertul, S. & Yilmaz M. (2009). Synthesis of Di-substituted Calix[4]arene-based Receptors for Extraction of Chromate and Arsenate Anions. *Tetrahedron*, Vol. 65, (Sept. 2009), pp. 7963–7968, ISSN: 00404020 DOI: 10.1016/j.tet.2009.07.062

Böhmer, V. (1995). Calixarenes, Macrocyles with (almost) Unlimited Possibilities. *Angewandte Chemie International Edition in English*, Vol. 34, No.7, (April 1995) pp. 713-745, DOI:0.1002/anie.199507131

Ding, X.-P., Tang, D.-B., Li, T., Wang, S.-F. & Zhou Y.-Y. (2011). A Novel Spectrofluorometric Method for the Determination of Methiocarb Using an Amphiphilic p-sulfonatocalix[4]arene. *Spectrochimica Acta Part A: Molecular and Biomolecular Spectroscopy* (in press), ISSN: 1386-1425

Elsellami, L. Chartron, V., Vocanson, F., Conchon, P., Felix, C., Guillard, C., Retailleau, L. & Houas, A. (2009). Coupling Process between Solid–liquid Extraction of Amino Acids by Calixarenes and Photo Catalytic Degradation. *Journal of Hazardous Materials,* Vol. 166, No. 2-3, pp. 1195–1200, ISSN: 0304-3894

Ferreira Machado, I.L., Vieira Ferreira, L.F. & Oliveira, A.S. (2010). Luminescence and Diffuse Reflectance Studies of Biacetyl Included within p-tert-Butylcalixarenes. *Journal of Luminescence,* Vol. 130, (July 2010), pp. 2251–2255, DOI:10.1016/j.jlumin.2010.06.029

García-Sosa, I. & Ramírez, F.de M. (2010). Synthesis, Solid and Solution Studies of Paraquat Dichloride Calixarene Complexes. Molecular Modelling. *Journal of the Mexican Chemical Society*, Vol. 54, No.3, (July-Sept. 2010), pp. 143-152, ISSN: 1870-249X

Gil, V. M. S. & Oliveira, N. C. (1990). On the Use of the Method of Continuous Variations. *Journal of Chemical Education,* Vol. 67, No. 6, (June 1990), pp. 473-478, DOI: 10.1021/ed067p473

Gutsche, C. D. *Calixarenes revisited,* Monographs in Supramolecular Chemistry, J. Frase Stoddart Series Ed. The Royal Society of Chemistry, London, 1998, ISBN: 0- 85404-502-3

Gutsche, C. D. *Calixarenes,* Monographs in Supramolecular Chemistry J. Frase Stoddart Series Ed. The Royal Society of Chemistry, London, 1989, ISBN: 0-85186-916-5

Halder, A., Nayak, S. K., Chattopadhyay, S. & Bhattacharya, S. (2010). UV–Vis and NMR Spectroscopic Investigations on Effective and Selective Non-Covalent Interactions between Fullerenes and Calix[6]arene. *Journal of Molecular Liquids,* Vol. 151, No. 2-3, (Feb. 2010), pp. 125–129, ISSN: 0167-7322.

Hill, Z. D. & Mac Carthy, P. (1986). Novel Approach to Job's Method. *Journal of Chemical Education,* Vol. 63, No. 2, (Feb. 1986), pp. 162–167, DOI: 10.1021/ed063p162

Joseph, R., Ramanujam, B., Acharya, A. & Rao, C. P. (2009). Fluorescence Switch-on Sensor for Cu^{2+} by an Amide Linked Lower Rim 1,3-bis(2-picolyl)amine Derivative of Calix[4]arene in Aqueous Methanol. *Tetrahedron Letters,* Vol. 50, No. 23, (June 2009), pp. 2735–2739, ISSN: 0040-4039

Karavan, M., Arnaud-Neu, F., Hubscher-Bruder, V., Smirnov, I. & Kalchenko, V. (2010). Novel Phosphorylated Calixarenes for the Recognition of f-Elements. *Journal of Inclusion Phenomena and Macrocyclic Chemistry*, Vol. 66, No.1- 2, pp. 113–123, ISSN: 0923-0750 (print version) ISSN: 1573-1111 (electronic version)

Kumar, M., Babu, J. N., Bhalla, V. & Kumar, R. (2010). Ratiometric/'On–Off' Sensing of Pb^{2+} Ion Using Pyrene-appended calix[4]arenes. *Sensors and Actuators B*, Vol. 144, No. 1, (Jan. 2010), pp.183–191, ISSN: 0925-4005

Kunsági-Máté, S., Szabó, K., Bitter, I., Nagy, G. & Kollár, L. (2004). Complex Formation between Water-soluble Sulfonated Calixarenes and C_{60} Fullerene. *Tetrahedron Letters*, Vol. 45, No. 7, (Feb 2004), pp. 1387–1390, ISSN: 0040-4039

Le Saulnier, L., Varbanov, S., Scopelliti, R., Elhabiri, M. & Bünzli, J-C G. (1999). Lanthanide Complexes with a p-tert-butylcalix[4]arene Fitted with Phosphinoyl Pendant Arms. *Journal of the Chemical Society, Dalton Transactions*, No. 22, pp. 3919-3925, DOI: 10.1039/A907693J

Lehn, J. M. (1990). Perspectives in Supramolecular Chemistry-from Molecular Recognition Towards Molecular Information Processing and Self-organization. *Angewandte Chemie International Edition in English*, Vol. 29, No. 11, (Nov. 1990), pp.1304-1319, DOI:10.1002/ANIE.199013041

Likussar, W. &. Boltz, D. F (1971). Theory of Continuous Variations Plots and a New Method for Spectrophotometric Determination of Extraction and Formation Constants. *Analytical Chemistry*, Vol. 43, No. 10, (Aug.1971), pp. 1265-1272, DOI: 10.1021/ac60304a006

Lumetta, G. J., Rogers, R. D., Gopalan, A. S. Ed.(s) (2000). Calixarenes for Separations DOI: 10.1021/bk-2000-0757.fw001 ACS Symposium Series, Vol. 757, ISBN:13: 9780841236608

Mahouachi, M., Ben Othman, A., Thuéry, P., Abidi, R., Jung, J. H., Kim, J. S., & Vicens, J. (2006). Novel calixarene-based Hyperbranched Molecules with N-multidentate Chelating Sites. *Journal of Nano & Bio Tech*, Vol. 2, No. 1, (March 2006), pp. 17-23

Mandolini, L., Ungaro, R. Ed. (s). *Calixarenes in Action* (2000). World Scientific Pub Co. Inc ImperialCollege Press, ISBN: 186094194X

Mohammed-Ziegler, I., Poór, B., Kubinyi, M., Grofcsik, A., Grün, A. & Bitter, I. (2003). Spectroscopic Study on the Complex Formation of Chromogenic Bridged Calixarenes with Aliphatic Amines. *Journal of Molecular Structure*, Vol. 650, No 1-3, (May 2003), pp. 39–44, ISSN: 0022-2860

Mokhtari, B., Pourabdollah, K. & Dallali, N. (2011a). A Review of Calixarene Applications in Nuclear Industries *Journal Radioanalytical and Nuclear Chemistry*, Vol. 287, No. 3, pp. 921-934, DOI:10.1007/s10967-010-0881-1

Mokhtari, B., Pourabdollah, K. & Dallali, N. (2011b). Analytical Applications of Calixarenes from 2005 up-to-date. *Journal of Inclusion Phenomena and Macrocyclic Chemistry*, Vol. 69, No. 1-2, pp 1–55, 0 DOI 10.1007/s10847-010-9848-7, ISSN: 09230750

Pacioni, N. L., Sueldo Occello, V. N., Lazzarotto, M. & Veglia, A. V. (2008). Spectrofluorimetric Determination of Benzoimidazolic Pesticides: Effect of p-sulfonatocalix[6]arene and Cyclodextrins. *Analytica Chimica Acta*, Vol. 624, No. 1, (Aug 2008), pp. 133–140, ISSN: 0003-2670

Pierro, T., Gaeta, C., Troisi, F. & Neri, P. (2009). Induced-fit Recognition by p-carboxylatocalix[4]arene Hosts. *Tetrahedron Letters*, Vol. 50, No.3, (Jan. 2009), pp. 350–353, ISSN: 0040-4039

Puntus, L. N., Chauvin, A-S., Varbanov, S. & Bünzli, J-C. G. (2007). Lanthanide Complexes with a Calix[8]arene Bearing Phosphinoyl Pendant Arms. *European. Journal of Inorganic. Chemistry,* No. 22, (Apr. 2007), pp. 2315-2326, ISSN: 1434-1948, ISSN: 1099-0682

Ramírez, F. de M., Charbonnière, L., Muller, G., Scopelliti, R. & Bünzli, J.-C. G. (2001). A p-tert-butylcalix[4]arene Functionalised at its Lower Rim with Ether-amide Pendant Arms Acts as an Inorganic–organic Receptor: Structural and Photophysical Properties of its Lanthanide Complexes. *Journal of the Chemical Society, Dalton Transactions,* (Oct. 2001), pp. 3205–3213, DOI: 10.1039/b105513p

Ramírez, F. M., Varbonov, S., Cécile, C., Muller, G., Fatin- Rouge, N., Scopelliti, R. & Bünzli, J.-C. G. (2002). A p-tert-butylcalix[6]arene Bearing Phosphinoyl Pendant Arms for the Complexation and Sensitisation of Lanthanide Ions. *Journal of the Chemical Society, Dalton Transactions,* No. 23, (Sept 2002), pp. 4505-4513, DOI: 10.1039/B206238K

Ramírez, F. M., Charbonnière, L., Muller, G. & Bünzli, J.-C. G. (2004). Tuning the Stoichiometry of Lanthanide Complexes with Calixarenes: Bimetallic Complexes with a Calix[6]arene Bearing Ether-amide Pendant Arms. *European Journal of Inorganic Chemistry,* (April 2004), pp.2348-2355, DOI: 10.1002/ejic.200300824

Ramírez, F. de M., Varbanov, S., Padilla, J. & Bünzli, J-C G. (2008) Physicochemical Properties and Theoretical Modeling of Actinide Complexes with a para-tert-butylcalix[6]arene Bearing Phosphinoyl Pendants. Extraction Capability of the Calixarene toward f Elements. *The Journal of Physical Chemistry B,* Vol. 112, No. 35, (Aug. 2008), pp. 10976–10988, DOI: 10.1021/jp710848m

Sahin, O. & Yilmaz, M., (2011). Synthesis and Fluorescence Sensing Properties of Novel Pyrene-armed Calix[4]arene Derivatives. *Tetrahedron,* Vol. 67, No. 19, (May 2011), pp. 3501-3508, ISSN: 0040-4020

Shimojo, K. & Goto, M. (2005). Synergistic Extraction of Nucleobases by the Combination of Calixarene and D2EHPA. *Separation and Purification Technology,* Vol. 44, No. 2, (July 2005), pp. 175–180, ISSN: 1383-5866

Shinkai, S. (1993). Calixarenes-The Third Generation of Supramolecules. *Tetrahedron,* Vol. 49, No. 40, pp. 8933-8968, ISSN: 0040-4020

Sliwa, W. & Girek, T. J. (2010). Calixarene Complexes with Metal Ions. *Journal of Inclusion Phenomena and Macrocyclic Chemistry,* Vol. 66, pp. 15–41, DOI: 10.1007/s10847-009-9678-7

Sliwa, W. (2002). Calixarene Complexes with Transition Metal, Lanthanide and Actinide Ions. *Croatica Chemica Acta,* Vol. 75, No. 1, pp. 131-153, ISSN: 0011-1643

Talanova, G. G. (2000). Phosphorus-Containing Macrocyclic Ionophores in Metal Ion Separations. *Industrial & Engineering Chemistry Research,* Vol. 39, No. 10, (Sept. 2000), pp. 3550 -3565, DOI: 10.1021/ie0001467

Zhou, Y., Xu, H., Yu, H., Chun, L., Lu, Q. & Wang, L. (2008). Spectrofluorometric Study on The Inclusion Behavior of p-(p-carboxylbenzeneazo) calix[4]arene with Norfloxacin. *Spectrochimica Acta Part A,* Vol. 70, No. 2, (July 2008), pp. 411–415, ISSN: 1386-1425

Zielenkiewicz, W., Marcinowicz, A., Poznanski, J., Cherenok, S. & Kalchenko, V. (2005). Complexation of Isoleucine by Phosphorylated Calix[4]arene in Methanol Followed by Calorimetry, NMR and UV–VIS Spectroscopies, and Molecular Modeling Methods. *Journal of Molecular Liquids,* Vol. 121, No.1, (July 2005), pp. 8 –14, ISSN: 0167-7322

2

Water-Soluble Calix[4]arene Derivatives: Binding Stoichiometry and Spectroscopic Evaluation of the Host-Guest Recognition Mechanism

Satish Balasaheb Nimse[1], Keum-Soo Song[2] and Taisun Kim[1]*
[1]*Institute for Applied Chemistry and Department of Chemistry, Hallym University, Chuncheon*
[2]*Biometrix Technology Inc., Chuncheon, Korea*

1. Introduction

If hydrophobic molecules are inserted into an aqueous medium, the water molecules order around the hydrophobic ones to build a quasi crystalline surface. In this way, the hydrogen bonding of the water molecules around a hydrophobic surface is maximized. If two hydrophobic molecules meet they will associate with their hydrophobic surfaces towards each other. The water molecules, previously attached to these surfaces, will be distributed back into the bulk solvent resulting in favourable entropy. The entropic gain is responsible for almost all associations in the medium water and hence extremely important for life (e.g. formation of membranes, micelles, and for protein folding where folding starts often with tryptophan residues forming a hydrophobic core). The hydrophobic effect is shown below (**Figure 1**).

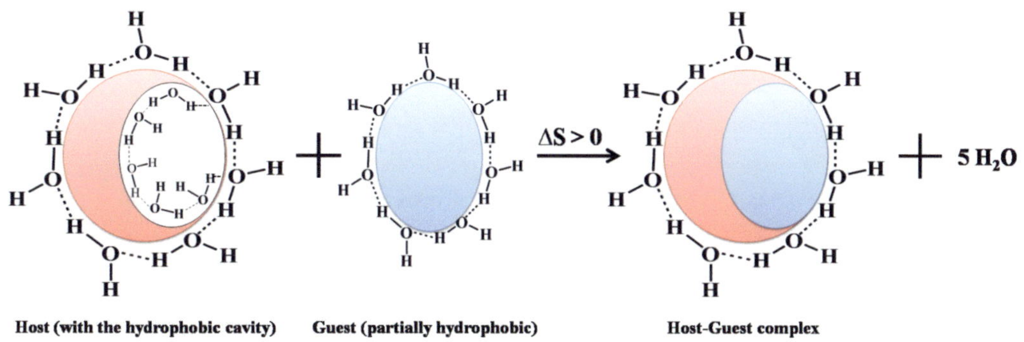

Fig. 1. Host-guest binding mechanism in aqueous medium.

Similarly, in most cases the protein-substrate binding is a result of the hydrophobic effect. However, there are evidences suggesting that the water molecules play an important role in the protein-substrate binding. Water molecules could participate in hydrogen bonding networks that link side chain and main chain atoms with the functional groups on the bases, and the phosphodiester backbone anionic oxygens.[1] Macromolecular crystallography provided the necessary supportive view, that water molecules act as major contributors to stability and specificity.[2,3,4]

Thermodynamic analyses of protein-DNA binding suggest that water released from protein-DNA interfaces is favourable to binding. Structural analyses of the remaining water at the interface in protein-DNA complexes indicate that a majority of these water molecules promote binding by screening protein and DNA electrostatic repulsions between electronegative atoms/like charges. A small fraction of the observed interfacial waters act as linkers to form extended hydrogen bonds between the protein and the DNA, compensating for the lack of a direct hydrogen bond.[5]

Is it by design or by default that water molecules are observed at the interfaces of some protein-DNA complexes? Both experimental and theoretical studies on the thermodynamics of protein-DNA binding overwhelmingly support the extended hydrophobic view that water release from interfaces supports binding. Structural and energy analyses indicate that the remaining waters at the protein-DNA complexes interfaces ensure liquid-state packing densities, screen the electrostatic repulsions between like charges (which seems to be by design), and in a few cases act as linkers between complementary charges on the biomolecules (which may well be by default). Protein-drug binding and DNA-small molecule binding also revealed the possibility of the role played by the water molecules in the receptors binding pockets. The binding of the cardiac toponin-I (cTnI) with the small molecule (Fluorescent probe) revealed the enzyme hydrophobic binding region as shown in **Figure 2**.[6]

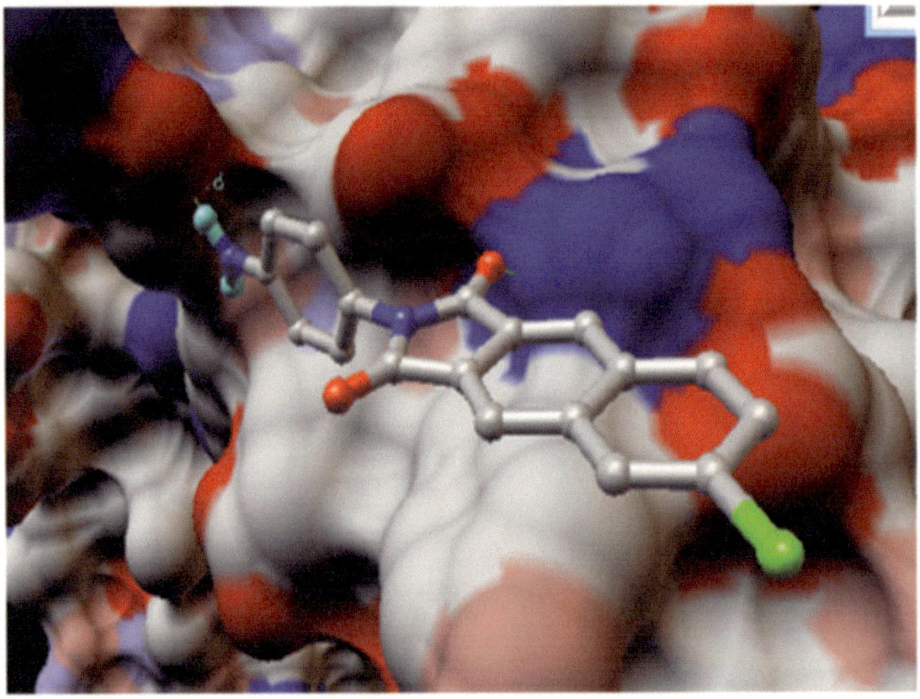

Fig. 2. Binding mode of cardiac toponin-I (cTnI) with the fluorescent probe. (*Reproduced from J. Am. Chem Soc.*133(38):14972-14974).

The protein enzymatic activity, being a surface function, depends on the recognition efficiency of negatively charged and polar amino acids of the substrate peptide.[7] The bulk-like environment in the close vicinity of the surface would enhance the interaction with the substrate (**Figure 3**). On the other hand, the structured water molecules are needed around the protein surface to be part of an efficient chemistry and possibly maintain a three dimensional structure.[8] From these observations, it is clear that the water molecules play a crucial role in the receptor-substrate binding, probably be due to the hydration effect or hydrophobic effect. Scientist has always tried to find the answers related to the biological receptor-substrate interactions using the host-guest chemistry of synthetic counterparts.

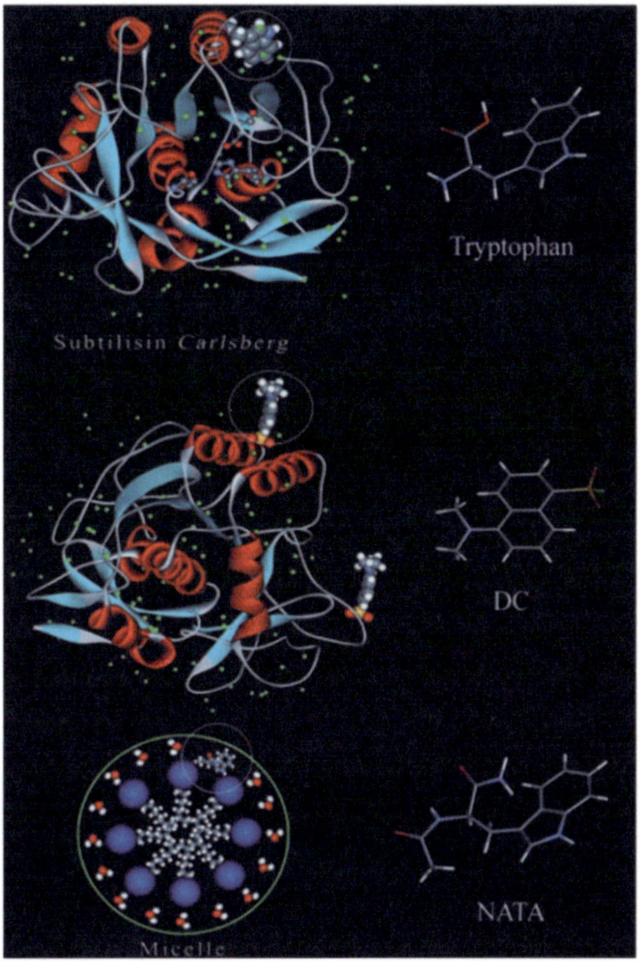

Fig. 3. High-resolution X-ray structure of the Subtilisin *Carlsberg* (SC) protein. This structure was downloaded from the Protein Data Bank and processed with WEBLAB-VIEWERLITE, Accelrys, San Diego, CA. (*Top*) Position of the protein single Trp residue. Note the bound water molecules around this residue. (*Middle*) Two of the nine potential binding sites for DC labeling are shown. (*Bottom*) Illustration of a micelle with a NATA molecule included. Molecular structures of the probes are presented on the right of each illustration. (*Reproduced from Proc. Nat. Acad. Sci.* 2002, 99(4): 1763–1768)

This chapter presents a survey of the current literature on water-soluble calix[4]arenes (hosts) complexes with various substrates (guests), elaborating the water-soluble calix[4]arenes applications. Moreover, a critique of various data interpretations, in the context of the water molecules role in host-guest binding and in general of the water-soluble calix[4]arene guest recognition principles, is also provided.

2. Stoichiometry of the water-soluble calix[4]arene complexes: The methods

2.1 Binding constant

The thermodynamic stability of a host-guest (e.g. metal–macrocycle) complex, in a given solvent (often water or methanol) at a given temperature, is gauged by the binding constant, *K*, measurement. The binding constant is the most widely used method for host-guest affinity assessment in solution, and it is of fundamental importance in supramolecular chemistry. The binding constant is merely the equilibrium constant for the reaction between a Host, H, and Guest, G, in water, described in the following equation:

$$H(H_2O)n + G(H_2O)n \rightleftharpoons [H.G] + n(H_2O)$$

$$K = \frac{[H.G]}{[H(H_2O)n][G(H_2O)n]}$$

Thus a large binding constant corresponds to a high equilibrium concentration of bound guest, and hence to a more stable host–guest complex.

If a sequential process of more than one guest is involved in the binding process, then two *K* values may be measured for the 1:1 and 1:2 complexes, respectively: K_1 and K_2.

$$H(H_2O)n + G(H_2O)n \xrightleftharpoons{K_1} [H.G] + n(H_2O)$$

$$[H.G](H_2O)n + G(H_2O)n \xrightleftharpoons{K_2} [H.G_2] + n(H_2O)$$

$$K_2 = \frac{[H.G_2]}{[[H.G](H_2O)n][G(H_2O)n]}$$

In these circumstances, an overall binding constant, β, may be defined for the complete process, with the individual *K* values known as the stepwise binding constants:

$$\beta = K_1 \; X \; K_2$$

Magnitudes of binding constants can widely change, so they are often reported as log *K*, hence:

$$log\beta = \log(K_1 \; X \; K_2) = \log K_1 + \log K_2)$$

The host-guest complex binding constant depends on the complex stoichiometry. As shown in the equations above, a key aspect of such calculations is the use of the correct stoichiometry model (i.e. the ratio of host to guest, which must be assumed or determined), so it is worthy spending some time in understanding the method to determine it.

2.2 Job plot (method of continuous variation)

There are different methods to determine the stoichiometry, e.g. Continuous Variation Methods (**Figure 4**),[9] the Slope Ratio Method,[10] the Mole Ratio Method,[11] and others. Being the Continuous Variation Method the most popular among these, this method has been adopted here to determine the stoichiometry.

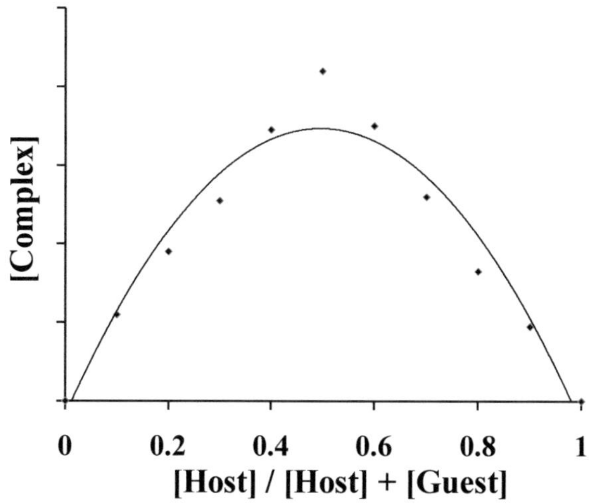

Fig. 4. Job plot for a 1:1 host-guest complex.

There is a strong bias in the host-guest chemistry literature towards the fitting of data to 1:1 stoichiometries, and it is a common mistake to neglect higher complexes. Binding stoichiometry may be confirmed in most kinds of titration experiments, allowing the complex concentration to be determined by making up a series of solutions with varying host-guest ratios such that the total concentration of host and guest remains constant. Monitoring the changing concentration of the host-guest complex in these samples allows a plot of [Complex] against ([Host]/([Host] + [Guest])) to be constructed (**Figure 4**). For a 1:1 complex, this kind of representation (referred to as a Job plot) should give a peak at 0.5 (**Figure 4**), a peak at 0.66 would correspond to a 2:1 stoichiometry and so on. The complex concentration is generally taken to be related to an observable quantity such as $\Delta\delta$ according to following equation

$$[\text{Complex}]\ \alpha\ \Delta\delta\ \text{X mole fraction of host}$$

In a spectrophotometric experiment, absorbance, at a properly chosen wavelength, is usually directly proportional to the complex concentration.

2.3 Methods for association constant measurements

Generally, the complex formation mechanism between a host and a guest is a basic and important process in supramolecular chemistry. Selectivity in the complexation is a crucial property in determining the molecular recognition ability of the host molecule, which discriminates among different guest species. The association constant's ratio of the corresponding complexation is usually treated as a measure of the selectivity. However, theoretically the association constants can be measured by any experimental technique yielding information about the concentration of a complex, [Host-Guest], as a function of the host or guest concentration changes. In practice, the methods described below are of common use. In every case a concentration range must be chosen to have equilibrium between significant amounts of complexed and free host and guest, limiting the range of binding constants that can be measured by a particular technique. If the binding by the target host is too strong, then a competing host is sometimes added, in order to reduce the apparent (measured) association constant according to the difference in guest affinity between the two hosts. The true affinity can then be extrapolated from the knowledge of the binding constant of the guest for the host with the lower affinity.

2.3.1 Potentiometric titrations

If the host molecules are susceptible to protonation (e.g. the aminocalix[4]arenes with their basic tertiary amine nitrogen), the protonation constants, and consequently the p*K*a values, may be readily determined using pH electrodes to monitor a simple acid–base titration. Initially, this will give the acid dissociation constant (p*K*a) of the hosts conjugate acid, $H.H^+$.[12] Addition of a guest cation will perturb the hosts basicity by competition with H^+ ions for the ligand lone pair(s) and hence will affect the titration curves shape. Analysis of the various equilibrium by a curve-fitting computer program (such as *sigmaplot* or *Hyperquad*), along with knowledge of the hosts p*K*a, allows the determination of the amount of uncomplexed host and subsequently the concentration of the complex and the stability constants for the host-guest complexation reaction, as shown in the following equation,

$$K = \frac{[\mathrm{H}^+][H]}{[G.H^+]}$$

2.3.2 Nuclear magnetic resonance titration

If the exchange of complexed and un-complexed guest is slow on the nuclear magnetic resonance (NMR) time scale, then the association constant may be approximately evaluated under the prevailing conditions of concentration, temperature solvent *etc.* by simple integration of the NMR signals for complexed and un-complexed host or guest. However, most host–guest equilibrium are fast on the (relatively slow) NMR spectroscopic time scale, and the chemical shift observed for a particular resonance (that is sensitive to the complexation reaction) is a weighted average between the chemical shift of the free and bound species.

In a typical NMR titration experiment, small aliquots of guest are added to a host solution of known concentration in a deuterated solvent, and the NMR spectrum of the sample monitored as a function of guest concentration, or host:guest ratio. Commonly, changes in chemical shift ($\Delta\delta$) are noted for various atomic nuclei present (e.g. ^{1}H in ^{1}H NMR) as a function of the guest binding influence on their magnetic environment. As a result, two kinds of information are gained. Firstly, the location of the most affected nuclei may give qualitative information about the guest binding regioselectivity (e.g. is the guest inside the host cavity?). More importantly, the treatment of the titration curve data (a plot of $\Delta\delta$ against added guest concentration, e.g. Figure 1.4) by different methods such as the Benesi-Hildebrand (Hanna-Ashbaugh) treatment,[13] the Rose-Drago,[14] the Scatchard (Foster-Fyfe) method,[15,16] and the non-linear curve fitting analysis (few examples of the software programs are EQNMR, AGRNMRL, GRAFIT, and GRAPHPAD PRISM)[17], give quantitative information about the association constant. NMR spectroscopic methods are useful for binding constants in the range $10–10^4$ M^{-1}. Recently, the diffusion NMR spectroscopy has become popular in supramolecular chemistry, due to its application in determining association constants in many systems.[18,19]

2.3.3 Fluorescence titration

Fluorescence titration measurements are based on the proportion of fluorescence intensity to fluorophore concentration (i.e. concentration of fluorescent species in solution; this is often a fluorescent guest, G). For a 1:1 complex with host, H, with stability constant $Ks=$ [HG]/[H][G] the fluorescence intensity F is given by the following equation:

$$F = k\mathrm{G}\,[\mathrm{G}] + k\mathrm{s}\,[\mathrm{HG}]$$

Where, the kG and ks represent proportionality constants for the guest and the 1:1 host-guest complex respectively. In the absence of host the fluorescence intensity, Fo, is given by:

$$F_0 = K^{\mathrm{o}}\,\mathrm{G}_{\mathrm{total}}$$

$$\text{Where } \mathrm{G}_{\mathrm{total}} = [\mathrm{G}] + [\mathrm{HG}].$$

Combining these two relationships gives the following equation, which provides the basis for almost all the fluorimetric methods for stability constant (K11) measurements:

$$\frac{F}{F_0} = \frac{(K_G/K_G^0) + (K_s/K_G^0)K_sH}{1 + K_sH}$$

This equation is greatly simplified when either the guest or host–guest complex are non-fluorescent (i.e. the fluorescence is 'turned on' by complexation, or, in the case of quenching, by the host), in which case either K_G or K_s become zero. For example, for $K_G = K^0{}_G$ 0 and $K_s = 0$, we obtain:

$$\frac{F_0}{F} = 1 + K_sH$$

A simple plot of F_o/F against [H] from the quenching host titration into a guest solution should yield a straight line of slope K_s.

2.3.4 UV-Vis Spectrophotometric titration

UV-Vis spectroscopic titration (or Spectrophotometric titration) involves monitoring the intensity of an electronic absorption band at a particular wavelength, characteristic of either the complex or free host or guest, and it is closely related to the fluorescence titration method. An absorbance intensity *vs.* concentration plot is generated by adding a guest to a solution of constant host concentration.[10,11,12,13,14] Software such as *Specfit®* can then be used, in association with an appropriate stoichiometry model, to evaluate the association constant. Both fluorescent and UV-Vis spectroscopic methods have the advantage over NMR methods of being more sensitive, hence lower concentrations of host and guest can be used. Unlike fluorescence methods, the observation of one or more clear isosbestic points is common in absorption spectroscopic titrations. An isosbestic point is reached when the observed absorption intensity remains constant throughout the titration. Furthermore, the observation of an isosbestic point is a good evidence for the free host conversion into a complex without any other significant intermediate species involved. The understanding of the statistical treatment of the obtained data to determine the association constants with the knowledge of primary statistics is the main feature of this method. When the complex stoichiometry is not 1 to 1, or when other premises are not satisfied, the data treatment should be changed or modified. Nonlinear least square data manipulation is one of the best approximations.

2.3.5 Calorimetric titration

Calorimetric titration, also known as isothermal titration calorimetry (ITC), involves accurate measurement of the heat (enthalpy) evolved from a carefully insulated sample as a function of added guest or host concentration.[20,21,22] The gradient of the ITC curve can be fitted to determine the binding constant and $\Delta G_{complex}$. Integration of the total area under the ITC plot gives the complexation enthalpy ($\Delta H_{complex}$)which allows for all the system thermodynamic parameters evaluation, being $\Delta G_{complex} = \Delta H_{complex} - T\Delta S_{complex}$. ITC is useful for determination of binding constants in range from *ca.*10^2 - 10^7 M^{-1}.

2.3.6 Mass spectrometry

Several electrospray-mass spectrometry (ESI-MS)-based methods are available for association constants (K_S) determination between a protein and a small substrate. Electrospray ionization is today the most widely used ionization technique in chemical and biochemical analysis. Interfaced with a mass spectrometer, it allows the investigation of the molecular composition of liquid samples. A large variety of chemical substances can be ionized with electrospray. Moreover, there is no limitation in mass which thus enables even the investigation of large non-covalent protein complexes. Its high ionization efficiency profoundly changed biomolecular sciences because proteins can be identified and quantified on trace amounts in a high throughput fashion.[23,24,25]

3. Molecular recognition by water-soluble calix[4]arenes

3.1 Cation recognition

Non-covalent interactions play a dominant role in many forefront areas of modern chemistry, from materials design to molecular biology. A detailed understanding of the physical origin and scope of such interactions has become a major goal of physical organic chemistry. The cation-π interaction is an important non-covalent kind of interaction, including hydrogen bonds, ion pairs (salt bridges), and the hydrophobic interaction.

3.1.1 Metal ion recognition

The first patent explicitly describing a calixarene for a practical application of p-tert-butylcalix[8]arene for the recovery of cesium from nuclear wastes, came in 1984. Numerous papers relating to the complexation of cesium by modified calixarenes have appeared since then.

Several other calixarenes for complexation of nuclides have also garnered attention (**Figure 5**), including a water-soluble calix[4]arene-bis-benzocrown-6 (**1**) for selective Cs^{+} complexation (1:1) in moderately salted media.[26] The water-soluble calix[4]arene-bis-benzocrown-6 (**1**) derivatives are also reported to separate the caesium–sodium by nanofiltration–complexation.[27] The voltammetric study on a water-soluble calix[4]arene (calix[4]arene-triacid-monoquinone (**2**), CTA, and calix[4]arene-triacid-diquinone (**3**)), which bind with the Ca^{2+}, Sr^{2+}, Ba^{2+} in basic aqueous solution, provided important information about the unique electrochemical behaviour of Ca^{2+}–CTA 1:1 complex at pH= 8.2.[28,29]

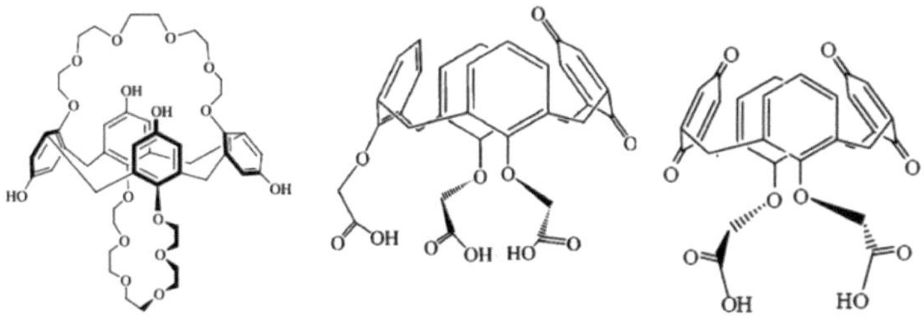

1 **2** **3**

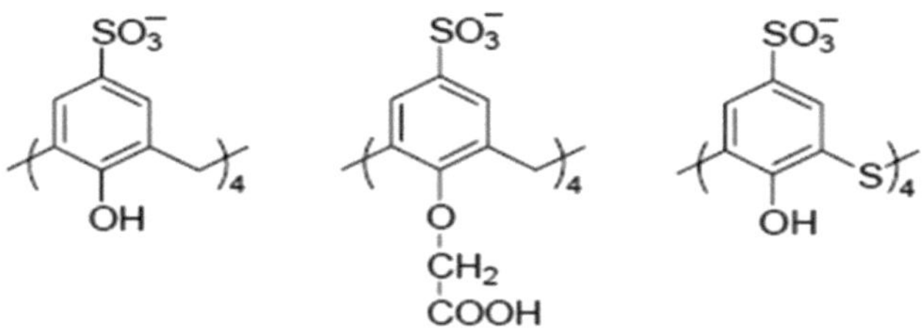

4 **5** **6**

Fig. 5. water-soluble calix[4]arene derivatives **1 - 6**

The 1:1 stoichiometric complexation of lanthanoid(III) nitrates (La-Gd, Tb) with water-soluble calix[4]arenesulfonate (**4**), and its structurally similar derivatives (**5**) and (**6**) is reported (**Table 1**).[30] The water-soluble calix[4]arenesulfonates (**5**) possessing four carboxylic groups at the lower rim of parent calix[4]arenesulfonate (**4**), displayed the enhanced binding abilities for Sm^{3+}. As compared with (**4**) and (**5**), *p*-sulfonatothiacalix[4]arene (**6**) gives not only the lower binding constants for all of lanthanoid(III) ions but also lower cations selectivity. Thermodynamically, the resulting complexes of lanthanoid(III) ions with (**4**) and its derivatives (**5**) and (**6**) are entirely entropy-driven in aqueous solution, typically showing larger positive entropy changes. These changes ($T\Delta S^{\circ}$), and somewhat smaller positive enthalpy changes (ΔH°), are directly contributed to the stability of the complexes as a compensative consequence.

It is interesting to notice that in all cases the solvated metal ions are the guests which form respective complexes with the water-soluble calix[4]arene derivatives (hosts) in the aqueous medium. Therefore, further studies are needed to evaluate the cations hydration shell effect on the complexation with water-soluble hosts.

Host	Guest (Cation)	Log Ks	$-\Delta G^{\circ}$	ΔH°	$T\Delta S^{\circ}$
4	La^{3+}	4.23	24.1 ± 0.3	9.2 ± 0.1	33.3 ± 0.4
	Nd^{3+}	4.08	23.3 ± 0.3	9.5 ± 0.2	32.8 ± 0.5
	Sm^{3+}	3.82	21.8 ± 0.2	10.4 ± 0.2	32.2 ± 0.4
	Eu^{3+}	3.83	21.9 ± 0.2	12.5 ± 0.2	34.4 ± 0.4
	Gd^{3+}	3.94	22.5 ± 0.3	9.8 ± 0.3	32.2 ± 0.6
5	La^{3+}	3.73 ± 0.03	21.3 ± 0.4	5.1 ± 0.5	26.5 ± 0.3
	Ce^{3+}	3.82 ± 0.01	21.8 ± 0.1	5.1 ± 0.3	26.9 ± 0.4
	Pr^{3+}	3.97 ± 0.04	22.7 ± 0.3	4.5 ± 0.4	27.2 ± 0.1
	Nd^{3+}	4.09 ± 0.03	23.4 ± 0.6	4.0 ± 0.1	27.4 ± 0.2
	Sm^{3+}	4.08 ± 0.02	23.3 ± 0.4	3.9 ± 0.1	27.2 ± 0.8
	Eu^{3+}	3.51 ± 0.04	20.1 ± 0.1	7.3 ± 0.3	27.4 ± 0.1
	Gd^{3+}	3.86 ± 0.05	22.0 ± 0.3	5.5 ± 0.2	27.5 ± 0.3
	Tb^{3+}	3.63 ± 0.01	20.9 ± 0.2	6.8 ± 0.7	27.7 ± 0.5
6	La^{3+}	3.45 ± 0.02	19.7 ± 0.1	7.2 ± 0.2	26.8 ± 0.3
	Ce^{3+}	3.41 ± 0.02	19.4 ± 0.2	7.0 ± 0.1	26.5 ± 0.2
	Pr^{3+}	3.42 ± 0.03	19.6 ± 0.3	6.9 ± 0.1	26.5 ± 0.3
	Nd^{3+}	3.40 ± 0.01	19.4 ± 0.1	6.8 ± 0.3	26.2 ± 0.1
	Sm^{3+}	3.37 ± 0.04	19.2 ± 0.2	7.2 ± 0.2	26.4 ± 0.4
	Eu^{3+}	3.26 ± 0.03	18.6 ± 0.4	7.5 ± 0.3	26.0 ± 0.3
	Gd^{3+}	3.30 ± 0.02	17.7 ± 0.6	9.0 ± 0.1	26.6 ± 0.1
	Tb^{3+}	3.33 ± 0.02	19.0 ± 0.1	7.7 ± 0.1	26.7 ± 0.5

Values are the averages of more than three independent measurements in pH = 2 acidic aqueous solution

Table 1. Complex stability constants (log *Ka*) and thermodynamic parameters (kJ mol^{-1}) for complexation of lanthanoid(III) nitrates with 4, 5, and 6 in acidic aqueous solution (pH = 2) at 25 °C.

3.1.2 Molecular cation recognition and hydrophobic cavity depth of water-soluble calix[4]arenes

The complexation of molecular cations by the water-soluble calix[4]arenes is widely studied. Shinkai and coworkers[31] were the first to investigate molecular cation complexation with p-sulfonatocalix[4]arenes **(7)** (**Figure 6**) as hosts and trimethylanilinium as a guest.

By measuring the ^{1}H NMR shift values over a temperature range of 0–80°C, they calculated ΔG°, ΔH° and ΔS° values and concluded that complexation with the cyclic tetramer (7.8, n=4) was driven by a favourable enthalpy change (stronger electrostatic interaction). It was emphasized that in studies with water soluble calixarenes an important feature that had to be taken into consideration was their aggregation properties.[32] A calix[4]arene with anionic groups (SO_3^- and CO_2^-) on both exo and endo rims, forms fairly strong complexes with cations such as $PhCH_2NMe_3^+$ (*K*s = 2500M^{-1}) **(15)**.[33] For cations derived from amines, the organic moiety introduces a significant steric factor, with the ammonium cation included in the host cavity.[34,35,36] A closely related study[37] involving a variety of ammonium guests, including acetylcholine and N-methylquinuclidinium, reached the same conclusion that the guest is in the cavity and that its ammonium portion is closely associated with the calixarene aromatic rings. This interaction was discussed as a π-cation interaction.[38,39,40] The N,N,N,-trimethylanilinium (TMA) cation (**14**) orientation was reported to have a dual binding mode (charged group vs. aromatic moiety inclusion) which occurs in a nonselective fashion with flexible water-soluble calix[4]arene hosts (**7a**, n=4). The binding mode can, however, be effectively controlled and turned into a selective process by preorganization of the calixarene cavity into the cone structure (**7b**, n=4). The presence of sulfonate groups at the upper rim provides, anchoring points for the positively charged guests, the sulfonate groups significantly deepening the cavity of host (**7**), thus improving its inclusion capability.

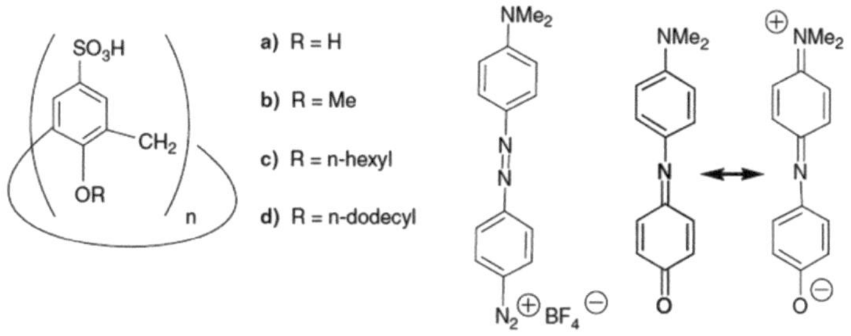

7 **8** **9**

Fig. 6. Water-soluble calix[4]arene host(s) **7** and guests **8, 9.**

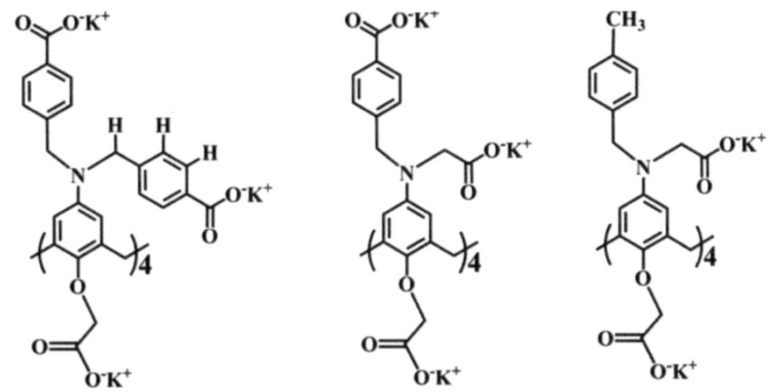

10 **11** **12**

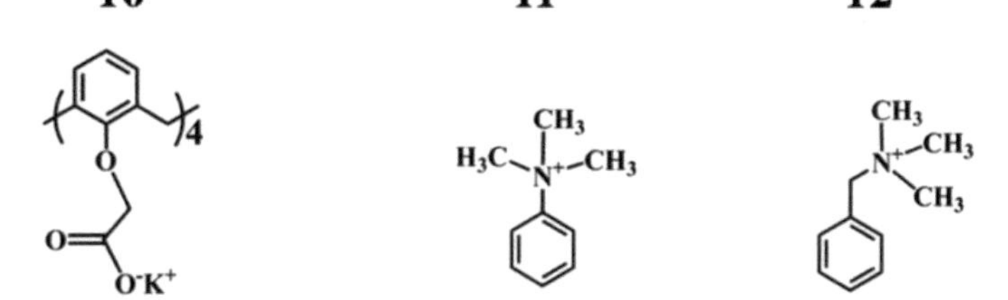

13 **14** **15**

Fig. 7. Hosts with deep hydrophobic cavities (**10 - 12**), and guests **14** (Phenyltrimethylammonium chloride), **15** (Benzyltrimethylammonium chloride).

The complexation of the water-soluble aminocalix[4]arenes containing deep hydrophobic cavities with cations have been reported.[41] However, the guest recognition and the orientation in the cavity of the host were reported to be dependent on the depth of the host hydrophobic cavity. The host **(11, 12)** interacts with both the cationic function and the aromatic moiety in the guests **(14, 15)**, but with a slight preference for the cationic functions. The host **(13)** selectively recognizes the trimethylammonium functions of the guests **(14** and **15)**.

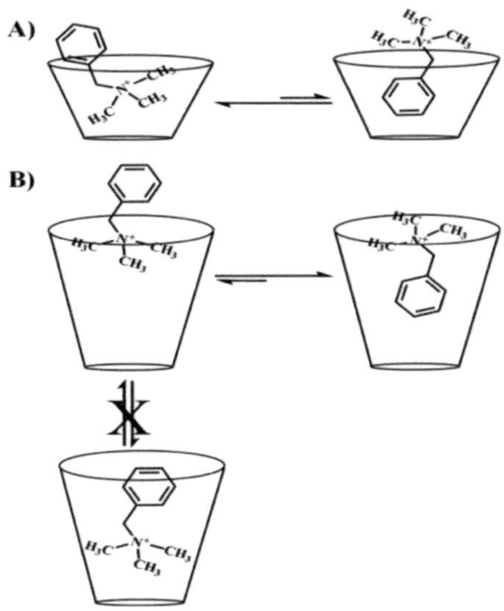

Fig. 8. A) Inclusion mode of the guest **15** by hosts **11-13**; B) Inclusion mode of the guest **15** by host **10**

However, the host **(10)** selectively recognizes the aromatic moiety of the ditopic trimethylammonium guests **(14** and **15)**. These results suggest that the water molecules around the calix[4]arene nucleus in the hosts **(11 - 13)** may assist the hydrophilic trimethylammonium function in entering the cavity. Furthermore, in case of the host **(10),** possessing a deep hydrophobic cavity, the trimethylammonium function cannot deeply enter into the calix[4]arene nucleus, being solvated by the water. As the guest molecules trimethylammonium function is engaged on the mouth of the host **(10)** deep hydrophobic cavity, the guest aromatic moiety is selected by the host **(10)** to form the inclusion complexes. These results suggest that the guest recognition and orientation in the cavity of the host are directly dependent on the host hydrophobic cavity depth.

The water-soluble iminecalix[4]arene **(16, Figure 9)** with deep hydrophobic cavity was also recognized for its selective recognition of the guest.[42,43] The negatively charged four carboxylate functions on the top of the deep hydrophobic cavity play a major role in the recognition of charged molecular species. The ^{1}H NMR titration experiments revealed that host **(16)** binds with cationic **(15, 21, 22)** and neutral guests **(17-20)** in water, with high binding constants in order of 10^4-10^5 M^{-1}. Cationic guest **(15)** showed the highest binding constant of 2.81×10^5 M^{-1} . These studies revealed that except for the -CH···π and π-π stacking interactions, the hydrophobic interactions proved to be crucial in the molecular recognition process in aqueous medium.

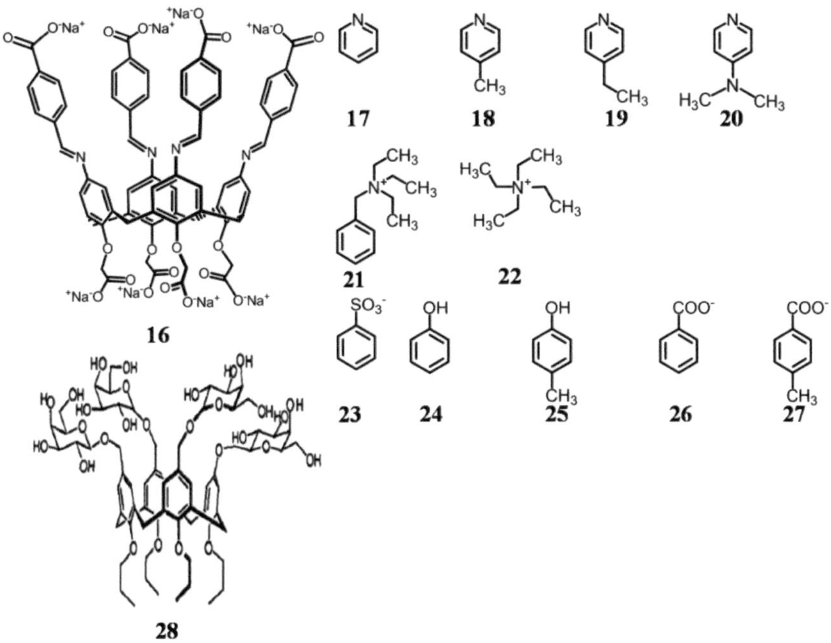

Fig. 9. Water-soluble iminecalix[4]arene **16**, **28** and guests **17-27.**

3.2 Anion recognition

Anion recognition (binding) plays an important role in a variety of chemical reactions and biochemical events as outlined in various reports.[44] This molecular recognition process has been the subject of numerous experimental and theoretical studies in recent years.[45,46]

3.2.1 Inorganic anions

The hydrogen-bond dynamics of water molecules solvating a Cl^-, Br^-, or I^- anion is slow compared with neat liquid water, indicating that the aqueous solvation shells of these ions are rigid. This rigidity can play an important role in the overall dynamics of chemical reactions in aqueous solution.[47]

Furthermore, the anions complexation can be more difficult than that of cations, and a variety of considerations come into play, including (a) the charge, (b) the size, which is often larger than the metal cation one, (c) the shape; whereas the metal cations are spherical, the anions frequently are not, (d) pH dependence, often more critical than in the case of metal cations and (e) solvation, which has a strong influence on the binding strength. There are enormous reports on the recognition of various anions (inorganic) by the calix[4]arene derivatives in the organic solvents but there are only few reports on the anion complexation by the water-soluble calix[4]arenes in the aqueous medium,[48] which opens a new direction for such studies.

Functionalisation of calix[4]arenes with carbohydrate moieties results in receptors which show considerable water solubility. A number of calixsugars have been developed[49] and their binding characteristics studied. Neutral guests such as carbohydrates and N-protected amino acids failed to bind. However, 1:1 complexation of dihydrogen phosphate was seen for **(28),** offering opportunities for the binding of larger, phosphate containing biological substrates.

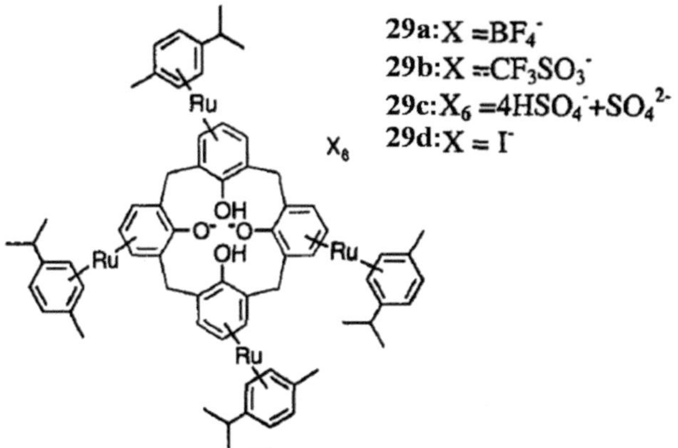

29

Fig. 10. Water-soluble π-metalated calix[n]arene **29** and complexes

A series of π-metalated calix[n]arenes were synthesised, among which compounds **29** are water-soluble due to the presence of six positive charges.[50] The calixarenes cavities are therefore electron-poor and able to complex anions both in the solid state and in water. The X-ray crystal structures of compounds **29a, 29c** and **29d** showed that a BF_4^-, SO_4^{2-}, and I^- anion is complexed in the calixarene cavity, respectively, tetrafluoroborate being the most deeply included one. Acetate, phosphate and sulfate anions are not bound by host **(29b),** due to their high hydrophilicity. An interesting inversion of the expected selectivity, on the basis of the free hydration energy order (Hofmeister series), is observed for halide ions due to size complementarity between the guest and the calixarene cavity.[51]

3.2.2 Molecular anion recognition and depth of hydrophobic cavity of water-soluble calix[4]arenes

Very few examples of anion complexation by water-soluble calixarenes have been reported so far. This is probably due to the fact that anion recognition is a rather new field in supramolecular chemistry and that anions are more highly hydrated than cations of comparable size and, therefore, their complexation in water is a remarkably difficult task. In the case of l-anilino-8-naphthalenesulfonate (ANS)[52] and 2-*p*-toluidino-6-naphthalenesulfonate (TNS) [53] the lipophilic residue of the guest is included inside the calixarene cavity.[54]

A cationic calix[4]arene derivative **(30)** binds both aliphatic **(31, 32)** and aromatic, sulfonate **(23)** and carboxylate **(26)** anions in aqueous solution with a Log *K* of 1.50, 1.48, 2.44, 2.32, respectively, as a result of concerted electrostatic and hydrophobic interactions. The sulfonate ion in guest **23** may show good electrostatic interaction with the cations on the top of the cavity. However, the sulfonate guest inclusion is affected by the host different mobility caused by the pH change. An interesting example of the anionic host **(10)** complexation with the anionic sulfonate **(23)** (Log *K*= 4.3, pH=7.3; Log *K*= 0, pH=5.8) has been recently reported.[55] The pH of the solution shows a significant effect on the dynamics of the gate (formed by eight benzylic functions) and portal on the hydrophobic cavity of the water-soluble aminocalix[4]arene host (**10**). At pH 5.8 the gate closes and prevents the entry of anionic guests. However, at pH 7.3 the gate opens and allows the entry of anionic guests (**23, 24**) to the hydrophobic cavity. Host **10** not only shows a similar behaviour towards guests **23** and **24** but also shows a preference for sulfonate derivatives. This preference can be assigned to the tripodal symmetry of sulfonate function, instead of dipodal in carboxylate, and its electron withdrawing effect. The tripodal symmetry gives extra room for negative charges of guest molecules on the cavity of host **10** reducing the electrostatic repulsion. The electron withdrawing effect prevails and increases the п-п stacking interactions between the guest (**23**) and the host (**10**). The deep hydrophobic cavity of the water-soluble aminocalix[4]arene role in the recognition of anionic guests cannot be neglected, despite the absence of favourable electrostatic interaction shown by host **30** towards guests **23** and **24**, host **10** showing strong binding with them.

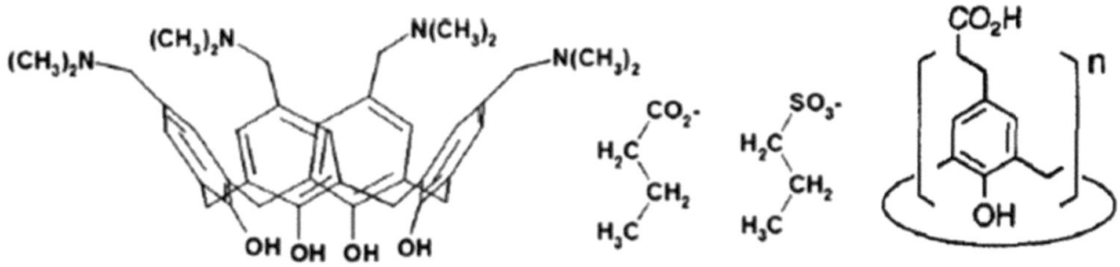

30 **31** **32** **33**

Fig. 11. Water-soluble calix[4]arene derivatives **30** (cationic), **33**.

3.3 Recognition of neutral molecules

The complexation of neutral molecules by water-soluble calixarenes was carried out in the eighties and has been already critically reviewed.[56,57,58] The pioneering work[59] on the complexation of aromatic hydrocarbons by hosts **33** (n=4) has however to be mentioned, since it disclosed a rough correlation between binding constants and host-guest complementarily. Calix[4]arenes are too small to host durene or naphthalene, calix[5]- or -[6]arenes preferring naphthalene, anthracene and phenanthrene.

Sciotto et al. have studied the interactions between alcohols, ketones, nitriles and p-sulfonatocalixarenes (**4**) and its derivatives by 1H NMR spectroscopy,[60,61] proving that the apolar aliphatic portions of the guests were included into the host hydrophobic cavity with the terminal polar groups directed towards the polar sulfonate groups of the host and to the solvent. The two most important factors for the complexation of the investigated hosts and guests are conformational properties of the receptors and electrostatic effects. Methanol is not included by p-sulfonatocalixarenes at all, probably due to the fact that the small methyl group inclusion inside the hydrophobic cavity would lead to a partial inclusion of polar OH group, causing the polar hydroxyl group to be less exposed to polar solvent.

The interactions of aromatic substrates (**34, 35, 36,** and **37**) (**Figure 12**) with **4** were studied by Schatz and co-workers via ^{1}H NMR titration experiments and molecular modelling studies combined with abinitio NMR shift calculation at neutral aqueous solutions.[62] All the guests are included into the hosts cavities, with a mechanism which is mainly driven by enthalpy term. In most cases, the five aromatic protons are pointing inside and the guest functional group is located outside the hosts cavities due to hydrophobic and π-π interactions. For (**34**), the complex binding mode is different, probably because the methyl group is included into the host cavity, contributing to the favorable C–H-π interactions and hydrophobic interactions.[63]

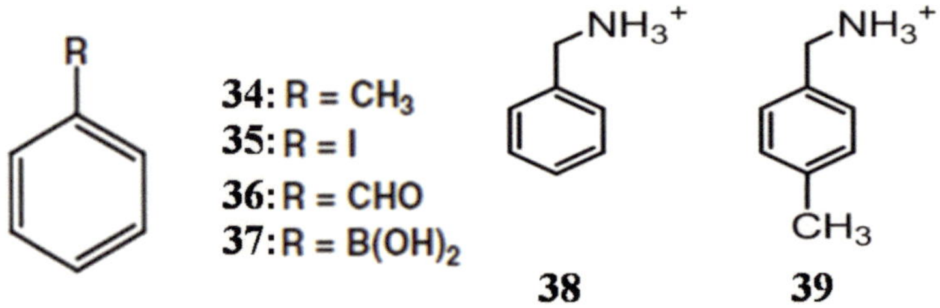

Fig. 12. Aromatic neutral guests (**34-37**), and cationic guests **38**, **39.**

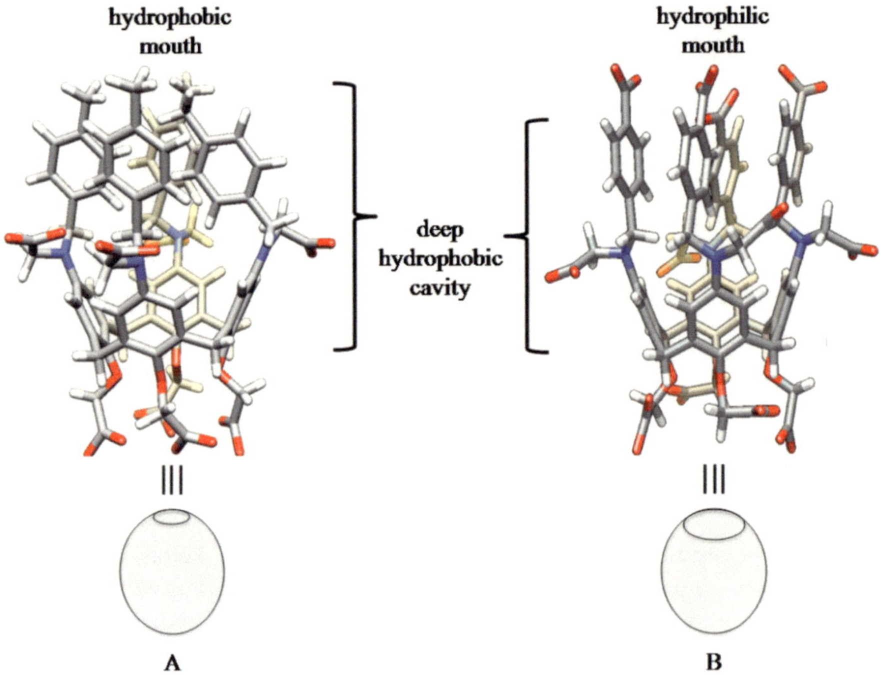

Fig. 13. Hosts **11** and **12,** A) host **12** (side view), B) host **11** (side view).

The new water-soluble aminocalix[4]arene hosts **11** and **12** with deep hydrophobic cavity facilitate hydrophilic mouth and hydrophobic mouth, respectively.[64] The ^{1}H NMR titrations revealed that host **12** shows high selectivity for neutral guests (**18** and **19**), with log *K* of 4.2 and 4.6, respectively. The host **11** shows log *K* of 4.9 for binding with guest **39**. Moreover, the host **11** binding ability for guest **38** is stronger by a factor of 1000 than that of the host **12**.

The NMR investigations indicate that host **11** and **12** can form 1:1 host–guest inclusion complexes with aromatic cationic guests and pyridine derivatives with high binding constants. Both hosts refused to recognize the hydrophilic anionic guests, possibly due to the electrostatic repulsion arising from carboxylate functions on the cavity of the host. The host **12**, with hydrophobic mouth, showed high binding constant for 4-methylbenzylammonium, as the carboxylate functions of the mouth showed strong electrostatic interactions with the ammonium function. However, the hydrophilic mouth of host **11** enhances the binding of 4-ethylpyridine. It is clear from the data that the cavity of both hosts has a preference for structurally flat guests containing methyl groups (either a CH_3 in *para* position of an aromatic ring or a presence of trimethylammonium group) and a very poor one for smaller but more hydrophilic primary ammonium groups, which indeed do not enter the hydrophobic cavity.

4. Conclusion

Mimicry of the molecular recognition features of naturally occurring proteins by synthetic receptors is one of the challenging research topics of supramolecular chemistry. The substrates and enzymes (host-guest) features can be studied by Potentiometry, NMR Spectroscopy, UV-Visible Spectroscopy, Fluorescence Spectroscopy, and Calorimetry. In some cases the ESI-MS can be employed to study the protein-protein, or protein-small molecule interactions. It is quite obvious that the exact host-guest complex stoichiometry is the most critical parameter in the evaluation of the host-guest interactions. The molecular recognition properties of the water-soluble calix[4]arene derivatives revealed that the hydrophobic cavity of these hosts play an important role in the guests recognition. Increasing the hydrophobic cavity depth, like in the water-soluble aminocalix[4]arene hosts, results in an increased binding of the guest into the hosts deep hydrophobic pockets. Synthetically tailored hosts based on the calix[4]arene framework can be used to probe the naturally occurring biomolecular reactions based on the non-covalent interactions.

5. Acknowledgement

This work was supported by the Ministry of Knowledge and Economy of South Korea. We also acknowledge Song Keum-soo and Kim Junghoon of Biometrix Technology Inc. Chuncheon, Korea for helpful discussions.

6. References

[1] Seeman NC, Rosenberg JM, Rich A. Sequence specific recognition of double helical nucleic acids by proteins. 1976. *Proc. Natl. Acad. Sci. USA* 73:804–8

[2] Janin J. Wet and dry interfaces: the role of solvent in protein-protein and protein-DNA recognition. 1999. *Structure* 7:R277–79

[3] Woda J, Schneider B, Patel K, Mistry K, Berman HM. 1998. An analysis of the relationship between hydration and protein- DNA interactions. *Biophys. J.* 75:2170–77

[4] Schwabe JW. The role of water in protein-DNA interactions. 1997. *Curr. Opin. Struct. Biol.* 7:126–34

[5] Reddy CK, Das A, Jayaram B. Do water molecules mediate protein-DNA recognition? 2001. *J. Mol. Biol.* 314:619–32

[6] Nandhikonda P, Heagy MD. An Abiotic Fluorescent Probe for Cardiac Troponin I. 2011. *J. Am. Chem. Soc.* 133(38):14972-14974

[7] Voet D, Voet JG. (1995) Biochemistry (Wiley, Somerset, NJ), 2nd Ed., pp. 398–400

[8] Pal S. K., Peon J, Zewail AH. Biological water at the protein surface: Dynamical solvation probed directly with femtosecond resolution. 2002. Proc. Nat. Acad. Sci. 99(4): 1763–1768

[9] Tsuchida R, 1935. *Bull. Chem. Soc. Jpn.*, 10:27

[10] Harvey AE, Manning DL, 1950. *J. Am. Chem. Soc.*, 72:4488

[11] Yoe JH, Jones AL, 1944. *Ind. Eng. Chem. Anal. Ed.*, 16:111.

[12] Bencini A, Bianchi A, Garcia-España E, Micheloni M, Ramirez JA. Proton coordination by polyamine compounds in aqueous solution. 1999. *Coord. Chem. Rev.* 188:97–156.

[13] Benesi HA, Hildebrand JH. 1949 *J. Am. Chem. Soc.* 71:2703-2707.

[14] Rose NJ, Drago RS. 1959. *J. Am. Chem. Soc.* 81: 6138-6141.

[15] Foster R, Fyfe CA. 1965. *J. Chem. Soc., Chem. Commun.* 642.

[16] Scatchard G. 1949 *Ann. N.Y. Acad. Sci.* 51: 660-672.

[17] Fielding L. Determination of Association Constants (Ka) from Solution NMR Data. 2000. *Tetrahedron,* 56:6151-6170.

[18] Cohen Y, Avram L, Frish L, 2005. *Angew Chem. Int. Ed.* 44:520–554

[19] Lucas LH, Larive CK, 2004. *Concepts Magn. Reson.*, 20A: 24–41.

[20] Ababou A, Ladbury JE. Survey of the year 2004: literature on applications of isothermal titration calorimetry. 2006. *J. Mol. Recognit.* 19:79–89

[21] Cliff MJ, Gutierrez A, Ladbury JE, A survey of the year 2003: literature on applications of isothermal titration calorimetry. 2004. *J. Mol. Recognit.* 17:513–523.

[22] Cliff M, Ladbury JE, A survey of the year 2002 literature on applications of isothermal titration calorimetry. 2003. *J. Mol. Recognit.* 16: 383–391.

[23] Rosu F, Gabelica V, Houssier C, Pauw ED. 2002. Determination of affinity, stoichiometry and sequence selectivity of minor groove binder complexes with double-stranded oligodeoxynucleotides by electrospray ionization mass spectrometry. *Nucl. Acids Res.* 30(16): e82.

[24] Wilm M. Principles of Electrospray Ionization. 2011. *Molecular & Cellular Proteomics,* 10: M111.009407.

[25] Wortmann A, Jecklin MC, Touboul D, Badertscher M, Zenobi, R. Binding constant determination of high-affinity protein–ligand complexes by electrospray ionization mass spectrometry and ligand competition. 2008. *J. Mass Spectrom.* 43:600–608.

[26] Pellet-Rostaing S, Chitry F, Spitz J-A, Sorin A, Favre-Re´guillon A, Lemaire M. 2003. *Tetrahedron,* 59: 10313.

[27] Pellet-Rostaing S, Chitry F, Spitz J-A, Sorin A, Favre-Réguillon A, Lemaire M. New water-soluble calix[4]arene-bis(benzocrown-6) for caesium–sodium separation by nanofiltration–complexation. 2003. Tetrahedron 59: 10313–10324

[28] Kang SK, Chung TD, Kim H. 2000. Electrochemical recognition of Ca^{2+} ion in basic aqueous media using quinone-derivatized calix[4]arene. *Electrochimica Acta.* 45:2939–2943

[29] Kim TH. Voltammetric Recognition of Ca2+ by Calix[4]arene Diquinone Diacid. 2010 *Bull. Korean Chem. Soc.,* 31: 3115-3117

[30] Liu Y, Wang H, Wang L-H, Zhang H-Y. Complexation thermodynamics of water-soluble calix[4]arene derivatives with lanthanoid(III) nitrates in acidic aqueous solution. 2004. *Thermochimica Acta* 414:65–70

[31] Shinkai S, Araki K, Manabe O. 1988. *J. Am. Chem. Soc.* 110, 7214.

[32] hinkai S, Arimura A, Araki V, Kawabata H, Satoh H, Tsubaki T, Manabe O, Sunamoto, J. 1989. *J. Chem. Soc. Perkin Trans. 1*, 2039.

[33] Arena G, Casnati A, Contino A, Lombardo GG, Sciotto D, Ungaro, R. 1999 *Chem. Eur. J.* 738-744.

[34] Shinkai S, Araki K, Matsuda T, Nishiyama N, Ikeda H, Takasu L, Iwamoto M. 1990. *J. Am. Chem. Soc.*, 112:9053- 9058

[35] Arena G, Casnati A, Mirone L, Sciotto D, Ungaro R. 1997. *Tetrahedron Letters* 38:1999.

[36] Arena G, Casnati A, Contino A, Sciotto D, Ungaro R, 1997. *Tetrahedron Letters*, 38:4685.

[37] Arnecke R, Böhmer V, Cacciapaglia R, Dalla Cort A, Mandolini L. 1997. *Tetrahedron* 53:4901.

[38] Arena G, Bonomo RP, Calì R, Gulino FG, Lombardo GG, Sciotto D, Ungaro R, Casnati A. 1995. *Supramol. Chem.* 4:287-295.

[39] Arena G, Contino A, Lombardo GG, Sciotto D. 1995. *Thermochimica Acta* 264:1-11.

[40] Arena G, Contino A, Musumeci S, Purrello R, 1990. *J. Chem. Soc. Dalton Trans.* 3383

[41] Nimse SB, Kim J, Song K, Kim J, Lee JT, Nguyen V, Ta V, Kim T. Selective recognition of the ditopic trimethylammonium cations by water-soluble aminocalix[4]arene. 2011. *Tetrahedron Letters* 52: 3751-3754.

[42] Nimse SB, Kim J, Ta V, Kim H, Song K, Jung C, Nguyen V, Kim, T. New water-soluble iminecalix[4]arene with a deep hydrophobic cavity. 2009. Tetrahedron Letters 52:7346-7350.

[43] Nimse SB, Song K, Kim J, Ta V, Nguyen V, Kim T. Synthesis and Modification of Novel Iminecalix[4]arene Derivatives. 2011. *Bull. Korean Chem. Soc.* 32: 1143-1145.

[44] Gale PA. 2004. *Coord. Chem. Rev.* 240:191

[45] Gale PA. 2001. *Coord. Chem. Rev.* 213:79.

[46] Atwood JL, Holman KT, Steed JW. 1996. *Chem. Commun.* 1401.

[47] Kropman MF, Bakker HJ. Dynamics of Water Molecules in Aqueous Solvation Shells. 2001 *Science* 291:2119-2120.

[48] Gupta VK, Ludwig R, Agarwal, S. Anion recognition through modified calixarenes: a highly selective sensor for monohydrogen phosphate. 2005. *Analytica Chimica Acta* 538: 213–218.

[49] Dondoni A, Marra A, Scherrmann M-C, Casnati A, Sansone F, Ungaro R. 1997. Chem. Eur. J. 3:1774-1782.

[50] Staffilani M, Hancock KSB, Steed JW, Holman KT, Atwood JL, Juneja RK, Burkhalter RS. 1997. *J. Am. Chem. Soc.* 119:6324-6335.

[51] Steed JW, Juneja RK, Atwood JL. 1994. *Angew. Chem., Int. Ed. Engl.* 33:2456-2457.

[52] van Dienst E, Snellink BHM, von Piekartz I, Engbersen JFJ, Reinhoudt DN. 1995. *J. Chem.Soc., Chem. Commun.* 1151-1152.

[53] Shi Y, Zhang Z, 1994. *J. Chem. Soc., Chem. Commun.* 375-376.

[54] Shi Y, Zhang Z.1994. *J. Incl. Phenom.* 18:137-147.

[55] Nimse SB, Song K, Kim J, Kim H, Nguyen V, Eoum W, Jung C, Ta, V, Kim, T. Aminocalix[4]arene: The Effect of pH on the Dynamics of Gate and Portals on the Hydrophobic Cavity. 2010. *Tetrahedron Letters* 51:6156-6160.

[56] Gutsche CD. *Calixarenes,* The Royal Society of Chemistry (Ed.: J. F. Stoddart), Cambridge, 1989.
[57] Shinkai S. in *Calixarenes, a Versatile Class of Macrocyclic Compounds,* Kluwer Academic Publishers (Eds.: J. Vicens, V. Böhmer), Dordrecht, 1991, pp. 173-198.
[58] Pochini A, Ungaro R. in *Comprehensive Supramolecular Chemistry, Vol. 2,* Pergamon Press (Ed.: F. Vögtle), Oxford, 1996, pp. 103-142.
[59] Gutsche CD, Alam I. 1988. *Tetrahedron* 4689-4694.
[60] Arena G, Casnati A, Contino A, Sciotto D, Ungaro R. Charge assisted hydrophobic binding of ethanol into the cavity of calix[4]arene receptors in aqueous solution. 1997. *Tetrahedron Letters* 38(26):4685–4688.
[61] Arena G, Contino A, Gulino FG, Magrí A, Sciotto D, Ungaro R. Complexation of small neutral organic molecules by water soluble calix[4]arenes. 2000. *Tetrahedron Lett*ers 41: 9327–9330.
[62] Baur M, Frank M, Schatz J, Schildbach F. Water-soluble calix[n]arenes as receptor molecules for non-polar substrates and inverse phase transfer catalysts. 2001. *Tetrahedron* 57:6985–6991.
[63] Guo D-S, Wang K, Liu y. Selective binding behaviors of p-sulfonatocalixarenes in aqueous solution. 2008. *Incl. Phenom. Macrocycl. Chem.* 62(1-2):1-21.
[64] Nimse SB, Nguyen V, Kim J, Kim H, Song K, Eoum W, Jung C, Ta V, Seelam SR, Kim T. Water-soluble aminocalix[4]arene receptors with hydrophobic and hydrophilic mouths. 2010. *Tetrahedron Letters* 51:2840-2845.

The Determination of the Stoichiometry of Cyclodextrin Inclusion Complexes by Spectral Methods: Possibilities and Limitations

Cristina Tablet, Iulia Matei and Mihaela Hillebrand
Dept. Physical Chemistry, University of Bucharest, Bucharest, Romania

1. Introduction

The inclusion complexes of many organic ligands, drugs or metal ions, in cyclodextrins (CDs) represent a class of the simplest supramolecular systems widely studied for the last several decades. The increasing interest for their investigation arises from both a theoretical and an applicative points of view. Considering the first one, their study contributes to the understanding of the molecular recognition and molecular interactions, emphasizing the role of different structural factors. From a more practical purpose, the encapsulation of different drugs in the CD cavity produces an increase in the solubility (Brewster & Loftsson, 2007) and allows for a more controlled oral, parental, ocular, nasal or rectal drug release (Challa et al., 2005). A special interest resides in the CDs potential as alternatives for conventional anti-obesity medications (Grunberger et al., 2007). The same goal is also realized using the supramolecular systems, such as hydrogels, obtained by the self-assembling of CDs with some polymers (Li, 2010; Zhang & Ma, 2010). One of the CDs applications that deserves both an experimental and theoretical focus is based on their interaction with the cellular or model membranes, resulting in cholesterol extraction (Abi-Mosleh et al, 2009). It was shown that the cholesterol removal occurs via inclusion complex formation, for which the stoichiometry plays an important role. Thus, it was stated on both experimental grounds and molecular dynamics calculations that the efficient stoichiometry for the extraction is 1:2 guest:host, requiring, for a good effect, the presence of CD dimers oriented in an appropriate way on the membrane layer (Lopez et al., 2011). Besides these, a remarkable amount of studies were devoted to CDs inclusion complexes, covering an extended basis for the discussion of their properties and applications (Arunkumar et al., 2005; Challa et al., 2005; Li & Loh, 2008; Loftsson et al., 2004; Loftsson & Duchene, 2007; Martin Del Valle, 2004; Sjetli, 1982; Vyas et al., 2008).

Continuing our studies on the CDs inclusion process (Oana et al., 2002; Matei et al., 2007; Tablet & Hillebrand, 2008, Tintaru et al., 2003), we report here some cases encountered in the study of some potentially bioactive compounds like coumarin and phenoxathiin derivatives, and of two drugs, atenolol and indapamide, presenting some peculiar structural factors which make their characterization more difficult. We will focus on the possibilities and limitations of some spectroscopic methods for the estimation of the stoichiometry and association constants for both cases, i.e. when the procedure is straightforward and when some problems were encountered. The guest molecules were chosen to elucidate some difficulties occurring during the analysis of the experimental data in establishing the real stoichiometry of the inclusion complexes.

This paper starts with a short description of the main features of CDs and their inclusion complexes. After a summary of the main mathematical models used for the estimation of the inclusion complexes properties, we will discuss our results on the specific aforementioned cases.

1.1 Cyclodextrins and the characterization of their inclusion complexes

Native CDs are macrocyclic oligosaccharides formed by the α-1,4-linkage of 6–8 glucose residues and named α-, β- and γ-CD, respectively. They have a toroidal structure and, based on molecular recognition principles, are able to include in their cavity different organic molecules and ions. Therefore, they will be hereafter named as Host, H, while the ligands are generally labelled as Guests, G. Differing from the hydrophobic character of the cavity, the presence of the primary and secondary OH groups ensures an hydrophilic exterior. Besides these three CDs, a large number of modified CDs were synthesized and used for experimental studies, aiming to a better understanding of the driving forces of the inclusion process. Furthermore there is an increasing interest on CDs, due to their multiple applications, especially in pharmacology and biotechnology. The characterization of a CD inclusion complex can be performed using different experimental methods and implicates several factors briefly summarized below.

1.1.1 Methodology

The spectral methods are based on monitoring the guest corresponding spectra, at a constant concentration, when increasing amounts of CDs are added. In absorption and fluorescence spectroscopy, the main effects in the guest spectra are changes in the intensity and/or band shifts. They may be accompanied by the appearance of isosbestic/isoemissive points, which indicate an equilibrium between the free and the complexed guest. Differently, the absence of isosbestic points can be indicative of the occurrence of high order associations in solution (Hamai et al., 1992). In the spectral range of the common guest molecules, there is no interference from the absorption bands of the CDs, located in the far UV region. Using NMR spectroscopy, the experimental data for characterizing the complexes are the variation in the chemical shifts of both guest and host protons (Tintaru et al., 2003). IR and Raman spectroscopies can be used as well for the characterization of the inclusion complexes.

A spectral method which brings about interesting information is the circular dichroism spectroscopy. Circular dichroism is essentially an absorption phenomenon occurring when an optically active molecule absorbs to different degrees the right and left components of a circularly polarized light beam. The magnitude of the dichroic signal depends on the difference between the molar extinction coefficients of the molecule for the right- and left-handed components. The changes that inclusion to CDs, chiral environments themselves, may produce in the circular dichroism spectrum of a guest molecule are of two types, depending on the nature of the guest: a) for a chiral guest, CD inclusion may lead to changes in its intrinsic dichroic signal; b) for an achiral guest, CD inclusion may lead to the appearance of an induced dichroic signal of the guest, by chirality transfer from the CD. As the circular dichroism technique offers data on the steric match between the two interacting partners, i.e. on the "geometry" of the interaction, the dimensions of the CD cavity mainly determine the changes observed in the spectrum of the guest upon CD incorporation. The dichroic band position is the same as the absorption one corresponding to the chromophore involved in the electronic transition.

The sign of the dichroic band of a guest molecule included in the CD cavity depends on the angle between the electronic transition moment and the symmetry axis of the CD. The rules of Harata and Kodaka state that the dichroic signal is positive for an axial inclusion (parallel orientation of the transition moment with respect to the CD axis) and negative for an equatorial inclusion (perpendicular orientation) (Harata & Uedaira, 1975; Kodaka, 1993). Thus, it is possible to obtain valuable information on the stoichiometry and the orientation of the guest molecule in the complex. Moreover, the intensity of the dichroic signal gives an indication on the magnitude of the interaction, namely on the induced asymmetry.

1.1.2 The stoichiometry

The stoichiometry of the complex is given by the number of G and H molecules contained in the supramolecular complex, the general notation being G_nH_m; the most common stoichiometry is 1:1 (GH), implying the inclusion of a single guest molecule, but other stoichiometries like G_1H_2, G_2H_1, G_2H_2, G_1H_3, G_3H_1, etc., can be encountered as well (Baglole et al., 2005; De Azevedo et al., 2000; Ge et al., 2011; Sancho et al., 2011; Shen et al., 1998) and some of them will be further discussed from a structural point of view. As the formation of the G_1H_2 complex can be the result of two successive equilibriums, the simultaneous presence of 1:1 and 1:2 complexes is also frequently mentioned.

Self-assembled, stable supramolecular systems can also be formed, containing a large number of H and G molecules. Such systems include the rotaxanes, catenanes and nanotubes (Li et al., 2011; Qu et al. 2005; Yui et al., 2009). In some cases, the obtained complexes form extended linear aggregates, revealed mostly from the unexpectedly large value of the fluorescence anisotropy, e.g. 2,5-diphenyl-oxazole with γ-CD (Agbaria & Gill, 1988), 2,5-diphenyl-1,3,4-oxadiazole, 2-phenyl-5-(4-biphenyl)-1,3,4-oxadiazole and 2,5-biphenyl-1,3,4-oxadiazole with γ-CD (Agbaria & Gill, 1994), 2,5-bis-(4-methylphenyl)-oxazole with β-CD and γ-CD (Yarabe et al., 2002), 1,4-diphenyl-1,3-butadiene with β-CD and γ-CD (De La Pena et al., 1997), trans-1,6-diphenyl-1,3,5-hexatriene with β-CD and γ-CD (Li & McGown, 1994), 4,4'-bis(2-benzoxazolyl) stilbene with β-CD and γ-CD (Wu et al., 2006) and coumarin 153 with γ-CD (Mandal et al., 2011).

1.1.3 The association constant

The quantitative measure of the guest–host interaction at a given temperature is represented by the value of the equilibrium constant governing the formation of the inclusion complex. It is also referred to as binding or association constant. The mathematical models for processing the experimental data in order to estimate the association constants will be discussed further for some of the most common cases.

1.1.4 The thermodynamic parameters

Performing the experiments at different temperatures and using the estimated associated constants in a Van't Hoff treatment allow for the determination of the thermodynamic parameters of the inclusion process, ΔH and ΔS (Tablet & Hillebrand, 2008). The sign and the absolute relative values of these quantities are further used in the discussion of the main forces involved in the inclusion process, i.e. electrostatic, hydrophobic, hydrogen bonds, etc.

1.1.5 Structural aspects

The structure of an inclusion complex in solution is difficult to be established. The guest can penetrate the CD cavity in several ways, through the wide or the narrow rim, in an axial or equatorial position with respect to the cavity long axis. Although for obtaining the previously mentioned features all the spectral methods (absorption, fluorescence, circular dichroism and NMR spectroscopy) can be used, information on the structure of the complexes can be experimentally obtained only from 2D-NMR and induced circular dichroism (ICD) spectra. The presence of the asymmetric environment of the cavity can induce a dichroic signal even for the achiral guests. According to the Harata-Kodaka rules, the positive/negative sign of the dichroic band indicates the axial/equatorial inclusion of the guest in respect to the cavity main axis. This information can be used as starting point to elaborate structural models that will be further optimized at different theoretical levels (molecular mechanics, semiempirical methods, DFT). The best test for judging the consistency of the model, although difficult to reach, is the agreement between the simulated ICD spectrum of the G_nH_m system and the experimental one.

1.2 Determination of the stoichiometry. Job's method

One of the first methods used for the determination of the stoichiometry of inclusion complexes was Job's method, also known as the continuous variation method (Job, 1928). The experiments use stock solutions with equimolecular concentrations of H and G components. The samples are prepared by mixing different volumes of these two solutions in such a way that the total concentration [H]+[G] remains constant and the molar fraction of the guest, X_G varies in the range 0–1. The variation of the experimental measured property, ΔP, in presence of the host in respect with the value for the free guest is plotted vs. X_G or X_H. The value of X_G for which the plot presents the maximum deviation gives the stoichiometry of the inclusion complex ($X_G = 0.5$ for 1:1 or 2:2 G:H complexes; $X_H = 0.33$ for 1:2 G:H complexes). Although, in most cases, in a Job plot ΔP represents the change of the absorbance of the guest during addition of the host, ΔA, (Rajaram et al., 2011), other properties correlated with the concentration of the complex, like the change in the NMR chemical shifts ($\Delta\delta$) or the enthalpy changes (ΔH) can be used as well (Chadha et al., 2011; Kacso et al., 2010; Thi et al., 2011).

Two typical schematic Job's plots for 1:1 and 1:2 inclusion complexes are given in Fig. 1, considering ΔP as the absorbance change, ΔA, for the HG complexes and the NMR proton shifts ($\Delta\delta$) for the HG_2 complexes. It can be seen that in the case of 1:1 complexes, the maximum deviation is obtained for $X_H = 0.5$, while for the second type of complexes the maximum is reached for $X_H \sim 0.37$. Literature data offers a lot of examples for the application of Job's method (Ge et al., 2011; Jadhav et al., 2007; Liu et al., 2001; Sainz-Rozas et al., 2005).

A development of Job's method was described by Landy *et al.* (Landy et al., 2007) for the determination of the stoichiometry of CD inclusion complexes and named Competitive Continuous Variation Plot. In fact, this new approach represents a coupling of Job's method with the competitive experiments, spectral displacements, well known in the study of biopolymer–ligand interactions. The basic idea was to monitor the changes of a given experimental property and to build a Job plot when a competitor ligand, for which the features of the inclusion complex were previously determined, is introduced in the system. The method is recommended for the cases in which either the low solubility prevents the usual experimental determinations or the spectral properties of the guest are not in the experimental accessible range.

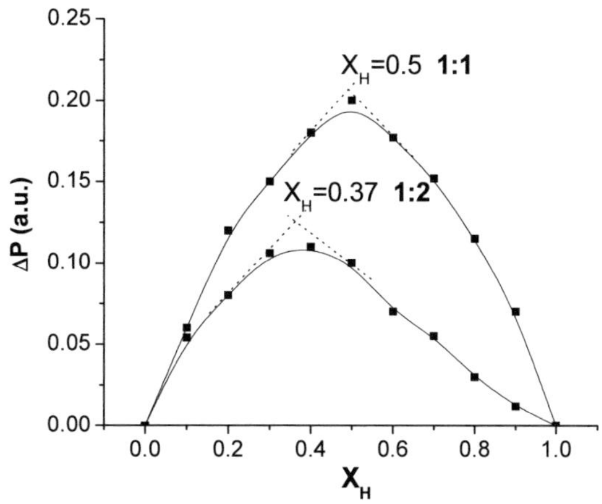

Fig. 1. Typical Job's plots for 1:1 and 1:2 complexes.

1.3 Determination of both the stoichiometry and the association constant

The determination of the stoichiometry in the host–guest interaction is strongly correlated with the estimation of the association constant. Excepting Job's method which gives indications only on the stoichiometry of the inclusion complexes, for all other methods the following procedure is applied. Several stoichiometries are assumed and the experimental data are fitted to the corresponding linear or nonlinear models. The description of all these models and their different applications are given in very well known books and reviews (Connors, 1987; Singh et al., 2010). Therefore, we will further present in Table 1 the main formula used in the analysis of the spectral experimental data, without the corresponding deductions. Starting with the equations of the assumed chemical equilibria, the general idea is to monitor the changes of an experimental property (P_{obs}) directly correlated with the concentration of the former or the new-formed species, at gradual host addition. The function P_{obs} = f(C_i, parameters), where C_i represents the equilibrium concentration of the species *i*, is called the binding isotherm. As for Job's plot, this property can be the absorbance (A), fluorescence quantum yield or fluorescence emission (Φ or F), ellipticity (θ) or NMR chemical shift (Δδ). Starting from the binding isotherm, the equations corresponding to some widely used linear (eqs. 1, 2, 5) (Benesi & Hildebrand, 1949; Scott, 1956) and nonlinear (eqs. 3, 4, 6–9) (Liu et al., 2001; Park et al., 2002) models are given in Table 1.

Stoichiometry	**Equations**
1:1	$\mathrm{G + H \rightleftharpoons GH}$ $\frac{1}{\Delta P_{obs}} = \frac{1}{(P_{GH} - P_{G_0})K_{11}[H]} + \frac{1}{(P_{GH} - P_{G_0})}$ (1) $\frac{[H][G]_0}{\Delta P_{obs}} = \frac{[G]_0}{P'_{GH}} + \frac{1}{K \cdot P'_{GH}}$ (2) $P_{obs} = \frac{P_{G_0} + P_{GH}K_{11}[H]}{1 + K_{11}[H]}$ (3) $\Delta P_{obs} = \frac{1}{2}([H] + [G] + \frac{1}{K_{11}}) - \sqrt{([H] + [G] + \frac{1}{K_{11}})^2 - 4[H][G])}$ (4)
1:2	$\mathrm{G + 2H \rightleftharpoons GH_2}$ $\frac{1}{\Delta P_{obs}} = \frac{1}{(P_{GH} - P_{G_0})K_{12}[H]^2} + \frac{1}{(P_{GH} - P_{G_0})}$ (5) $P_{obs} = \frac{P_{G_0} + P_{GH_2}K_{12}[H]^2}{1 + K_{12}[H]^2}$ (6)
1:1+1:2	$\mathrm{G + H \rightleftharpoons GH;\ GH + H \rightleftharpoons GH_2}$ $P_{obs} = \frac{P_{G_0} + P_{GH}K_{11}[H] + P_{GH_2}K_{11}K_{12}[H]^2}{1 + K_{11}[H] + K_{11}K_{12}[H]^2}$ (7)
2:1	$\mathrm{G + H \rightleftharpoons GH;\ GH + G \rightleftharpoons G_2H}$ $P = P_{G_2H}\frac{1}{2}([G]_0 - [G] - K_{11}[H][G])$ (8) where $[G] = \frac{-(K_{11}[H] + 1) + \sqrt{(K_{11}[H] + 1)^2 + 8K_{11}K_{21}[H][G]_0}}{4K_{11}K_{21}[H]}$
2:2	$\mathrm{G + H \rightleftharpoons GH;\ GH + GH \rightleftharpoons G_2H_2}$ $P = P_{G_2H_2}\frac{1}{2}([G]_0 - [G] - K_{11}[H][G])$ (9) where $[G] = \frac{-(K_{11}[H] + 1) + \sqrt{(K_{11}[H] + 1)^2 + 8K_{11}^2K_{22}[H]^2[G]_0}}{4K_{11}^2K_{22}[H]^2}$

Table 1. Nonlinear and linear fitting models for the determination of the stoichiometry and association constant of a CD inclusion complex.

An interesting case is the formation of inclusion complexes in which the guest is included as a dimer. There are two types of stoichiometry for such complexes: 2:1, obtained by the inclusion of a second guest molecule in a 1:1 complex already formed, or 2:2, resulted from the association of two 1:1 complexes. Over the time, Hamai has reported extensive studies on this regard (Hamai, 1990, 1999, 2005, 2010). Fluorescence is an excellent tool to reveal the formation of these complexes because the dimer, called excimer in excited state, has a distinct band localized at longer wavelength than the monomer. Monitoring the dependence of its fluorescence intensity *vs.* its concentration we can distinguish between the 2:1 and 2:2 stoichiometries using the eqs. 8 and 9 from Table 1. There are two ways to find the K_{21} and K_{22} values. The first one is to drive the experiment at small guest concentrations, when the dimer does not exist, and thus to obtain the K_{11} value. Then, with this value, we can simulate curves according to eqs. 8 and 9 for various values of K_{21} and K_{22}. The best fit gives the value of the association constant. The second one is to fit the data directly with the said equations and to obtain K_{11} and K_{21} or K_{22}.

When several complex types, i.e. complexes with different stoichiometry, are present in the system, the necessity to introduce several fitting parameters reduces the reliability of the fits. Therefore, for spectral measurements, one recommended method (Davies & Deary, 1999; Sainz-Rozas et al., 2005) is to work with sets of data read at different wavelengths and to perform a multivariable analysis of the whole set of data, imposing the condition that the association constants are the same, independent on the wavelength.

A special case when it is impossible to unambiguously differentiate by fitting procedures between the 1:1 and the mixture of 1:1+1:2 complexes was discussed by Pistolis and Malliaris (Pistolis & Malliaris, 1999). They found that this happens when the ratio of the corresponding equilibrium constants K_{11}/K_{12} depends on the extinction coefficients of the species present in the system, the free guest, the 1:1 complex and the 1:2 complex, according to eq. 10, written in respect to the extinction coefficients:

$$\frac{K_{11}}{K_{12}} = \frac{(\varepsilon_{GH_2} - \varepsilon_G)^2}{(\varepsilon_{GH} - \varepsilon_G)(\varepsilon_{GH_2} - \varepsilon_{GH})} \tag{10}$$

The same relationship holds also for the analysis of fluorescence data, with the fluorescence quantum yields of the three species, Φ_G, Φ_{GH}, Φ_{GH_2}, replacing the extinction coefficients. The authors recommend that in such cases additional experiments must be carried out, for example fluorescence time-resolved or anisotropy experiments.

The most used equations are the Benesi-Hildebrand linear or double reciprocal equations. However, their reliability was the subject of many discussions, especially to differentiate the formation of 1:1 and 1:2 complexes. Besides the usual approximations included in the deduction of the Benesi-Hildebrand equation, Wang (Wang & Yu, 2007) used computer simulations to establish some required experimental conditions for obtaining consistent results with the Benesi-Hildebrand equations, rules that can also be applied for the guest-CD systems.

Shortly, they stated that the CD concentration should be at least an order of magnitude larger than the guest's, the minimum concentration ratio of the two partners should be sufficiently large and the ratio 1/(K[G]) should be large, around 20. Analyzing the electronic absorption data, they also emphasized the role of the differences in the extinction coefficients for the 1:1 and 1:2 complexes compared to the free guest.

A slight different methodology for the association constants estimation considers the time-resolved fluorescence experiments. The study of the decay fluorescence curves allows for the estimation of the stoichiometry, and, consequently of the association constants. In the case of the 1:1 complexes, the decay fit by two exponentials is expected, corresponding to the presence of two species in the system, namely the complexed and uncomplexed guest. Considering the ratio of the two pre-exponential coefficients (B), the following relation is obtained:

$$\frac{B_{bound}}{B_{free}} = \frac{C_{bound} kr_{bound} \varepsilon_{bound}}{C_{free} kr_{free} \varepsilon_{free}} \tag{11}$$

where C, kr and ε represent the concentration, the radiative rate constant and the extinction coefficient, respectively, for the bound and free species (Monti et al., 1993).

Since kr is constant and we can consider $\varepsilon_{bound} = \varepsilon_{free}$, in excess of CD eq. 11 becomes:

$$\frac{B_{bound}}{B_{free}} = K[CD] \tag{12}$$

The linearity of the plot of B_{bound}/B_{free} *vs.* the CD concentration confirms the formation of a complex with 1:1 stoichiometry and allows for the estimation of the association constant (Rajaram et al., 2011).

Some examples, emphasizing different situations encountered in the CD inclusion complexes study, starting with a guest for which the stoichiometry and the association constants were unambiguosly established and continuing with cases of increasing complexity, are reported.

2. Experimental methods and computational details

α-, *β*-, 2-HP-*β* and *γ*-CDs (Aldrich) were used as received. 2-[2'-quinoxalinyl]-phenoxathiin was synthesised as described in Ref. (Nicolae et al., 1998). Indapamide was purchased from Helcor (Romania). Two samples of atenolol were used, one purchased from Helcor and the other from IPCA (India). The guest–CD samples were prepared from stock solution of both components, keeping in all cases the guest concentration constant (10^{-6}–10^{-5} M for fluorescence measurements and 10^{-5}–10^{-4} M for absorption and circular dichroism measurements). The spectra were recorded on a Jasco FP-6300 spectrofluorimeter, Jasco J-815 CD spectropolarimeter and Jasco V-560 UV-VIS spectrophotometer.

All the necessary computational steps to find the most stable complexes in vacuo and in water were detailed in a previous paper (Matei et al., 2009).

3. Some particular cases encountered in the estimation of the stoichiometry of guest–cyclodextrin inclusion complexes

3.1 2-[2'-quinoxalinyl]-phenoxathiin (QP)

An unequivocal example for the determination of the stoichiometry is given by the inclusion complex formed by QP with 2-HP-*β*-CD. QP is a fluorescence probe sensitive to the medium polarity and ability to form hydrogen bonds. In presence of 2-HP-β-CD, a decrease in the emission from QP is observed (Fig. 2A). The changes in the fluorescence intensity of guests upon CD inclusion are usually rationalized by comparing the emission properties of the complexed guest with those of the free guest in different solvents (Wagner et al., 2003). The fluorescence quantum yield of QP in propanol, solvent of polarity similar to that of the CD cavity, is smaller than in dimethylformamide–aqueous solution, the medium in which the experiment was performed. On this basis, the experimentally observed fluorescence decrease was ascribed as due to the lower polarity experienced by QP inside the CD cavity, as compared to aqueous solution.

In this case, the fluorescence–concentration dependence reflects reliable experimental data; the entire binding isotherm was obtained even without using the maximum possible host concentration. Fitting the data with eq. 3 evidenced the 1:1 stoichiometry of the complex (Fig. 2B) and the value of its association constant (inset of Fig. 2B). The results obtained for the 2-HP-β-CD complex of QP are in accordance with our results previously obtained for its β-CD complex (Matei et al, 2007).

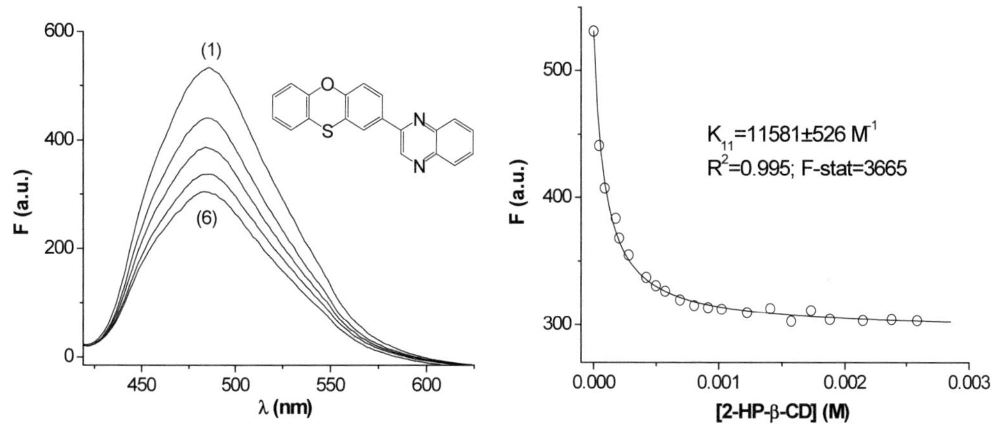

Fig. 2. (A) The fluorescence spectrum of QP (10^{-5} M in dimethylformamide:water 1:9 v:v) in absence (1) and presence (2–6) of increasing amounts of 2-HP-β-CD (up to 3×10^{-3} M). (B) Determination of the 1:1 stoichiometry of the complex by means of eq. 3. Inset: parameters of the fit.

3.2 7-Diethylamino-3-carboxycoumarin (DEAC)

The CD inclusion complexes were often considered as a starting point for choosing good fluorophores to be used in protein studies (Abou-Zied & Al-Hinai, 2006). The changes in the photophysical properties of the guests upon inclusion in the CD cavity can be correlated to their sensitivity on the local polarity, possibility to be involved in hydrogen bonds, etc. Our previous studies on 3-carboxy-coumarin derivatives (Varlan & Hillebrand, 2011) showed that this class of compounds, present in aqueous solution of pH = 7.4 as the corresponding carboxylate ions, are suitable for protein studies. Among the carboxycoumarin derivatives, DEAC represents an interesting guest to be studied in the presence of CD, due to the existence of a second substituent with donor character (the diethylamino group), (Jung et al., 2009; Zhang, et al., 2008).

The fluorescence spectrum of DEAC in the presence of γ-CD, the largest native cyclodextrin, is given in Fig. 3. The increase of the γ-CD concentration induces an enhancement of the emission intensity accompanied by a blue shift of the band (~7 nm), without the appearance of an isoemissive point. All this data clearly indicate that the DEAC molecule has passed from the bulk solution to the less polar cavity of the CD, where it has a higher quantum yield and emits at shorter wavelength, as stated by Ramakrishna and Ghosh (Ramakrishna & Ghosh, 2002).

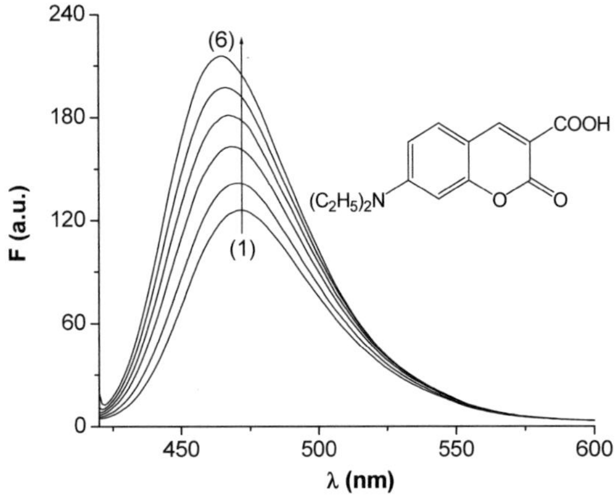

Fig. 3. The fluorescence spectrum of DEAC (2×10^{-6} M) in the presence of increasing amounts of γ-CD. λ_{ex} = 410 nm.

In order to find the stoichiometry of the complexes, the dependence of the fluorescence intensity *vs.* the γ-CD concentration was analyzed. The experimental points could be fitted with good statistical parameters to both eqs. 3 and 7 corresponding to the formation of 1:1 and of a mixture of 1:1+1:2 complexes (Fig. 4), the parameters being given in Table 2. As it can be seen from the R^2 values, the better fit corresponds to the mixture of 1:1+1:2 complexes. This is also supported by the lower and more random distribution of the fits residuals, included as insets in Fig. 4. Another point to be stressed is that when the ratio of intensities of the bound and free guest in a 1:1 complex is near 1, as in the case of DEAC (F_{11}/F_0=1.19), it is very important to have experimental data in the first domain of concentration, otherwise the complexation process will be misinterpreted as a solely 1:1 complex formation.

Stoichiometry	K_{11} (M^{-1})	K_{12} (M^{-1})	F_{11}/F_0	F_{12}/F_0	R^2	F-stat
1:1	1256±112	–	1.64±0.01	–	0.971	831
1:1+1:2	15450±2987	421±36	1.19±0.01	1.72±0.08	0.998	5721

Table 2. Fitted parameters for the DEAC-γ-CD interaction: association constants (K), normalized fluorescence of the complex (F/F_0); R^2 – correlation coefficient; F-stat – Fisher statistic coefficient.

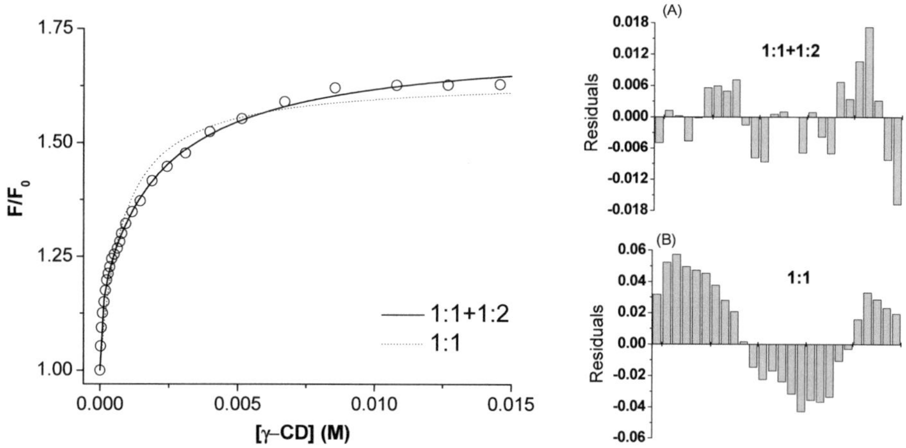

Fig. 4. Normalized experimental data fits with eqs. 7 (solid line) and 3 (dotted line) for the determination of the stoichiometry of the DEAC-γ-CD complex. Inset: The distribution of the residuals for the (A) 1:1+1:2 and (B) 1:1 fits.

3.3 Indapamide

Indapamide is an antihypertensive, diuretic drug of the sulphonamide class (Ciborowski et al., 2004; Ghugare et al., 2010; Radi & Eissa, 2011). We have studied its complexation with *α*-, *β*-, 2-HP- *β*- and *γ*-CD, by means of absorption spectroscopy. The isolated guest presents two absorption bands, located at 240 nm and 280 nm. In presence of CD, the absorbance of these bands increases, without any band shift or appearance of isosbestic points (Fig. 5). Absorbance increase by complexation has been reported by several authors (El-Kemary, 2002) and considered as evidence for the formation of an inclusion complex. The shape of the spectra of the complexes is similar, irrespective of the CD type, but the magnitude of the absorbance increase depends on the CD type.

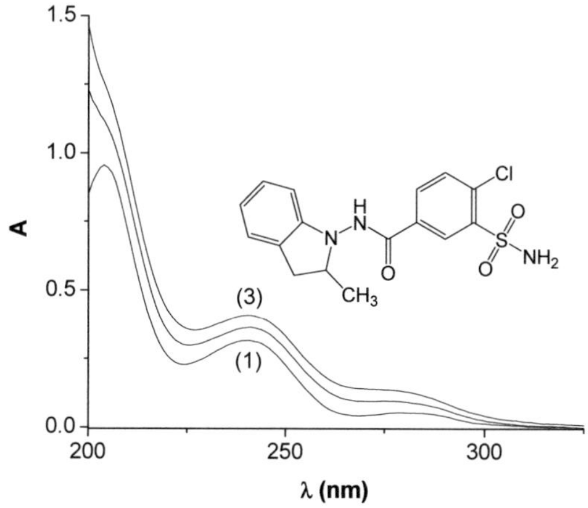

Fig. 5. The absorption spectrum of indapamide (10^{-5} M in methanol:water 1:9 v:v) in absence (1) and presence (2, 3) of increasing concentrations of 2-HP-*β*-CD (up to 2×10^{-2} M).

In the first attempt to determine the stoichiometry of the complexes, the Benesi-Hildebrand model was applied. As previously discussed, a linear dependency of the type $1/(A\text{-}A_0)$ *vs.* $1/[CD]^n$, with n = 1 or 2, indicates the presence of complexes of 1:1 or 1:2 stoichiometry, respectively. For indapamide, the plot $1/(A\text{-}A_0)$ *vs.* $1/[CD]$ shows a positive deviation, irrespective of the CD type (inset of Fig. 6A), which eliminates the hypothesis of the formation of solely 1:1 complexes. This is in accordance with the lack of isosbestic points. The plot $1/(A\text{-}A_0)$ *vs.* $1/[CD]^2$, although characterized by a good correlation coefficient ($R^2 = 0.990$), has unacceptably high standard errors and standard deviations of the fits (Fig. 6A). The Benesi-Hildebrand model cannot offer conclusive data on the presence of the 1:2 stoichiometry.

Applying the nonlinear model describing the formation of a 1:2 complex (eq. 6, dotted line), we obtained good results for all CDs, with small errors (<15%), good correlation coefficients ($R^2 > 0.990$) and Fisher statistic coefficients (F ~ 1500–7000) (Fig. 6B). The predicted association constants are: $K_{\alpha\text{-CD}} = 2447 \pm 89\ M^{-1}$, $K_{\beta\text{-CD}} = 25550 \pm 783\ M^{-1}$, $K_{2\text{-}HP\text{-}\beta\text{-CD}} = 3330 \pm 370\ M^{-1}$ and $K_{\gamma\text{-CD}} = 3897 \pm 481\ M^{-1}$.

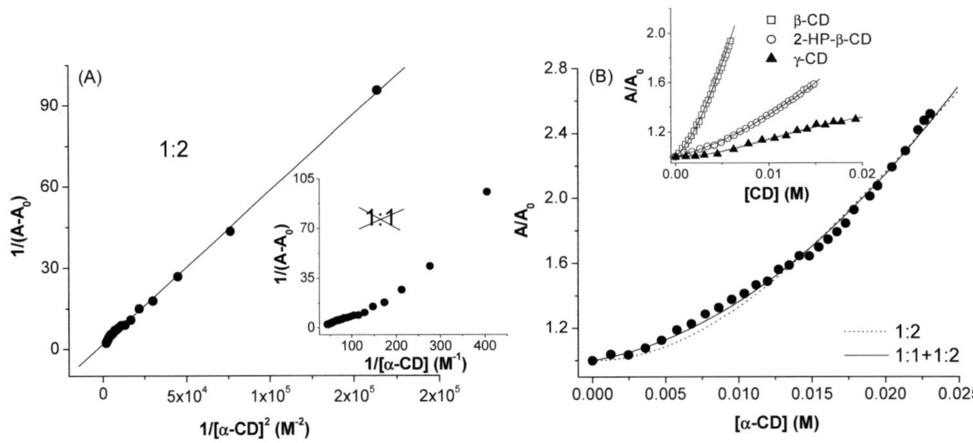

Fig. 6. (A) Benesi-Hildebrand plots for the investigation of the formation of indapamide–α-CD complexes of 1:2 and 1:1 (inset) stoichiometry. (B) The dependence of the normalized absorption of indapamide on the CD concentration. Fits with eqs. 6 and 7.

However, the examination of the first segment of the curves, corresponding to low CD concentrations, reveals some deviations of the experimental points, reflected in the shape of the fit residuals. This prompted us to check for the presence of a mixture of 1:1+1:2 complexes (eq. 7, solid line). These fits are characterized by higher correlation coefficients ($R^2 > 0.995$), as well as smaller and more randomly distributed residuals for the first segment of the curve. Still, in this case the standard errors have high values for K_{12} and A_{12}, due to the uncertainty introduced in the fit by the lack of experimental points on the last segment of the curve, at high CD concentrations.

In the attempt to discern between the two cases, i.e. the 1:2 stoichiometry and the mixture of 1:1+1:2 complexes, we have generated fitting curves on a broader range of CD concentrations, using the values of the association constants and absorbances of the complexes obtained with eqs. 6 and 7, respectively (Fig. 7A). This technique has been employed before, for the stoichiometries determination of some simvastatin–CD complexes (Matei et al., 2009). From Fig. 7A we can observe that up to a CD concentration of ~2.5×10^{-2} M, the two curves are identical, the difference between them appearing only at high CD concentrations. Therefore, in the absence of experimental points in this range, it is impossible to asses without a doubt the stoichiometry of the inclusion complexes. As these experimental data are of crucial importance for the determination of the stoichiometry, the working conditions must be selected in such a way to be as close as possible to the CD solubility limit, i.e. α: 1.5×10^{-1} M, β: 1.6×10^{-2} M, 2-HP-β: 3.3×10^{-1} M, γ: 1.8×10^{-1} M (Connors, 1987).

We performed such an experiment, using indapamide and high concentrations of α-CD (Fig. 7B). This experiment was revelatory and allowed us to discard the formation of mixtures of 1:1+1:2 complexes. Thus, when the experimental points at high CD concentrations were added to the previous experimental data, they aligned on the generated curve corresponding to the formation of 1:2 complexes, revealing that this is the real stoichiometry.

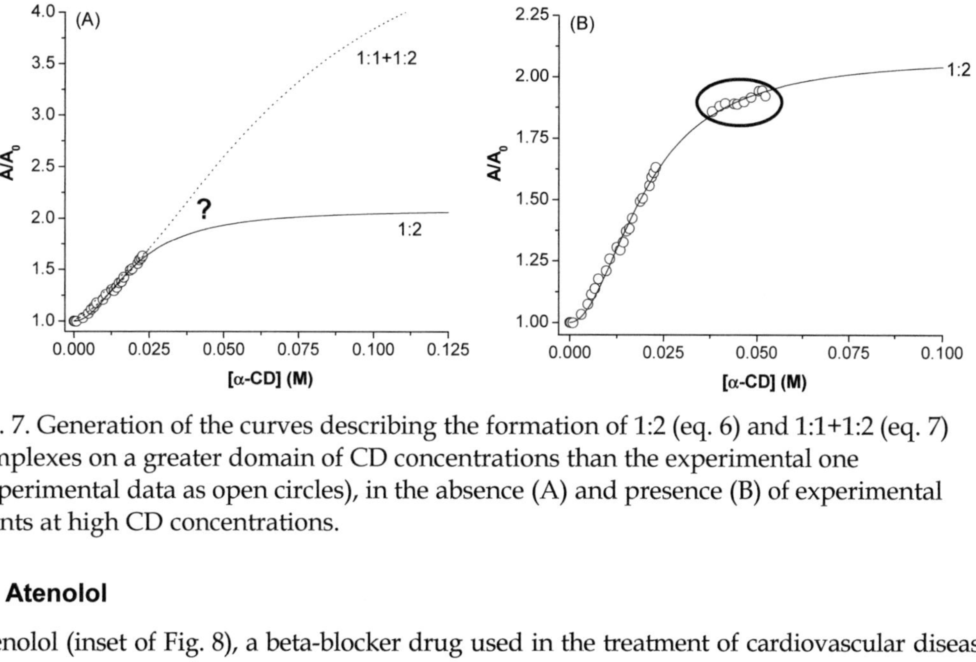

Fig. 7. Generation of the curves describing the formation of 1:2 (eq. 6) and 1:1+1:2 (eq. 7) complexes on a greater domain of CD concentrations than the experimental one (experimental data as open circles), in the absence (A) and presence (B) of experimental points at high CD concentrations.

3.4 Atenolol

Atenolol (inset of Fig. 8), a beta-blocker drug used in the treatment of cardiovascular diseases (Bontchev et al., 2000; Castro et al., 1998; Esteves de Castro et al., 2007; Moloney et al., 1998; Pandeeswaran & Elango, 1009; Pulgarin et al., 1998; Ranta et al., 2002), is a very flexible molecule, consisting of fragments with different features: an amido-substituted aromatic ring, a flexible three-carbon chain (Siqintuya et al., 2007) and a dimethyl-substituted amino group.

3.4.1 Photophysical properties of atenolol

The photophysical properties of atenolol, measured prior to the study of its CD inclusion complexes, showed very interesting features. The absorption spectra of atenolol in water, methanol and acetonitrile are presented in Fig. 8A. An intense band ($\varepsilon \sim 10^4$ $M^{-1}cm^{-1}$) is recorded at 225 nm and assigned to a π-π* transition correlated to the presence of the aromatic ring (Pillot et al., 1997). In the range of 265–290 nm, a second band is observed, characterized by a lower ε value (~10^3 $M^{-1}cm^{-1}$), at the limit of a weak π-π* and a forbidden n-π* transition. According to literature data, this band was considered a benzenic band bathochromically shifted due to the amide substitution (Gratzer, 1967).

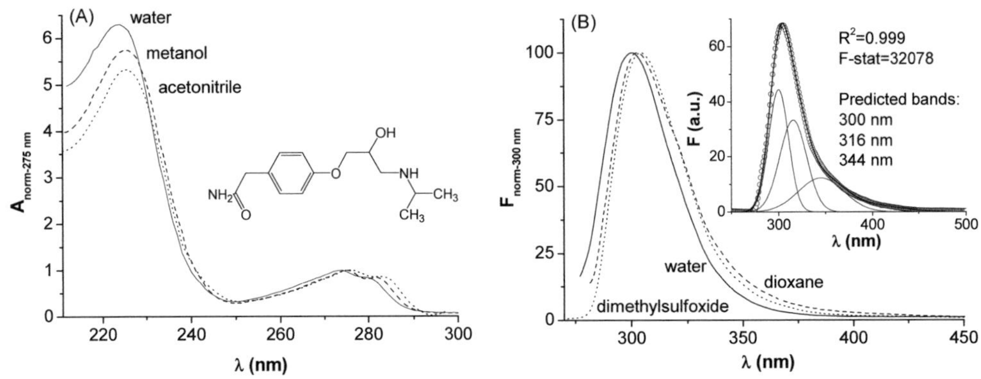

Fig. 8. Absorption (A) and fluorescence (B) spectra of atenolol in different solvents. Inset: Deconvolution of the fluorescence spectrum of atenolol in dimethylformamide. λ_{ex} = 275 nm.

The fluorescence spectrum of atenolol was recorded in nonpolar, polar aprotic and polar protic solvents considering several excitation wavelengths, in the range of the two aforementioned bands. An intense emission band, hereafter labelled B1, slightly influenced by the solvents, was obtained in the range 299–306 nm (Fig. 8B), characterized by a fluorescence quantum yield of 0.11 in water and 0.20 in acetonitrile. A careful examination of the band shape revealed an asymmetry at the longer wavelength range, better evidenced by a deconvolution process, as it can be seen from the inset of Fig. 8B. Besides the main band (300 nm), two other bands were found, one at 316 nm, very close to the first band, and another at 344 nm. This new band, located at 344 nm, much lower in intensity than the former one, will be further called B2. Performing a systematic scanning of the role of different experimental factors (concentration, excitation wavelength, etc.) on the shape of the fluorescence bands, we have found that B2 strongly increases in intensity by dilution, presents in fact two maxima (Fig. 9A) and that it is very sensitive to the excitation wavelength, being much enhanced for λ_{ex} = 250 nm. The ratio of the two bands composing B2 remains constant upon dilution, suggesting a vibrational structure of the band. By comparison with the fluorescence spectrum of a related compound, 4-phenyl-1-N,N-dimethylaminobutane (Xie et al., 2004), B1 was assigned to the emission of the excited aromatic system and B2 to a species in which the excitation is localized on the amino chromophore.

For obtaining supplementary data on the emission process, the fluorescence spectra were recorded at several temperatures in the range 25–75°C using different excitation wavelengths. By cooling back to 25°C, we have observed a reversible decrease of the intensity of the B1 band, which allowed for the estimation of the activation energy of the nonradiative processes. In the limit of experimental errors, the obtained values showed that the process is not influenced by the excitation wavelength (E_a ~ 1.2 kcal/mol). Analyzing the behaviour of B2 in the same temperature range, a different result was obtained, *i.e.* a larger value of the activation energy of the process, 5.38 kcal/mol, for λ_{ex} = 250 nm.

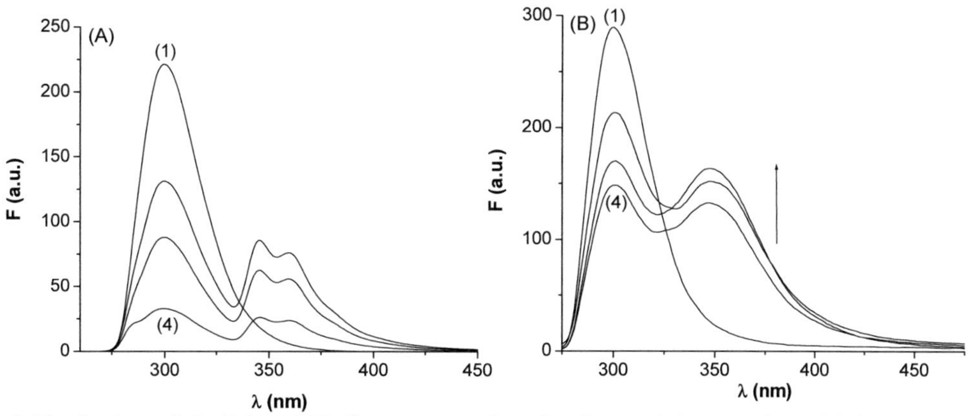

Fig. 9. Evolution of the B1 and B2 fluorescence bands of atenolol in methanol (A) upon dilution with methanol and (B) upon irradiation at 254 nm (three steps of 25 minutes each).

All these data show that atenolol exists in solution as several conformers differently influenced by the solvent, the excitation energy and/or the temperature. Furthermore, considering the pKa value of 9.6 of atenolol (Kasim et al., 2004), we can not rule out the presence of different amounts of protonated/nonprotonated species, especially in water and protic solvents.

In order to obtain more information on the species present in solution, the fluorescence spectrum of atenolol was recorded after irradiation with a mercury lamp at 254 nm. The results are displayed in Fig. 9B and show unambiguously that the irradiation favours the accumulation of the species emitting at 350 nm.

In conclusion, the experimental data on the emission process of atenolol showed the presence of two emitting species, influenced by the concentration, excitation wavelength, temperature and irradiation of the system. All these data must be considered in the further discussion of the atenolol–CD inclusion complexes, especially when the fluorescence spectroscopy is used as the method of investigation.

3.4.2 Characterization of the atenolol-cyclodextrin inclusion complexes

Several spectral methods (FTIR, DSC, SEM, etc.) have been employed for the characterization of the CD inclusion complexes of atenolol in solid state (Borodi et al., 2008; Ficarra et al., 2000a, 2000b). In the following, we will present our results on the interaction of atenolol with α-, β- and γ-CD in solution, studied by means of fluorescence, circular dichroism and absorption spectroscopies. Recording the fluorescence spectra of atenolol in the presence of CDs, we observed slight changes in the intensity of B1 and the strong increase of a band in the same spectral region and with the same shape as the B2 band of uncomplexed atenolol (Fig. 10). This increase indicates that the inclusion process favours the same process as previously discussed for uncomplexed atenolol, *i.e.* the emission correlated to the amino group evidenced in several experimental conditions. This could be due to the inclusion of the isopropylamine fragment in the CD cavity. The fluorescence spectra are strongly dependent on the excitation wavelength (Fig. 11).

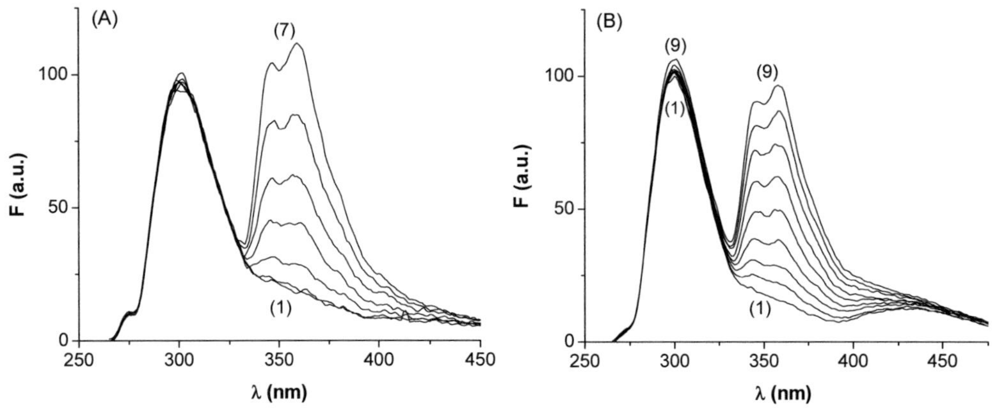

Fig. 10. The fluorescence spectrum of atenolol (2×10^{-5} M in methanol:water 1:9 v:v) in absence (1) and presence (2–9) of increasing amounts of CD: (A) β (up to 5.5×10^{-4} M) and (B) γ (up to 7.3×10^{-4} M). λ_{ex} = 250 nm.

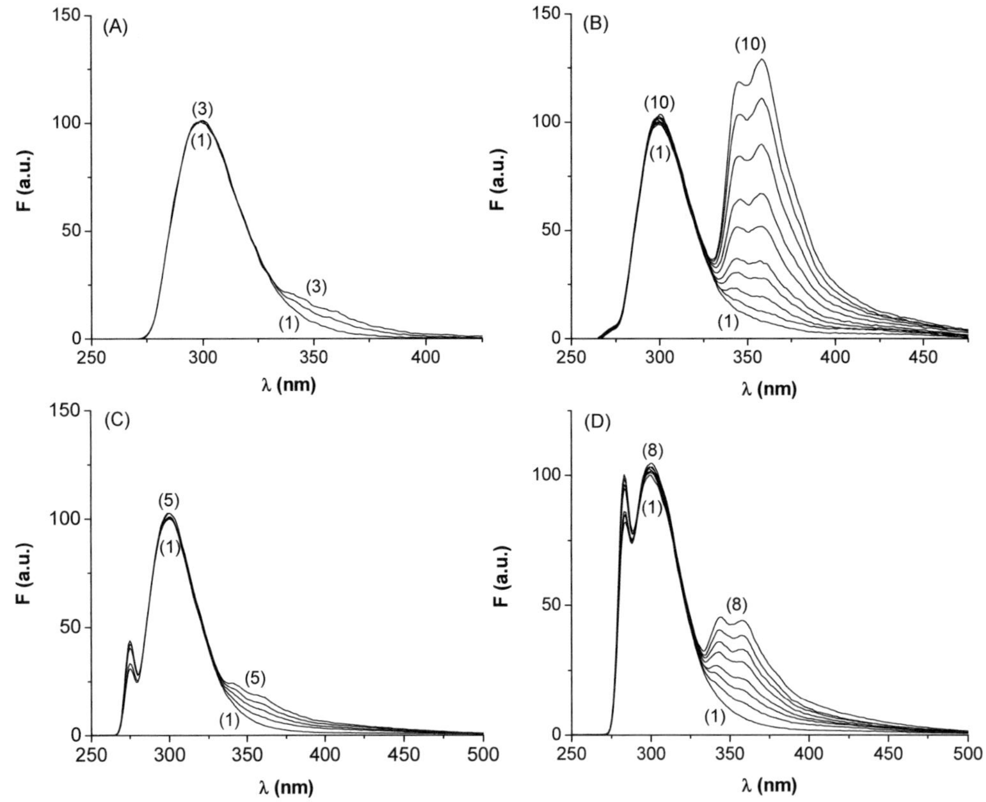

Fig. 11. The fluorescence spectrum of atenolol (2×10^{-5} M in methanol:water 1:9 v:v) in absence (1) and presence (2–10) of increasing amounts of α-CD (up to 7.4×10^{-4} M), at various λ_{ex} (nm): (A) 225, (B) 250, (C) 275 and (D) 282.

The 1:2 stoichiometry of the inclusion complexes in methanol:water has been determined by fitting the experimental data with eq. 6. In the case of the atenolol–*α*-CD complex, the readings have been made on both B1 and B2, at λ_{ex} = 282 nm (Fig. 12). In an attempt to obtain a more consistent value of the association constant, for B2, the emission intensities were read at three wavelengths within the band (345, 358 and 380 nm). The obtained data for all CDs are summarized in Table 3. For λ_{ex} = 225 and 275 nm, the fits resulted in high standard errors, while for λ_{ex} = 250 nm, due to high data scattering, no reliable results could be obtained. Considering that this band is also evidenced in absence of CD and most prominently at λ_{ex} = 250 nm, it must be stressed that the great deviations may be due to the superposition of several effects.

The influence of the temperature on the equilibriums present in solution is the same, irrespective of the CD type and λ_{ex} (Fig. 13), and it is similar to that discussed for uncomplexed atenolol in different solvents. Upon raising the temperature, we observed an increase in the intensity of B1 and a decrease of B2. Similar data were obtained for all CDs. The trend of B1 is an usually encountered for fluorescent molecules one, and can be explained by an increased magnitude of the nonradiative deactivation processes. Differently, the behaviour of B2 could be rationalized in terms of a conformational change leading to an atenolol molecule in a highly fluorescent conformation. This process could be favoured by the decreased viscosity of the medium, leading to an increased mobility of the molecular fragments. Interesting information can be obtained from the behaviour of B1 and B2 upon cooling. While B1 temperature variation is reversible, the intensity of B2 doesn't return to its original value upon decreasing the temperature. This irreversibility could indicate that the amino group is included in the CD cavity and only successively fixed in a fluorescent conformation.

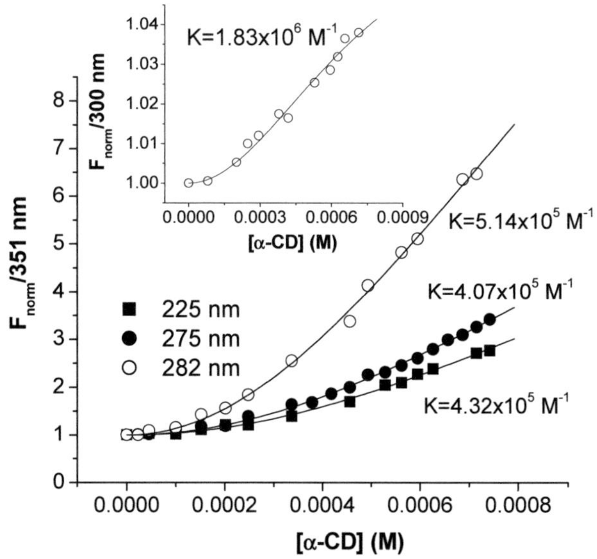

Fig. 12. Plots for the determination of the stoichiometry and association constant of the atenolol–*α*-CD complex in methanol:water 1:9 v:v using fluorescence data read on B2 at three excitation wavelengths (225, 275 and 282 nm) and B1 (inset) at 282 nm.

Band	$K_{12}\times10^{-6}$ (M^{-1})	F_{12}/F_0	R^2; F-stat
	α-CD		
B1, 300 nm	1.83±0.43	1.08	0.987; 739
B2, 345 nm	0.43±0.10	15.22	0.997; 5291
358 nm	0.51±0.09	29.13	0.998; 7786
380 nm	0.81±0.11	24.71	0.997; 6133
	β-CD		
B2, 345 nm	3.67±0.77	3.47	0.991; 1056
359 nm	4.91±0.90	5.67	0.988; 887
380 nm	5.54±0.75	6.48	0.992; 1312
	γ-CD		
B2, 345 nm	0.94±0.19	5.63	0.992; 2168
359 nm	1.02±0.19	10.44	0.992; 2252
380 nm	1,88±0,30	9,19	0,988; 1484

Table 3. Parameters of the 1:2 atenolol–CD inclusion complexes in methanol:water 1:9 v:v. λ_{ex} = 282 nm.

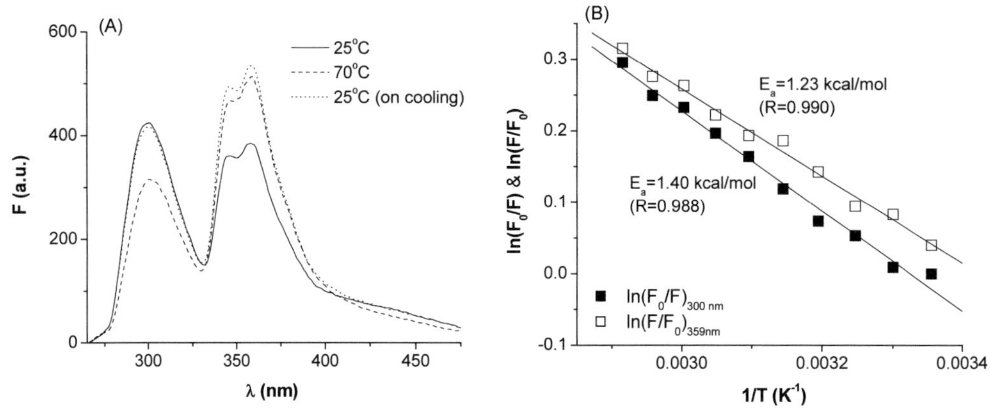

Fig. 13. The temperature dependence of the fluorescence intensity of the atenolol–*γ*-CD system in methanol:water 1:9 v:v (A) and the activation energies of the respective processes (B). λ_{ex} = 250 nm.

Differing from the spectra in methanol:water, using dimethylformamide as solvent we observed an enhanced decrease of the B1 band intensity, together with a significant increase of B2 (Fig. 14). Despite the significant intensity change of B1, the readings on this band could not be used for the stoichiometry determination. On band B2, the fits, according to eq. 6, indicated the presence of 1:2 complexes (inset of Fig. 14).

To obtain more data on the atenolol complexation process, several other methods were used, including circular dichroism and absorption spectroscopies, together with molecular modeling. Therefore, the stoichiometry of the inclusion complex of atenolol with β-CD has been determined *via* circular dichroism spectroscopy. While in absence of CD no signal is recorded for atenolol, upon CD addition a negative dichroic signal appears at 275 nm (Fig. 15A). The corresponding calculated transition moment is located in the plane of the aromatic ring, perpendicular to the long molecular axis (*vide infra*). The appearance of an induced circular dichroism signal of atenolol confirms its inclusion into the asymmetric CD cavity and indicates that the aromatic ring is perturbed by CD incorporation. Moreover, its negative sign indicates the perpendicular orientation of the transition moment with respect to the symmetry axis of β-CD.

The data for the system atenolol-β-CD were fitted with eq. 3, revealing the formation of complexes of 1:1 stoichiometry (Fig. 15B). One can observe the greater scattering of the experimental points, characteristic to the measurements by circular dichroism. The data were also analyzed using the Scott model (eq. 2, inset of Fig. 15B), which yielded a K_{11} value in good accordance with the results of the nonlinear model, although the fit was of somewhat lower quality. The value of the association constant also correlates to that obtained by us (Fig. 16) and by Borodi *et al.* (Borodi et al., 2008) (110±22 M^{-1}, Scott's model) from UV-vis absorption data.

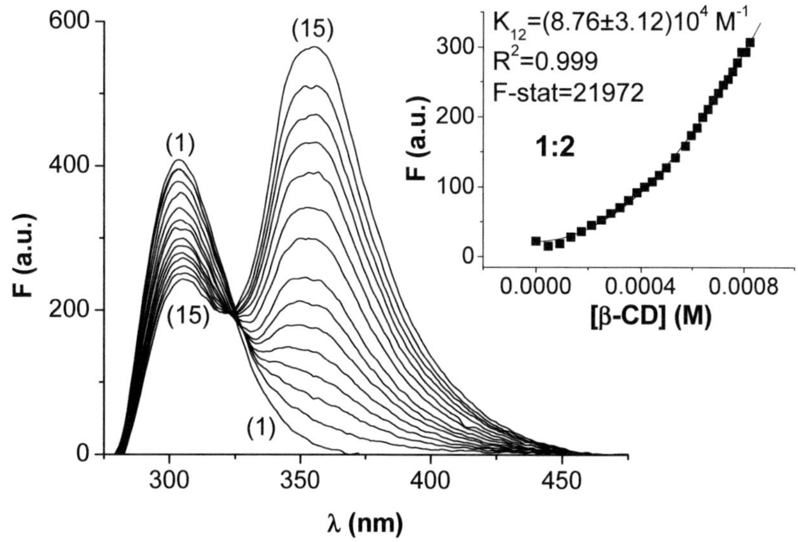

Fig. 14. The fluorescence spectrum of atenolol (2×10^{-5} M in dimethylformamide) in the absence (1) and presence (2–30) of increasing amounts of β-CD (up to 8×10^{-4} M). λ_{ex} = 275 nm. The DMF spectrum has been subtracted. Inset: Plot of the fluorescence intensity of B2 *vs*. the β-CD concentration.

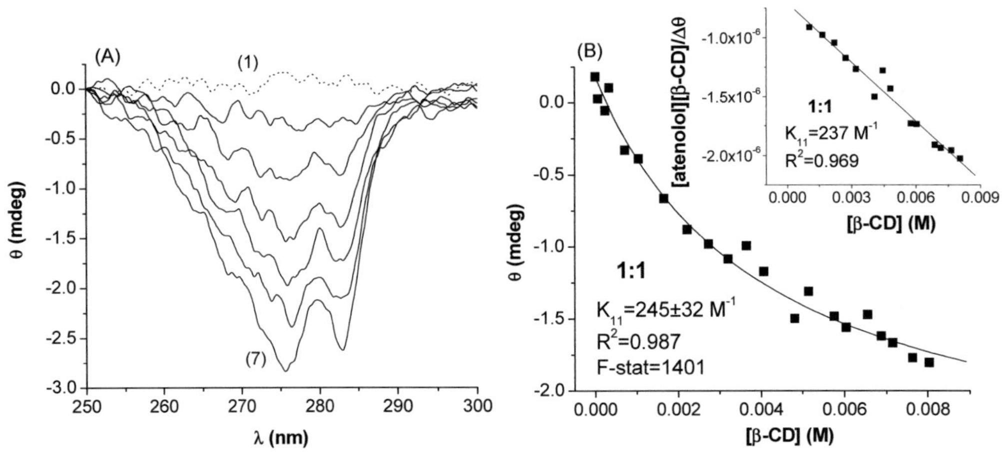

Fig. 15. (A) The circular dichroism spectra of atenolol (5×10^{-4} M in pH 7.4 phosphate buffer) in absence (1) and presence (2–7) of increasing concentrations of *β*-CD (up to 2×10^{-2} M). (B) Determination of the stoichiometry and association constant of the atenolol–*β*-CD complex.

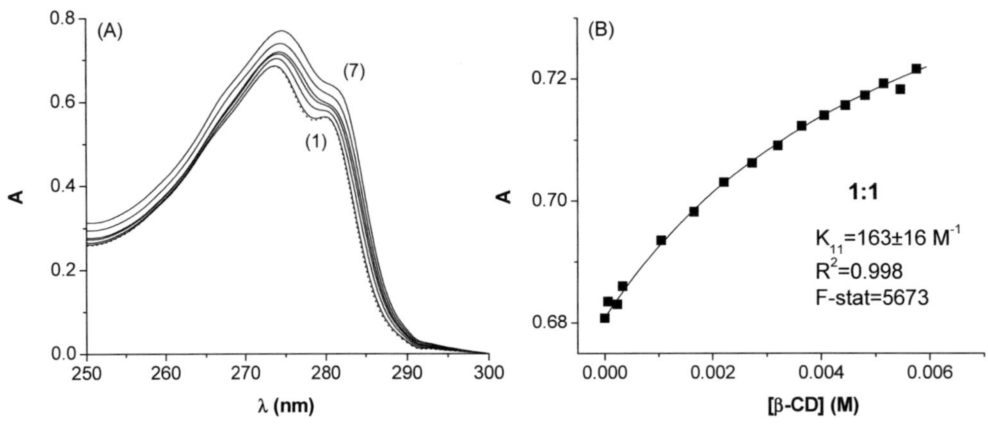

Fig. 16. (A) The absorption spectra of atenolol (5×10^{-4} M in pH 7.4 phosphate buffer) in absence (1) and presence (2–7) of increasing concentrations of *β*-CD (up to 2×10^{-2} M). (B) Determination of the stoichiometry and association constant of the atenolol–*β*-CD complex.

As stated above, molecular mechanics calculations were performed using the MM+ force field in order to gain theoretical support for two experimental results:

a. the negative signal of the dichroic band of atenolol in the 1:1 complex.

This is rationalized in terms of the equatorial orientation of the corresponding transition moment of atenolol calculated at the TDDFT level (represented in grey in Fig. 17A) with respect to the β-CD symmetry axis;

b. the increased and temperature irreversible emission correlated to the amino group observed upon the formation of the 1:2 complex.

This behaviour can be explained on the basis of the inclusion of the isopropylamino moiety of atenolol in one of the two CD cavities of the 1:2 complex (Fig. 17B). The molecule is "fixed" by the cavity in a conformation where the excited state is predominantly localized on the amino group.

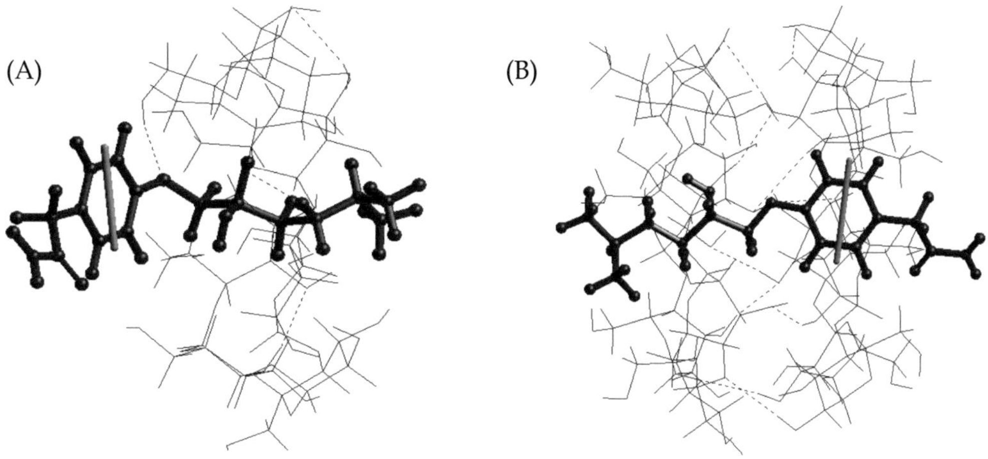

Fig. 17. Proposed structures for the (A) 1:1 and (B) 1:2 atenolol–β-CD inclusion complexes, *via* molecular modeling. The dotted lines represent hydrogen bonds. The transition moment of atenolol is plotted in grey.

4. Conclusions

The estimation of the stoichiometry of a CD inclusion complex represents the first step in the characterization of the complex, leading to the determination of reliable association constants and offering a hint of the supramolecular structure. Unfortunately, the unequivocal estimation of the stoichiometry is not always straightforward and in some cases a single experiment is not sufficient.

In the four discussed examples we have described some cases we have encountered, in order of increasing complexity. In the first case we have had no problems in determining the stoichiometry, the 1:1 inclusion complex formed by the phenoxathiin derivative being clearly defined, with all the other models leading to absurd results. For the two following guests, DEAC and indapamide, the uncertainties arose in the determination of the stoichiometry were solved in two ways, starting with the careful examination of the results obtained by fitting the data to different models.

For DEAC, the slightly better statistical parameters, R^2 and Fisher statistic coefficient, for the 1:1+1:2 stoichiometry, as compared to 1:1, was a first indication of the real stoichiometry. The presence of a mixture of complexes became clear by examining the residuals of the two corresponding fits. Thus, we have rejected the hypothesis of the 1:2 stoichiometry, for which the residuals were grouped in positive and negative values for different regions of the plot, and accepted the simultaneous presence of a mixture of two complexes, 1:1+1:2, for which the residuals were lower and randomly distributed, attesting the inherent experimental errors and not an inadequate model.

When the values of the statistical parameters are not sufficient to determine the adequate model, a theoretical simulation of the property *vs.* concentration curve for the assumed stoichiometry is necessary. In the case of the indapamide–CD systems, we succeeded to establish the presence of a 1:2 mixture of complexes by coupling an improvement of the experimental conditions, *i.e.* extending the concentration of the host up to the limit of solubility, with theoretical curves built assuming different stoichiometries.

In the last case, the atenolol–CD inclusion complexes represented more difficult systems and some uncertainties still remained. The problems are due to the high complexity of the fluorescence spectrum of the free drug, very sensitive to the experimental conditions such as the solvent, excitation wavelength, temperature, *etc.* We have observed that the emission band that is enhanced in intensity in the presence of CDs, and therefore assigned to the inclusion complex formation, is also present for some experimental conditions and to different extents in the spectrum of the free guest. Therefore, it is difficult to state that the fluorescence intensity measured in the presence of CDs is uniquely due to the inclusion complex and not to another species pre-existent in the system. The presence of several conformational equilibriums and/or of inter-/intra-molecular interactions in the free atenolol solution can be influenced by the CD addition. The second problem encountered was the very slight variation in the main emission band intensity, which prevented its use for quantitative estimations. With all these reservations, we considered that the stoichiometry of the inclusion complex, as revealed by the fluorescence measurements, is 1:2. In the circular dichroism spectra, working in other concentration domain and measuring a ground state property, we evidenced the presence of a 1:1 complex but the association constants are different as compared to those obtained by fluorescence. Getting different values for the association constants, by the use of several experimental methods, is a widely discussed topic in literature (Valeur et al., 2007), various explanations being given, the different range of concentrations used being the most frequent (Radi & Eissa, 2011). Another explanation invoked especially for the cases in which association parameters measured using fluorescence, on one side, and absorption and circular dichroism spectroscopies, on the other, are compared consists in the different features of the involved guest state, the excited state for the first method and the ground state for the other two. Last but not least, the isothermal calorimetric titration is a method also suitable for completing the information on the inclusion process, the method allowing for the determination, in a single experiment, of the stoichiometry, association constant and enthalpy change during the process. The experimental data can be fitted to several models, including one or more independent classes of binding sites or sequential binding [Xing et al., 2009].

As a general conclusion, to establish the real stoichiometry of G:H systems, the use of multiple methods is recommended together with considering several required conditions, summarized in the scheme below.

SPECTRAL METHODS

SPECIFIC REQUIREMENTS

Absorption

Experimental data must be analysed:
- In the spectral region free from band overlap
- On the band showing the largest change in intensity

Fluorescence

- A very careful study of the photophysical properties of the free guest is a must (emission wavelength, quantum yield, presence of several species, influence of solvent, temperature, *etc.*)
- Perform experiments using several excitation wavelengths if the presence of several species is assumed

Circular dichroism

- Spectra must be recorded with a large number of accumulations
- Identify the position of the dichroic signals, their sign and intensity

Correlation with the theoretical results:
- The sign of the band indicates the orientation of the guest transition moment
- Comparison of the experimental and simulated spectra

GENERAL REQUIREMENTS

- Use several fitting models
- Examine carefully the statistical parameters of the fits
- Compare when possible with theoretical simulations

5. Acknowledgement

This work was supported by the grant CEEX-VIASAN-7/2008 entitled "Polymorphic forms and the encapsulation of bioactive substances into cyclodextrins for improving drug quality (CALIMED)" and by the strategic grant POSDRU/89/1.5/S/58852, Project "Postdoctoral programme for training scientific researchers" cofinanced by the European Social Fund within the Sectorial Operational Program Human Resources Development 2007-2013.

6. References

Abi-Mosleh, L., Infante, R.E., Radhakrishnan, A., Goldstein, J.L. & Brown, M.S. (2009). Cyclodextrin overcomes deficient lysosome-to-endoplasmic reticulum transport of cholesterol in Niemann-Pick type C cells. *Proceedings of the National Academy of Sciences*, Vol. 106, No. 46, (November 2009), pp. 19316-19321, ISSN 1091-6490

Abou-Zied, O.K. & Al-Hinai, A.T. (2006). Caging Effects on the Ground and Excited States of 2,2′-Bipyridine-3,3′-diol Embedded in Cyclodextrins. *Journal of Physical Chemistry A*, Vol. 110, No. 25, (June 2006), pp. 7835-7840, ISSN 1089-5639

Agbaria, R.A. & Gill, D. (1988). Extended 2,5-diphenyloxazole-gamma-cyclodextrin aggregates emitting 2,5-diphenyloxazole excimer fluorescence. *Journal of Physical Chemistry*, Vol. 92, No. 5, (March 1988), pp. 1052-1055, ISSN 0022-3654

Agbaria, R.A. & Gill, D. (1994). Non-covalent polymers of oxadiazole derivatives induced by γ-cyclodextrin in aqueous solutions- fluorescence study. *Journal of Photochemistry and Photobiology A: Chemistry*, Vol. 78, No. 2, (March 1994), pp. 161-167, ISSN 1010-6030

Arunkumar, E., Forbes, C.C. & Smith, B.D. (2005) Improving the properties of organic dyes by molecular encapsulation. *European Journal of Organic Chemistry*, Vol. 2005, No. 19, (August 2005), pp. 4051-4059, ISSN 1099-0690

Baglole, K.N., Boland, P.G. & Wagner, B.D. (2005). Fluorescence enhancement of curcumin upon inclusion into parent and modified cyclodextrins. *Journal of Photochemistry and Photobiology A: Chemistry*, Vol. 173, No. 3, (July 2005), pp. 230-237, ISSN 1010-6030

Benesi, A.H. & Hildebrand, J.H. (1949). A spectrophotometric exploration of the interplay of iodine with scented hydrocarbons. *The Journal of American Chemical Society*, Vol. 71, No. 8, (August 1949), pp. 2703-2707, ISSN 0002-7863

Bontchev, P.R., Pantcheva, I.N.& Gochev, G.P. (2000). Complexes of copper(II) with the β-blocker atenolol. *Transition Metal Chemistry*, Vol. 25, No. 2, (April 2000), pp. 196-199, ISSN 1572-901X

Borodi, G., Bratu, I., Dragan, F., Peschar, R., Helmholdt, R.B. & Hernanz, A. (2008). Spectroscopic investigations and crystal structure from synchrotron powder data of the inclusion complex of beta-cyclodextrin with atenolol. *Spectrochimica Acta, Part A: Molecular and Biomolecular Spectroscopy*, Vol. 70, No. 5, (October 2008), pp. 1041-1048, ISSN 1386-1425

Brewster, M.E. & Loftsson, T. (2007). Cyclodextrins as pharmaceutical solubilizers. *Advanced Drug Delivery Reviews*, Vol. 59, No. 7, (July 2007), pp. 645-666, ISSN 1872-8294

Castro, B., Gameiro, P., Guimaraes, C., Lima, J. & Reis, S. (1998). Fluorimetric and solubility studies of nadolol and atenolol in SDS micelles. *Journal of Pharmaceutical and Biomedical Analysis*, Vol. 18, No. 4-5, (December 1998), pp. 573-577, ISSN 0731-7085

Chadha, R., Gupta, S., Shukla, G., Jain, D.V.S. & Singh, S. (2011). Characterization and in vivo efficacy of inclusion complexes of sulphadoxine with β-cyclodextrin: calorimetric and spectroscopic studies. *Journal of Inclusion Phenomena and Macrocyclic Chemistry*, (January 2011), DOI 10.1007/s10847-010-9919-9, ISSN 1573-1111

Challa, R., Ahuja, A., Ali, J. & Khar, R.K. (2005). Cyclodextrins in Drug Delivery: An Updated Review. *AAPS PharmSciTech*, Vol. 6, No. 2, (October 2005), pp. E329-E357, ISSN 1530-9932

Ciborowski, M., Catala Icardo, M., Garcia Mateo, J.V. & Martinez Calatayud, J. (2004). FI-chemiluminometric study of thiazides by on-line photochemical reaction. *Journal of Pharmaceutical and Biomedical Analysis*, Vol. 36, No. 4, (November 2004), pp. 693-700, ISSN 0731-7085

Connors, K.A. (1987). *Binding Constants*, John Wiley & Sons, ISBN 0471830836, New York.

Davies, D.M. & Deary, M.E. (1999). Stability of 1:1 and 2:1 α-cyclodextrin–p-nitrophenyl acetate complexes and the effect of α-cyclodextrin on acyl transfer to peroxide anion nucleophiles. *Journal of the Chemical Society, Perkin Transactions 2*, No. 5, (May 1999), pp. 1027-1034, ISSN 1364-5471

De Azevedo, M.B.M., Alderete, J.B., Lino, A.C.S., Loh, W., Faljoni-Alario, A. & Duran, N. (2000). Violacein/β-cyclodextrin inclusion complex formation studied by measurements of diffusion coefficient and circular dichroism. *Journal of Inclusion Phenomena and Macrocyclic Chemistry*, Vol. 37, No. 1-4 (May 2000), pp. 67-74, ISSN 1573-1111

De La Pena, A.M., Agbaria, R.A., Sanchez, M., Pena, I & Warner, M. (1997). Spectroscopic studies of the interaction of 1,4-diphenyl-1,3-butadiene with alpha-, beta-, and gamma-cyclodextrins. *Applied Spectroscopy*, Vol. 51, No. 2, (February 1997), pp. 153-159, ISSN 1943-3530

El-Kemary, M.A., El-Gezawy, H.S., El-Baradie, H.Y. & Issa, R.M. (2002). Spectral and photophysical studies of inclusion complexes of 2-amino-4,6-dimethyl pyrimidine with β-cyclodextrin. *Spectrochimica Acta, Part A: Molecular and Biomolecular Spectroscopy*, Vol. 58, No. 3, (February, 2002), pp. 493-500, ISSN 1386-1425

Esteves de Castro, R.A., Canotilho, J., Barbosa, R.M. & Simoes Redinha, J. (2007). Infrared spectroscopy of racemic and enantiomeric forms of atenolol. *Spectrochimica Acta, Part A: Molecular and Biomolecular Spectroscopy*, Vol. 67, No. 5, (August 2007), pp. 1194-1200, ISSN 1386-1425

[a] Ficarra, R., Ficarra, P., Di Bella, M.R., Raneri, D., Tommasini, S., Calabro, M.L., Villari, A. & Coppolino, S. (2000). Study of the inclusion complex of atenolol with β-cyclodextrins. *Journal of Pharmaceutical and Biomedical Analysis*, Vol. 23, No.1, (August 2000), pp. 231-236, ISSN 0731-7085

[b] Ficarra, R., Ficarra, P., Di Bella, M.R., Raneri, D., Tommasini, S., Calabro, M.L., Gamberini, M.C. & Rustichelli, C. (2000). Study of β-blockers:β-cyclodextrins inclusion complex by NMR, DSC, X-ray and SEM investigation. *Journal of Pharmaceutical and Biomedical Analysis*, Vol. 23, No. 1, (August 2000), pp. 33-40, ISSN 0731-7085

Ge, X., He, J., Yang, Y., Qi, F., Huang, Z., Lu, R., Huang, L. & Yao, X. (2011). Study on inclusion complexation between plant growth regulator 6-benzylaminopurine and β-cyclodextrin: Preparation, characterization and molecular modelling. *Journal of Molecular Structure*, Vol. 994, No. 1-3, (May 2011), pp. 163-169, ISSN 0022-2860

Ghugare, P., Dongre, V., Karmuse, P., Rana, R., Singh, D., Kumar, A. & Filmwala, Z. (2010). Solid state investigation and characterization of the polymorphic and pseudopolymorphic forms of indapamide. *Journal of Pharmaceutical and Biomedical Analysis*, Vol. 51, No. 3, (February 2010), pp. 532-540, ISSN 0731-7085

Gratzer, W.B. (1967). *Proceedings of the Royal Society of London. Series A. Mathematical, Physical and Engineering Sciences*. Vol. 297 (February 1967), pp. 163-170, ISSN 1364-5021

Grunberger, G., Artiss, J.D. & Jen, K.L.C. (2007). The benefits of early intervention in obese diabetic patients with FBCx TM-a new dietary fibre. *Diabetes/Metabolism Research and Reviews*, Vol. 23, No. 1, pp. 56-62, ISSN 1520-7560

Hamai, S. (2005). Excimer formation of 1-chloronaphthalene in alkaline aqueous solutions containing γ-cyclodextrin or maltosyl-γ-cyclodextrin. *Journal of Materials Chemistry*, Vol. 15, (April 2005), pp. 2881-2888, ISSN 0959-9428

Hamai, S. (1990). Association modes of a 1:1 inclusion compound of β-cyclodextrin with 1-cyanonaphthalene in aqueous solutions: self-association, association with alcohols, and association with a 1:1 β-cyclodextrinanisole inclusion compound. *Journal of Physical Chemistry*, Vol. 94, No. 6, (March 1990), pp. 2595-2600, ISSN 0022-3654

Hamai, S. (1999). Fluorescence polarization studies of inclusion complexes between β-cyclodextrin and 1-chloronaphthalene in aqueous and aqueous D glucose solutions. *Journal of Physical Chemistry B*, Vol. 103, No. 2, (December 1998), pp. 293-298, ISSN 1520-5207

Hamai, S. (2010). Inclusion of methyl 2-naphthalenecarboxylate and dimethyl 2,3-, 2,6-, and 2,7-naphthalenedicarboxylates by cyclodextrins in aqueous solution. *Bulletin of the Chemical Society of Japan*, Vol. 83, No. 12, (December 2010), pp. 1489-1500, ISSN 1348-0634

Hamai, S., Ikeda, T., Nakamura, A., Ikeda, H., Ueno, A. & Toda, F. (1992). Inclusion of Azulene and Alcohol by β-Cyclodextrin in Aqueous Solution. *The Journal of American Chemical Society*, Vol. 114, No. 15, (July 1992), pp. 6012-6016, ISSN 0002-7863

Harata, K. & Uedaira, H. (1975). The circular dichroism spectra of the beta-cyclodextrin complex with naphthalene derivatives. *Bulletin of the Chemical Society of Japan*, Vol. 48, No. 2, (February, 1975), pp. 375-378, ISSN 1348-0634

Jadhav, G.S., Vavia, P.R. & Nandedkar, T.D. (2007). Danazol-β-cyclodextrin binary system: A potential application in emergency contraception by the oral route. *AAPS PharmSciTech*, Vol. 8, No. 2, (May 2007), pp. E1-E10, ISSN 1530-9932

Job, P. (1928). Recherches sur la formation de complexes mineraux en solution et sur leur stabilite. *Annales de Chimie*, Vol. 9, pp. 113-203, ISSN 0365-1444

Jung, H.S., Kwon, P.S., Lee, J.W., Kim, J.I., Hong, C.S., Kim, J.W., Yan, S., Lee, J.Y., Lee, J.H., Joo, T. & Kim, J.S. (2009). Coumarin-derived Cu^{2+}-selective fluorescence sensor: synthesis, mechanisms, and applications in living cells. *The Journal of American Chemical Society*, Vol. 131, No. 5, (January 2009), pp. 2008-2012, ISSN 0002-7863

Kacso, I., Borodi, G., Farcas, S.I., Hernanz, A. & Bratu, I. (2010). Host–guest system of Vitamin B10 in β-cyclodextrin: characterization of the interaction in solution and in solid state. *Journal of Inclusion Phenomena and Macrocyclic Chemistry*, Vol. 68, No. 1-2, (March 2010), pp. 175-182, ISSN 1573-1111

Kasim, N.A., Whitehouse, M., Ramachandran, C., Bermejo, M., Lennernas, H., Hussain, A.S., Junginger, H.E., Stavchansky, S.A., Midha, K.K., Shah, V.P. & Amidon, G.L. (2004). Molecular properties of WHO essential drugs and provisional biopharmaceutical classification. *Molecular Pharmaceutics*, Vol. 1, No. 1 (December 2003), pp. 85-96, ISSN 1543-8384

Kodaka, M. (1993). A general rule for circular dichroism induced by a chiral macrocycle. *The Journal of American Chemical Society*, Vol. 115, No. 9, (May 1993), pp. 3702-3705, ISSN 0002-7863

Landy, D., Tetart, F., Truant, E., Blach, P., Fourmentin, S. & Surpateanu, G. (2007). Development of a competitive continuous variation plot for the determination of inclusion compounds stoichiometry. *Journal of Inclusion Phenomena and Macrocyclic Chemistry*, Vol. 57, No. 1-4, (April 2007), pp. 409-413, ISSN 1573-1111

Li, G. & McGown, L.B. (1994). Molecular nanotube aggregates of β- and γ-cyclodextrins linked by diphenylhexatrienes. *Science* Vol. 264, No. 5156, (April 1994), pp. 249-251, ISSN 1095-9203

Li, J. (2010). Self-assembled supramolecular hydrogels based on polymer–cyclodextrin inclusion complexes for drug delivery. *NPG Asia Materials,* Vol. 2, No. 3, (July 2010), pp. 112-118, ISSN : 1476-4660

Li, J. & Loh, X.J. (2008). Cyclodextrin-based supramolecular architectures: Syntheses, structures, and applications for drug and gene delivery. *Advanced Drug Delivery Reviews,* Vol. 60, No. 9, (June 2008), pp. 1000-1017, ISSN 0169-409X

Li, J.J., Zhao, F. & Li, J. (2011). Polyrotaxanes for applications in life science and biotechnology. *Applied Microbiology and Biotechnology,* Vol. 90, No. 2, (April 2011), pp. 427-443, ISSN 1432-0614

Liu, Y., Chen, Y., Li, L., Zhang, H.Y. & Guan, X.D. (2001). Bridged bis(β-cyclodextrin)s possessing coordinated metal center(s) and their inclusion complexation behavior with model substrates: enhanced molecular binding ability by multiple recognition. *Journal of Organic Chemistry,* Vol. 66, No. 25, (December 2001), pp. 8518-8527, ISSN 1520-6904

Liu, Y., Li, B., Wada, T. & Inoue, Y. (2001). Molecular recognition studies on supramolecular systems. 31. Circular dichroism spectral studies of molecular and chiral recognition of aliphatic alcohols by various 6-modified β-cyclodextrins. *Tetrahedron,* Vol. 57, No. 33, (August 2001), pp. 7153-7161, ISSN 0040-4020

Loftsson, T. & Duchene, D. (2007). Cyclodextrins and their pharmaceutical applications. *International Journal of Pharmaceutics,* Vol. 329, No. 1-2, (February 2007), pp. 1-11, ISSN 0378-5173

Loftsson, T., Brewster, M.E. & Masson, M. (2004). Role of Cyclodextrins in Improving Oral Drug Delivery. *American Journal of Drug Delivery,* Vol. 2, No. 4, (October 2004), pp. 261-275, ISSN 1175-9038

Lopez, C.A., de Vries, A.H., Marrink, S.J. (2011). Molecular mechanism of cyclodextrin mediated cholesterol extraction. *PLoS Computational Biology,* Vol. 7, No. 3, (March 2011), e1002020, ISSN 1553-7358

Mandal, A.K., Das, D.K., Das, A.K., Mojumdar, S.S. & Bhattacharyya, K. (2011). Study of γ-cyclodextrin host–guest complex and nanotube aggregate by fluorescence correlation spectroscopy. *Journal of Physical Chemistry B,* Vol. 115, No. 35, (September 2011), pp. 10456-10461, ISSN 1520-5207

Martin Del Valle, E.M. (2004). Cyclodextrins and their uses: a review. *Process Biochemistry,* Vol. 39, No. 9, (May 2004) pp. 1033-1046, ISSN 1359-5113

Matei, I., Nicolae, A. & Hillebrand, M. (2007). Fluorimetric and molecular mechanics study of the inclusion complex of 2-quinoxalinyl-phenoxathiin with β-cyclodextrin. *Journal of Inclusion Phenomena and Macrocyclic Chemistry,* Vol. 57, No. 1-4, (January 2007), pp. 597-601, ISSN 1573-1111

Matei, I., Soare, L., Tablet, C. & Hillebrand, M. (2009). Characterization of simvastatin and its cyclodextrin inclusion complexes by absorption and circular dichroism spectroscopies and molecular mechanics calculations. *Revue Roumaine de Chimie,* Vol. 54, No. 2, (February 2009), pp. 133-141, ISSN 0035-3930

Moloney, G.P., Craik, D.J., Iskander, M.N. & Nero, T.L. (1998). Synthesis, NMR studies and conformational analysis of oxazolidine derivatives of the β-adrenoreceptor antagonists metoprolol, atenolol and timolol. *Journal of the Chemical Society, Perkin Transactions 2*, No. 2, (February 1998), pp. 199-206, ISSN 1364-5471

Monti, S., Kohler, K. & Grabner, G. (1993). Photophysics and photochemistry of methylated phenols in β-cyclodextrin inclusion complexes, *Journal of Physical Chemistry*, Vol. 97, No. 49, (December, 1993), pp. 13011-13016, ISSN 0022-3654

Nicolae, A., Gavriliu, D., Maior, O. & Draghici, C. (1998). Pheoxathiin chemistry. Synthesis based on 2-ω-bromo-acetylphenoxathiin. *Southern Brazilian Journal of Chemistry*, Vol. 6, No. 7, (1998), pp. 33-46, ISSN 0104-5431

Oana, M., Tintaru, A., Gavriliu, D., Maior, O. & Hillebrand, M. (2002). Spectral study and molecular modeling of the inclusion complexes of β-cyclodextrin with some phenoxathiin derivatives. *Journal of Physical Chemistry B*, Vol. 106, No. 2, (December 2001), pp. 257-263, ISSN 1520-5207

Pandeeswaran, M. & Elango, K.P. (2009). Spectroscopic studies on the molecular complex of the drug atenolol with iodine. *Journal of Solution Chemistry*, Vol. 38, No. 12, (December 2009), pp. 1558-1572, ISSN 1572-8927

Park, J.W., Song, H.E. & Lee, S.Y. (2002). Face selectivity of inclusion complexation of viologens with β-cyclodextrin and 6-O-(2-Sulfonato-6-naphthyl)-β-cyclodextrin. *Journal of Physical Chemistry B*, Vol. 106, No. 43, (June 2002), pp. 7186-7192, ISSN 1520-5207

Pillot, J.P., Birot, M., Bonnefon, E., Dunogues, J., Rayez, J.C., Rayez, M.T., Liotard, D. & Desvergne, J.P. (1997). First evidence of visible-range absorbing Si-B chromophores. *Chemical Communications*, No. 16, (August 1997), pp. 1535-1536, ISSN 1359-7345

Pistolis, G. & Malliaris, A. (1999). Limitations on the determination of the stoichiometry and equilibrium constants of weak complexes by computer fitting methods: experimental verification. *Chemical Physics Letters*, Vol. 310, No. 5-6, (September, 1999), pp. 501-507, ISSN 0009-2614

Pulgarin, J.M., Alanon Molina, A. & Fernandez Lopez, P. (1998). Simultaneous determination of atenolol, propranolol, dipyridamole and amiloride by means of non-linear variable-angle synchronous fluorescence spectrometry. *Analitica Chimica Acta*, Vol. 370, No. 1, (August, 1998), pp. 9-18, ISSN 0003-2670

Qu, D.H., Wang, Q.C., Ma, X. & Tian, H. (2005). A [3]rotaxane with three stable states that responds to multiple-inputs and displays dual fluorescence addresses. *Chemistry - A European Journal*, Vol. 11, No. 20, (October 2005), pp. 5929-5937, ISSN 1521-3765

Radi, A.E. & Eissa, S. (2011). Electrochemical study of indapamide and its complexation with β-cyclodextrin. *Journal of Inclusion Phenomena and Macrocyclic Chemistry*, DOI 10.1007/s10847-010-9906-1, ISSN 1573-1111

Rajaram, R., Sundararajalu, K.N. & Meenakshisundaram, S. (2011). Unusual Excited State Characteristics of 6-aminobenzothiazole with β-cyclodextrin. *Journal of Fluorescence*, Vol. 21, No. 2, (October 2010), pp. 521-529, ISSN 1573-4994

Ramakrishna, G. & Ghosh, H.N. (2002). Efficient electron injection from twisted intramolecular charge transfer (TICT) state of 7-diethyl amino coumarin 3-carboxylic acid (D-1421) dye to TiO_2 nanoparticle. *Journal of Physical Chemistry A*, Vol. 106, No. 11, (February 2002), pp. 2545-2553, ISSN 1089-5639

Ranta, V., Toropainen, E., Talvitie, A., Auriola, S. & Urtti, A. (2002). Simultaneous determination of eight β-blockers by gradient high-performance liquid chromatography with combined ultraviolet and fluorescence detection in corneal permeability studies in vitro. *Journal of Chromatography B: Analytical Technologies in the Biomedical and Life Sciences*, Vol. 772, No. 1, (May 2002), pp. 81-87, ISSN 1570-0232

Sainz-Rozas, P.R., Isasi, J.R. & Gonzalez-Gaitano, G. (2005). Spectral and photophysical properties of 2-dibenzofuranol and its inclusion complexes with cyclodextrins. *Journal of Photochemistry and Photobiology A: Chemistry*, Vol. 173, No. 3, (July 2005), pp. 319-327, ISSN 1010-6030

Sancho, M.I., Gasull, E., Blanco, S.E.& Castro, E.A. (2011). Inclusion complex of 2-chlorobenzophenone with cyclomaltoheptaose (β-cyclodextrin): temperature, solvent effects and molecular modeling. *Carbohydrate Research*, DOI 10.1016/j.carres.2011.05.002, ISSN 0008-6215

Scott, R.L. (1956). Some comments on the Benesi-Hildebrand equation. *Recueil des Travaux Chimiques*, Vol. 75, No. 7, (July 1956), pp. 787-789, ISSN 0165-0513

Shen, X., Belletete, M., Durocher, G. (1998). Spectral and photophysical studies of the 1:3 (guest/host) rotaxane-like inclusion complex formed by a 3H-indole and beta-cyclodextrin. *Journal of Physical Chemistry B*, Vol. 102, No. 11, (February 1998), pp. 1877-1883, ISSN1520-5207

Singh, R., Bharti, N., Madan, J. & Hiremath, S.N. (2010). Characterization of cyclodextrin inclusion complexes – A review. *Journal of Pharmaceutical Science and Technology*, Vol. 2, No. 3, (March 2010), pp. 171-183, ISSN 0975-5772

Siqintuya, Sueishi, Y., Yamamoto, S. (2007). Solvent-dependent intramolecular exciplex formation of N-benzyl-N-methylamine and N,N-dibenzylamine. *Journal of Photochemistry and Photobiology A: Chemistry*, Vol. 186, No. 1, (February 2007), pp. 41-46, ISSN 1010-6030

Szejtli, J. (1982). *Cyclodextrins and their inclusion complexes*, Akadémiai Kiadó, ISBN 9630528509, Budapest, p. 296

Tablet, C. & Hillebrand M. (2008). Theoretical and experimental study of the inclusion complexes of the 3-carboxy-5,6-benzocumarinic acid with cyclodextrins. *Spectrochimica Acta, Part A: Molecular and Biomolecular Spectroscopy*, Vol. 70, No. 4, (September 2008), pp. 740-748, ISSN 1386-1425

Thi, T.D., Nauwelaerts, K., Baudemprez, L., Van Speybroeck, M., Vermant, J., Augustijns, P., Annaert, P., Martens, J., Van Humbeeck, J. & Van den Mooter, G. (2011). Comparison between 2-hydroxypropyl-β-cyclodextrin and 2-hydroxypropyl-γ-cyclodextrin for inclusion complex formation with danazol. *Journal of Inclusion Phenomena and Macrocyclic Chemistry*, (January 2011), DOI 10.1007/s10847-010-9917-y, ISSN 1573-1111

Tintaru, A., Hillebrand, M. & Thevand, A. (2003). NMR Study of the inclusion complexes of carboxy-phenoxathiin derivatives with cyclodextrin. *Journal of Inclusion Phenomena and Macrocyclic Chemistry*, Vol. 45, No. 1-2, (February 2003), pp. 35-40, ISSN 1573-1111

Valeur, B., Berberan-Santos, M.N. & Martin, M.M. (2007). Photophysics and Photochemistry of Supramolecular Systems, In: *Analytical Methods in Supramolecular Chemistry*, Schalley, C., pp. 221-226, Wiley-VCH, ISBN 978-3-527-31505-5, Weinheim

Varlan, A. & Hillebrand, M. (2011). Spectral study of coumarin-3-carboxylic acid interaction with human and bovine serum albumins. *Central European Journal of Chemistry*, Vol. 9, No. 4, (August 2011), pp. 624-634, ISSN 1644-3624

Vyas, A. Saraf, S. & Saraf, S., (2008). Cyclodextrin based novel drug delivery systems, *Journal of Inclusion Phenomena and Macrocyclic Chemistry*, Vol. 62, No. 1-2, (May 2008), pp. 23-42, ISSN 1573-1111

Wagner, B.D., Fitzpatrick, S. & McManus, G. (2003). Fluorescence suppression of 7-methoxycoumarin upon inclusion into cyclodextrins. *Journal of Inclusion Phenomena and Macrocyclic Chemistry*, Vol. 47, No. 3-4, (December 2003), pp. 187-192, ISSN 1573-1111

Wang, R. & Yu, Z. (2007). Validity and reliability of Benesi-Hildebrand method, *Acta Physico-Chimica Sinica*, Vol. 23, No. 9, (September 2007), pp. 1353-1359, ISSN 1872-1508

Wu, A., Shen, X. & Gao, H. (2006). Cyclodextrin nanotube induced by 4,4'-bis(2-benzoxazolyl) stilbene, *International Journal of Nanoscience*, Vol. 5, No. 2-3, (April & June 2006), pp. 213-218, ISSN 1793-5350

Xie, G., Nakamura, M., Sueishi, Y. & Yamamoto, S. (2004). Separation into polar and hydrogen-bonding factors of the effects of alcohols on the emission spectrum of 4-phenyl-1-N, N-dimethylaminobutane in THF. *Journal of Photochemistry and Photobiology A: Chemistry*, Vol. 162, No. 1, (February 2004), pp. 73-79, ISSN 1010-6030

Xing, S., Zhang, Q., Zhang, C., Zhao, Q., Ai, H. & Sun, D. (2009). Isothermal titration calorimetry and theoretical studies on host-guest interaction of ibuprofen with α-, β- and γ–cyclodextrin. *Journal of Solution Chemistry*, Vol. 38, No. 5, (May 2009), pp. 531-543, ISSN 1572-8927

Yarabe, H.H., Agbaria, R.A., Rugutt, J.K., McCarroll, M.E., Gooden, R.A., Werner, T.C. & Warner, I.M. (2002). Spectroscopic studies of cyclodextrin complexes with 2,5-bis-(4-methylphenyl)oxazole. *Applied Spectroscopy*, Vol. 56, No. 8, (August 2002), pp. 1048-1054, ISSN 1943-3530

Yui, N., Katoono, R. & Yamashita, A. (2009). Functional cyclodextrin polyrotaxanes for drug delivery. *Advances in Polymer Science*, Vol. 222, (March 2009), pp. 55-77, ISSN 0065-3195

Zhang, H., Yu, T., Zhao, Y., Fan, D., Chen, L., Qiu, Y., Qian, L., Zhang, K. & Yang, C. (2008). Crystal structure and photoluminescence of 7-(N,N'-diethylamino)-coumarin-3-carboxylic acid. *Spectrochimica Acta, Part A: Molecular and Biomolecular Spectroscopy*, Vol. 69, No. 4, (April, 2008), pp. 1136-1139, ISSN 1386-1425

Zhang, J. & Ma, P.X. (2010). Host-guest interactions mediated nano-assemblies using cyclodextrin-containing hydrophilic polymers and their biomedical applications. *Nano Today*, Vol. 5, No. 4, (August 2010), pp. 337-350, ISSN 1748-0132

Part 2

Stoichiometry of Metal Complexes

4

Coordination Chemistry of Palladium(II) Ternary Complexes with Relevant Biomolecules

Ahmed A. El-Sherif*
Department of Chemistry, Faculty of Science, Cairo University, Cairo, Egypt

1. Introduction

*Cis*platin, *cis*-Diamminedichloroplatinum (II), is one of the most effective anticancer agents (Rosenberg, 1969). It has demonstrated a remarkable chemotherapeutic potential in a large variety of human solid cancers, such as, testicular, ovarian, bladder, lung and stomach carcinomas (Wong and Giandomenico, 1999; Guo and Sadler, 2000). The successful use of platinum (II) complexes as potent anticancer drugs has attracted the interest of many scientists. It was observed that the nature and arrangement of the ligands can affect the mode of action and metabolism of the drug while crossing the cell membrane and inside the cell. Despite the widespread use of *cis*-platin as an anticancer drug there is still scope for improvement, with respect to: i) reduced toxicity; ii) increased clinical effectiveness; iii) broader spectrum of action; iv) elimination of side effects (e.g., nausea, hearing loss, vomiting, etc); v) increased solubility and vi) ability to use them in combination with other drugs, limited by severe toxicities so far. Replacement of the chloro ligands by carboxylate groups in carboplatin, *cis*-diamine(1,1cyclobutanedicarboxylate)platinum(II), is a widely used second-generation platinum anticancer drug showing less side effects than *cis*-platin. The development of several new anticancer platinum drugs including Carboplatin, Nedaplatin, Lobaplatin and Oxaliplatin (Scheme 1) still have draw-backs and offer no more clinical advantages over the existing cisplatin (Gill, 1984; Galanski et al., 2005; Momekov et al., 2005). Furthermore, the development of acquired resistance to cis-platin is frequently observed during chemotherapy (Heim, 1993).

There is also much interest in Pd(II) analogues because they are usually isostructural with those of Pt(II), which show a very similar coordination process and geometry. However, Pd(II) systems attain equilibrium much more quickly than Pt(II) systems (~10^4-10^5 faster kinetics). The slow formation kinetics for Pt(II) complexes generally rules out the determination of stability constants. Therefore, Pd(II) complexes are frequently used as model complexes to study the interaction of Pt(II) with DNA and to mimic the binding properties of various platinum(II) species (Tercero-Moreno et al., 1996). It was also suggested that the faster aquation of palladium(II) compared with platinum(II) *in vitro*, makes the former a better model for studying Pt(II) reactions *in vivo* (Nelson, et al.,1976) with biological molecules, since these reactions always start with the aquation of the platinum(II) complexes. Several palladium complexes have been reported (Gill, 1984) with

*Corresponding Author

bidentate amine ligands which have shown anticancer activity comparable to or greater than cisplatin. Moreover, a series of labile Pd(II) complexes have proved to be useful as models to obtain a reasonable picture of the thermodynamics of the reactions for closely related Pt(II) complexes. It has also been suggested that these palladium complexes may be useful for the treatment of tumors of the gastrointestinal region where cisplatin fails. Mono-dentate ligands can bind in both cis- and *trans* arrangements around the metal and the isomers stability depend on several factors. Consequently, bidentate ligands are more reliable for the preparation of *cis*-complexes, in particular with palladium(II) and platinum(II) (Misra et al., 1998; Byabartta et al., 2001; Santra et al., 1999; Pal, et al., 2000; Rauth, et al., 2001; Roy et al., 1996; Das, et al., 1997; Das, et al., 1998). The reaction of DNA bases with Pd(II)/Pt(II) complexes of chelating N,N'-donors having *cis*-MCl_2 configuration constitutes a model system which may allow for exploration of the mechanism of the anti-tumor activity of cisplatin. Considering the importance of palladium complexes as potential anticancer drugs, we report here the coordination chemistry of mixed-ligand palladium complexes of bidentate amines with biologically active ligands.

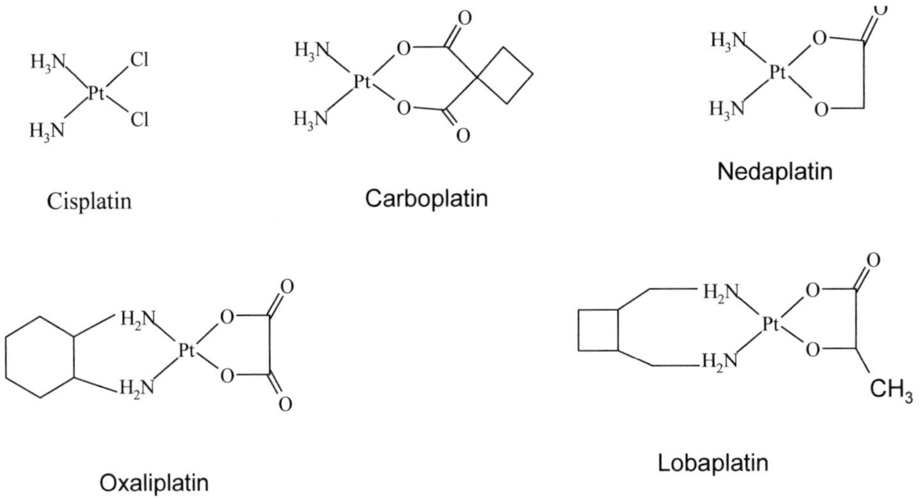

Scheme 1. Platinum-based drugs currently in clinical use.

2. Methods used for detection of aqueous solution complexes

Ion-selective electrodes were used for determination of the position of dynamic equilibrium system and the most common one is the glass electrode or hydrogen gas electrode which can be used for hydrogen ion measurements. Metal-ion selective electrodes or metal-amalgam electrodes can also be used for certain metal ions, but they are seldom as precise or convenient as the hydrogen ion electrode.

A great advantage with the use of ion-selective electrode measurements is that series of data can be easily collected through a titration procedure. From an initial analytical composition, stepwise changes with a burette are made with intervening electrode recordings. The elapsed time between these changes must be certained to be sufficient for equilibrium to be attained. A good method to check for this pre-requisite is to make repeated high-resolution electrode readings at predetermined time intervals, since this will make sluggish attainments of equilibrium clearly visible.

In addition, other experimental techniques are sometimes available. For example, if the metal ion or the ligand is coloured, and the colour changes (in intensity and/or frequency) upon complexation, spectrophotometry can be used. If the metal ion is diamagnetic, or if the ligand contains a suitable nucleus, nuclear magnetic resonance (NMR) is a striking method. This latter method, which ideally gives one separated signal for each unique chemical surrounding, can provide information not only on the free metal ion or ligand concentration, but also on the number of species and their respective concentration for a given analytical composition. Furthermore, since the positions of these signals are susceptible to protonation/deprotonation reactions, they can also be used to gain information on acid/base reactions of ligands and their complexes. Stopped-flow technique can be applied for fast reactions.

2.1 Determination of stability constants of mixed ligand complexes

The solution equilibria between metal ions and ligands may be described by two word-continuous competitions: The proton and a range of metal ions compete for a range of donor sites, the contest being ruled by concentration and pH conditions. The determination of equilibrium constants is an important process for many branches of chemistry (Motekaitis and Martell, 1988) Equilibrium constants can be determined from potentiometric data and/or spectrophotometric data. Developments in the field of computation of equilibrium constants from experimental data were reviewed by Leggett (Legget, 1985) and Meloun et al.[(Meloum, et al., 1994). Since then, many more programs have been published, mainly so as to be able to use microcomputers for the computations. The most commonly used programs for solution equilibrium constant determination are given in Table 1 (Motekaitis and Martell, 1988; Sabatini et al., 1974; Gans et al.,1976; Gans et al.,1985; Zekany and Nagypal, 1985; Sabatini et al., 1992; Gordon, 1982; Chandler et al., 1984; Perrin and Stunzi, 1985 ; Beltrán et al., 1993; Frassineti et al., 1995; Gampp et al.,1985; Tauler, et al., 1991). All of these programs use least-square refinements to reduce the differences between calculated and experimental data to get the best model from the best fit. The sum of square of residuals between experimental and calculated values are normally very small, it is typically between 10^{-6}-10^{-9}. Potentiometry generally used for measurements of formation constants of metal complexes is based on pH-metric titration of the ligand in absence and presence of metal ions. The formation constants derived by the least squares analysis of potentiometric data can describe completely the solution equilibria. The measurements are usually carried out at a constant ionic strength higher than the metal ion concentration. Therefore, no appreciable change in the ionic strength of the solution medium occurs. In general for the reaction:

$$L(M) + p(L_1) + q(L_2) + r(H) \rightleftharpoons [(M)_l(L_1)_p(L_2)_q(H)_r] \quad (1)$$

The overall stability constant, β_{lpqr}, can be calculated from:

$$\beta_{lpqr} = [(M)_l(L_1)_p(L_2)_q(H)_r]/[M]^l[L_1]^p[L_2]^q[H]^r \quad (2)$$

(charges are omitted for simplicity)

where M, L_1, L_2 and H stand for $[Pd(diamine)(H_2O)_2]^{2+}$ ion, ligand(1), ligand(2) and proton, respectively. For OH^- the coefficient (r) for H = -1.

Program	Data type[a]	Reference
PKAS	V	(Motekaitis and Martell, 1988)
MINIQUAD	V	(Sabatini et al., 1974)
MINIQUAD75	V	(Gans et al.,1976)
SUPERQUAD	V	(Gans et al.,1985)
PSEQUAD	V, A	(Zekany and Nagypal, 1985)
HYPERQUAD	V, A	(Sabatini et al., 1992)
TITAN	V	(Gordon, 1982)
SCOGS2a	V	(Chandler et al., 1984)
SCOGS2b	V	(Perrin and Stunzi, 1985)
STAR	A	(Beltrán et al., 1993)
HYPNMR	N	(Frassineti et al., 1995)
SPECFIT	A(E)	(Gampp et al.,1985)
SPFAC	A(E)	(Tauler, et al., 1991)

[a]Additional data types used in calculations: E, ESR and N, NMR

Table 1. The most commonly used programs for calculating equilibrium constants from potentiometric (V) and spectrophotometric (A) data.

2.2 Determination of stability constants of Pd(II) complexes

As mentioned earlier, determination of formation constants of the Pd(II) complexes is made more difficult than in the case of other metals as a result of the unstable nature of $[Pd(H_2O)_4]^{2+}$ in aqueous solution. Some authors have used $[PdCl_4]^{2-}$, as the metal ion source, but in this case the inclusion of the Cl^- as a ligand as well as other ligands in the calculation of formation constants becomes necessary (Bóka, et al., 2001). Elding (Elding, 1972) calculated log β_{14} for $[PdCl_4]^{2-}$ to be ~ 10. Therefore, $[Pd(NH_3)_2(H_2O)_2]^{2+}$ and $[Pd(diamine)(H_2O)_2]^{2+}$ were considered as the starting metal ions for Pd(II) and the acid-base equilibria of the diaquo complexes were first determined. Secondary ligands were then introduced and the formation constant of the mixed ligand complex calculated using one of the above mentioned programs. Hydrolytic reactions of Pt(II) and Pd(II) complexes are important issues because they are related to the action of the *cis*-platinum(II) anti-cancer drugs. The very high thermodynamic stability constants of the chelated diamine complexes of palladium(II) result in the complete formation of the species $[Pd(diamine)(H_2O)_2]^{2+}$ even under very acidic conditions (pH <2), while the relatively high ratios of the stepwise stability constants suppress the bis(bidentatediamine) complex formation in equimolar solution (Nagy and Sóvágó, 2001). As a consequence, all the Pd(II) species are present in the form of $[Pd(bidentatediamine)]^{2+}$, and therefore, the ternary complex, Pd(bidentate diamine)-ligand, can be treated as a binary complex.

2.3 Preparation of $[Pd(diamine)(H_2O)_2]^{2+}$ complex

$[Pd(diamine)Cl_2]$ complexes were prepared, by reaction of $[PdCl_4]^{2-}$ with diamine in the molar ratio 1:1. For equilibrium studies, $[Pd(diamine)Cl_2]$ was converted into the diaqua complex $[Pd(diamine)(H_2O)_2](NO_3)_2$ by stirring the chloro-complex with two equivalents of $AgNO_3$ overnight, and removing the AgCl precipitate by filtration through a 0.1 µm pore membrane filter. Great care was taken to ensure that the resulting solution was free of Ag^+ ions and that the chloro-complex had been converted into the aqua species, the filtrate made up to the desired volume in a standard volumetric flask. Also, the ligands in the form of hydrochlorides were converted to the corresponding hydronitrate in the same way as described above.

2.4 Speciation distribution as a function of pH

Speciation (based on concentrations of metal ions and complexing species) refers to a program (Pettit) which calculates and plots the species distribution of a series of complexes over a specified pH range. In this program, the input data of total concentrations of metal and ligand, pH range and the best fit set of β values are used to compute equilibrium concentrations of all the available complex species over the given pH range. All types of complexes can be calculated, including mixed complexes, protonated, hydroxo and polynuclear species. The graphical output can thus provide a visual record of the most predominant complex species at any pH especially within the physiological pH range.

2.5 Determination of the acid-base equilibria of $[Pd(diamine)(H_2O)_2]^{2+}$ complex

The hydrolysis reactions of Pt(II) complexes are among the most important issues which should be considered under physiological conditions. As a consequence, hydrolysis of cisplatin and its derivatives has been thoroughly studied in both solution and solid state (Martin, 1983; Martin, 1999; Faggiani et al., 1977; Faggiani et al., 1977). It is clear from these studies that hydrolysis of cisplatin and other *cis*-diamine platinum(II) species can not be described by the formation of simple monomeric dihydroxo complexes, but various dinuclear (Faggiani et al., 1978) and trinuclear species are also formed (Faggiani et al., 1977; Faggiani et al., 1977). The very slow formation kinetics, however, hampers the determination of stability constants of platinum(II), but the corresponding palladium(II) complexes can be used as appropriate model compounds (Tercero-Moreno et al., 1996).

The main species formed during the hydrolysis of $[Pd(diamine)(H_2O)_2]^{2+}$ ion are 10-1, 10-2, 20-1 and 20-2. The first two species are due to deprotonation of the two coordinated water molecules, as given by Eqs. 3 and 4.

$$\underset{100}{[Pd(N\text{-}N)(H_2O)_2]^{2+}} \xrightleftharpoons{pK_{a1}} \underset{10\text{-}1}{[Pd(N\text{-}N)(H_2O)(OH)]^{+}} + H^{+} \qquad (3)$$

$$\underset{10\text{-}1}{[Pd(N\text{-}N)(H_2O)_2(OH)]^{+}} \xrightleftharpoons{pK_{a2}} \underset{10\text{-}2}{[Pd(N\text{-}N)(OH)_2]} + H^{+} \qquad (4)$$

The third species, (20-1), is the hydroxo bridged-dimer formed as result of the combination of the monoaqua hydroxo species (10-1) with the diaqua species (100) $[Pd(diamine)(H_2O)_2]^{2+}$ as given by Eq. 5.

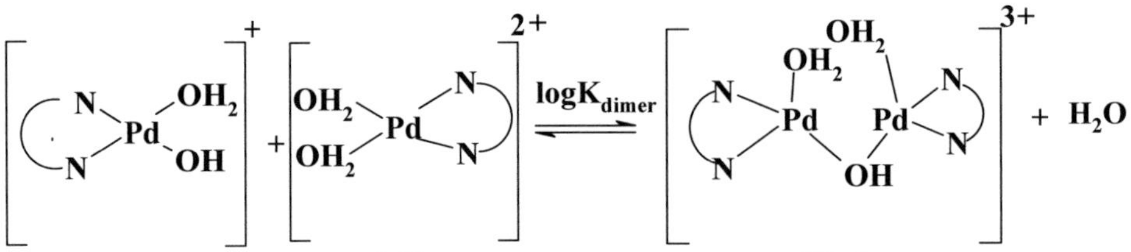

(5)

10 -1 100 20 -1

The fourth species, 20-2, is the dimeric di-μ-hydroxo complex of two 10-1 species according to Eq.6.

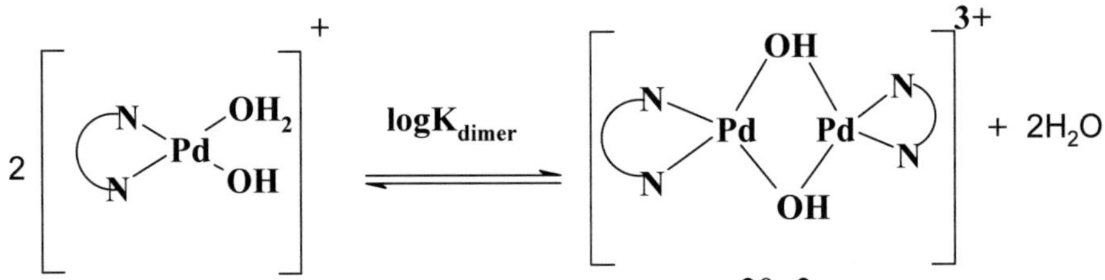

(6)

10 -1 20 -2

According to the data in Table 2 (Britten et al., 1982; Lim et al., 1976; Hohmann, et al., 1991; Shoukry, et al., 1999; El-Sherif, et al., 2003 ; Shehata, 2001), the pK_{a1} and pK_{a2} values in the bipyridine as a non-leaving group were found to be 3.91 and 8.39, respectively and are lower than the corresponding values of all the Pd^{II}-diamine complexes. The $[Pd(Pic)(H_2O)_2]^{2+}$ values are intermediate because Pic has one pyridine ring. This can be attributed to the increased positive charge on Pd atom due to the π-acceptor properties of the aromatic moiety of Pyridine ring, leading to an increase in the electrophilicity of the Pd ion and consequently to a decrease in the pK_a of the coordinated water molecule. The equilibrium constant for the dimerization reactions (5) and (6) can be calculated with Eqs. 7 and 8 respectively.

$$\log_{10} K_{dimer} = \log \beta_{20\text{-}1} - \log \beta_{10\text{-}1} \tag{7}$$

$$\log_{10} K_{dimer} = \log \beta_{20\text{-}2} - 2 \log \beta_{10\text{-}1} \tag{8}$$

The concentration distribution diagram for $[Pd(AMBI)(H_2O)_2]^{2+}$ and its hydrolysed species as a representative example of hydrolysis of $[Pd(diamine)(H_2O)_2]$ is shown in Fig.1. The concentration of the monohydroxo species, 10-1 and the dimeric species, 20-2 increase with increasing pH, predominating in the pH range 4.8 to 7.8 with formation percentages of ca. 44% and 54% for the monohydroxo (10-1) and dimeric species (20-2), respectively, i.e., they are the main species present in solution in the physiological pH range. A further increase in pH is accompanied by an increase in the dihydroxo species, which is the main species above a pH of ca. 11. In the high pH range the inert dihydroxo complex would be the predominant species, so that the reactivity of DNA to bind the Pd(amine) complex will considerably decrease.

Complex[a]	Pk_{a1}	pK_{a2}	Reference
Cis-$[Pt(NH_3)_2(H_2O)_2]^{2+}$	5.6	7.3	(Britten et al., 1982)
$[Pt(en)(H_2O)_2]^{2+}$	5.8	7.6	(Lim et al., 1976)
$[Pd(en)(H_2O)_2]^{2+}$	5.6	7.3	(Hohmann, et al., 1991)
$[Pd(1,2\text{-}DAP)(H_2O)_2]^{2+}$	5.62	9.35	(Shoukry, et al., 1999)
$[Pd(Pic)(H_2O)_2]^{2+}$	4.81	8.46	(El-Sherif, et al., 2003)
$[Pd(BPY)(H_2O)_2]^{2+}$	3.91	8.39	(Shehata, 2001)

[a]en, 1,2-DAP, Me_2en, Pic and BPY represent ethylenediamine, 1,2-diaminopropane, N,N'-dimethylethylenediamine, picolylamine and 2,2'-bipyridyl, respectively.

Table 2. Comparison of acid dissociation constants of some Pt and Pd-diaquo complexes.

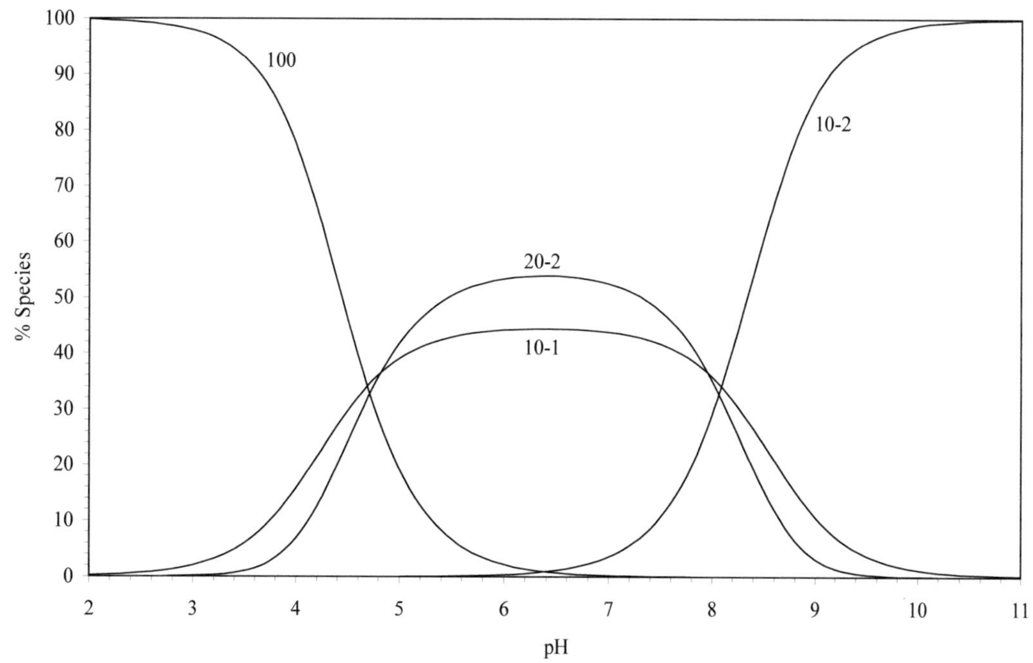

Fig. 1. Concentration distribution of various species as a function of pH in the $Pd(AMBI)(H_2O)_2$ system at concentration of 1.25×10^{-3} mol-dm^{-3}, I = 0.1 mol-dm^{-3} ($NaNO_3$) and T = 25 ± 0.1 ^0C).

3. Interactions of [Pd(diamine)(H_2O)$_2$] with bio-relevant ligands

3.1 Interactions of [Pd(diamine)(H_2O)$_2$] with amino acids

The potential donor atoms in the amino acids are (the amino-N, the carboxylato- O, as well as the other donor atoms which may be present in the side chains). Pd(II) and Pt(II) form stable complexes with the N-, O-, S-donor atoms present in amino acids, with thermodynamic preference for S- and N- donors over O-donors. Though the thermodynamic preference of the metal ion for a particular donor atom is a very important parameter in determining the choice of donor atoms, at the pH value used for the experiment, these donor atoms may be protonated. Additionally, the effect of chelate ring size may also be a factor in determining the adopted coordination mode.

3.1.1 Acid-base equilibria of amino acids

All amino acids undergo two reversible proton dissociation steps in fairly well separated pH ranges, proceeding according to equilibrium reaction (9).

$$\underset{(H_2L^+)}{^{+}NH_3CH(R)COOH} \underset{}{\overset{pH=2\text{-}3}{\rightleftharpoons}} \underset{(HL^{\pm})}{^{+}NH_3CH(R)COO^-} \overset{pH=8\text{-}10}{\rightleftharpoons} \underset{(L^-)}{NH_2CH(R)COO^-} \quad (9)$$

Besides these two functional groups, most of the essential amino acids contain further functional groups in the side chains of amino acids.

3.1.2 Interactions of [Pd(diamine)(H_2O)$_2$] with amino acids containing no functional group in the side chain

3.1.2.1 Complexes formed when only one metal coordination site is available

Multi-NMR studies (Appleton et al., 1986; Appleton, 1997) of complexes as $[M(NH_3)_3(H_2O)]^{2+}$, M = Pt(II) or Pd(II) with amino acids (AA) showed the initial formation of metastable isomer e.g. $[Pd(NH_3)_3(HGly\text{-}O)]^{2+}$ is formed at low pH~3, which coordinate through the carboxylate oxygen. Since glycine nitrogen ($pK_a \sim 9.6$) is protonated under these conditions and the carboxyl group ($pK_a \sim 2.3$) partially deprotonated, carboxylate oxygen is more available for reactions than the amine nitrogen. This complex was slowly converted to $[Pd(NH_3)_3(HGly\text{-}N)]^{2+}$ isomer and the conversion can be slowed at lower pH. β-alanine has an additional methylene group. Its corresponding complex, Hβala-O, did not isomerise at pH = 4.5, but slowly isomerise at higher pH to the complex with β-ala-N. Appleton et al. (Appleton et al., 1986) using multinuclear NMR showed that γ-aminobutyric acid complex, $[Pt(NH_3)_3(\gamma aba\text{-}O)]^{2+}$, standing at pH = 10 caused only slow displacement of the carboxylate-bound ligand by hydroxide. Generally, the O-bound isomer is thermodynamically more stable relative to N-bound form for Pd(II) relative to Pt(II), reflecting a kind of hardness Pd(II) compared to Pt(II) (Appleton, 1997).

3.1.2.2 Complexes formed when two metal coordination sites are available

It has been well established that N,O-chelation is a characteristic coordination mode for glycine bound to palladium(II) (Freeman and Colomb, 1964). The complex-formation equilibria for amino acids may be represented as shown in scheme 2.

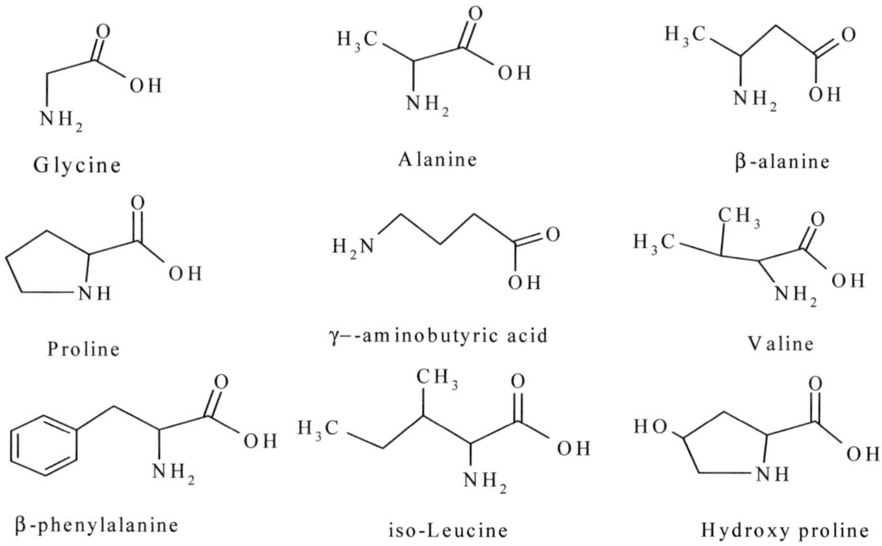

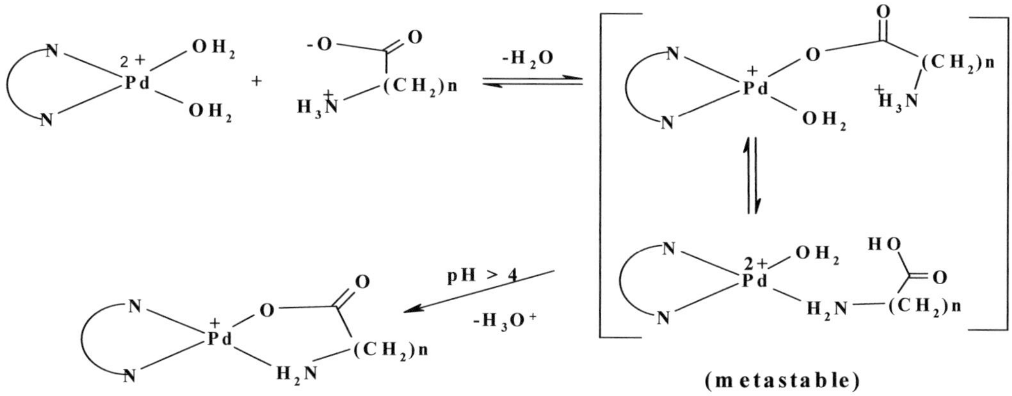

Scheme 2. Coordination mode of amino acids

The complexes of general fomula [Pd(diamine)(AA)], where AA = glycine, alanine, valine, proline, phenylalanine, γ-aminobutyric acid, β-alanine and proline are investigated. The potentiometric titration curves of the [Pd(diamine)] with amino acids, lie significantly below the amino acid alone ones. This reveals that the formation of complex species occurs through release of hydrogen ions.

The stability constants of amino acids with [Pd(amine)(H_2O)$_2$] are showed in Tables 3 and 4 (Shoukry et al., 1999; Lim, (1978); Mohamed. and Shoukry, 2001; El-Sherif et al., 2010; Shehata et al., 2008; Shehata et al., 2009; El-Sherif, 2006). The amino acids with no functional groups in the side chains generally form 1:1 complexes with $[Pd(diamine)(H_2O)_2]^{2+}$. Their complexes are very stable, with stability constants of log β_{110} ~ 10-12. They coordinate through both the amino group and the carboxylate oxygen, forming stable five-membered chelate ring.

The stability constant of 1:1 complex with imidazole have a smaller value than those of amino acids, further supporting that amino acids are coordinating as bidentate ligands.

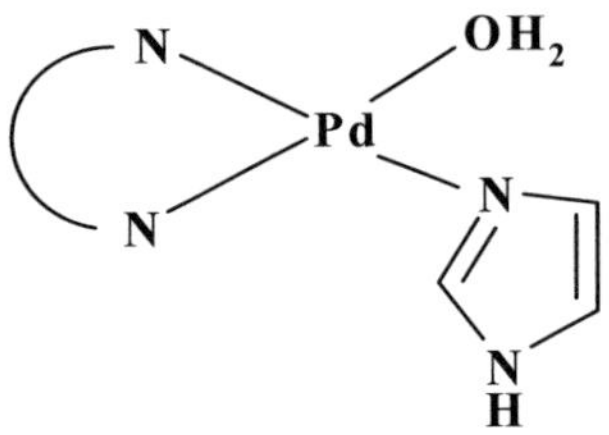

$[Pd(N\text{-}N)(imidazole)]^{+2}$

(110)

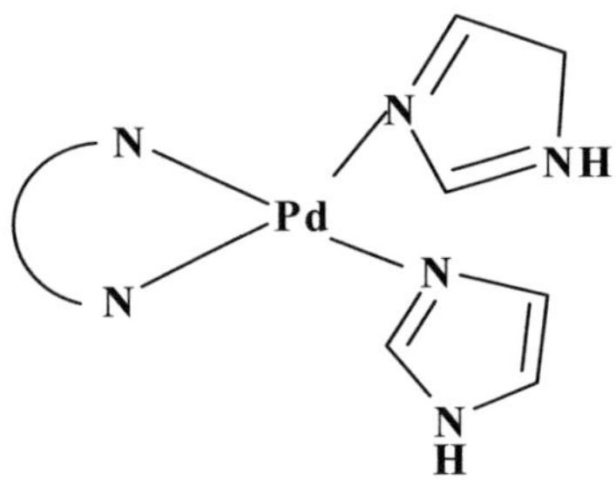

$[Pd(N\text{-}N)(imidazole)_2]^{+2}$

(120)

The stability constants log β_{110} of $[Pd(AEPY)alanine]^{2+}$ (10.46) > $[Pd(AEPY)\text{-}\beta\text{-}alanine]^{2+}$ (9.81) > [Pd(AEPY)-γ-aminobutyric acid] (7.81). This trend is attributed to extra stability of five-membered chelate rings for alanine complexes compared to six and seven-membered rings for β-alanine and γ-aminobutyric acid, respectively (Shehata et al., 2009).

3.1.3 Interactions of $[Pd(diamine)(H_2O)_2]$ with amino acids containing sulphur atom in the side chain

Sulphur containing amino acids (e.g. cysteine, methionine and S-methylcysteine) easily react with Pd(II) because of the great tendency of sulphur (a soft Lewis base) to form bonds with these metals (soft Lewis acids).

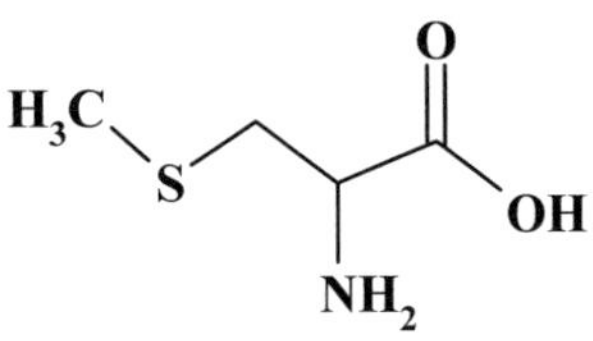

S-Methyl cysteine

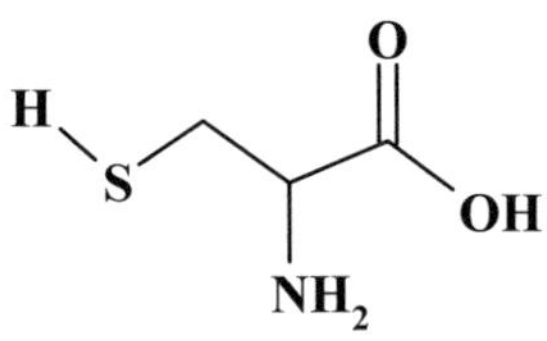

Cysteine

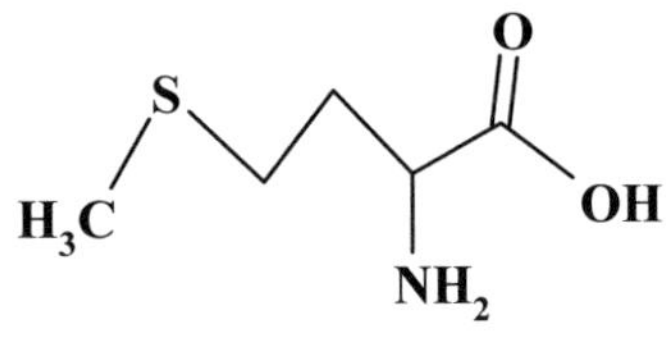

Methionine

The interaction of Pt(II) and Pd(II) with methionine in aqueous solution primarily occurs through the sulphur atom and chelates only in a further step, binding through the amino group (Norman et al., 1992).

The stability constants of S-methyl cysteine (SMC) and methionine with Pd(II) (tables 3 and 4) are lower than those of ordinary amino acids, suggesting that they are not coordinated as glycine complexes. The stability constants with SMC are generally higher than those with methionine due to the formation of more stable 5-membered ring. The reaction between $[Pd(diamine)(H_2O)_2]^{2+}$ and S-containing amino acids is showed in scheme 3. At low pH values the coordination site is through S-atom, slowly forming bidentate ligand followed by deprotonation of the carboxylic group.

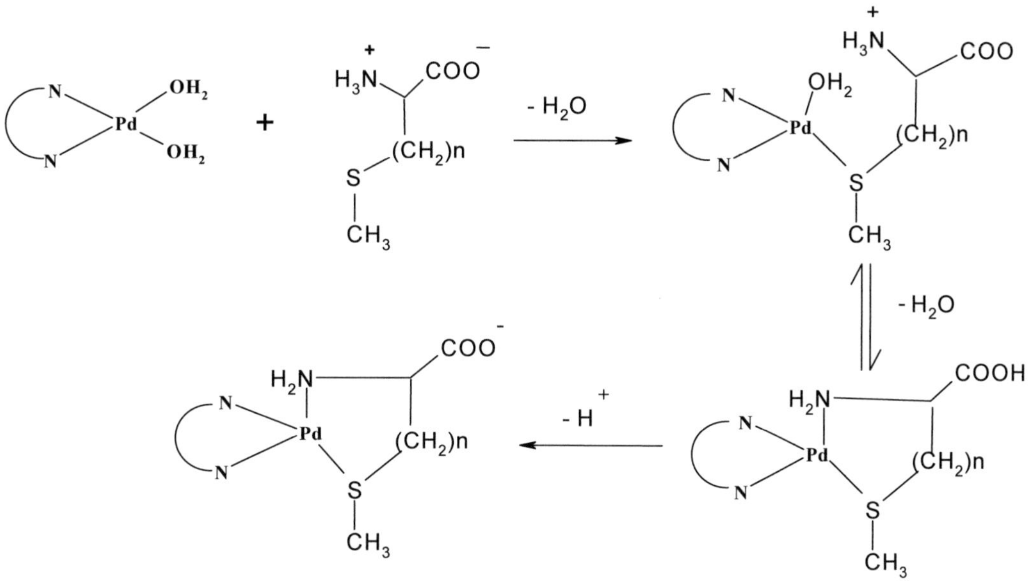

Scheme 3. Interaction of $[Pd(diamine)(H_2O)_2]^{2+}$ with S-containing amino acids.

3.1.4 Interactions of $[Pd(diamine)(H_2O)_2]$ with amino acids containing hydroxy group in the side chain

Serine and threonine are α-amino acids with β-OH group in the side-chain. They contain only two dissociable protons in the measurable pH range ($-NH_3^+$ and -COOH), as the alcoholic hydoxy group is so weakly acidic ($pK_a > 14$), that it does not undergo dissociation in the measurable pH range. The β-alcoholate group in the side chain of the amino acids serine and threonine have been found to play an essential role in the action mechanism of a number of proteolytic enzymes, e.g. chymotrypsin and subtilisin (Bernhard, 1986).

Serine Threonine

$[Pd(diamine)(H_2O)_2]^{2+}$ promotes the ionization of the alcohol group of serine and threonine, the presence of the species 11-1 indicates the ionization of the OH side-chain. The pK_a of the ionization can be calculated using Eq.10

$$pK_a = \log \beta_{110} - \log \beta_{11-1} \quad (10)$$

The pK_a of ionization for serine and threonine are 8.26 and 7.53 with Pd(1,2-DAP), respectively (Shoukry et al.,1999). Values of 8.51 and 8.05 were obtained with Pd(en), Table 3 (Shoukry, et al., 1999; Lim, 1978; Mohamed and Shoukry, 2001; El-Sherif et al., 2010; Shehata, et al., 2008). This large acidification of ~ 6 log units indicates a large contribution of the OH group in the coordination process at higher pH and participation of the OH group in complex formation is not contributing significantly in the physiological pH range. The pK_a value of the alcoholate group incorporated in the Pd(II)-AMBI-serine complex is 8.21 (El-Sherif, 2006). This value is lower than that of the Pd(N,N´-dimethylethylenediamine)-serine complex (8.43) (Mohamed and Shoukry, 2001). This may be due the π-acceptor property of the pyridine ring, which increases the electrophilicity of the Pd(II) ion and consequently decreases the pK_a value of the coordinated alcoholate group.

System	p	q	r[b]	en[c]	$(Me)_2$en[d]	1,2-DAP[e]	1,3-DAP[f]	SMC[g]
Glycine	1	1	0	11.21	11.79	11.01	11.12	10.13
Alanine	1	1	0	11.22	10.89	11.42	11.22	10.21
β-Phenylalanine	1	1	0	-	10.09	11.06	-	9.97
β-Alanine	1	1	0	-	-	-	-	9.75
	1	1	1					13.37
Valine	1	1	0	-	11.59	11.36	-	9.82
Proline	1	1	0	12.16	11.14	11.55	-	10.62
Iso-leucine	1	1	0		-	-	-	10.44
Methionine	1	1	0	9.14	11.27	10.37	10.31	8.75
S-Methylcysteine	1	1	0	9.38	-	10.83	10.64	8.94
Cysteine	1	1	0	-	-	-	-	14.32
	1	1	1					22.67
Serine	1	1	0	11.01	10.92	12.00	-	9.87
	1	1	-1	2.50	2.49	3.74		0.67
Threonine	1	1	0	10.96	-	11.76	10.57	9.76
	1	1	-1	2.91		3.83	2.11	0.38
Ornithine	1	1	0		13.34	13.65	-	11.23
	1	1	1		20.85	19.86		20.21
Lysine	1	1	0		11.19	11.49	-	10.87
	1	1	1		21.19	20.44		20.69
Histidine	1	1	0		14.45	14.75	-	11.50
	1	1	1					
Histamine	1	1	0		12.61	13.22	-	10.92
	1	1	1		17.03			
Aspartic acid	1	1	0		10.70	-	-	-
	1	1	1					
Glutamic acid	1	1	0		10.56	-	9.72	10.61
	1	1	1				13.60	13.99

[a]N-N = aliphatic diamine, [b]p, q and r are stoichiometric coefficients corresponding to $[Pd(diamine)(H_2O)_2]$, ligand and H^+ respectively, [c]en = ethylenediamine, data taken from reference (Lim, 1978), [d]Me_2en = N,N'-dimethylethylenediamine, data taken from reference (Mohamed and Shoukry, 2001), [e]1,2-DAP=1,2-diaminopropane, data taken from reference (Shoukry, et al., 1999); [f]1,3-DAP=1,3-diaminopropane, data taken from reference (El-Sherif et al., 2010); [g]SMC=S-Methyl-L-cysteine, data taken from reference (Shehata, et al., 2008).

Table 3. Formation constants ($\log \beta_{110}$) of $[Pd(diamine)(H_2O)_2]^a$ with amino acid at 25 ^{0}C and 0.1 mol dm^{-3} $NaNO_3$.

System	p	q	r[b]	Pic[c]	AEPY[d]	AMBI[e]
Glycine	1	1	0	9.95	10.33	9.71
Alanine	1	1	0	10.89	10.46	9.98
β-Phenylalanine	1	1	0	11.05	9.86	11.01
β-Alanine	1	1	0	-	9.81	-
	1	1	1		13.37	
Valine	1	1	0	10.33	10.22	9.91
Proline	1	1	0	11.16	10.81	10.85
Iso-leucine	1	1	0	11.76	10.56	11.10
Methionine	1	1	0	9.49	9.08	9.12
S-Methylcysteine	1	1	0	10.52	9.16	10.15
Cysteine	1	1	0	-	15.11	-
	1	1	-1		19.20	
Tyrosine	1	1	0	14.61	-	-
Tryptophan	1	1	0	10.95	-	-
Serine	1	1	0	11.35	10.34	10.61
	1	1	-1	3.05	2.04	2.40
Threonine	1	1	0	10.40	10.29	-
	1	1	-1	-	2.19	
Ornithine	1	1	0	13.13	13.27	10.21
	1	1	1	20.54	20.53	18.68
Lysine	1	1	0	-	10.62	-
	1	1	1		19.49	
Histidine	1	1	0	13.36	13.37	13.14
	1	1	1		16.32	19.15
Histamine	1	1	0	13.19	12.85	10.34
	1	1	1			
Aspartic acid	1	1	0	10.02	-	-
	1	1	1			
	1	1	2			
Glutamic acid	1	1	0	-	9.19	-
	1	1	1		13.27	
	1	1	2		15.79	

[a]N-N = aromatic diamine, [b]p, q and r are stoichiometric coefficients corresponding to [Pd(diamine)(H_2O)$_2$], ligand and H^+ respectively, [c]Pic = picolylamine, data taken from reference (El-Sherif et al., 2003), [d]AEPY = 2-aminoethylpyridine, data taken from reference (Shehata, et al., 2009), [e]AMBI=2-aminomethylbenzimidazole, data taken from reference (El-Sherif, 2006).

Table 4. Formation constants (log β_{110}) of [Pd(diamine)(H_2O)$_2$][a] with amino acid at 25 ^{0}C and 0.1 mol dm^{-3} $NaNO_3$.

The pK_a value (9.20) for the Pd(SMC)-serine complex as reported in Table 3 is higher than the corresponding values of the Pd(N, N′-dimethylethylenediamine)-serine (8.43) [52] and Pd(Picolylamine)-serine complexes (8.30) (El-Sherif et al., 2003). This is due to the strong *trans* labilization effect of sulfur on the coordinated alcoholate group, and in turn hinders the induced proton ionization. This will increase the pK_a value of the alcoholate group in the case of the Pd(SMC)-serine complex.

3.1.5 Interactions of [Pd(diamine)(H_2O)$_2$] with amino acids containing amino group in the side chain

Ornithine and lysine are α- amino acids having an extra terminal- amino group. They coordinate with [Pd(diamine)(H_2O)$_2$]$^{2+}$ as bidentate either by the two amino groups (N,N-donor set) or glycine-like, through the α-amino and carboxylate groups (N,O-donor set). The way of coordination is depending on three factors:

1. The chelate ring size.
2. The steric effects.
3. The pH of the solution.

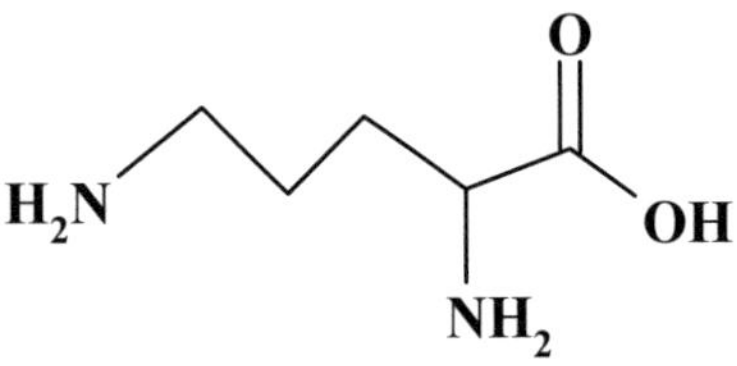

Ornithine

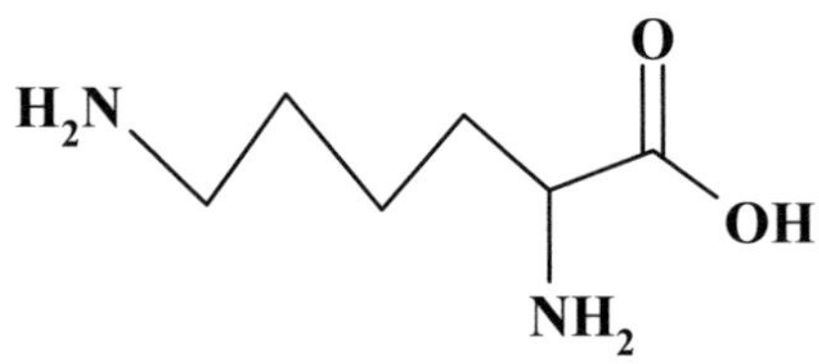

Lysine

The stability constant of the Pd(DAP)-Ornithine complex (logβ_{110} = 13.65) is higher than those of α- amino acids. This may indicate that ornithine most likely chelates by the two amino groups at higher pH, this is being supported by the great affinity of palladium to nitrogen donor centres. Unlike ornithine, The stability constant of the Pd(DAP)-lysine complex (logβ_{110} = 11.49) is extremely fair with those of α- amino acids. This may indicate that lysine most likely chelates by the amino and carboxylate groups (glycine-like), because chelates formed through binding with the two amino groups will form unstable eight-membered ring. The concentration distribution diagram of [Pd(AMBI)(ornithine)] complex is given in Fig. 2. It clearly shows that lysine starts to form the protonated species (111) at low pH and predominates between pH (4-9) and attains maximum concentration of ~ 98%, i.e it is the main complex species in physiological pH range. The complex species (110) predominates after pH ~ 9. The (10-1) hydrolysed species is present in very low concentration and the (10-2) species starts to form at higher pH, ca. ~ 10. Therefore, in the physiological pH range the OH^- ion doesn't compete with ornithine in the reaction with the palladium (II) complexes.

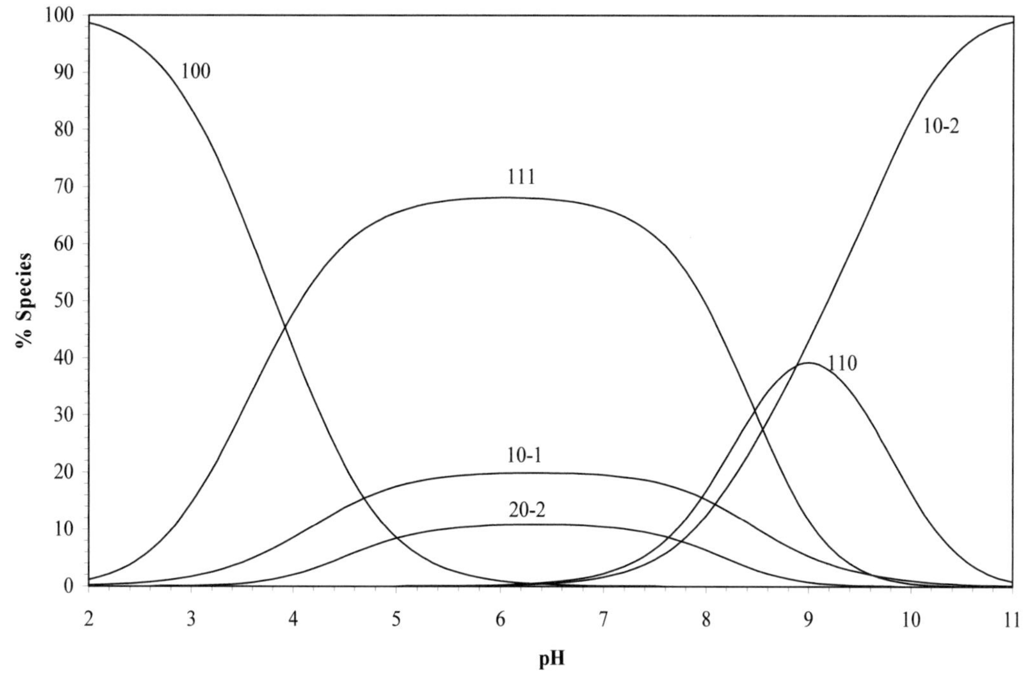

Fig. 2. Concentration distribution of various species as a function of pH in the Pd(AMBI)-Ornithine system at concemtrations of $1.25x10^{-3}$ mol-dm^{-3} for $Pd(AMBI)^{2+}$ and ornithine, I = 0.1 mol-dm^{-3} ($NaNO_3$) and T = 25 ± 0.1 ^{0}C).

3.1.6 Interactions of $[Pd(diamine)(H_2O)_2]$ with amino acids containing carboxylic acid group in the side chain

Aspartic and glutamic are α- amino acids having two carboxylic and one amino group as potential chelating sites. They coordinate with $[Pd(diamine)(H_2O)_2]^{2+}$ as bidentate either by the two carboxylate groups or by the amino and one carboxylate group. The stability constant of the aspartic and glutamic acid complexes is in the range of those for amino acids. This may reveal that both amino acids coordinate by the amino and one carboxylate group.

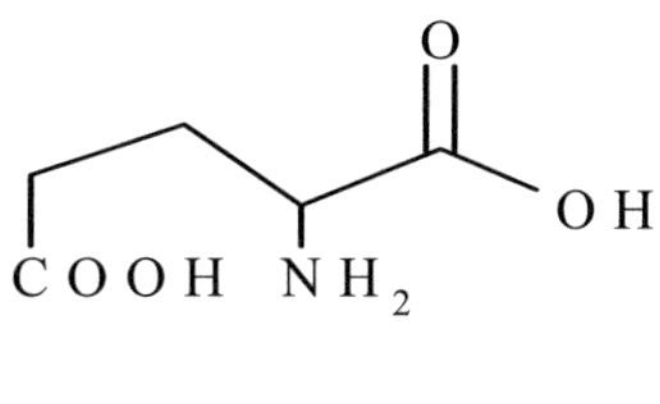

Glutamic acid

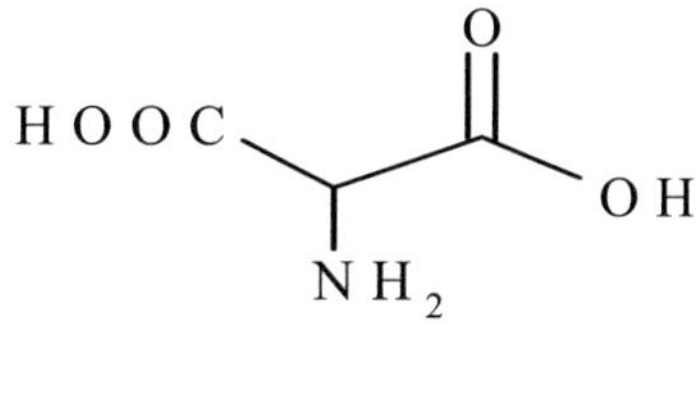

Aspartic acid

3.1.7 Interactions of $[Pd(diamine)(H_2O)_2]$ with amino acids containing imidazole group in the side chain

The protonated histidine contains three dissociable protons, which can dissociate in the following sequence: carboxylic acid, imidazolium N(3)-H and side chain NH_3^+. The imidazole N(1)-H is very weekly acidic (pK_a = 14.4), and thus it does not dissociate in the measurable pH range (Burger, 1990).

Histidine has three binding sites, provided imidazole, amino and carboxylate groups. It coordinates with $[Pd(diamine)(H_2O)_2]^{2+}$ as bidentate either by the α-amino group and imidazole groups (N,N-donor set) or glycine-like, through the α-amino and carboxylate groups (N,O-donor set).

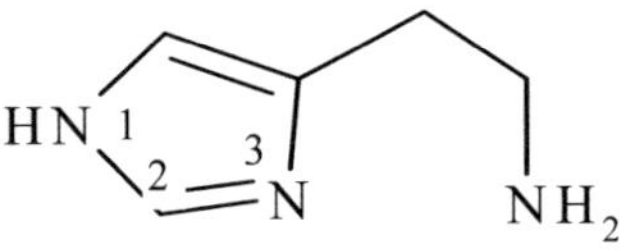

Histamine

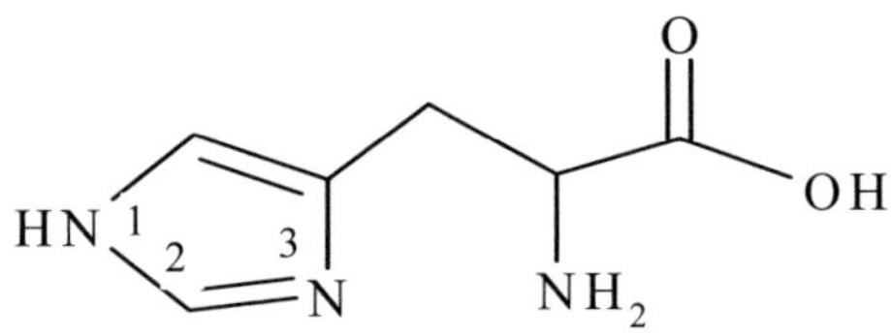

Histidine

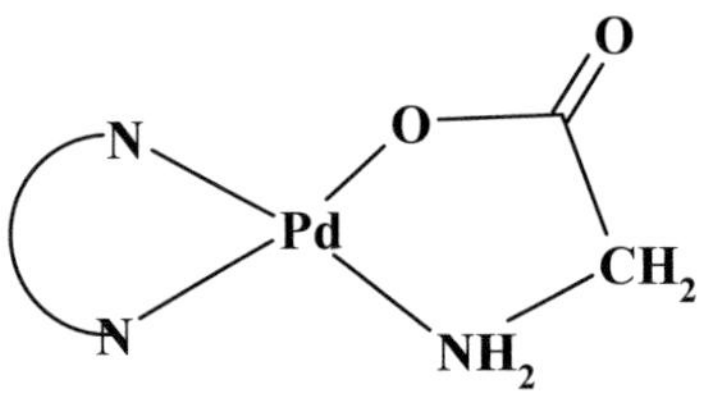

(Glycine-like)

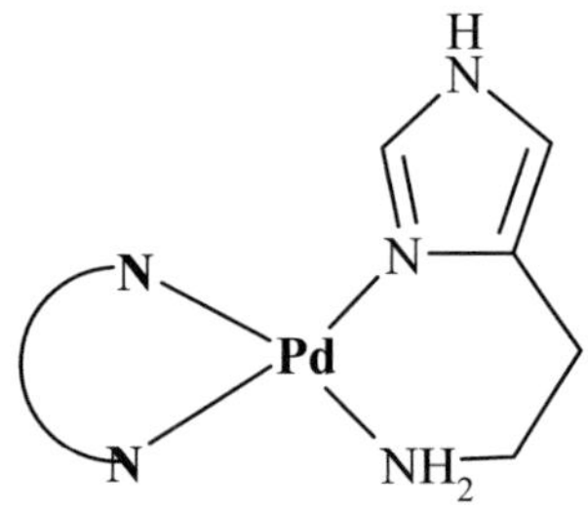

(Histamine-like)

The formation constant value of the (110) species is in fair agreement with that of histamine complex, but higher than those of α-amino acids. This indicates that histidine interacts with $[Pd(diamine)(H_2O)_2]$ in the same way as histamine does i.e. through the amino and imidazole.

Histidine has shown to form both protonated (111) and deprotonated (110) complex species. The acid dissociation constant of the protonated species is given by the following Eq. (11).

$$pK^H = \log \beta_{111} - \log \beta_{110} \qquad (11)$$

In the reaction with $[Pd(AEPY)(H_2O)_2]^{2+}$ species only two of the above three binding sites are involved in complex formation. The stability constants of the histidine complexes ($\log\beta_{110}$ = 13.37) is higher than that of histamine ($\log\beta_{110}$ = 12.85) by 0.52 log β units. Moreover, it is higher than those of amino acids (e.g. $\log\beta_{110}$ of glycine = 10.33) by 3.04 log units, indicating that both kinds of chelation are involved glycine-like (N,O) at lower pH and histamine-like (N,N) at higher pH. In general, histidine forms more stable complex than histamine due to the negative charge of histidine compared to neutral histamine. Furthermore, palladium may form back bonding to the π–system of imidazole ring, which brings more stable complexes.

3.2 Interactions of [Pd(diamine)(H_2O)$_2$] with peptides

Amide bonds or groups provide the linkage between adjacent amino acids. A protein is composed of a chain of (n) amino acids contains (n-1) peptide (amide) bonds in the backbone. The tetrahedral amino nitrogen in an amino acid with pK_a ~ 9.7 loses its basicity upon reaction to give trigonal nitrogen in an amide bond. Amide groups are planar due to 40% double-bond character in the C-N bond, and the *trans* form is strongly favoured (Sigel and Martin, 1982).

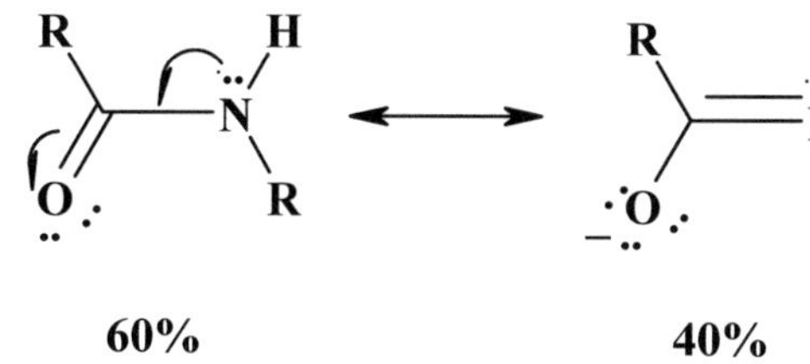

The presence of the peptide linkage decreases the basicity of the amino group and the acidity of the carboxylic group.

An amide group offers two potential binding atoms, the oxygen and nitrogen atoms. Throughout most of pH range, in the absence of metal ions, the amide group is neutral. It is being a very weak acid for proton loss from the trigonal nitrogen to give a negatively charged species. This very weak acidity makes quantitative equilibrium measurements very difficult. For acetamide it was reported that pK_a = 15.1, and the pK_a for glycylglycinate is 14.1.

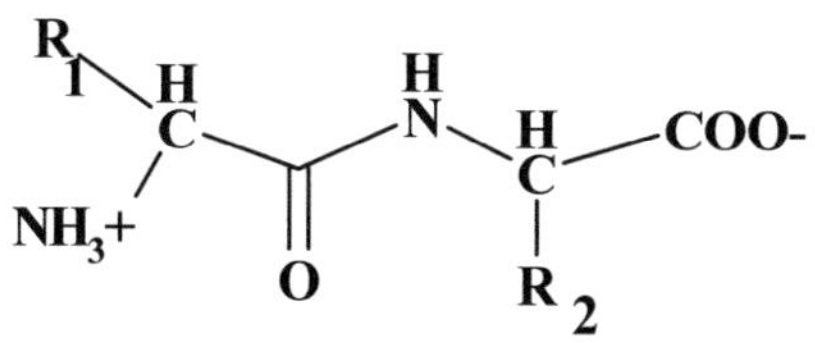

There are at least four donor groups in the dipeptide (Sigel and Martin, 1982) (amino-N, carboxylate-O, amide-N and carbonyl-O), all are capable of metal ion coordination. Because of the neutrality of the amide group, the terminal amino and carboxylate groups are the most effective binding sites for metal ions in peptides. The coordination of amide group can occur after deprotonation. Other groups may additionally be present in the side chains R_1 and R_2.

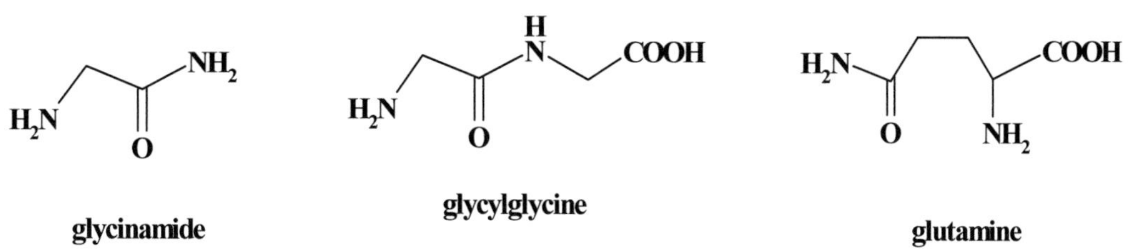

Peptides form complexes with stochiometric coefficients 110 and 11-1 according to Scheme (4). Peptides with Pd(II) are known for promoting ionization of the peptide linkage with pK_a value calculated by Eq.10.

It is found that, most metal ions form complexes with peptides by coordinating with carbonyl oxygen of the peptide group. Only certain specific metal ions are able to promote the deprotonation of the peptide nitrogen and become coordinated with it. Among these metals are Co(II), Ni(II), Cu(II) and Pd(II). The affinity for nitrogen bonding sites over oxygen bonding sites increases from cobalt to palladium corresponding to the stability of their deprotonated complexes. This is consistent with the idea that the deprotonated amide nitrogen is a "soft" base.

It is clear that, the stability of the complex with glycylglycine (log β_{110}) is generally higher than glycinamide as indicated in Tables 5 and 6 (Shoukry et al., 1999 ; El-Sherif, 2003 ; Lim, 1978 ; Mohamed and Shoukry 2001 ; El-Sherif et al., 2010 ; Shehata et al., 2008 ; Shehata et al., 2009; El-Sherif, 2006) due to the negative charge of glycylglycinate compared to neutral glycinamide. The electrostatic interaction between dipositively charged palladium complex and the negatively charged glycylglycine would result in a general free formation energy lowering.

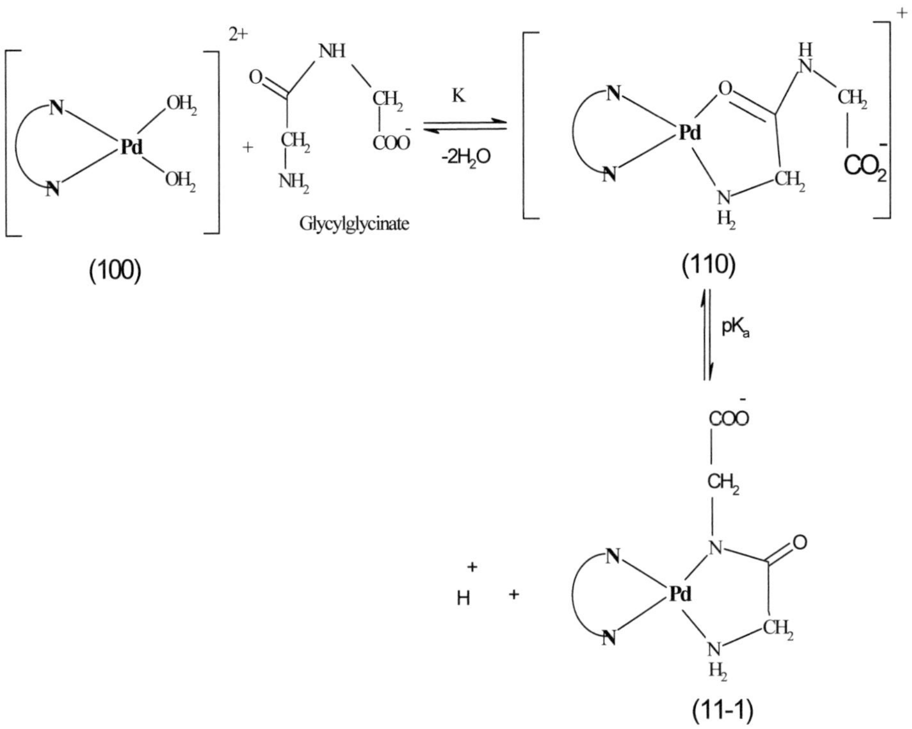

Scheme 4. Mode of coordination of [Pd(diamine)(H_2O)$_2$] with peptides

The pK_a value for glycinamide complex is lower than those for other peptides. This is due to the bulky substituent group on the other peptides that may hinder the structural changes when going from species 110 to 11-1 (peptide ionization). Glutamine complex has the highest stability, probably due to the presence of α-NH_2 that can coordinate first (glycine-like). The α-NH_2 of glutamine is more basic than those of other peptides resulting in more stable complexes compared to other peptides. The concentration distribution diagrams of Pd(diamine)-peptide complexes indicate that all peptides form the complex species (110) at low pH with the species (11-1) as the main product at higher pH.

System	p	q	r[b]	en[c]	$(Me)_2en$[d]	1,2-DAP[e]	1,3-DAP[f]	SMC[g]
Glycinamide	1	1	0	8.64	7.40	8.58	8.63	7.56
	1	1	-1	2.47	3.03	5.35	5.23	-3.38
Glutamine	1	1	0	10.76	10.73	11.02	9.24	8.73
	1	1	-1	9.03	5.82	2.12	-0.32	1.08
Glycylalanine	1	1	0	-	7.63	-	-	-
	1	1	-1		0.84			
Glycylglycine	1	1	0	9.60	7.75	9.41	8.01	7.73
	1	1	-1	3.76	2.69	6.02	4.24	2.61
Asparagine	1	1	0	10.46	12.31	12.79	-	8.92
	1	1	-1	6.46	4.71	6.38		2.08
Glycylleucine	1	1	0	-	8.36	7.73	-	7.69
	1	1	-1		0.01	3.30		1.98
Glycylvaline	1	1	0	-	-	-	-	7.66
	1	1	-1					2.00

[a]N-N = aliphatic diamine [b]p, q and r are stoichiometric coefficients corresponding to $[Pd(diamine)(H_2O)_2]$, ligand and H^+ respectively, [c]en = ethylenediamine, data taken from reference (Lim, 1978), [d]Me_2en = N,N'-dimethylethylenediamine, data taken from reference (Mohamed and Shoukry 2001), [e]1,2-DAP=1,2-diaminopropane, data taken from reference (Shoukry et al., 1999); [f]1,3-DAP=1,3-diaminopropane, data taken from reference (El-Sherif et al., 2010); [g]SMC=S-Methyl-L-cysteine, data taken from reference (Shehata et al., 2008).

Table 5. Formation constants (log β_{110}) of $[Pd(diamine)(H_2O)_2]$[a] with peptides at 25 ^0C and 0.1 mol dm^{-3} $NaNO_3$.

System	p	q	r[b]	Pic[c]	AEPY[d]	AMBI[e]
Glycinamide	1	1	0	9.30	8.01	8.63
	1	1	-1	5.73	4.16	5.23
Glutamine	1	1	0	10.02	9.11	9.24
	1	1	-1	0.36	0.47	-0.32
Glycylalanine	1	1	0	8.31	-	-
	1	1	-1	3.08		
Glycylglycine	1	1	0	8.29	8.20	8.01
	1	1	-1	4.37	3.56	4.24
Asparagine	1	1	0	10.06	9.42	8.81
	1	1	-1	2.65	1.90	-0.42
Glycylleucine	1	1	0	8.22	7.75	-
	1	1	-1	3.06	2.18	
Glycylvaline	1	1	0	7.73	-	-
	1	1	-1	2.39		
Leucylalanine	1	1	0	7.73	-	-
	1	1	-1	2.39		

[a]N-N = aromatic diamine, [b]p, q and r are stoichiometric coefficients corresponding to $[Pd(diamine)(H_2O)_2]$, ligand and H^+ respectively, [c]Pic = picolylamine, data taken from reference (El-Sherif, 2003), [d]AEPY = 2-aminoethylpyridine, data taken from reference (Shehata et al., 2009), [e]AMBI=2-aminomethylbenzimidazole, data taken from reference (El-Sherif, 2006). .

Table 6. Formation constants (log β_{110}) of $[Pd(diamine)(H_2O)_2]$[a] with peptides at 25 ^0C and 0.1 mol dm^{-3} $NaNO_3$.

Fitting the potentiometric data for the Pd(DAP)-glutathione system indicated the formation of complex species with the stoichiometric coefficients 110 and 111. Glutathione has various binding sites, namely oxygen atom of carboxylic group, nitrogen atom of amino group and sulphur atom of sulfhydryl group. The stability constant of the (110) complex (log β = 15.92) is higher than the ones of α-amino acids (log $\beta_{[Pd(DAP)(glycine)]}$ = 11.12). This indicates that glutathione interacts with Pd(II) ion by the amino and deprotonated SH groups and not by the amino and caboxylate group like simple α-amino acids. This is in good agreement with the fact that Pd(II) has a high affinity for S-donor ligands. The concentration distribution diagram of [Pd(DAP)(glutathione)] given in Fig. 3, shows the formation of the protonated complex 111 with a formation degree of 81% at pH 3.1. At pH 6, the complex species (110) predominates with a concentration of 99 % i.e. the reaction of $[Pd(DAP)]^{2+}$ goes to completion in the physiological pH range. This may suggest that GSH will compete with DNA for the reaction with the Pd(II) complex.

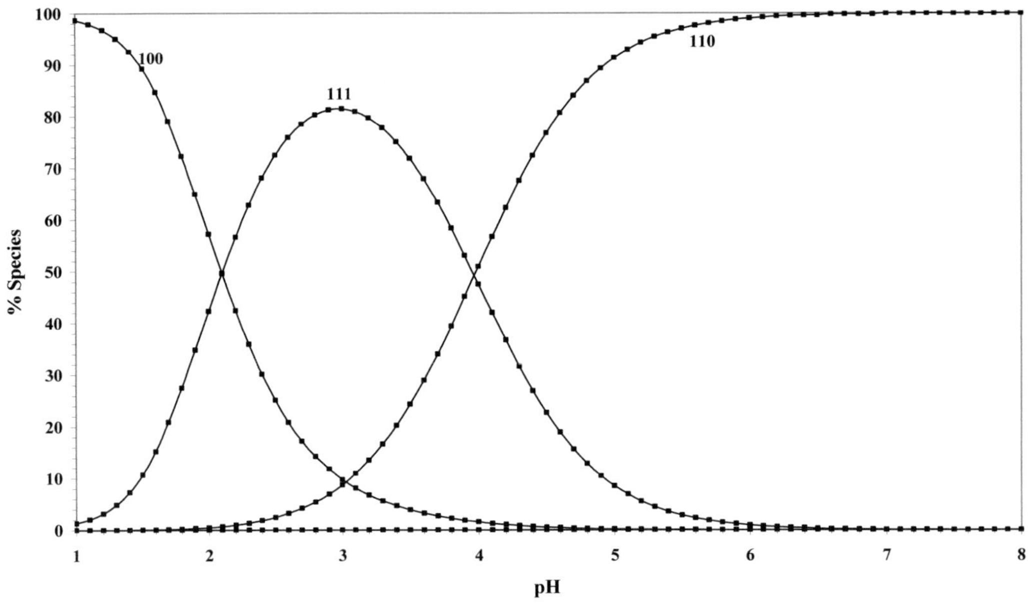

Fig. 3. Concentration distribution of various species as a function of pH in the Pd(DAP)-Glutathione system at concentrations of 1.25×10^{-3} mol-dm^{-3} for $Pd(DAP)^{2+}$ and glutathione, I = 0.1 mol-dm^{-3} ($NaNO_3$) and T = 25 ± 0.1 ^{0}C).

3.3 Interactions of $[Pd(diamine)(H_2O)_2]$ with DNA constituents

3.3.1 Nucleosides, nucleotides and nucleic acid

Nucleosides are composed of a purine or pyrimidine base attached to the sugar ribose via the N-9 and C-1 atoms, respectively. In nucleotides, the sugar is linked to a phosphate group.

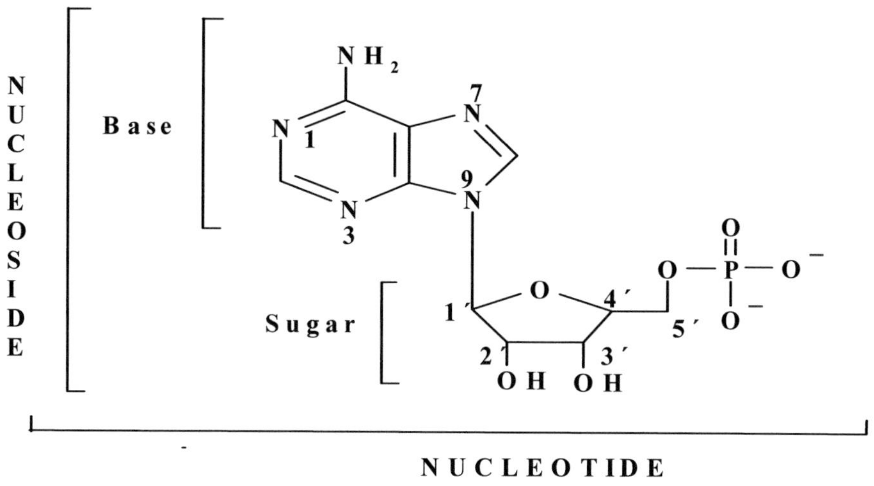

Adenosine monophosphate

The nucleic acids are polymers built up from nucleotides via phosphodiester bond formation between the 3′-OH group of one nucleotide and the 5′-OH group of the adjacent nucleotide. The sequence of the nucleotides is extremely important as it constitutes the genetic code in DNA. Different nucleotides vary in the nature of the purine and pyrimidine bases (Hay, 1985).

3.3.2 Ternary complexes involving DNA constituents and [Pd(diamine)(H_2O)$_2$]

The accepted models for DNA complex formation with [Pd(diamine)(H_2O)$_2$]$^{2+}$ are consistent with the formation of 1:1 and 1:2 complexes, as shown in Tables 7 and 8 (Shoukry et al.,1999; El-Sherif et al., 2003; Lim, 1978; Mohamed and Shoukry, 2001; El-Sherif, et al., 2010; Shehata, et al., 2008); Shehata, et al., 2009; El-Sherif, 2006). Generally, from Table 8, the complexes with DNA constituents are more stable (higher log β values) with bipyridine than with all other amine ligands. They are probably stabilized by intramolecular stacking between the bipyridine aromatic ring and the purine rings (Fisher and Sigel, 1980). The stability of the corresponding complexes with picolylamine has intermediate log β values, probably because in this case there is only one pyridine ring.

The pyrimidines, uracil and thymine have only basic nitrogen donor atoms (N3-C4O group).

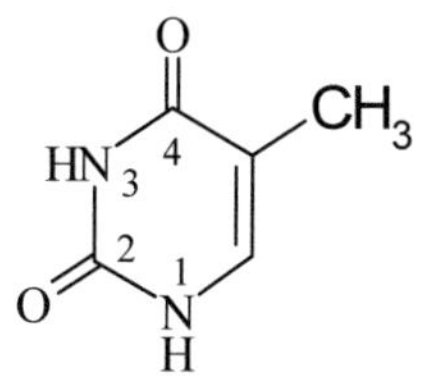

Thymine

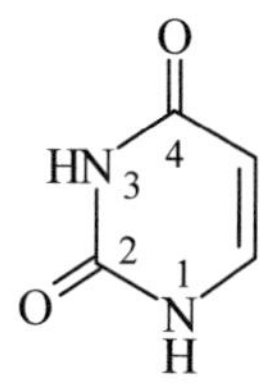

Uracil

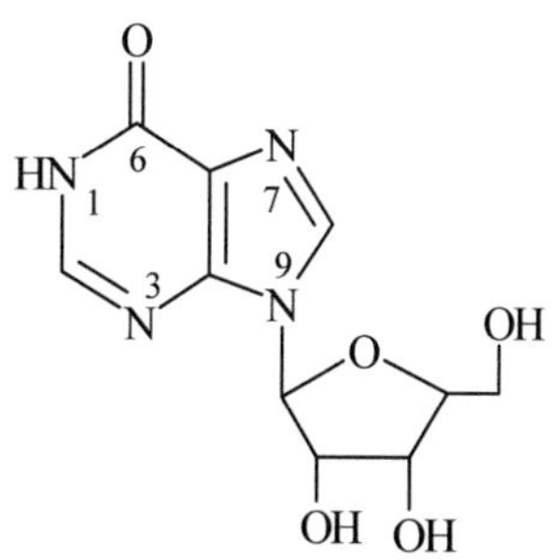

Inosine

System	p	q	r[b]	en[c]	$(Me)_2en$[d]	1,2-DAP[e]	1,3-DAP[f]	SMC[g]
Uracil	1	1	0	8.35	8.35	8.74	8.61	8.18
	1	2	0	14.88	14.88	15.43	14.76	12.40
Uridine	1	1	0	8.70	8.70	-	-	8.10
	1	2	0	14.37	14.37			12.21
Thymine	1	1	0	-	8.56	8.90	9.02	8.63
	1	2	0		15.14	15.80	15.65	13.28
Thymidine	1	1	0	8.84	8.75	8.92	-	9.27
	1	2	0	14.69	14.53	14.84		14.10
Cytosine	1	1	0	-	-	-	-	5.73
	1	2	0					8.54
Cytidine	1	1	0	-	-	-	-	4.93
	1	2	0					8.44
Inosine	1	1	0	6.83	8.03	-	7.62	6.81
	1	1	1	-	12.40		9.69	10.16
	1	2	0	11.26	12.74			10.84
UMP	1	1	0	-	-	-	-	8.35
	1	1	1					13.62
	1	2	0					14.17
IMP	1	1	0	8.76	8.76	-	-	7.25
	1	1	1	15.26	15.26			10.60
	1	1	2	18.50	18.50			-
	1	2	0	12.31	12.31			10.51
	1	2	1		21.69			-
	1	2	2		28.45			-
GMP	1	1	0	-	-	-	-	8.20
	1	1	1					11.35
	1	2	0					14.52
Adenine	1	1	0	-	12.15	11.14	-	9.14
	1	1	1		-			11.96
	1	2	0					12.57
CMP	1	1	0	-	-	-	-	5.34
	1	1	1					7.67
	1	2	0					11.59
TMP	1	1	0		-	-	-	8.41
	1	1	1					13.53
	1	2	0					13.84

[a]N-N = aliphatic diamine [b]p, q and r are stoichiometric coefficients corresponding to $[Pd(diamine)(H_2O)_2]$, ligand and H^+ respectively, [c]en = ethylenediamine, data taken from reference (Lim, 1978), [d]Me_2en = N,N′-dimethylethylenediamine, data taken from reference (Mohamed and Shoukry 2001), [e]1,2-DAP=1,2-diaminopropane, data taken from reference (Shoukry et al., 1999); [f]1,3-DAP=1,3-diaminopropane, data taken from reference (El-Sherif, et al., 2010); [g]SMC=S-Methyl-L-cysteine, data taken from reference (Shehata et al., 2008).

Table 7. Formation constants (log β_{110}) of $[Pd(diamine)(H_2O)_2]^a$ with DNA constituents at 25 ^{0}C and 0.1 mol dm^{-3} $NaNO_3$.

System	p	q	r[b]	Pic[c]	AEPY[d]	BPY[e]	AMBI[f]
Uracil	1	1	0	9.17	8.03	10.96	9.08
	1	2	0	15.98	14.47	17.17	12.98
	1	1	1		-	13.50	
	1	2	1		-	22.15	
Uridine	1	1	0	9.00	-	9.71	9.43
	1	2	0	14.96		16.88	13.11
	1	1	1			13.29	
	1	2	1			22.65	
Thymine	1	1	0	8.96	-	-	8.89
	1	2	0	15.62			12.94
Thymidine	1	1	0	9.17	8.25	-	9.12
	1	2	0	15.21	13.72		12.93
Cytosine	1	1	0	-	5.98	-	-
	1	2	0		8.91		
	1	1	1		10.86		
Adenosine	1	1	0	-	2.84		
	1	2	0		5.25		
Guanosine	1	1	0	-	10.48		
	1	2	0		19.03		
Adenine	1	1	0	-	9.47	11.95	-
	1	2	0		14.05	16.59	
	1	1	1		18.56	15.97	
	1	2	1		-	25.76	
	1	2	2		-	30.25	
Inosine	1	1	0	-	7.78	9.71	10.02
	1	2	0		11.64	14.89	-
	1	1	1		11.89	12.55	12.06
	1	2	1		-	20.11	-
	1	2	2		-	25.37	-
	1	1	2		-	-	14.40
IMP	1	1	0	10.42	9.18	10.17	10.05
	1	2	0	-	16.35	14.80	-
	1	1	1	16.46	13.93	16.65	15.81
	1	2	1	-	-	21.49	-
	1	2	2	-	-	28.50	-
	1	1	2	18.73	-	20.98	17.79
GMP	1	1	0	10.83	9.23	-	10.40
	1	2	0	-	13.44		-
	1	1	1	17.35	15.16		16.57
	1	2	1	-	-		-
	1	2	2	-	-		-
	1	1	2	21.01	-		19.78
CMP	1	1	0	-	5.89	11.95	-
	1	2	0		8.57	16.59	
	1	1	1		10.86	15.97	
	1	2	1		-	25.76	
	1	2	2		-	30.25	

[a]N-N = aromatic diamine, [b]p, q and r are stoichiometric coefficients corresponding to [Pd(diamine)(H_2O)$_2$], ligand and H^+ respectively, [c]Pic = picolylamine, data taken from reference (El-Sherif, 2003), [d]AEPY = 2-aminoethylpyridine, data taken from reference (Shehata et al., 2009), [e]BPY = 2,2′-bipyridyl, data taken from reference (Shehata, 2001), [e]AMBI=2-aminomethylbenzimidazole, data taken from reference (El-Sherif, 2006)

Table 8. Formation constants (log β_{110}) of [Pd(diamine)(H_2O)$_2$][a] with DNA constituents at 25 ^{0}C and 0.1 mol dm^{-3} $NaNO_3$.

The thymine complex is more stable than the uracil one, most probably owing to the high basicity of the N3 group of thymine resulting from the extra electron donating methyl group. As a result of the high pK_a values of pyrimidines ($pK_a \approx 9$) and the fact that they are monodentates, the complexes are formed only above pH 6, supporting the view that the negatively charged nitrogen donors of pyrimidine bases are important binding sites in the neutral and slightly basic pH ranges. The purines like inosine have two metal ion binding centres N1 and N7 nitrogens. Inosine can be protonated at N7 forming a (N1H-N7H) monocation. The pK_a of N1H is 8.43 (El-Sherif, 2006) and the pK_a of N7H is 1.2 (Martin, 1985). It was reported that, in the acidic pH range, N1 remained protonated, while the metal ion is coordinated to N7 i.e. these N-donors are pH dependent binding sites and there is a gradual change from N7- binding to N1-binding with increase of pH (Maskos, 1985). The results showed that inosine form the complexes 110 and 111. The speciation diagrams of Pd(diamine)-inosine complexes indicated that the species 111 is formed in acidic pH range and it corresponds to the N7 coordinated complex, while N1 nitrogen is in protonated form. Inosine is slightly more acidic than the pyrimidine bases, a property which can be related to the existence of a higher number of resonance forms for the inosine anion. Based on the existing data, uracil and thymine ligate in the deprotonated form through the N3 atom.

Several solid Pd(II) complexes of guanosine and inosine have suggested to exhibit N7-O6 chelation (Pneumatikakis, 1984 ; Pneumatikakis et al., 1988). Also, according to *ab initio* SCF calculations, N7-O6 chelation is the energetically favored bonding mode (Del Bene, 1984) ; Anwader et al., 1987).

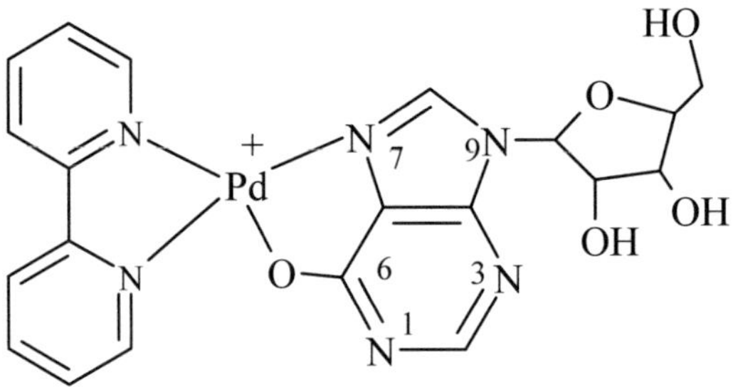

The IR spectrum of $[Pd(BPY)(Inosine)]NO_3$ showed a shift of the ν(C=O) stretching vibration from 1700 cm^{-1} and 1676 cm^{-1} in the free inosine (which corresponds to keto-enol forms) to 1639 in the complex (Shehata, 2001). This clearly indicates the involvement of C=O in coordination. At higher pH, the N1H is deprotonated and the negative charge on N1 resonates with C=O, increasing the negative charge on the oxygen atom. This is in consistent with the large acidification of the N1H.

Inosine-5'-monophosphate (5'-IMP) forms a stronger complex with $[Pd(diamine)(H_2O)_2]$ than does inosine. The extra stabilization can be attributed to the triply negatively charged 5'-IMP^{3-} ion. The purines, inosine-5′-monophosphate and guanosine-5′-monophosphate form 110, 111 and 112 complexes. The protonated species are easily detected with aromatic amine (BPY, Pic and AMBI) rather than with aliphatic amines (en, Me_2en, 1,2-DAP and 1,3-DAP). This may be interpreted on the basis that the protonated species are stabilized through the back bonding to the π–system of aromatic rings, which makes more stable complexes. For Pd(AMBI)-complexes, the pK_a values of the protonated species of the IMP complex (112) are 1.98 (log β_{112} - log β_{111}) and 5.76 (log β_{111} - log β_{110}). The corresponding values for GMP are 3.21 and 6.17. The former pK_a value for IMP and GMP corresponds to the N1H group while the second is assignable to the -$PO_2(OH)$ group. The N1H groups were acidified upon complex formation by 7.23 (9.21-1.98) and 6.07 (9.28-3.21) pK units for IMP and GMP, respectively. Acidification of the N1H group upon complex formation is consistent with previous reports for IMP and GMP complexes (Sigel et al. 1994). In the fully protonated species (112), the two protons bound to N1 and the phosphate groups, exist at pH ~ 3 or lower. In the (111) complex species, which reaches its maximum concentration of 88 % at pH ~ 4.8 (Fig. 4), the single proton binds to phosphate. Therefore, monoprotonated species (111) is an N1-coordinated. The stability constant difference between the (112) and (111) complexes is 3.21, due to the pK_a of the N1 deprotonation process. The phosphate group was not acidified upon complex formation since it is too far from the coordination center. A proposed coordination process of $Pd(AMBI)^{2+}$ with 5'-GMP is reported in Scheme 5.

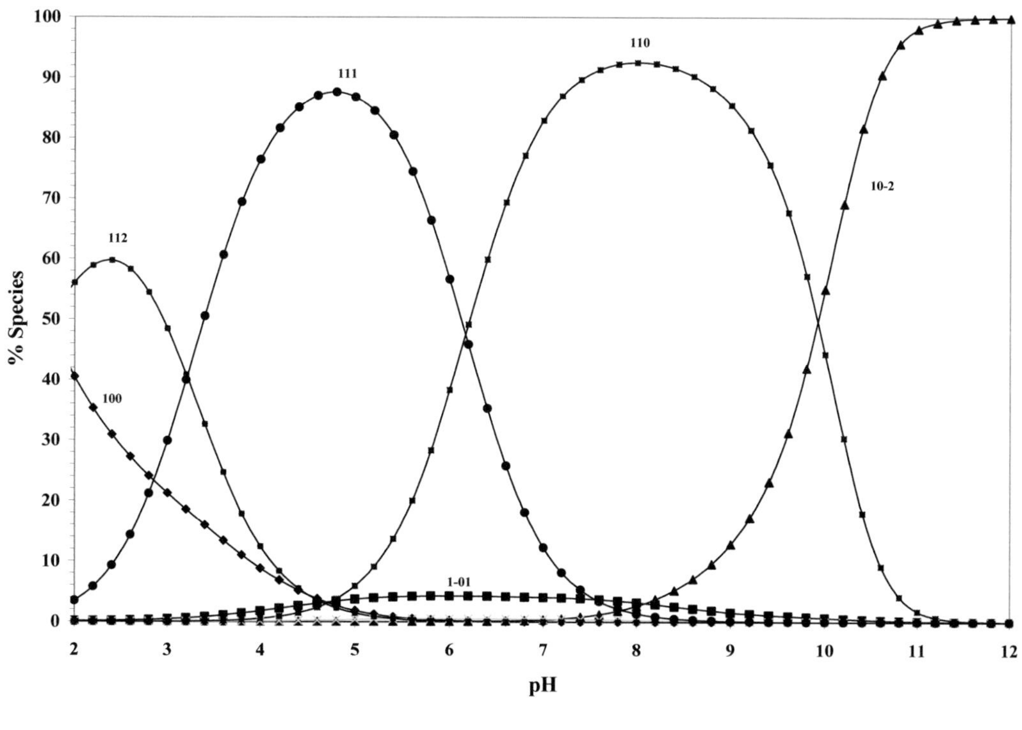

Fig. 4. Concentration distribution of various species as a function of pH in the Pd(AMBI)-5′-GMP system at concentrations of $1.25x10^{-3}$ mol-dm^{-3} for $Pd(AMBI)^{2+}$ and 5′-GMP, I = 0.1 mol-dm^{-3} ($NaNO_3$) and T = 25 ± 0.1 ^{0}C).

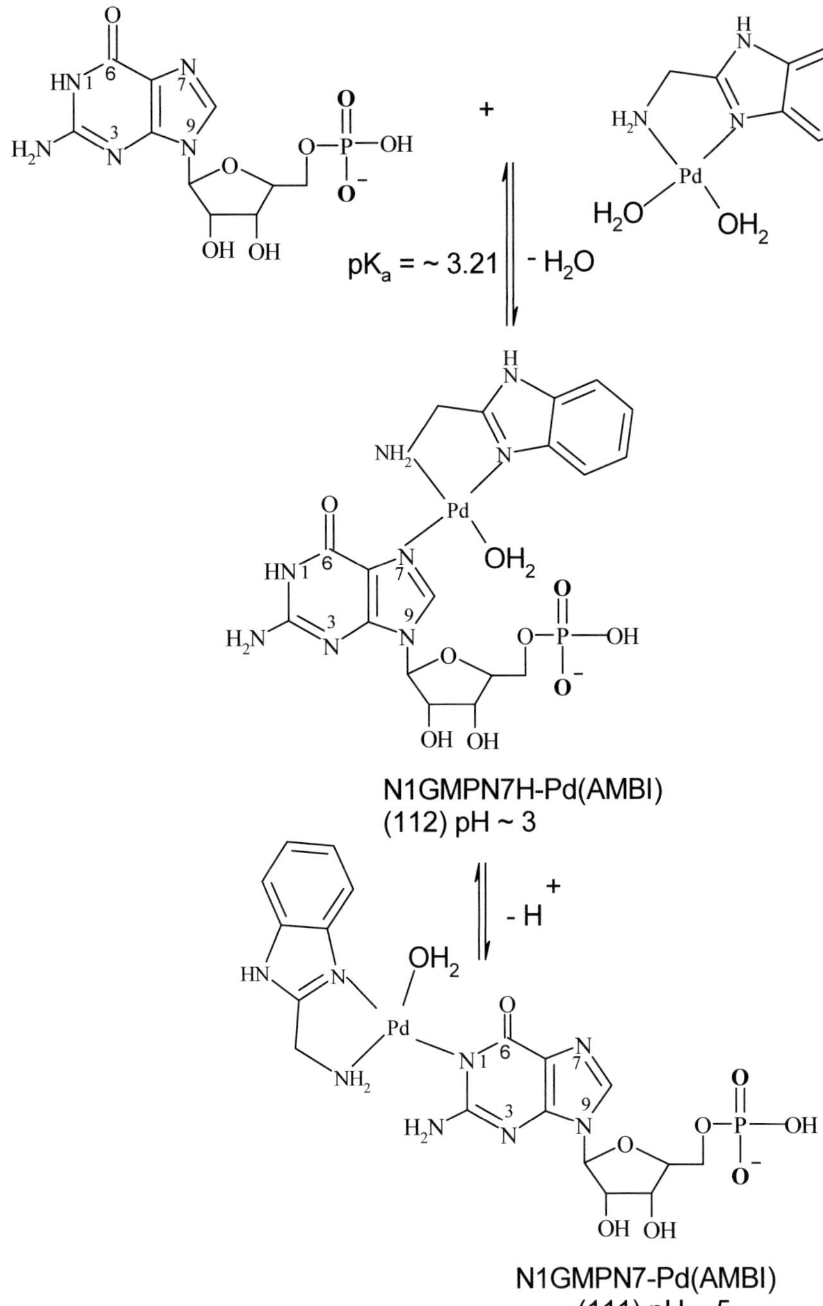

Scheme 5. Proposed coordination process of $Pd(AMBI)^{2+}$ with 5'-GMP

The IMP and GMP complexes are more stable than those of the pyrimidines. The extra stabilization can be explained on the basis of different columbic forces operating between the ions resulting from the negatively charged phosphate group. Hydrogen bonding between the phosphate and the exocyclic amine is also thought to contribute to the higher stability of the nucleotides over that of the nucleosides (Reedik, 1992).

3.3.3 Comparison of thermodynamic and kinetic data

It is interesting to compare the the stability constants obtained from earlier kinetic results of Pd(diamine) with DNA and those estimated from potentiometric measurements. Much of the kinetic work was done in an acidic pH range in order to simplify the speciation of the system. Under these conditions, $Pd(Pic)^{2+}$ for example, binds to IMP through the N7 site, leaving the N1 site and the phosphate groups protonated. The stability constant (K) of the species formed under this condition is calculated using Eq. 12.

$$\log K = \log \beta_{112} - \log \beta_{012} \qquad (12)$$

The log K value was found to be 3.52. This is comparable with the value obtained from the kinetic investigation (log K = 2.09) (Rau et al., 1997). The difference can be related to different experimental conditions (the kinetic study was performed at 10 ^{0}C with an ionic strength of 0.5 M), techniques employed and the acidity range selected for the kinetic measurements, where more than one Pd^{II} complex and/or IMP acid-base forms may contribute to the kinetic result.

It was previously shown that N-donor ligands such as DNA constituents have an affinity for $[Pd(AEPY)(H_2O)_2]^{2+}$, which may have important biological implications. However, the preference of Pd(II) to coordinate to S-donor ligands was demonstrated as shown in Tables 3 & 4. These results suggest that Pd(II)-N adducts can easily be converted into Pd-S adducts. Consequently, the equilibrium constant for such conversion is of biological significance. If we consider inosine as a typical DNA constituent (presented by HL) and cysteine as a typical thiol ligand (presented by H_2B), the equilibria involved in the complex-formation and displacement reactions are:

$$HL \rightleftharpoons H^+ + L^-$$

$$\underset{(100)}{[Pd(AEPY)]^{2+}} + L^- \rightleftharpoons \underset{(110)}{[Pd(AEPY)L]^+} \qquad (13a)$$

$$\beta_{110}^{[Pd(AEPY)L]+} = [Pd(DAP)L]^+ / [Pd(AEPY)]^{2+} [L^-] \qquad (13b)$$

$$H_2B \rightleftharpoons 2H^+ + B^{2-}$$

$$\underset{(100)}{[Pd(AEPY)]^{2+}} + B^{2-} \rightleftharpoons \underset{(110)}{[Pd(AEPY)B]} \qquad (14a)$$

$$\beta_{110}^{[Pd(AEPY)B]} = [Pd(AEPY)B] / [Pd(AEPY)]^{2+} [B^{2-}] \qquad (14b)$$

$$[Pd(AEPY)L]^+ + B^{2-} \underset{}{\overset{K_{eq}}{\rightleftharpoons}} [Pd(AEPY)B] + L^- \qquad (15)$$

The equilibrium constant for the displacement reaction given in equation (15) is given by:

$$K_{eq} = [Pd(AEPY)B]\,[L^-] \,/\, [Pd(AEPY)L]^+[B^{2-}] \qquad (16)$$

Substitution from eq. (13b) and (14b) in eq. (16) results in :

$$K_{eq} = \beta_{110}{}^{[Pd(AEPY)B]} / \beta_{110}{}^{[Pd(AEPY)L]+} \qquad (17)$$

The 100 species, $[Pd(AEPY)(H_2O)_2]^{2+}$, is represented in the above equations as $[Pd(AEPY)]^{2+}$ for simplicity reasons. $\log\beta_{110}$ values for $[Pd(AEPY)(L)]^+$ and [Pd(AEPY)B] complexes taken from Tables 4 and 8 amount to 7.78 and 15.11, respectively, and by substitution in equation (17) it was found that log K_{eq} = 7.33. In the same way the equilibrium constants for the displacement of coordinated inosine by glycine and S-methylcysteine are log K_{eq} = 2.55 and 1.38, respectively. These values clearly indicate how sulfhydryl ligands such as cysteine and by analogy glutathione are effective in displacing the DNA constituent, i.e., the main target in tumour chemotherapy. Chelated cyclobutanedicarboxylate (log K_{eq} = 7.11) may undergo displacement reaction with inosine. Log K_{eq} for such a reaction was calculated as described above and amounts to 0.68. The low value of the equilibrium constant for reaction is of biological significance since it is in line with the finding that carboplatin interacts with DNA through ring opening of chelated CBDCA and not through displacement of CBDCA.

3.4 Ternary complexes involving CBDCA

Cyclobutane-1,1-dicarboxylic acid (H_2CBDCA) is a diprotic acid with pK_{a1} and pK_{a2} of 2.75 and 5.48, respectively at 25 ^{0}C and 0.1M ionic strength (El-Sherif, et al., 2010 ; Shehata, et al., 2009). The acid-base equilibria are schematized as follows:

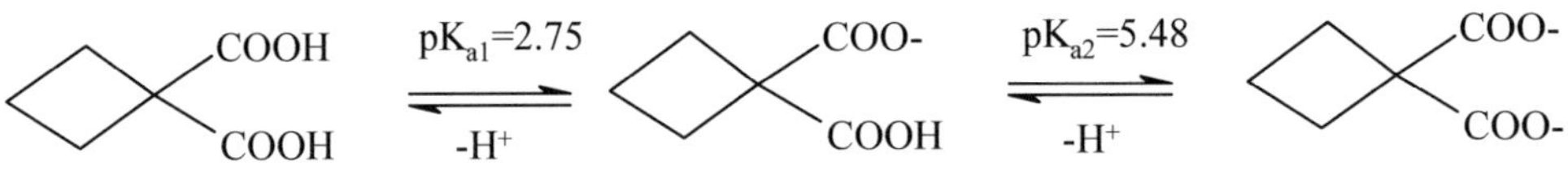

3.4.1 Ternary complexes involving CBDCA and $[Pd(diamine)(H_2O)_2]$

The potentiometric data for H_2CBDCA complex-formation with $[Pd(diamine)(H_2O)_2]^{2+}$ were fitted considering the formation of 110 and the monoprotonated complex species 111 (Table 9) (Shoukry et al., 1999; El-Sherif et al., 2003 ; Shehata, 2001; El-Sherif et al., 2010; El-Sherif, 2006) according to Scheme (6).

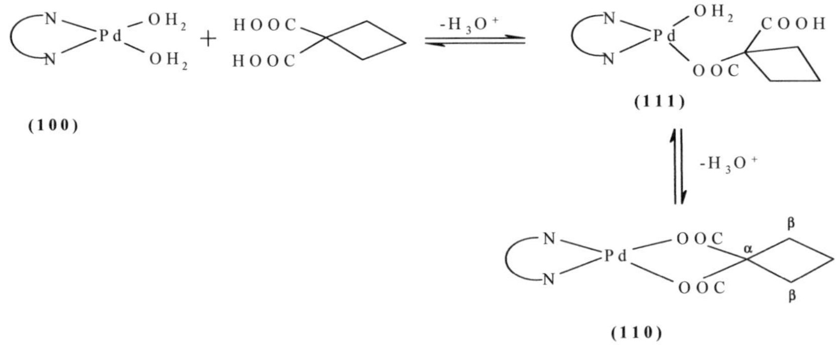

Scheme 6. Coordination mode of CBDCA with $[Pd(diamine)(H_2O)_2]$

Complex	log β_{110}	log β_{111}	Reference
1,2-DAP[a]	6.05	-	(Shoukry et al., 1999)
1,3-DAP[b]	7.16	-	(El-Sherif et al., 2010)
Pic[a]	8.09	10.91	(El-Sherif et al., 2003)
AMBI[a]	7.55	10.53	(El-Sherif, 2006)
BPY[a]	8.47	11.37	(Shehata, 2001)

[a]1,2-dap,1,3-DAP, Pic, AMBI and BPY are 1,2-diaminopropane, 1,3-diaminopropane Picolylamine, 2-aminomethylbenzimidazole, and 2,2'-bipyridyl respectively at 25 °C and I = 0.1 M.

Table 9. Stability constants of [Pd(diamine)(CBDCA)].

The stability constants of the CBDCA complex with $[Pd(aromaticdiamine)(H_2O)_2]^{2+}$ is higher than those for $[Pd(aliphaticdiamine)(H_2O)_2]^{2+}$. Moreover, the protonated species were not observed in similar palladium complexes of CBDCA and aliphatic amines (Shoukry et al., 1999; El-Sherif et al., 2010) using potentiometric technique. The higher stability of CBDCA complexes with $[Pd(aromaticdiamine)(H_2O)_2]$ and the stabilization of the protonated species may be attributed to the π-acceptor properties of the pyridine rings. The pK_a of the protonated species of Pd(BPY) with CBDCA is 2.92; lower value than the one measured for $HCBDCA^-$, indicating acidification upon first chelation to Pd through one carboxylate group by 2.56 pK units (5.48-2.92). The pK_a value of this protonated species was estimated previously from UV-Vis. measurements to be ca. 2.5 at 25 °C and 0.1 M ionic strength (Shoukry et al., 1998). The involvement of the carboxylic oxygen in coordination is confirmed by the shift of the asymmetric and symmetric stretching frequencies of COO^- to lower and higher frequencies, respectively. υ_{as} and υ_s, which can be found at 1706 and 1293 cm^{-1} in H_2CBDCA are shifted to 1645 and 1354 cm^{-1} in the [Pd(BPY)(CBDCA)] complex. This corresponds to a unidentate chelation mode (Nakamoto, 1997).

3.4.2 Ring-opening of [Pd(DAP)(CBDCA)] and the formation of [Pd(DAP)(CBDCA-O)(DNA)]

The potentiometric data for the system consisting of $[Pd(diamine)(H_2O)_2]^{2+}$, CBDCA and DNA constituents were fitted assuming different models. The accepted model for the investigated DNA constituents is consistent with the formation of the 1110, 1111 and 1112 species (Table 10) (El-Sherif et al., 2003; Shehata, 2001; Mohamed and Shoukry, 2001). The results were further verified by comparing the experimental potentiometric data with the theoretically calculated curve. This supports the formation of the quaternary complex. It is interesting to notice that the quaternary complex of inosine is more stable than those of pyrimidines. This may be explained on the premise that the cyclobutane ring forms a close hydrophobic contact with the purine ring of inosine. Such contacts may contribute to the stabilization of the quaternary complexes. These studies bring to the conclusion that CBDCA is attached through one carboxylate oxygen while 5′-GMP is attached through N7 of the purine base. The same finding was obtained from an NMR investigation of the ring opening reaction of carboplatin with phosphate, chloride, and 5′-guanosine monophosphate (5′-GMP) in aqueous solution at 310 K using ^1H, ^{15}N and ^{31}P NMR spectroscopy (Frey et al., 1993). In each case a ring-opened species containing monodentate CBDCA was detected during reaction development. A structure of cis-$[Pt(NH_3)_2(CBDCA\text{-}O)(5'\text{-}GMP)]$ is proposed, taking into account the equivalence of all six cyclobutane ring protons. There is a close hydrophobic contact between the cyclobutane ring of monodentate CBDCA and the purine ring of coordinated 5´-GMP. The reaction of carboplatin with 5´-GMP (k_{obs} 4.1 × 10^{-6} s^{-1}) was faster than that with phosphate (k_{obs} 4.3 × 10^{-7} s^{-1}) and chloride (k_{obs} 1.2 × 10^{-6} s^{-1}), or water alone (< 5 × 10^{-9} s^{-1}), suggesting that direct attack of nucleotides on carboplatin may be importance crucial step in the mechanism of action for this drug. Estimation of the concentration distribution of the various species in solution provides a useful picture of metal ion binding. To illustrate the main features observed in the species distribution plots in these systems, the speciation diagram obtained for the Pd(Pic)-CBDCA-IMP system as a representative example of [Pd(Pic)(CBDCA-O)(DNA)] is shown in Fig. 5. The Pd(Pic)-CBDCA species (1100) predominates at pH = 4.3 with maximum concentration of 73%. The Pd(Pic)-IMP species (1010) reaches the maximum concentration of 16 % at pH = 7.4. The quaternary species Pd(Pic)-CBDCA-IMP (1110) attains a maximum of 80 % in the pH range 7.6-9. This reveals that in the physiological pH range the ring opening of chelated CBDCA by DNA is quite feasible.

System	l	P	q	r[a]	$(Me)_2en$ [b]	Pic[c]	BPY[d]
Uracil	1	1	1	0	16.18	14.18	18.31
	1	1	1	1	-	-	24.76
	1	1	1	2	-	-	27.05
Uridine	1	1	1	0	15.17	14.18	20.14
	1	1	1	1	-	-	26.74
	1	1	1	2	-	-	28.62
Thymine	1	1	1	0	15.71	14.34	-
	1	1	1	1	-	-	
	1	1	1	2	-	-	
Thymidine	1	1	1	0	16.26	-	-
	1	1	1	1			
	1	1	1	2			
Adenine	1	1	1	0	-	-	17.06
	1	1	1	1			23.24
	1	1	1	2			27.08
Inosine	1	1	1	0	12.29	-	16.64
	1	1	1	1	17.72		22.77
	1	1	1	2	-		25.58
GMP	1	1	1	0	-	15.07	-
	1	1	1	1		21.58	
	1	1	1	2		-	
IMP	1	1	1	0	-	14.65	16.00
	1	1	1	1		20.86	22.42
	1	1	1	2		-	27.92
	1	1	1	3		-	31.49

[a] l, p, q and r are the stoichiometric coefficients corresponding to Pd(diamine)(H2O)2], cyclobutane-1,1'-dicarboxylate, DNA and H+, respectively. [b]Me_2en = N,N'-dimethylethylenediamine, data taken from reference (Mohamed and Shoukry, 2001), [c]Pic = picolylamine, data taken from reference (El-Sherif et al., 2003), [d]BPY = 2,2'-bipyridyl, data taken from reference (Shehata, 2001).

Table 10. Formation constants (log β_{1110}) for mixed ligand complexes of $[Pd(diamine)(H_2O)_2]$ with cyclobutanedicarboxylic acid and some DNA units at 25 ^0C and 0.1M ionic strength.

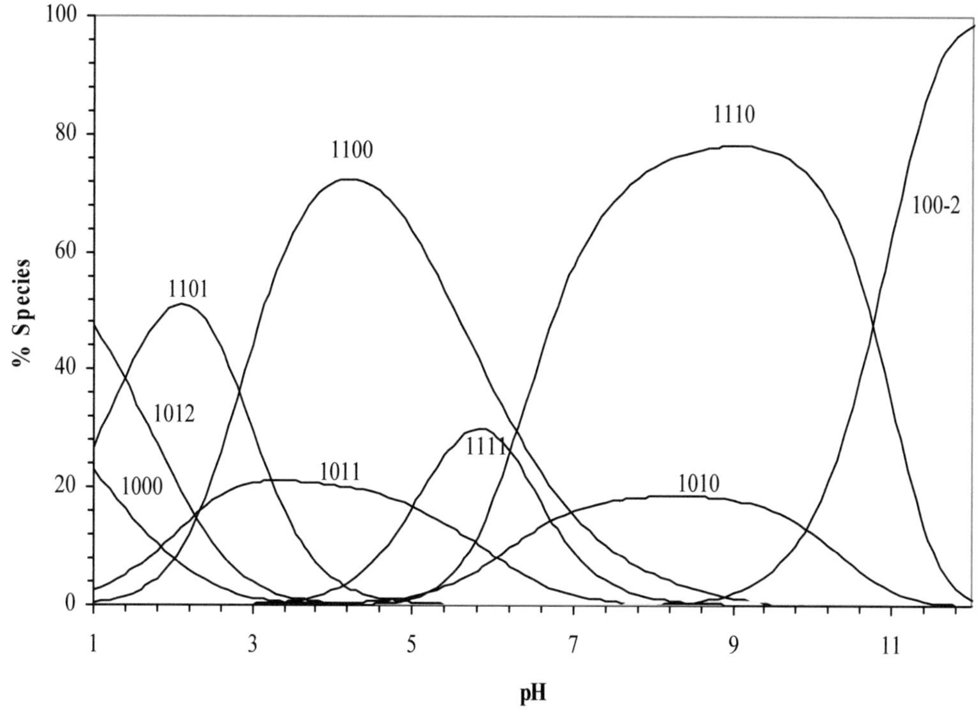

Fig. 5. Concentration distribution of various species as a function of pH in the Pd(Pic)-CBDCA-IMP system at concentrations of 1.25x10^{-3} mol-dm^{-3} for $Pd(Pic)^{2+}$; CBDCA and IMP, I = 0.1 mol-dm^{-3} ($NaNO_3$) and T = 25 ± 0.1 ^{0}C).

4. Effect of solvent on the stability constants

Traditionally, water has been considered as the solvent that best represents biological conditions. Although this is a general assumption, a lower polarity has been detected in some biochemical micro-environments, such as active sites of enzymes and side chains in proteins (Rees, 1980 ; Rogersa et al., 1985; Akerlof and Short, 1953). It was suggested that these properties approximately correspond to those (or can be simulated by those) existing in the water/dioxane mixtures. Consequently, a study of the Pd(Pic)-CBDCA and Pd(1,3-DAP)-CBDCA complex formation, taken as a typical example for [Pd(aliphaticdiamine)CBDCA] and [Pd(aromaticdiamine)CBDCA] respectively, in dioxane-water solutions of different compositions could be of biological significance. In order to characterize the formation equilibria of the Pd(diamine)-CBDCA complex in dioxane-water solutions, all other equilibria involved, namely acid-base equilibria of CBDCA and $[Pd(diamine)(H_2O)_2]^{2+}$, have to be studied in the same solvent. The equilibrium constants are reported in Table 11 (El-Sherif et al., 2003, 2010). The hydrolysis of $Pd(diamine)^{2+}$ complex in dioxane-water solution leads to the formation of mono- and dihydroxy species. The dihydroxo bridged dimer was not detected. The pK_a values of CBDCA and those of the coordinated water molecules in $[Pd(diamine)(H_2O)_2]^{2+}$ increase linearly with increasing of dioxane concentration. This may be correlated with the ability of a relatively low dielectric solvent to increase the electrostatic attraction between the proton and the ligand anion in case of CBDCA and between a proton and the hydrolysed form of Pd(II) species. The variation in the stability constant of the $[Pd(diamine)(H_2O)_2]^{2+}$ complex with CBDCA as a function of solvent composition, is shown in Fig. 6. The stability constant for the Pd(diamine)-CBDCA complex increases linearly with increasing dioxane concentration. This is explained in terms of complex formation involving oppositely charged ions as in the Pd(diamine)-CBDCA complex, which is favoured by the low dielectric constant of the medium, i.e. with increasing dioxane concentration. The results show that the CBDCA complex with $Pd(diamine)^{2+}$ will be more favoured in biological environments of lower dielectric constant.

% Dioxane	p	q	r[a]	Pic[b]	1,3-DAP[c]
12.5	1	1	0	8.93	8.13
25	1	1	0	9.36	8.57
37.5	1	1	0	9.89	8.98
50	1	1	0	10.58	9.48
62.5	1	1	0	10.99	10.13

[a]p, q and r are stoichiometric coefficients corresponding to $[Pd(diamine)(H_2O)_2]$, ligand and H^+ respectively, [b]Pic = picolylamine, data taken from reference (El-Sherif et al., 2003), [c]1,3-DAP = 1,3-diaminopropane, data taken from reference (El-Sherif et al., 2010).

Table 11. Effect of dioxane on the formation constant (log β_{110}) of $[Pd(diamine)(H_2O)_2]$ with CBDCA at 25 ^{0}C and 0.1 mol dm^{-3} $NaNO_3$.

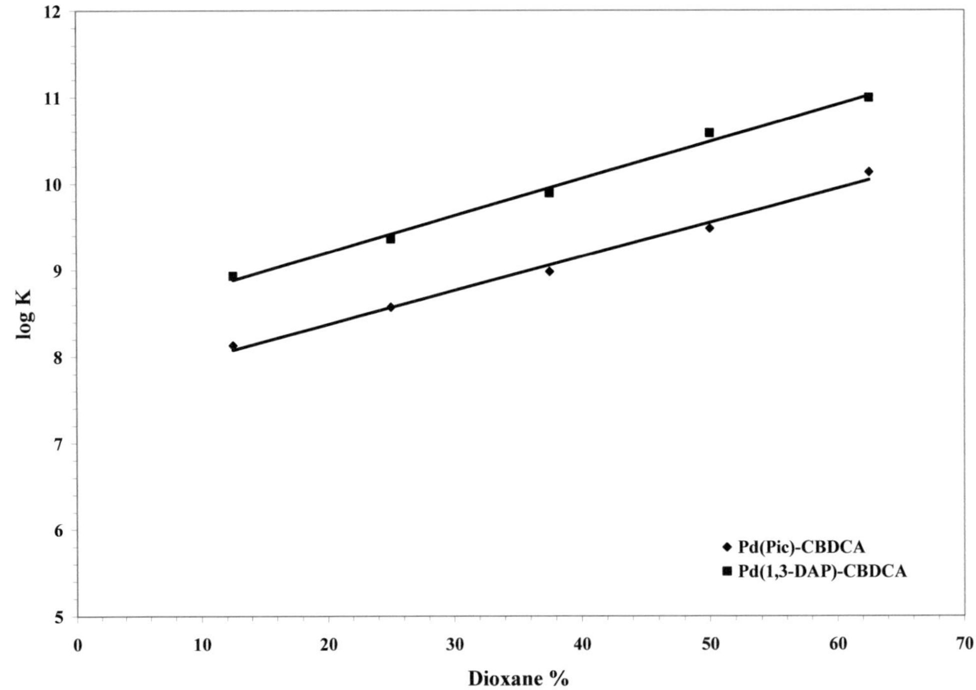

Fig. 6. Effect of dioxane concentration on the stability of the Pd(diamine)-CBDCA system and logK refers to the 110 species.

5. Effect of chloride on the stability constants

Carboplatin or *Cis*-diamine(1,1-cyclobutanedicarboxylate)platinum(II), is a clinically successful second generation platinum complex. When Pt antitumor drugs are injected into the blood, it is crucial that they reach their final target, the intracellular DNA, without reacting with other nucleophiles within the cytoplasm. In human blood plasma the chloride content is quite high (~ 100 mM), so that hydrolysis of *cis*-[$PtCl_2(NH_3)_2$] is less likely to occur than within the cell where the chloride concentration is as low as 4 mM (Rosenberg, 1980). The high chloride concentration allows the neutral complex, *cis*-[$PtCl_2(NH_3)_2$], to flow almost unchanged through the blood. It then diffuses through the cell membrane and finally hydrolyzed to give more reactive aquated species as shown in scheme 7. Due to the lower chloride concentration the aquated complexes can react with DNA.

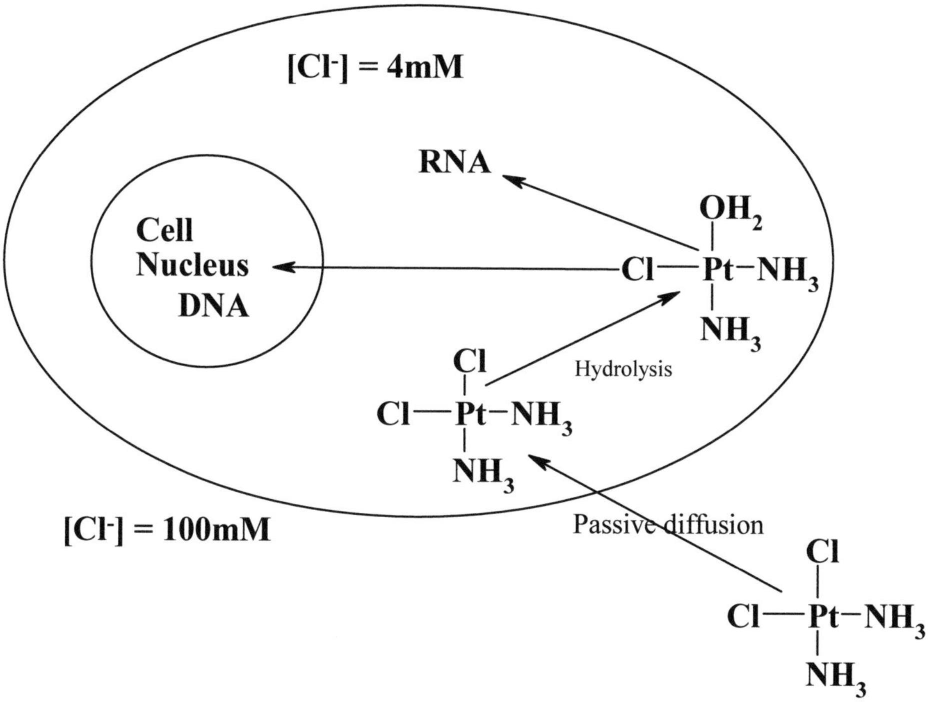

Scheme 7. The cellular uptake of cisplatin and its targets.

A realistic extrapolation of the present study to biologically relevant conditions will require information on the effect of the chloride concentration on the reported stability constants. The reactivity of CBDCA toward the different Pd(II) species increases markedly when chloride ions of Pd(AMBI)Cl_2 are replaced successively by one and two water molecules. A similar qualitative conclusion has been reached in the case of Pt(en)Cl_2 by Lim and Martin (Lim and Martin, 1976), based on equilibrium distribution of Pt(en) and on rates of reactions of pyridine with Pt(dien) complexes.

The equilibrium constants for Pd(AMBI)-CBDCA complex obtained for different chloride ion concentrations, keeping the ionic strength constant at 0.30 mol-dm^{-3}, are summarized in

Table 12 (El-Sherif et al., 2003; El-Sherif, 2006). The stability constants of the Pd(AMBI)-CBDCA complex, tend to decrease while increasing the chloride ion concentration. This can be accounted for on the basis that the concentrations of the active species, the mono- and the diaqua complexes, decrease with increasing [Cl^-]; this will in turn affect the stability of the complexes formed. The variation in stability constant of the Pd(diamine)$^{2+}$ complex with CBDCA as a function of Cl^- ion concentration, is shown in Fig. 7.

[Cl^-]/M	p	q	r[a]	Pic[b]	AMBI[c]
0.05	1	1	0	3.95	3.55
0.10	1	1	0	3.56	3.15
0.15	1	1	0	3.30	2.80
0.20	1	1	0	3.00	2.40
0.25	1	1	0	2.62	-

[a]p, q and r are stoichiometric coefficients corresponding to [Pd(diamine)$(H_2O)_2$], ligand and H^+ respectively, [b]Pic = picolylamine, data taken from reference (El-Sherif et al., 2003), [c]AMBI = 2-aminomethylbenzimidazole, data taken from reference (El-Sherif, 2006).

Table 12. Effect of chloride on the formation constant (log β_{110}) of [Pd(diamine)$(H_2O)_2$] with CBDCA at 25 ^{0}C and 0.3 mol dm^{-3} (KCl + $NaNO_3$).

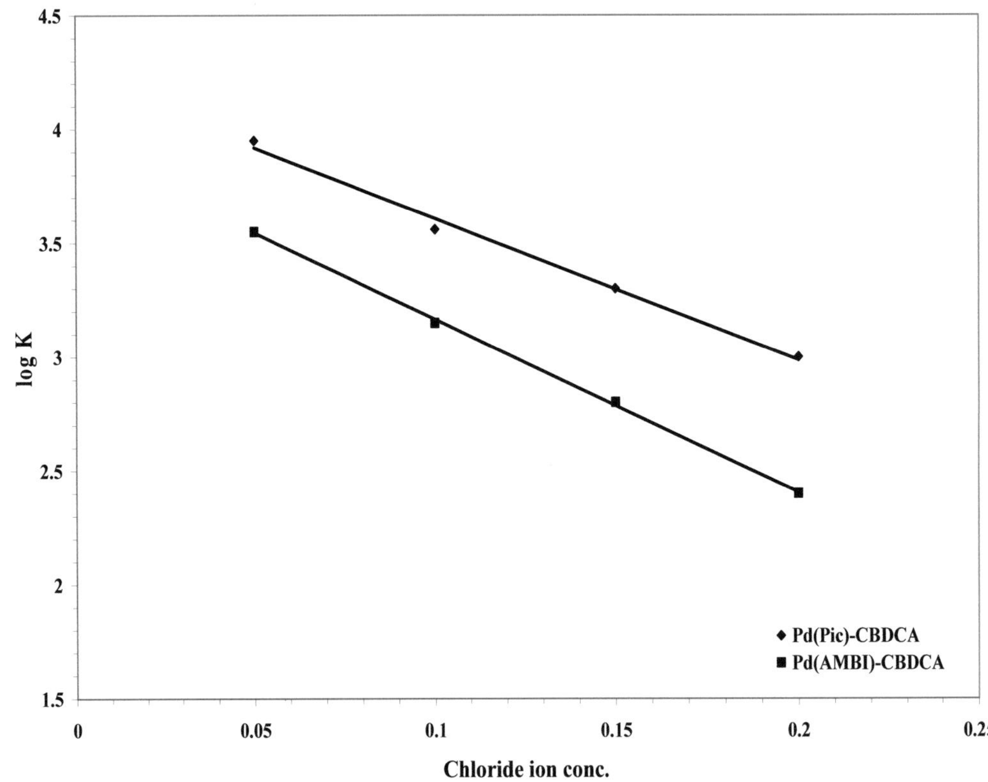

Fig. 7. Effect of chloride ion concentration on the stability of the Pd(diamine)-CBDCA system and logK refers to the 110 species.

6. Biological activity of mixed ligand Pd(II) complexes with biologically active ligands

Four new palladium(II) and platinum(II) complexes of formula $[M(BPY)(AA)]^+$ (where BPY is 2,2′-bipyridylamine, AA is an anion of glycine or L-alanine, and M is Pd(II) or Pt(II) have been synthesized (Paul et al., 1993) and characterized with amino acids bound as bidentate ligands. These complexes are 1:1 electrolyte in conductivity water. Among the studied complexes, the two L-alanine complexes show ID_{50} values against lymphocytic leukemia cells lower than cis-diammine dichloroplatinum(II), whereas the two glycine complexes show ID_{50} values higher than cisplatin. The interaction of calf thymus DNA with the above complexes shows significant spectral changes in the presence of [Pt(BPY)(gly)]Cl, [Pd(BPY)(ala)]Cl, and [Pt(BPY)(ala)]Cl and the binding mode between these complexes and DNA seems to be noncovalent.

Nine palladium(II) complexes of the formula $[Pd(BPY)(AA)]^{n+}$ (where BPY is 2,2′-bipyridylamine, AA is an anion of L-cysteine, L-aspartic acid, L-glutamic acid, L-methionine, L-histidine, L-arginine, L-phenylalanine, L-tyrosine, L-tryptophan, n = 0 or1) have been synthesized by the interaction of $[Pd(BPY)Cl_2]$ with an appropriate sodium salt of amino acids in water. The Pd(II)-complexes have shown growth inhibition against L1210 lymphoid leukemic, P388 lymphocytic leukemic sarcoma 180 and Ehrlich ascites tumor cells. Some of these complexes show ID_{50} values comparable to *cis*-platin (Puthraya et al.,1986).

The amino acids (AA) complexes of $[Pt(phen)(AA)]NO_3 \cdot xH_2O$ and $[Pd(phen)(AA)]NO_3 \cdot x H_2O$ have been prepared by the interaction of palladium and platinum complexes, $[Pt(phen)Cl_2]$ and $[Pd(phen)Cl_2]$ with salts of amino acids in methanol and characterized by ^1H NMR and IR spectroscopy which confirmed the formation of a very large variety of compounds (Jin et al., 2000). All of these new compounds have been isolated and tested for cytotoxicity on Molt-4, a human leukaemia cell line. The IC_{50} values of $[Pt(phen)(Pro)]Cl \cdot 2H_2O$ and $[Pd(phen)(Asp)]Cl \cdot 1.5H_2O$ are 9.8 and 7.31 μM, respectively, exhibiting a significant activity which is close to *cis*-$[PtCl_2(NH_3)_2]$.

Palladium(II) complexes of type $[Pd(phen)(AA)]^+$ (where AA is an anion of glycine, L-alanine, L-leucine, L-phenylalanine, L-tyrosine, L-tryptophan, L-valine, L-proline, or L-serine), have been synthesized. These palladium(II) complexes have been characterized by ultraviolet-visible, infrared, and ^1H NMR spectroscopy. They have also been screened for cytotoxicity in P388 lymphocytic cells. Only two complexes, $[Pd(Phen)(Gly)]^+$ and $[Pd(phen)(Val)]^+$, showed a comparable cytotoxictty with cisplatin (Mital, et al., 1991).

Five new palladium(II) complexes of the formula $[Pd(AMBI)(AA)]^{n+}$ (where AMBI = 2-aminomethyl benzimidazole, AA is an anion of glycine, alanine, cysteine, methionine and threonine) have been synthesized (El-Sherif, 2011). These palladium(II) complexes have been ascertained by elemental, molar conductance, infrared and ^{1}HNMR spectroscopy. The isolated Pd(II)-complexes were screened for their antibacterial and cytotoxic activities and the results are reported and discussed. The activity of these compounds against Staphylococcus pyogenes decreased in the order Tavanic (standard) > [Pd(AMBI)(Met)]~ [Pd(AMBI)(Cys)] > [Pd(AMBI)(Ser)] > [Pd(AMBI)(Ala)] > [Pd(AMBI)(Gly)] and against E. coli decreased in the order Tavanic ~ [Pd(AMBI)(Met)] > [Pd(AMBI)(Cys)] > [Pd(AMBI)(Ser)] > [Pd(AMBI)(Ala)] > [Pd(AMBI)(Gly)] under experimental conditions. Cytotoxic study of the compounds against colon carcinoma (HCT116) and larynx carcinoma

(HEP2) cells indicate that, [Pd(AMBI)(Met)]Cl.H_2O complex shows significant activity against (HCT116) cells with IC_{50} value of 0.74 μg/ml, while [Pd(AMBI)(Cys)] complex shows significant activity against (HEP2) with IC_{50} value of 0.60 μg/ml. These results confirm the chemotherapeutically significance of these compounds (El-Sherif, 2011).

7. Conclusions

In this review, a detailed survey of the formation equilibria of $[Pd(diamine)(H_2O)_2]^{2+}$ with ligands of biological significance is presented. The main conclusions may be summarized as follows:

1. The stability constants of the hydroxo complexes are higher for $[Pd(aromaticdiamine)(H_2O)_2]^{2+}$ than $[Pd(aliphaticdiamine))(H_2O)_2]^{2+}$, suggesting that the presence of aromatic residues increases the affinity of palladium(II) for hydrolysis.
2. Combining of stability constants data of such diaqua-complexes with amino acids, peptides and DNA constitutents, it would be possible to calculate the equilibrium distibution of the metal species in biological fluids where all types of ligands are present simultaneously. This would constitute a powerful starting point for understanding the mode of action of such metal species under physiological conditions.
3. Amino acids form highly stable complexes, with the substituent on the α- carbon atom possessing a significant effect on the stability of the formed complex. The thioether group in S-methylcysteine increase the stability constant of its complex due to the highest coordination potentiality of the sulphur atom. The imidazole group in histidine increases the stability of the complex due to high affinity of PdII to the nitrogen donor group. On the other hand the extra carboxylic group in aspartic acid does not contribute to the stability of the formed complex, as the extra-carboxylic group is not competing with the amino group in complex formation.
4. The present study clearly shows clearly that $[Pd(diamine)(H^2O)_2]^{2+}$ complex can form strong bonds with peptides and promote easy deprotonation of the peptide. The relative magnitudes of the pK_a values of the Pd(II) complexes with peptides have interesting biological implications. Under normal physiological condition (pH 6-7), the peptides would coordinate to $[Pd(diamine)(H^2O)_2]^{2+}$ in entirely different ways. Glutaminate exists solely in its protonated form, whereas the other peptides are present entirely in the deprotonated form. Furthermore, the slight difference in the side chain of the peptides seem to produce dramatic differences in their behaviour toward the Pd(II) complex.
5. Anti-tumour Pt(II) amines are usually administrated as cisdichloro complexes. This form persists in human blood plasma because of its high chloride content (0.1 M). The net zero charge on the complex facilitates its passage through cell walls. Within many cells the chloride ion concentration is much lower (only ca. 4 mM), giving more reactive aquated species. Due to the lower chloride concentration, the complex diffuses through the cell membrane and is then hydrolyzed to give the more reactive aquated complexes which can then react with DNA
6. The reactivity of CBDCA toward the different Pd(II) species increases markedly when chloride ions of $Pd(diamine)Cl_2$ are replaced successively by one and two water molecules. A similar qualitative conclusion has been reached in the case of $Pt(en)Cl_2$ by Lim and Martin, based on equilibrium distribution of en Pt(II) and on rates of reactions of pyridine with dien Pt(II) complexes (Lim, and Martin, 1976).

7. Pd(diamine)-CBDCA complex formation is more favoured in biological environments of lower dielectric constant.
8. Hopefully that these data will bring a significant contribution in carrying out mechanistic studies in biological media.

8. Aknowledgement

The author thanks the Chemistry Department, Cairo University, Faculty of Science, Egypt for financial support and Prof. Dr. M.M. Shoukry for his efforts and co-operation. The author is also grateful to the chairman of Chem. Department (Prof. Dr. M. Badway) and the Dean of Faculty of Science (Prof. Dr. Gamal Abd El-Nasar for their constant encouragement for this work.

9. Abbreviations

Pic = Picolylamine (2-Aminomethylpyridine); BPY = 2,2'-bipyridyl; 1,3-DAP = 1,3-diaminopropane; 1,2-DAP = 1,2-diaminopropane; AEPY = 2-aminoethyl pyridine; UMP = Uridine-5'-monophosphate; TMP = Thymidine-5'-monophosphate; GMP = Guanosine-5'-monophosphate; CMP = Cytidine-5'-monophosphate; IMP = Inosine-5'-monophosphate; Phe = Phenylalanine; Ala = Alanine.

10. References

Akerlof, G. Short, O.A. (1953) The dielectric constant of dioxane-water mixtures between 0 and 80 degrees-correction. J Am Chem Soc. 75, 6357.

Anwader, E.H.S., Probst, M.M. and Rode. B.M. (1987) Investigations of Zn(II) complexes with DNA/RNA bases by means of quantum chemical calculations. Inorg Chim Acta. 137, 203-208.

Appleton, T.G. (1997) Donor atoms preferences in complexes of Pt(II) and Pd(II) with amino acids and related molecules. Coord Chem Rev 166, 313-359.

Appleton, T.G., Hall, J.R. and Ralph, S.F. (1986) ^{15}N and ^{195}Pt NMR-study of the effect of chain-length, n, on the reactions of amino-acids, $^{+}NH_3(CH_2)NCO_2$ (N = 1, 2, 3), with platinum(II) ammine complexes. Aus J Chem. 39(9), 1347-1362.

Beltrán, J.L., Codony, R. and Prat, M.D. (1993) Evaluation of stability constants from multi-wavelength absorbance data: program STAR. Anal Chim Acta. 276, 441.

Bernhard, S.A. (1986). The structure and function of enzymes, Benjamin WA, New York, ch. 8.

Burger, K., in Burger, K. (Ed.) (1990) Bio-coordination chemistry: coordination equilibria in biological active systems, Ellis Horwood Ltd., England.

Bóka, B., Nagy, Z. and Sóvágo, I. (2001) Solution equilibria and structural characterisation of the palladium(II) and mixed metal complexes of peptides containing methionyl residues. Journal of Inorganic Biochemistry 83, 77-89.

Britten, J.F., Lock, C.J.L., Pratt, W.M.C. (1982) The structures of chloro(diethylenetriamine) platinum(II) chloride and (diethylenetriamine)nitratoplatinum(II) nitrate and some comments on the existence of Pt^{II}-OH_2 and Pt^{II}–OH bonds in the solid state. Acta Crystallogr Sect B 38(8), 2148-2155.

Byabartta, P., Santra, P.K., Misra, T.K., Sinha, C. and Kennard, C.H.L., (2001) Synthesis, spectral characterisation, redox studies of isomeric dichloro-bis-[1-alkyl-2-(naphthyl-(α/β)-azo)imidazole]ruthenium(II). Single crystal X-ray structure of blue-green dichloro-bis-[1-ethyl-2-(naphthyl-α-azo)imidazole] ruthenium(II). Polyhedron. 20, 905.

Chandler, J.P., Thomson. R.E., Spivey, H.O. and Li, EL-F (1984) An improved computer program for calculating formation constants of ligand complexes from pH data. Anal Chim Acta. 162, 399-402.

Das, D., Nayak, M.K. and Sinha, C. (1997). Chemistry of azoimidazoles. Synthesis, spectral characterization and redox studies of N(1)-benzyl-2-(arylazo) imidazolepalladium(II) chloride. Transition Met Chem. 22,172-175.

Das, D. and Sinha, C. (1998). Synthesis, spectral and electrochemical characterization of (dithiocarbamato) (arylazoimidazole)Palladium(II) perchlorates. Transition Met Chem. 23, 309-311

Del Bene, J.E. (1984) Molecular orbital study of the lithium (1+) of the DNA bases J Phys Chem. 88, 5927-5931.

El-Sherif, A.A., (2006) Mixed-Ligand Complexes of 2-(aminomethyl)benzimidazole palladium(II) with various biologically relevant ligands. J Solution Chem. 35, 1287-1301.

El-Sherif, A.A., Shoukry, M.M., El-Bahnasawy, R.M. and Ahmed, D.M. (2010) Complex formation reactions of palladium(II)-1,3-diaminopropane with various biologically relevant ligands. Kinetics of hydrolysis of glycine methyl ester through complex formation. Cent Eur J Chem. 8(4), 919-927.

El-Sherif, A.A. (2011) Synthesis and characterization of some potential antitumor palladium(II) complexes of 2-aminomethylbenzimidazole and amino acids. J Coord. Chem, 64(12) 2035-2055.

El-Sherif, A.A., Shoukry, M.M. and van Eldik, R. (2003) Complex-formation reactions and stability constants for mixed-ligand complexes of diaqua(2-picolylamine)palladium(II) with some bio-relevant ligands. J. Chem Soc Dalton Trans, 1425-1432.

Faggiani, R., Lippert, B., Lock, C.J.L., and Rosenberg, B. (1977) Hydroxo-bridged platinum(II) complexes. 1. Di-.mu.-hydroxo-bis[diammineplatinum(II)] nitrate, $[(NH_3)_2Pt(OH)_2Pt(NH_3)_2](NO_3)_2$. Crystalline structure and vibrational spectra. J Am Chem Soc. 99, 777.

Faggiani, R., Lippert, B., Lock, C.J.L., and Rosenberg, B., (1977) Hydroxo-bridged platinum(II) complexes. 2. Crystallographic characterization and vibrational spectra of cyclo-tri-.mu.-hydroxo-tris[cis-diammineplatinum(II)]nitrate. Inorg Chem. 16, 1192-1196.

Faggiani, R., Lippert, B., Lock, C.J.L. and Rosenberg, B. (1978) Hydroxo-bridged platinum(II) complexes. 3. Bis[cyclo-tri-.mu.-hydroxo-tris(cis-diammineplatinium(II)] trisulfate hexahydrate. Crystallographic characterization and vibrational spectra. Inorg Chem. 17, 1941-1945.

Fisher, B.E. and Sigel, H. (1980) Ternary complexes in solution. Intramolecular hydrophobic ligand-ligand interactions in mixed ligand complexes containing an aliphatic amino acid. J Am Chem Soc. 102, 2998-3008.

Frassineti, C., Ghelli, S., Gans, P., Sabatini, A., Moruzzi, M.S. and Vacca, A. (1995) Nuclear magnetic resonance as a tool for determining protonation constants of natural polyprotic bases in solution. Anal Biochem. 231, 374-382.

Freeman, H.C. and Golomb, M.L. (1964) The crystal structure of trans-bisglycinatoplatinum(II) $Pt(NH_2CH_2COO)_2$. Acta Cryst Sect B 25(6),1203-1206.

Frey, U., Ranford, J.D. and Sadler P.J. (1993) Ring-opening reactions of the anticancer drug carboplatin: NMR characterization of cis-$[Pt(NH_3)_2$(CBDCA-O)(5'-GMP-N7)] in solution. Inorg Chem. 32, 1333-1340.

Galanski, M., Jakupec, M.A. and Keppler, B.K. (2005) Update of the preclinical situation of anticancer platinum complexes: Novel design strategies and innovative analytical approaches. Curr Med Chem. 12, 2075-2094.

Gampp, H., Maeder, M., Meyer, C.J and Zuberbühler, A. (1985) Calculation of equilibrium constants from spectroscopic data-II:Specfit: two user-friendly in basic and standard fortran. Talanta 32, 251-264.

Gans, P. Sabatini, A. and Vacca, A. (1976), An improved computer program for the computation of formation constants from potentiometric data. Inorg Chim Acta. 18, 237-239.

Gans, P., Sabatini, A. and Vacca, A. (1985) SUPERQUAD, an improved general program for computation of formation constants from potentiometric data. J Chem Soc, Dalton Trans. 1195.

Gill, D.S. (1984) in Platinum Coordination Complexes in Cancer Chemotherapy, Hacker, M.P., Douple, E.B., Krakoff, I.H., Eds. Nijhoff, Boston, pp. 267-278.

Guo, Z. Sadler, P.J. (2000) Medicinal inorganic chemistry. Adv. Inorg. Chem 49: 183-306.

Gordon, W.E. (1982) Data analysis for acid-base titration of an unknown solution. Anal Chem. 54 (9), 1595-1601.

Hay, R.W. (1985) "Bio-inorganic chemistry", Ellis Horwood Ltd., John Wiley and Sons NY.

Heim, M.E. (1993) in: B.K. Keppler, (Ed.), Metal complexes in cancer chemotherapy, VCH, Weinheim, p. 9.

Hohmann, H., Hellquist, B. and van Eldik, R. (1991) Effect of steric hindrance on kinetic and equilibrium data for substitution reactions of diaqua(N-substituted Eehylenediamine)palladium(II) with chloride in aqueous solution. Inorg Chim Acta. 188, 25-32.

Jin, V.X. and Ranford, J.D. (2000) Complexes of platinum(II) or palladium(II) with 1,10-phenanthroline and amino acids. Inorg Chim Acta. 304, 38.

Legget, D.J. (Ed.) (1985) Computational methods for the determination of formation constants, Plenum Press, New York.

Lim, M.C. (1978) Mixed-ligand complexes of Pd(II). Part(3). Diaqua(ethylenediamine)Pd(II)-complexes of L-amino acids. JCS Dalton. 726-728.

Lim, M.C., Martin, R.B. (1976) The Nature of cis-ammine Pd(II) and antitumor in aqueous solutions. J Inorg Nucl Chem 38, 1911-1914

Maskos, K. (1985) Spectroscopic studies on Cu(II)-Inosine system, J Inorg Biochem. 25,1-14.

Martin, R.B. (1983) in Platinum, Gold and other chemotherapeutic agents: Chemistry and Biochemistry, ed. Lippard, S.J., ACS Symposium Series, Wiley, New York, 209, 231.

Martin, R.B. (1985) Nucleoside sites for transition metal-ion binding, Accounts Chem Research 18(2), 32-38.

Martin, R.B. (1999) Platinum complexes: Hydrolysis and binding to N(7) and N(1) of purines, in Cisplatin. ed. Lippert, B., Wiley-VCH, Weinheim. 183-205.

Misra, T.K., Das, D., Sinha, C., Ghosh, P.K. and Pal. C.K. (1998) Chemistry of azoimidazoles: Synthesis, spectral characterization, electrochemical studies, and X-ray crystal structures of isomeric dichloro bis[1-alkyl-2-(arylazo)imidazole] complexes of ruthenium(II). Inorg Chem. 37,1672-1678.

Mital, R., Srivastava, T.S., Parekh, H.K., Chitnis, M.P. (1991) Synthesis, characterization, DNA binding, and cytotoxic studies of some mixed-ligand palladium(II) and platinum(II) complexes of α-diimine and amino acids. J Inorg Biochem. 41, 93-103.

Mohamed, M.M.A. and Shoukry, M.M. (2001) Complex formation reactions of (N,N'-dimethylethylenediamine) palladium(II) with various biologically relevant ligands. Polyhedron. 20, 343-352.

Momekov, G. Bakalova, A. and Karaivanova, M. (2005) Novel approaches towards development of non-classical platinum-based antineoplastic agents: Design of platinum complexes characterized by an alternative DNA-binding pattern and/or tumor-targeted cytotoxicity. Curr Med Chem. 12(19), 2177-2191.

Motekaitis, R.J. and Martell, A.E. (1988). The determination and use of stability constants, VCH, Ne.w York.

Meloum, M., Havel, and J., Hgfeldt, E. (1994) Computation of solution equilibria, Ellis Horwood, Chichester.

Nagy, Z. and Sóvágó, I. (2001) Thermodynamic and structural characterization of the complexes formed in the reaction of $[Pd(en)(H_2O)_2]^{2+}$ and $[Pd(pic)(H_2O)_2]^{2+}$ with N-alkyl nucleobases and N-acetylamino acids. J Chem Soc, Dalton Trans. 2467.

Nakamoto, K. (1997) Infrared and raman spectra of inorganic and coordination compounds, 5th edit., part B applications in coordination, organometallic, and bioinorganic chemistry, Wiley Interscience, New York.

Nelson, D.J., Yeagle, P.L., Miller, T.L. and Martin, R.B., (1976) Carbon-13 magnetic resonance spectra of nucleosides and their Pd(II) complexes, Bioinorg Chem. 5, 353-358.

Norman, R.E., Ranford, J.D., Sadler, P.J. (1992) Studies of platinum(II) methionine complexes: metabolites of cisplatin. Inorg Chem 31, 877.

Pal, S. Das, D. Chattopadhyay, P., Sinha, C., Panneerselvam, K. and Lu, T.H. (2000) Spectral and structural studies of metal complexes of isatin 3-hexamethyleneiminylthiosemicarbazone prepared electrochemically. Polyhedron 19, 1263.

Paul, A.K., Mansuri-Torshizi, H., Srivastava, T.S., Chavan, S.J., Chitnis, M.P. (1993) Some potential antitumor 2,2'-dipyridylamine Pt(II)/Pd(II) complexes with amino acids: Their synthesis, spectroscopy, DNA binding, and cytotoxic studies. J Inorg Biochem. 50, 9.

Perrin, D.D. and Stunzi, H. in Leggett, D.J. (Ed.) (1985) Computational methods for the determination of formation constants. Plenum Press, New York, p.71.

Pettit, L., University of Leeds, personal communication, UK.

Pneumatikakis, G. (1984) 1:1 complexes of Pd(II) and Pt(II) with caeffine and their interaction with nucleosides. Inorg Chim Acta. 93, 5-11.

Pneumatikakis, G., Yannopoulos, A. Markopoulos and J. Angelopoulos, C. (1988) Monotheophylline and monotheophyllinato complexes of Pd(II) and their interactions with nucleosides. Inorg Chim Acta. 152, 101-106.

Puthraya, K.H., Srivastava, T.S., Amonkar, A.J., Adwankar, M.K., Chitnis, M.P. (1986) Some potential anticancer Pd(II) complexes of 2,2'-bipyridine with amino acids. J Inorg Biochem. 26, 45-54.

Rau, T., Shoukry, M.M., and van Eldik, R. (1997) Complex formation and ligand substitution reactions of (2-Picolylamine)palladium(II) with various biologically relevant ligands. Characterization of (2-picolylamine)(1,1-cyclobutanedicarboxylato)palladium(II). Inorg Chem. 36, 1454-1463.

Rauth, G.K., Pal, S., Das, D., Sinha, C., Slawin, A.M.Z., and Woollins, J.D. (2001) Synthesis, spectral characterization and electrochemical studies of mixed-ligand complexes of platinum(II) with 2-(arylazo)pyridines and catechols. Single-crystal X-ray structure of dichloro{2-(phenylazo) pyridine}platinum(II). Polyhedron. 20, 63.

Reedik, J. (1992) The relevance of hydrogen bonding in the mechanism of action of platinum antitumor compounds. Inorg Chim Acta. 198-200, 873-881.

Rees, D.C. (1980) Experimental evaluation of the effective dielectric constant of proteins. J Mol Biol. 141, 323-326.

Rogersa, N.K., Mooreb, G.R. and Sternberga M.J.E. (1985) Electrostatic interactions in globular proteins: calculation of the pH dependence of the redox potential of cytochrome C551. J Mol Biol. 182,613-616.

Rosenberg, B. (1980) In metal ions in biological systems, Sigel H, Ed., Dekker, New York 11,127-196.

Rosenberg, B. Van Camp, L. Trasko, J.E. and Mansour, V.H. (1969) Platinum compounds: a new class of potent antitumour agent. Nature. 222,385-386.

Roy, R., Chattopadhyay, P., Sinha, C. and Chattopadhyay, S. (1996) Synthesis, spectral and electrochemical studies of arylazopyridine complexes of palladium(II) with dioxolenes. Polyhedron. 15, 3361-3269.

Sabatini, A., Vacca, A. and Gans, P. (1992) Mathematical algorithms and computer programs for the determination of the equilibrium constants from potentiometric and spectrophotometric measurements. Coord Chem Rev. 120, 389-405.

Sabatini, A., Vacca, A. and Gans, P. (1974) Miniquad-A general computer programme for the computation of formation constants from potentiometric data. Talanta 21, 53-77.

Santra PK, Misra TK, Das D, Sinha C, Slawin AMZ, Woollins JD (1999), Chemistry of azopyrimidines. Part II. Synthesis, spectra, electrochemistry and X-ray crystal structures of isomeric dichloro bis[2-(arylazo)pyrimidine] complexes of ruthenium(II). Polyhedron. 18, 2869.

Shehata, M.R. (2001) Mixed ligand complexes of diaquo(2,2′-bipyridine)plladium(II) with cyclobutane-1,1-dicarboxylic acid and DNA constituents. Transition Met Chem. 26, 198-204.

Shehata, M.R., Shoukry, M.M., Abdel-Shakour, F.H. and van Eldik, R. (2009) Equilibrium studies on complex-formation reactions of $Pd[(2\text{-}(2\text{-aminoethyl})pyridine)(H_2O)_2]^{2+}$ with ligands of biological significance and displacement reactions of DNA constituents. Eur J Inorg Chem.3912-3920.

Shehata, M.R., Shoukry, M.M., Nasr, F.M.H. and van Eldik, R. (2008) Complex-formation reactions of dicholoro(S-methyl-L-cysteine)palladium(II) with bio-relevant ligands. Labilization induced by S-donor chelates. Dalton Trans 779-786.

Shoukry, A., Rau, T., Shoukry, M., and van Eldik, R., (1998) Kinetics and mechanisms of the ligand substitution reactions of bis(amine)(cyclobutane-1,1-dicarboxylato) palladium(II). J Chem Soc Dalton Trans. 3105-3112.

Shoukry, M.M., Shehata, M.R., Abdel-Razik, A., Abdel-Karim, A.T. (1999) Equilibrium studies of mixed ligand complexes involving (1,2-diaminopropane)-Palladium(II) and Some bioligands. Monatsh Fur Chem. 130, 409-423.

Sigel, H. and Martin, R.B. (1982) Coordinating properties of the amide bond. Stability and structure of metal ion complexes of peptides and related ligands. Chem Rev 82, 385-426.

Sigel, H., Massoud, S.S., Corfu, N.A. (1994) Comparison of the extent of macrochelate formation in complexes of divalent metal ions with guanosine (GMP^{2-}), inosine (IMP^{2-}), and adenosine 5́-monophosphate (AMP^{2-}). The crucial role of N-7 basicity in metal ion-nucleic base recognition. J. Am. Chem. Soc. 116, 2958–2971

Tauler, R. Casassas, E. and Izquierdo-Ridorsa, A. (1991) Self-modelling curve resolution in studies of spectrometric titrations of multi-equilibria systems by factor analysis. Anal Chim Acta. 248, 447-458.

Tercero-Moreno, J.M., Matilla-Hernandez, A., Gonzalez-Garcia, S. and Niclos-Gutierrez, J. (1996) Hydrolytic species of the ion cis-diaqua(ethylenediamine) palladium(II) complex and of cis-dichloro(ethylenediamine) palladium(II): fitting its equilibrium models in aqueous media with or without chloride ion. Inorg Chim Acta. 253, 23.

Wong, E. and Giandomenico, C.M. (1999) Current Status of Platinum-Based Antitumor Drugs. Chem. Rev. 99, 2451.

Zekany, L. and Nagypal, I. (1985) in Leggett, D.J. (Ed.), Computational methods for the determination of formation constants. Plenum Press, New York, P. 71.

5

Heavy Metal Ion Extraction Using Organic Solvents: An Application of the Equilibrium Slope Method

Tjoon Tow Teng, Yusri Yusup and Ling Wei Low
Universiti Sains Malaysia
Malaysia

1. Introduction

The separation procedure of a chemical species from a matrix is essentially based on the transportation of the solute between the two involved phases, generally an organic and an inorganic one. Specifically, solvent extraction uses the concept of unique solute distribution ratios between two immiscible solvents. However, there are several situations where solutes have been observed to completely move from the inorganic to the organic phase (Anthemidis and Ioannou, 2009).

Organic solvent extraction is the transport of solutes, e.g. heavy metal ions, from an inorganic (or aqueous) phase to an organic phase. Solvents used comprise of an extractant + diluent combination. The roles of each are as follows: 1) the extractant, as a specific metal ion extractant; 2) the diluent, as a solvent condition controller, i.e. hydrophobicity, which can affect the molecules extractability (Watson, 1999; Cox, 2004). Occasionally, a phase modifier can be added to solve the problem of emulsion formation, aside from improving the phase demarcation process in an aqueous organic system (Cox, 2008).

Solvent extraction is widely applied to processes of metal ions recovery, ranging from aqueous solutions in hydrometallurgical treatment to environmental applications. It is also considered a useful technique to increase the initial concentration of the solute, commonly used in the separation processes of analytical applications (Reddy et al., 2005).

In the biomedical field, supported liquid membrane methodology was used for trace analytes determination by facilitating chromatogram differentiation between samples, water and blood plasma (Jonsson and Mathiasson, 1999). It is also used to enrich human wastes (e.g. urine) with heavy metals prior to concentration determination using atomic absorption spectroscopy (AAS) (Lindegrade et al., 1992; Djane et al., 1997a; Djane et al., 1997b).

1.1 Organic solvents

Numerous organic solvents have been utilized to remove heavy metals (Leopold et al., 2010; Rafighi et al., 2010; Chang et al., 2011; Fu et al., 2011; Mishra and Devi, 2011). Most of them are, in part, made from petroleum. Recently, solvents such as vegetable oil (Venkateswaran et al., 2007; Chang et al., 2010), were exploited as alternatives to replace the commonly used petroleum-based organic solvents. Additionally, a family of "specialist" extractants, known as the organo-phosphorous compounds, are also employed as metal extractants (Sainz-Diaz et al., 1996).

Some examples of solvents applied in heavy metals extraction are:

a. Di-2-ethylhexylphosphoric acid (D2EHPA), extensively used as an extractant for the separation of Cu(II) from aqueous solutions (Gherrou et al., 2002; Ren et al., 2007; Cox, 2008). Other applications of this popular extractant include the removal of Cd(II) (Kumar et al., 2009), Zn(II) (Vahidi et al., 2009), Fe(III) and Ti(IV) (Silva et al., 2008);
b. Tributylphosphate (TBP), used to act as a phase modifier in Cu(II) extraction (Cheng, 2000). The extractant and phase modifier are diluted at certain ratios in the petroleum-based organic diluents such as kerosene and chloroform (Ak et al., 2008; Ren et al., 2008), cumene (Svendsen et al., 1990), dichloromethane (Memon et al., 2003), isododecane (Mortes and Bart, 2000), n-dodecane (Simonin et al., 2003), n-decanol (Lin et al., 2005), n-heptane (Morais and Mansur, 2004), and n-hexane (Valenzuela et al., 2002);
c. LIX 84 and Cyanex 272, applied to extract Cu(II), Ni(II), and Al(III) (Mohapatra et al., 2007; Agrawal et al., 2008);
d. Cyanex 921, used to extract Cu(II) from HCl (Mishra and Devi, 2011);
e. Miscellaneous organic solvents such as I) 1-phenyl-3-heptyl-1,3-propanedione, II) 1-phenyl-4-ethyl-1,3-octanedione, III) 1-(4′-dodecyl) phenyl-3-tert-butyl-1,3-propanedione in kerosene, used to extract Cu(II) (Fu et al., 2011).

2. Stoichiometry of heavy metals extracted using organic solvents: Equilibrium slope method

The equilibrium slope method has been used by many researchers to determine the stoichiometry of various metal–organic complexes in organic solvents (Nagaosa and Yao, 1997; Wang and Nagaosa; 2001; Mansur et al., 2002; Kumar et al., 2009). Most of its applications deal with extracting metal ions from aqueous solutions. It has proven a very useful technique of its ease of use, and its accuracy when validated by other methods, such as numerical and quantitative analysis from Fourier Transform Infrared Spectroscopy (FTIR).

2.1 General equilibrium slope methodology

Following this methodology, the extractant form in the organic solvent would need to be estimated first. Subsequently, the formulation of a balanced reaction equation would be derived. A general form of the reaction equation is shown below (Eq. 1). Some applied assumptions include that the solubility of the extractant and the metal-extractant complex in the aqueous phase is small, and that the extracted metal ions are not associated to one another.

$$M^{n+}{}_{(aq)} + xHR_{(org)} \overset{K_{eq}}{\leftrightarrow} MR_{x(org)} + xH^{+}{}_{(aq)} \tag{1}$$

where,

- M = metal ion
- R = hydrocarbon group
- n = oxidation number
- x = stoichiometric coefficient
- $_{org}$ = organic phase
- K_{eq} = equilibrium constant

The equilibrium constant, K_{eq}, can be experimentally determined. In turn, K_{eq} is a function of D_{eq}, which is the equilibrium distribution ratio of the metal ion concentration in the organic and the aqueous phase (Eq. 2).

$$D_{eq} = \left(\frac{M^{n+}{}_{(org)}}{M^{n+}{}_{(aq)}}\right)_{eq} \quad (2)$$

During the experiment, the ionic strength and the correlated activity coefficient, a, is needed to be kept constant by adding inert chemicals or substances such as salts. A plot of lg D_{eq} against pH_{eq} can be drawn to determine the valency of the extracted metal ion. This information can also be used to ensure the experiment validity by cross-checking the actual valency of the studied metal ion to the slope of the drawn plot. In addition, a plot of lg D_{eq} versus lg [extractant], will reveal the value of the stoichiometric coefficient of the extractant, x.

2.2 Application of the equilibrium slope methodology

In this section a separated study on the equilibrium slope method applied to different metal ions reported in literature is presented.

2.2.1 Cu (II)

Cu(II) extraction from aqueous solutions using different organic solvents have been studied extensively. Combination of extractants and solvents used to extract Cu(II) from an aqueous solution in literature include D2EHPA + soybean oil (Chang et al., 2010; Chang et al., 2011), LIX 84 + kerosene (Agrawal et al., 2008), Cyanex 921 + kerosene (Leopold et al., 2010; Mishra and Devi, 2011), and Cyanex 272 + kerosene (Mohapatra et al., 2007; Agrawal et al., 2008; St John et al., 2010). The solvents employed are mostly non-polar in nature.

The steps required to determine the stoichiometric coefficient of the extractant are somewhat similar between the extractant + solvent combinations. Thus, the general technique, in sequence, is listed below.

The relevant reaction equation can be written as Eq. (3), where K_{eq} is defined as Eq. (4) and Eq. (5).

$$Cu^{2+}{}_{(aq)} + xHR_{(org)} \overset{K_{eq}}{\leftrightarrow} CuR_{x(org)} + xH^{+}{}_{(aq)} \quad (3)$$

where,

$$K_{eq} = \frac{[CuR_x][H^+]^x}{[Cu^{2+}][HR]^x} \quad (4)$$

$$D_{eq} = \left(\frac{Cu^{2+}{}_{(org)}}{Cu^{2+}{}_{(aq)}}\right)_{eq} \tag{5}$$

By substituting Eq. (5) into Eq. (4),

$$K_{eq} = D_{eq}\frac{[H^+]^x}{[HR]^x} \tag{6}$$

$$K_{eq}[HR]^x = D_{eq}[H^+]^x \tag{7}$$

$$lgK_{eq} + xlg[HR] = lgD_{eq} + xlg[H^+] \tag{8}$$

Since,

$$xlg[H^+] = -xpH_{eq} \tag{9}$$

Hence,

$$lgD_{eq} = xpH_{eq} + lgK_{eq} + xlg[HR] \tag{10}$$

A plot of lg D_{eq} versus pH_{eq} is illustrated in Fig. 1. A summary of published slope and intercept values is listed in Table 1. It can be deduced that the stoichiometric coefficient would generally equal to the charge of the metal ion extracted.

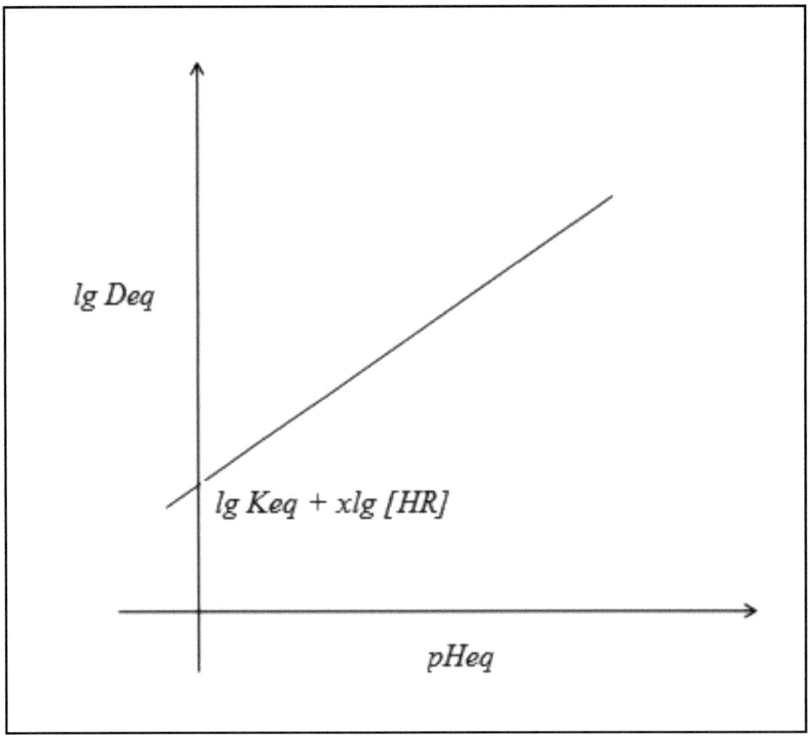

Fig. 1. lg D_{eq} versus pH_{eq}

Extractant + solvent	x	lg K_{eq}+ x lg$[HR]$	Extractant formula with metal	Reference
D2EHPA + soybean	1.99	-7.12	$CuR_2(HR)_2$	Chang et al. (2011)
LIX 84 + kerosene	1.5133	-0.9 (estimated)	CuR_2	Agrawal et al. (2008)
Cyanex 921 + kerosene	2.249	-1.6105	CuR_2	Mishra and Devi (2011)
Cyanex 272 + kerosene	1.75	-1 (estimated)	CuR_2	Agrawal et al. (2008)

Table 1. Slope and intercept of lgD_{eq} versus pH_{eq}

An average of 1.88 ≈ 2 for the slope has been observed by researchers using non-polar solvents. According to Chang et al. (2011), the Cu(II) ions were solvated by two simple molecules of D2EHPA, a supposition that stem from the slope obtained using the equilibrium slope method. In conclusion, the number of molecules of the extractant $(HR)_x$ (or R) determined by all researchers was unanimously 2, even when using different extractant and diluent combinations.

2.2.2 Ni (II)

Since Ni(II) has the same oxidation number as Cu(II) and not much work has been published on the extraction of this metal ion, then it can be assumed that Ni(II) would behave as Cu(II) would. A precaution when using this assumption is the type of solvent + extractant combination, which would give variable results on slope and intercept values. These values, in turn, depend on empirical or experimental values. The general reaction equation is written as Eq. (11) and the equilibrium constant as Eq. (12).

$$Ni^{2+}{}_{(aq)} + xHR_{(org)} \overset{K_{eq}}{\leftrightarrow} NiR_{x(org)} + xH^{+}{}_{(aq)} \tag{11}$$

$$K_{eq} = \frac{[NiR_x][H^+]^x}{[Ni^{2+}][HR]^x} \tag{12}$$

The results obtained is similar to what has been developed for Cu(II). This is supported by Tanaka and Alam (2011), which obtained a slope of 2 for pH between 1 and 4. Moreover, they found that for Ni(II), the lg D_{eq} versus pH diagram would exhibit 3 regions: I) pH < 4; II) 5 < pH ≤ 8; and III) pH > 8 (refer to Figure 2). It was also discovered by the latter researchers that at higher initial concentrations of LIX84I, another extractant, would extend the line with slope 2 until a pH of approximately 5.

In the pH < 4 region, the slope of the lg D versus pH curve would be 2 and the Ni(II) ions would exist as free ions. Thus, the extraction process would result from the ion exchange interaction between Ni(II) and $2H^+$ (same as Cu(II)). For 5 < pH ≤ 8, the slope would be virtually zero and the organic phase would be saturated with the Ni(II) ions. However, Ni(II) ions can still be extracted through proton exchange by forming the compound, NiR_2 (similar to Cu(II)). Still, the pH needs to be adjusted to achieve this. In the third region, pH > 8, the slope would essentially be negative (in this case of extracting Ni(II) from ammonium solutions) because of the formation of nickel-ammine complexes occurring concurrently with the decrease in free Ni(II) ion concentrations (Agrawal et al., 2008).

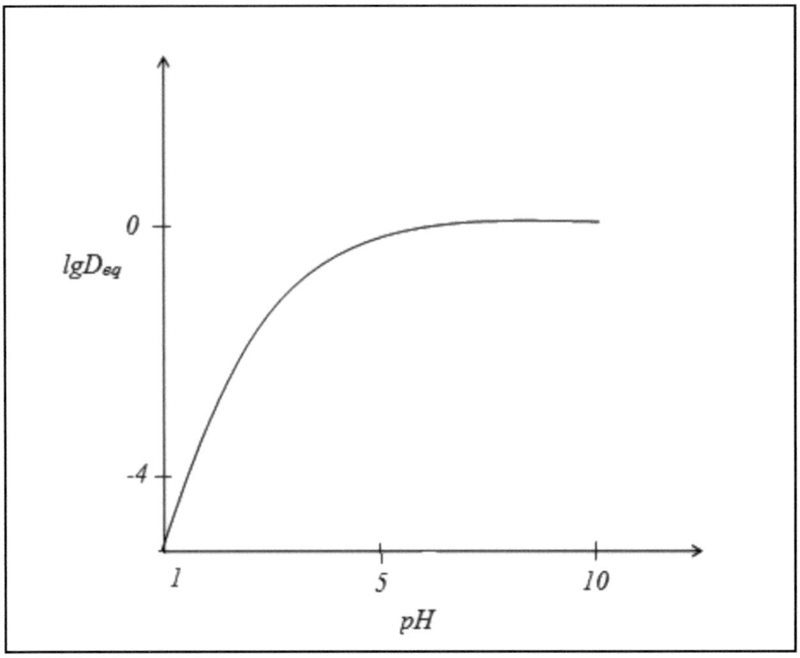

Fig. 2. lg D_{eq} as a function of pH at equilibrium

2.2.3 Cd(II)

A dimer formation between Cd(II) ions and an organic group has been suggested by many researchers (Kumar et al., 2009). Thus, the mechanism of extraction of Cd(II) with organic solvents would also behave the same as Cu(II) and Ni(II), as previously discussed . Since the researchers postulated a molecular form of the resulting organic complex, they could formulate a specific chemical reaction equation, written as Eq. (13). In the specific case of using D2EHPA + kerosene to extract this metal ion, the researchers have found a slope of 1.9143 and y-intercept of 4.5132 between the pH range of 1 and 5.

$$M^{n+}{}_{(aq)} + (n+p)/2\overline{(H_2R_2)_{org}} \overset{K_{eq}}{\leftrightarrow} \overline{(MR_n(HR)_p)_{org}} + nH^+_{aq} \tag{13}$$

where,

p = number of molecules of extractant engaged in reaction

Parrus et al. (2011) plotted a lg D_{eq} versus lg [extractant] graph to determine the number of organic molecules attached to Cd(II) following the application of the equilibrium slope method using 1-(2-pyridyl)-tridecan-1-one and 1-(2-pyridyl)-pentadecan-1-ol oximes in chloroform. They found that the slopes are, on average, 2, corroborating the postulate of the previous researchers on the molecular structure of the Cd(II) organic complex.

2.2.4 Cr(III)

Using the general reaction equation given by Eq. (1) and the steps applied on Cu(II), the relevant resulting equations are written below (Eq. 14-19).

$$Cr^{3+}{}_{(aq)} + xHR_{(org)} \overset{K_{eq}}{\leftrightarrow} CrR_{x(org)} + xH^{+}{}_{(aq)} \tag{14}$$

where,

$$K_{eq} = \frac{[CrR_x][H^+]^x}{[Cr^{3+}][HR]^x} \tag{15}$$

$$D_{eq} = \left(\frac{Cr^{3+}{}_{(org)}}{Cr^{3+}{}_{(aq)}}\right)_{eq} \tag{16}$$

By substituting Eq. (16) into Eq. (15),

$$K_{eq} = D_{eq}\frac{[H^+]^x}{[HR]^x} \tag{17}$$

$$K_{eq}[HR]^x = D_{eq}[H^+]^x \tag{18}$$

Hence,

$$lgD_{eq} = xpH_{eq} + lgK_{eq} + xlg[HR] \tag{19}$$

Researchers (Al-Zoubi et al., 2011) have found that for their situation, i.e. a combination of Cu(II) and Cr(III) ions in an aqueous solution, only Cu(II) is the extractable species. A linear relationship was still observed for Cu(II) and Cr(III) with a slope of 2 and 0.68, respectively.

2.2.5 Zn(II)

Baba and Adekola (2011) proposed the general reaction equation, Eq. (1), for metals Zn, Cd, Co, Fe, Pb, Ca, and Mg when using D2EHPA. They stated that the extraction process depends on solution composition, equilibrium, pH, and type of diluents, while the increase in proton concentrations would further promote this reaction. Mellah and Benarchour (2006) proposed a specific reaction equation for Zn(II) when extracting it using D2EHPA written as Eq. (20) based on the assumptions that extractant molecules exist as dimers in the solvent (kerosene in their work). They obtained a slope of 1.7152 and 1.7153 for 0.1 M and 0.2 M of D2EHPA, respectively.

$$Zn^{2+}{}_{(aq)} + 1.5(H_2R_2)_{(org)} \overset{K_{eq}}{\rightarrow} ZnR_2(HR)_{org} + 2H^{+}{}_{(aq)} \tag{20}$$

Since the general reaction equation is applicable for Zn(II) and shown by Baba and Adekola (2011) as well, a slope of approximately 2 would be evident from the lg D_{eq} versus pH plot. The latter authors reported a slope of 1.86. Li et al. (2003) has also reported a close to 2 value of 1.92 when extracting Zn(II) using Cyanex 272

2.2.6 U(VI)

Even though the oxidation number of U(VI) is more than 2, in the work published by St John et al. (2010) it was found that the slope of the lg D_{eq} versus pH plot is 2.10. This is due to U(VI) forming a complex with O_2 that results in the formation of UO_2^{2+}, thus the equilibrium slope of 2.

2.2.7 Co(II)

The reaction equation and the related equilibrium constant for the extraction of Co(II) using Cyanex 272 are written as Eq. (21-25) (Parhi et al., 2008). A slope of 2.0282 was obtained, proving that the extracted species was CoR_2.

$$Co^{2+}{}_{(aq)} + xHR_{(org)} \overset{K_{eq}}{\leftrightarrow} CoR_{x(org)} + xH^{+}{}_{(aq)} \quad (21)$$

where,

$$K_{eq} = \frac{[CoR_x][H^+]^x}{[Co^{2+}][HR]^x} \quad (22)$$

$$D_{eq} = \left(\frac{Co^{2+}{}_{(org)}}{Co^{2+}{}_{(aq)}}\right)_{eq} \quad (23)$$

By substituting Eq. (23) into Eq. (22),

$$K_{eq}[HR]^x = D_{eq}[H^+]^x \quad (24)$$

Hence,

$$lgD_{eq} = xpH_{eq} + lgK_{eq} + xlg[HR] \quad (25)$$

In another study by Rafighi et al. (2010), a different reaction equation was proposed (Eq. 26) Plots of lg D_{eq} versus lg [extractant] showed slopes of 1 and 2, pertaining to the number of organic molecules attached to Co(II).

$$Co^{2+}{}_{(aq)} + HR^{1(2)}{}_{(org)} + Cl^{-}{}_{(aq)} \leftrightarrow CoR^{1(2)}Cl.3H_2O_{(org)} + H^{+}{}_{(aq)} \quad (26)$$

2.2.8 Al(III)

In a paper by Mohapatra et al. (2007), Al(III) was extracted using Na-Cyanex 272 and Na-D2EHPA. The slopes of the lg D_{eq} versus pH are 1.85 and 2.40 for the two solvents, respectively. The reaction equation is written below (Eq. 27-31). Notice the stoichiometric coefficient of H^+ is 3.

$$Al^{3+} + n[HR]_2 \overset{K_{eq}}{\leftrightarrow} AlH_{2n-3}R_{2n} + 3H^+ \quad (27)$$

$$K_{eq} = \frac{[AlH_{2n-3}R_{2n}][H^+]^3}{[Al^{3+}][HR]_2^n} \quad (28)$$

$$K_{eq} = \frac{D_{eq}[H^+]^3}{[HR]_2^n} \quad (29)$$

where,

$$D_{eq} = \frac{[AlH_{2n-3}R_{2n}]}{[Al^{3+}]} \quad (30)$$

Hence,

$$lgD_{eq} = lgK_{eq} + nlg[HR]_2 - 3\lg[H^+] \quad (31)$$

3. Other methods to determine stoichiometry of heavy metals extraction using organic solvents

There are other methods that can be used to validate the stoichiometry of the organic complexes produced from the heavy metal extraction process using organic solvents. These methods include numerical analysis and quantitative analysis using FTIR.

Numerical analysis requires that a multiple regression analysis be conducted using a first order function, written as Eq. (32).

$$y = \beta_0 + \sum_{i=1}^{k} \beta_i x_i + \varepsilon \quad (32)$$

where,

- β_0 = constant for intercept
- β_i = constant for linear variables
- y = dependent variable
- x_i = independent variable
- ε = error term

This is followed by a best fit exercise using the least square method. As an example, albeit a very specific one and since this analysis is highly empirical in nature, constants can be estimated, along with the corresponding standard deviation, t and probability (P) values, for the variable terms of a regression model of log D_{eq}. At a 5% significance level, all variable terms, when found to have $P < 0.05$, are thus considered statistically significant. Hence, a first-order polynomial model that correlates log D_{eq} with all the variable terms can be developed.

The adequacy or goodness of fit of the regression model can be analyzed using analysis of variance (ANOVA) at a 5% significance level. Low P ($P < 0.05$) value of the regression model indicates that it is statistically significant. To test the global fit of the model, the coefficient of determination (r^2) can also be evaluated. Small deviations between the r^2 and adjusted r^2 values would imply that there is less chance for the inclusion of any insignificant terms in the model and that the model is highly significant.

Since Eqs. (32) and (10) are of the same forms, their constants for each variable term can be compared conveniently. By evaluating the constants of $\log[(HR)_2]$ from Eq. (4), i.e. $(2 + m)/2$, with that from the regression model, the m value can be determined and, thus, brings about the stoichiometric ratio.

Chang et al. (2011) has used this method to confirm that the slope of the lg D_{eq} versus pH is 2 (= 1.988).

Quantitative analysis using FTIR requires an FTIR analysis of the metal ion-loaded organic solvent. This is detailed in the paper by Sainz-Diaz et al. (1996). For the case of Cu(II) and D2EHPA, it leverages the fact that there is a highly polar phosphoryl bond (P=O) in the D2EHPA compound and could easily react with Cu(II). Knowing that the absorbance of the P=O band is at 1235 cm^{-1} at multiple concentrations of D2EHPA standard solutions, a calibration curve can be obtained. This calibration curve can be used to determine the concentration of D2EHPA that did not react with Cu(II). By finding the difference between the reacted and unreacted concentrations of D2EHPA, the concentration of Cu-D2EHPA (organic complex) can be estimated. A plot of the Cu-D2EHPA versus the organic concentration of Cu will reveal the slope that corresponds to the constant stochiometic ratio of D2EHPA.

4. Conclusion

Liquid extraction of heavy metals is widely applied in many fields ranging from the environmental to the biomedical discipline. In the environmental field, some of the more prominent applications include: removal and recovery of heavy metals and dyes from wastewater. In the biomedical field, liquid extraction has been used in the determination of heavy metals in human waste (e.g. urine). However, trace analytes extraction is still a great challenge in the pharmaceutical and medical industry.

In this chapter, the equilibrium slope method and its utility in estimating the stoichiometry of the resulting organic complexes has been reviewed for multiple heavy metal ions. The number of protons involved generally dictates the slope of the lg D_{eq} versus pH plot. A slope of 2 is common for many heavy metals, thus attributing that the general organic complexes obtained from these extraction processes are in the form of dimers.

In brief other methods, numerical and FTIR quantitative analysis have been discussed and might be helpful to further corroborate the results of the equilibrium slope method.

5. References

Agrawal, A.; Manoj, M.K., Kumari, S., Bagchi, D., Kumar, V. & Pandey, B.D. (2008). Extractive separation of copper and nickel from copper bleed stream by solvent extraction route. *Minerals Engineering*, Vol.21, pp. 1126-1130.

Ak, M.; Taban, D. & Deligoz, H. (2008). Transition metal cations extraction by ester and ketone derivatives of chromogenic azocalix arenes. *Journal of Hazardous Materials*, Vol.154, pp. 51-52.

Al-Zoubi, W.; Kandil, F. & Chebani, M.K. (2011). Solvent extraction of chromium and copper using Schiff base derived from terephthaldialdehyde and 5-amino-2-methoxy phenol. *Arabian Journal of Chemistry*, Article in Press DOI:10.1016/j.arabjc. 2011.06.023

Anthemidis, A.N. & Ioannou, K.G. (2009). Recent development in homogenous and dispersive liquid-liquid extraction for inorganic elements determination. A review. *Talanta*, Vol.80, pp. 413-421.

Baba, A.A. & Adekola, F.A. (2011). Beneficiation of a Nigerian sphalerite mineral: solvent extraction of zinc by Cyanex 272 in hydrochloric acid. *Hydrometallurgy*, Vol. 109, pp. 187-193.

Chang, S.H.; Teng, T.T. & Norli, I. (2010). Extraction of Cu(II) from aqueous solutions by vegetable oil-based organic solvents. *Journal of Hazardous Materials*, Vol.181, pp. 868-872.

Chang, S.H.; Teng, T.T. & Norli, I. (2011). Efficiency, stoichiometry and structural studies of Cu(II) removal from aqueous solutions using di-2-ethylhexylphosphoric acid and tributhylphosphate diluted in soybean oil. *Chemical Engineering Journal*, Vol.166, pp. 249-255.

Cheng, C.Y. (2000). Purification of synthetic laterite leach solution by solvent extraction using D2EHPA. *Hydrometallurgy*, Vol.56, pp. 369-386.

Cox, M. (2004). *Solvent extraction in hydrometallurgy*, In: J. Rydberg, M. Cox, C. Musikas, G.R. Choppin (Eds.), Solvent Extraction Principles and Practice, Marcel Dekker Inc., The United States of America, pp. 457–462.

Cox, M. (2008). *Liquid–liquid extraction and liquid membranes in the perspective of the twenty-first century*, In: M. Aguilar, J.L. Cortina (Eds.), Solvent Extraction and Liquid Membranes Fundamentals and Applications inNewMaterials, CRC Press, the United States of America, pp. 1–19.

Djane, N.K.; Bergdahl, I.A.; Ndung's, K.; Schutz, A.; Johansson, G. & Mathiasson, L. (1997a). Supported liquid membrane enrichment combined with atomic absorption spectrometry for the determination of lead in urine. *Analyst*, Vol.122, pp.1073-1077.

Djane, N.K.; Ndung'u, K.; Malcus, F.; Johansson, G. & Mathiasson, L. (1997b). Supported liquid membrane enrichment using an organophosphorus extractant for analytical trace metal determinations in river waters. *Fresenius' Journal of Analytical Chemistry*, Vol.358, pp.822

Fu, W.; Chen, Q., Hu, H., Niu, C. & Zhu, Q. (2011). Solvent extraction of copper from ammoniacal chloride solutions by sterically hindered β-diketone extractants. *Separation and Purification Technology*, Vol.80, pp. 52-59.

Gherrou, A.; Kerdjoudj, H., Molinari, R. & Drioli, E. (2002). Removal of silver and copper ions acidic thiourea solutions with a supported liquid membrane containing D2EHPA as carrier, *Separation and Purification Technology*, Vol.28, pp. 235–244.

Jonsson, J.A. & Mathiasson, L. (1999). Liquid membrane extraction in analytical sample preparation II: Applications. *Trends in Analytical Chemistry*, Vol.18, pp. 325-334.

Kumar, V.; Kumar, M., Jha, M.K., Jeong, J. & Lee, J. (2009). Solvent extraction of cadmium from sulfate solution with di(2-ethylhexyl)phosphoric acid diluted in kerosene. *Hydrometallurgy*, Vol.96, pp. 230–234.

Leopold, A.A.; Coll, M.T., Fortuny, A., Rathore, N.S. & Sastre, A.M. (2010). Mathematical modelling of cadmium (II) solvent extraction from neutral and acidic chloride media using Cyanex 923 extractant as a metal carrier. *Journal of Hazardous Materials*, Vol.182, pp. 903-911.

Li, D.Q.; Wang, L.G. & Wang, Y.G. (2003). Synergistic extraction of Zinc(II) with mixtures of CA-100 and Cyanex 272. *Separation Science and Technology*, Vol.38, pp. 2291–2306.

Lin, S.H.; Kao, H.C., Su, H.N. & Juang, R.S. (2005). Effect of formaldehyde on Cu(II) removal from synthetic complexed solutions by solvent extraction. *Journal of Hazardous Materials*, Vol.120, pp. 1–3.

Lindegrad, B.; Jonsson, J.A. & Mathiasson, L. (1992). Liquid membrane work-up of blood plasma samples applied to gas chromatographic determination of aliphatic amines. *Journal of Chromatography*, Vol.573, pp.191-200.

Mansur, M.B.; Slater, M.J. & Biscaia Jr, E.C. (2002). Equilibrium analysis of the reactive liquid-liquid test system $ZnSO_4$/D2EHPA/n-heptane. *Hydrometallurgy*, Vol.63, pp. 117-126.

Mellah, A. & Benachour, D. (2006). The solvent extraction of zinc and cadmium from phosphoric acid solution by di-2-ethylhexyl phosphoric acid in kerosene diluent. *Chemical Engineering and Processing*, Vol.45, pp. 684-690.

Memon, S.; Akceylan, E., Sap, B., Tabakci, M., Roundhill, D.M. & Yilmaz, M. (2003). Polymer supported calyx arene derivatives for the extraction of metals and dichromate anions. *Journal of Polymer and Environment*, Vol.11, pp. 67–69.

Mishra, S. & Devi, N. (2011). Extraction of copper (II) from hydrochloric acid solution by Cyanex 921. *Hydrometallurgy*, Vol.107, pp. 29-33.

Mohapatra, D.; Kim, H.I., Nam, C.W. & Park, K.H. (2007). Liquid-liquid extraction of aluminium (III) from mixed sulphate solutions using sodium salts of Cyanex 272 and D2EHPA. *Separation and Purification Technology*, Vol.56, pp. 311-318.

Morais, B.S. & Mansur, M.B. (2004). Characterization of the reactive test system ZnSO4/D2EHPA in n-heptane, *Hydrometallurgy*, Vol.74, pp. 11–18.

Mortes, M. & Bart, H.J. (2000). Extraction equilibria of zinc with bis(2 ethylhexyl)phosphoric acid. *Journal of Chemical Engineering Data*, Vol.45, pp. 82–85.

Nagaosa, Y. & Yao, B.H. (1997). Extraction equilibria of some transition metal ions by bis(2-ethylhexyl)phosphoric acid. *Talanta*, Vol.44, pp. 327-337.

Parhi, P.K.; Panigrahi, S., Sarangi, K. & Nathsarma, K.C. (2008). Separation of cobalt and nickel from ammoniacal sulphate solution using Cyanex 272. *Separation and Purification Technology,* Vol. 59, pp. 310-317.

Parus, A.; Wieszczycka, K., Olszanowski, A. (2011). Solvent extraction of cadmium (II) from chloride solutions by pyridyl ketoximes. *Hydrometallurgy,* Vol.105, pp. 284-289.

Rafighi, P.; Yaftian, M.R. & Noshiranzadeh, N. (2010). Solvent extraction of cobalt (II) ions; cooperation of oximes and neutral donors. *Separation and Purification Technology,* Vol.75, pp. 32-38.

Reddy, B.R.; Priya, D. N., Rao, S.V. & Radhika, P. (2005). Solvent extraction and separation of Cd(II), Ni(II) and Co(II) from chloride leach liquors of spent Ni-Cd batteries using commercial organo-phosphotus extractants. *Hydrometallurgy,* Vol. 77, pp. 253-261.

Ren, Z.; Zhang, W., Meng, H., Liu, Y.M. & Dai, Y. (2007). Extraction equilibria of copper(II) with D2EHPA in kerosene from aqueous solutions in acetate buffer media. *Journal of Chemical Engineering Data,* Vol.52, pp. 438–441.

Ren, Z.Q.; Zhang, W., Dai, Y., Yang, Y. & Hao, Z. (2008). Modeling of effect of pH on mass transfer of copper(II) extraction by hollow fiber renewal liquid membrane. *Industrial Engineering Chemistry and Research,* Vol.47, pp. 4256–4262.

Sainz-Diaz, C.I.; Klocker, H., Marr, R. & Bart, H.J. (1996). New approach in the modelling of the extraction equilibrium of zinc with bis-(2ethylhexyl) phosphoric acid. *Hydrometallurgy,* Vol.42, pp. 1-11.

Silva, G.C.; Cunha, J.W.S.D., Dweck, J. & Afonso, J.C. (2008). Liquid–liquid extraction (LLE) of iron and titanium by bis-(2-ethyl-hexyl)phosphoric acid D2EHPA). *Mineral Engineering,* Vol.21, pp. 416–419.

Simonin, J.P.; Hendrawan, H., Dardoize, F. & Clodic, G. (2003). Study of salt effects on the kinetics of extraction of cobalt(II) and zinc(II) at trace level by D2EHPA in ndodecane. *Hydrometallurgy,* Vol.69, pp. 23–25.

St John, A.M.; Cattrall, R.W. & Kolev, S.D. (2010). Ectraction of uranium (VI) from sulphate solutions using a polymerinclusion membrane containing di-(2-ethylhexyl) phosphoric acid. *Journal of Membrane Science,* Vol.364, pp. 354-361.

Svendsen, H.F.; Schei, G. & Osman, M. (1990). Kinetics of extraction of Zn by di(2-ethylhexyl)phosphoric acid in cumene. *Hydrometallurgy,* Vol.25, pp. 197–212.

Tanaka, M. & Alam, S. (2010). Solvent extraction equilibria of nickel from ammonium nitrate solution with LIX84I. *Hydrometallurgy,* Vol.105, pp. 134-139.

Vahidi, E.; Rashchi, F. & Moradkhani, D. (2009). Recovery of zinc from an industrial zinc leach residue by solvent extraction using D2EHPA. *Mineral Engineering,* Vol.22, pp. 204–206.

Valenzuela, F.; Vega, M.A., Yanez, M.F. & Basualto, C. (2002). Application of amathematical model for copper permeation from a Chilean mine water through a hollow fiber-type supported liquid membrane. *Journal of Membrane Science,* Vol.204, pp. 385–387.

Venkateswaran, P.; Gopalakrishnan, A.N. & Palanivelu, K. (2007). Di(2- ehtylhexyl) phosphoric acid–coconut oil supported liquid membrane for the separation of copper ions from copper plating wastewater. *Journal of Environmental Science,* Vol.19, pp. 1446–1453.

Wang, T. & Nagaosa, Y. (2001). Solvent extraction equilibrium of copper (II) with diisodecylphosphoric acid in heptanes and dodecane. *Analytical Science,* Vol.17, pp. 401-404.

Watson, J.S. (1999). *Separation Methods for Waste and Environmental Applications,* Marcel Dekker Inc., The United States of America.

Part 3

Stoichiometry in Lipids and Polymers Architecture

6

Lipid Composition in Miscible and Immiscible Phases

Walter F. Schmidt[1*], Michael A. Crawford[2], Swati Mookherji[1] and Alva D. Mitchell[1]
[1]*Agriculture Research Service, United States Department of Agriculture, Beltsville, MD,*
[2]*Imperial College, Department of Cancer and Surgery, Division of Reproductive Physiology, Obstetrics and Gynecology, London,*
[1]*USA*
[2]*UK*

1. Introduction

Lipids play a vital role in the architecture of cell membranes. About one third of the known cellular proteins are located in the membrane lipid and these are largely the transporters, signalers, receptors and defense systems. The fatty acid component in membranes across species and in different cell types is species, organ and sub cellular specific. In human cell types, the inner cell membrane is dominated by arachidonic acid whilst that of the photo receptor and neural synapse is strikingly rich in docosahexaenoic acid. The biophysical basis for this molecular specificity in not understood.

Differences in lipid composition and lipids membrane packing must inevitably affect cell function. Dietary deficiency of docosahexaenoic acid (DHA) in pregnant rats has been shown to reduce fetal neurogenesis and neuronal cell migration [19]. Deficiency in infants can restrict visual and cognitive development [18]. Close structural analogs of DHA do not displace DHA from active sites even when such analogs are present at higher concentrations than DHA in the diet or in cell systems [3]. Thus the chemical structure of lipids at active sites is conserved at the molecular level by dietary lipids but lipids generated biochemically somehow do not displace or dilute them.

NMR spectroscopy, X-ray crystallography, and computational chemistry are essential tools in discriminating the molecular shape of biomolecules. Although NMR experiments using Deuterium-Labeled NMR have long been used to probe phospholipid bilayers [17], far fewer experiments yielding structural information have been generated for lipids than for proteins and carbohydrates. Natural abundance ^{13}C-NMR experiments with DHA demonstrated that highly unsaturated lipids pack more closely than more saturated lipids [2]. However, identifying the specific inter-molecular sites critical to lipid packing was not discernable.

Discrete chemical compositions of mixtures at the molecular level within definable unit cell molar volumes have been reported for stearic acid (SA) in the presence of structurally

*Corresponding Author

different solvents [13]. Although above a specific concentration, SA was "insoluble" in methyl oleate (MeOA); the immiscible phase was not SA, but a more densely packed MeOA/SA phase [14]. We report herein that an immiscible lipid phase on adding SA also occurs with structurally diverse lipids (e.g. DHA, pig fat and seal oil) and the thermal properties of the second phase are a fingerprint marker of its initial lipid identity. Differential scanning calorimetry (DSC) experiments distinguish the kinetic components from the thermodynamic components of these lipid physical properties.

2. Materials and methods

2.1 Materials

Stearic acid (SA) and methyl oleate (MeOA) were obtained from Sigma Aldrich (St. Louis, MO, USA). Pig fat and seal oil were provided by Alva Mitchell (ARS, Beltsville, MD) and fish DHA and DHA-PC samples were provided by Michael Crawford (UK).

2.2 Differential Scanning Calorimetry (DSC)

DSC measurements were performed using TA Instrument's Q200 calorimeter and a universal 4.5 data analysis software from TA Instrument. Approximately 15-20 mg of lipid samples were sealed in aluminum DSC pans and subjected to either traditional DSC or modulated DSC (MDSC) analysis. A sealed empty pan was used as reference. For DSC analysis, the sample was equilibrated at 65°C and kept isothermally for 30 minutes at that temperature and then cooled to 25°C at a rate of 1°C min^{-1}. The sample was then heated to 65°C at the same rate, and this cycle was repeated for 3 more times. For modulated DSC, the experiment lasted for 10 hrs. The sample was cooled down stepwise by initially equilibrating it at 65°C and the temperature was modulated at the rate of +/-2°C every 200 sec. The first cooling step was 48°C and then it was cooled down by 2°C and this process continued until the temperature reached 40°C. At each step the sample was kept in isothermal condition for 100 minutes.

2.3 Raman spectroscopy and imaging microscopy

Samples (ca. 1-10mg) were placed on an aluminum tape lined glass slide. Raman spectra were collected using a LabRam Aramis confocal Raman microscope (Horiba Jobin Yvon, Edison, New Jersey) with a 10×, 50×, and 100× objectives. The spectra were collected over the range of 200–4000cm^{-1} Raman shift using a HeNe laser (633 nm) for excitation. The confocal hole, and slit aperture were 500_m and 100_m, respectively. Maps were generated using a grating of 1200 g/mm, exposure time of 5 s with 20 accumulations per data point. In maps, spectral range was reduced to 600- 1800 cm^{-1}. For Raman imaging, and map of mixtures, a microscopic field of view was selected to include two lipid phases simultaneously. In map processing of mixtures following frequency ranges were selected: 1035–1162 cm−1 (for C C group), 1403–1459cm−1 (for C H group), and 1476–1772 cm−1 (for C C and C O group). On the region chosen for mapping, the program plots the localized distribution and intensity of these specific peaks.

2.4 Molecular mechanics

The chemical structure of individual lipid molecules was generated on HyperChem 8.0 (Gainesville, FL). The packing among lipid molecules was optimized using MM+ force fields

(Zhdanov et al., 2003). The conjugate gradient (Fletcher-Reeves) method was used to energy minimize distances among lipid molecules. Convergence condition limits were a RMS gradient of 0.01 kcal/Å mol. The packing among the lipids was the smallest cubical molecular volume in which stoichiometry could maintain the macroscopic mole ratios determined experimentally.

3. Results and discussion

3.1 DSC

The thermodynamic component of miscibility and immiscibility has not previously been addressed. The DSC curves of structurally different lipids (MeOA, DHA, seal oil, pig fat), cycling through the temperatures 25°C to 65 °C four times, are presented (Figure 1a). Once a threshold concentration of SA was added to MeOA, the DSC curve showed a readily distinguishable phase transition in each cycle in which the lipid becomes cloudy (Figure 1b). MeOA was also the major component in the second phase as confirmed by Raman Spectroscopy [14]. The SA concentration in the clear phase remained identical to that of the threshold concentration and the higher concentration of SA occurred only in the second phase.

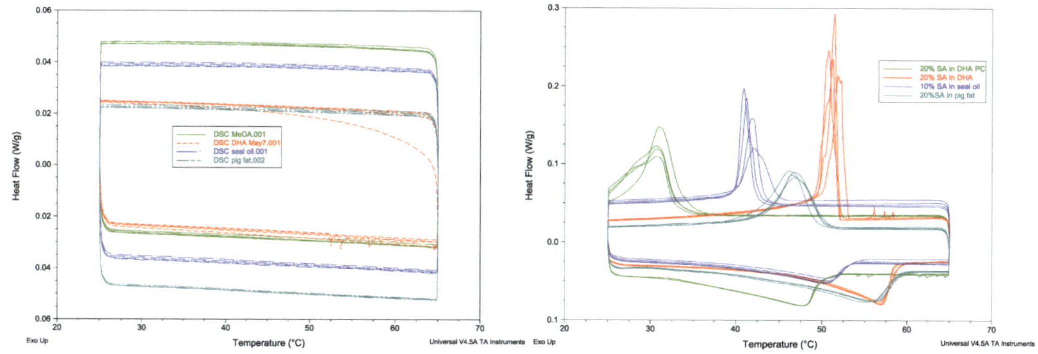

(a) (b)

Fig. 1. (a) The natural lipids have no identifiable phase transition in the Differential Scanning Calorimetry (DSC) curves. (b) Discretely different phase transitions of same lipids upon including 10-20% Stearic acid (SA).

Lipids are assumed amorphous because thermal properties of miscible lipid phases are unaffected by chemical structure. Differential scanning calorimetry (DSC) (Figure 1a) of methyl oleate (MeOA), docosahexaenoic acid (DHA), pig fat and seal oil are presented. Heating and cooling cycles were repeated four times yielding minimal thermal information. Phase transitions were absent likewise for high purity single component fatty acid methyl ester (MeOA) as for a complex mixture of natural triacylglycerides (seal oil). Mixtures of these lipids with 5% stearic acid (SA) remained fully miscible and no phase transition is observed. DSC of SA in DHA-phosphotidylcholine (DHA-PC), seal oil, pig fat, and DHA (Figure 2b) demonstrates an immiscible phase forms, and thermal properties among structurally different lipids are discretely different from each other.

A cube can have the average length of a lipid molecule (e.g. MeOA). The lipid composition in that space can have a same stoichiometry at the molecular level as is determined at the macroscopic level. Four rows of five MeOA molecules are the most that can fit into a cubic volume. Since 5% SA equals 1/20, the structurally simplest molar volume at this mole ratio contains 21 molecules (Figure 2). For comparison, the same unit cell can be oriented such that the single SA molecule is in an X, Y, or Z direction. The cross sectional area of each of the surfaces is similar. Computational chemistry optimized the packing and the spacing within and between cubic unit cell volumes of adjacent lipid molecules and adjacent unit cells, i.e. van der Waals distances from each other.

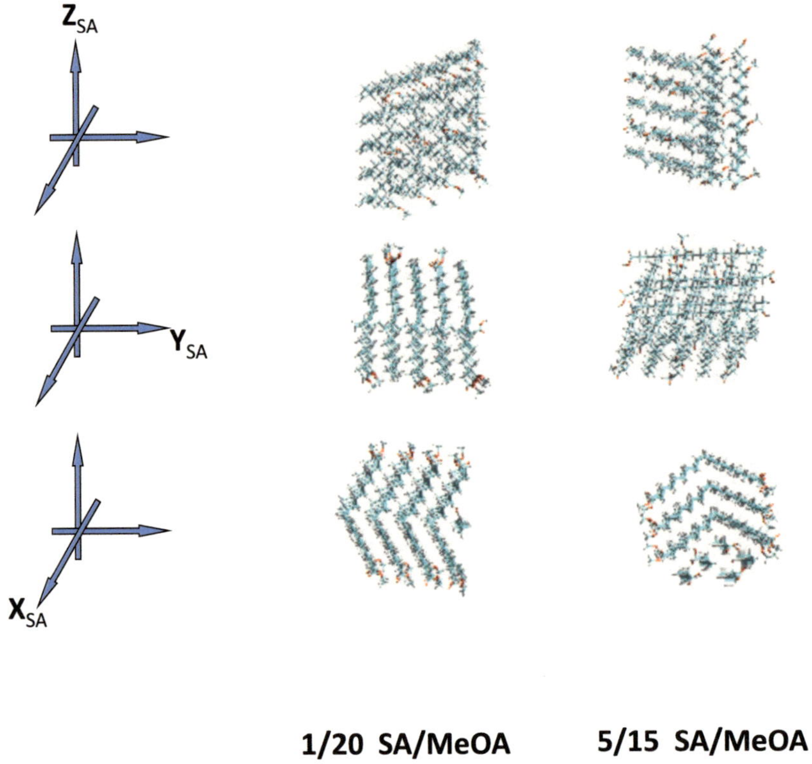

Fig. 2. Stoichiometry in packing of SA lipid unit cell volumes of Methyl Oleate (MeOA) and Docosahexaenoic acid (DHA). DHA packs more efficiently in unit cell volume than MeOA.

A discrete lipid stoichiometry requires predicable and efficient packing. Three unit cell volumes are presented in 3-D views: Stearic Acid (SA) in Methyl Oleate (MeOA) (1/20), SA in MeOA (5/15), and SA in Docosahexaenoic Acid (DHA) (4/20). The Cartesian axes align with SA orientation within the cubic unit cell volume (views = X_{SA}, Y_{SA} and Z_{SA}). SA enhances the packing density of lipids within the unit cell volumes.

Lipid packing is a barrier to the flow of lipids from unit cell to unit cell and also into/out of aggregates of lipids. Steric hindrance precludes aggregates from unpacking. Void volume is the space that enables the mobility of lipids within the unit cell volume. Mathematically, the void volume in optimally packed equally sized spheres is 26% of the total volume; poorly packed spheres have up to 34% of the total volume empty [1]. In contrast void volume within a cubic unit cell can be 10% of the total volume.

Once a SA molecule filled the void volume in the lipid unit cell volume, diffusion into neighboring unit cells would be inhibited. By increasing the concentration of SA, the only structural space available would be from packing existing unit cells more efficiently. A 1/3 = 5/15 ratio of SA/MeOA packed efficiently into unit cells (Figure 2a). The mass of the unit cells contained 20 lipids whereas the 1/20 unit cells contained 21 lipids, so the kinetic energy of the 5/15 lipid had 5% less mass per unit cell than the 1/20 unit cell volume lipid. The kinetic energy of the smaller unit cell volume at a given temperature will be about 5% faster than the larger one. When a unit cell is anisotropic, the molecular dynamics will be anisotropic. X_{SA}, Y_{SA} and Z_{SA} directions label the axis corresponding to the axis of the SA molecules in the unit cell volume. In the X_{SA} direction, the unit cell was more tightly packed in the 5/15 ratio than in the 1/20 ratio unit cell; in the other two dimensions, the packing differences were almost indistinguishable from each other.

For mixing to occur, unit cell volumes need to exchange places with other lipid unit cell volumes (Figure 3). The void volume between unit cells was largest in the X_{SA} direction in the 5/15 unit cell. Mixing occurs with the neighboring unit cell in which X_{SA} direction of both are aligned. In this proposed mechanism, during one clockwise rotation of the 5/15 unit cell volume, five molecules of MeOA and 4 molecule of SA can very efficiently exchange site with a neighboring 1/20 unit cell volume. Thus, the 5/15 unit cell moved 25 Å (the length of a unit cell) in a Y direction and the 1/20 unit cell moved 25 Å in a (-Y) direction. Rotational motion resulted in translational motion.

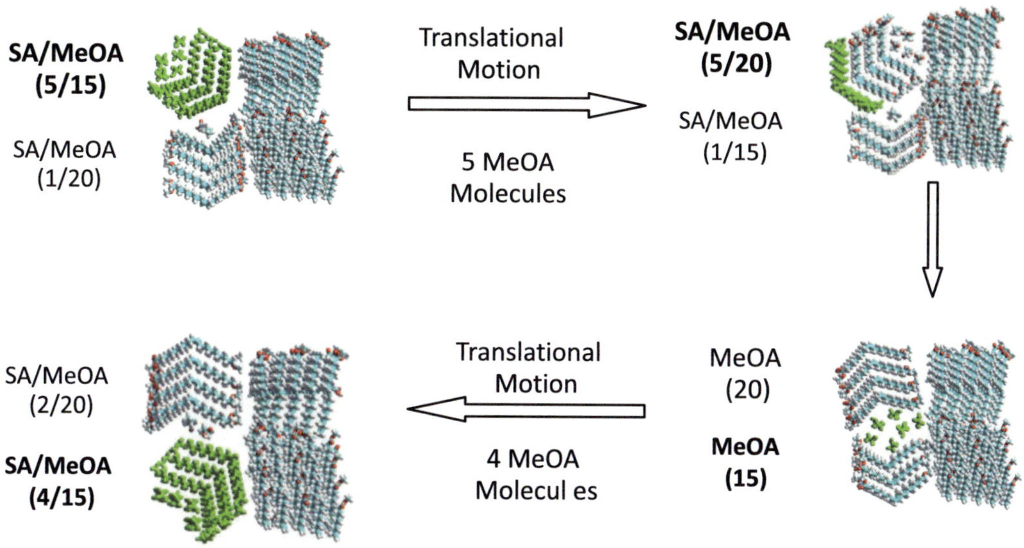

Fig. 3. Proposed mixing between two Unit Cell Volumes, each with a different lipid composition stoichiometry.

Lipid translational motion requires sufficient empty space/volume for this to occur. When three unit cell volumes of (1/20) mix with one unit cell volume of (5/15) SA/MeOA, the more dense packing in the (5/15) unit cell creates the space for SA exchange between two neighboring unit cells. Mixing of lipids between unit cells can appear to be diffusion of unit cell volumes, when in fact only a fraction of the total lipid molecules would be moving.

Uniformity in the distribution of unit cell volumes is not the same as uniformity of lipid composition "unit cell to unit cell." Translational motion of a specific chemical composition between two unit cells enables dispersing the unit cell with the higher SA concentration throughout the lipid. Lipids may be composed of at least two distinct unit cell volumes, non-uniform at the molecular level, yet macroscopically fully interspersed/mixed. Alternatively, lipids immiscible at the molecular level can also be non-uniformly dispersed throughout the lipid.

The DSC detected phase transitions during both cooling and heating cycles (Figure 4). On cooling the 2/20 SA/MeOA mixture from 65°C to 51°C, no thermal evidence of a phase transition was found. A very sharp DSC phase transition (width: 2 °C) began at 48 °C on the second cycle and the temperature lowered to 45 °C by the fourth cycle. A rapid exothermal phase transition indicates the products of this phase transitions were rather uniform, and suggests the mechanism causing it is uncomplicated. The simplest interpretation of the data is: two phases formed two discrete uniform unit cell volumes from one single uniform lipid liquid phase. The single uniform unit cell volumes could for example be same size and shape as the 5/15 unit cell volume. However, because of stoichiometry, for every 1.5 molecules of SA/15 MeOA present, the volume of 3.5 molecules of SA had been replaced with void volumes (1.5 +3.5 = 5). Alternatively, the unit cell volume could also be some volume intermediate between the two. Void volume adds to the average unit cell volume, and adds nothing to its mass. The sudden loss of volume with no loss in mass most probably is the structural basis for the rapid phase transition.

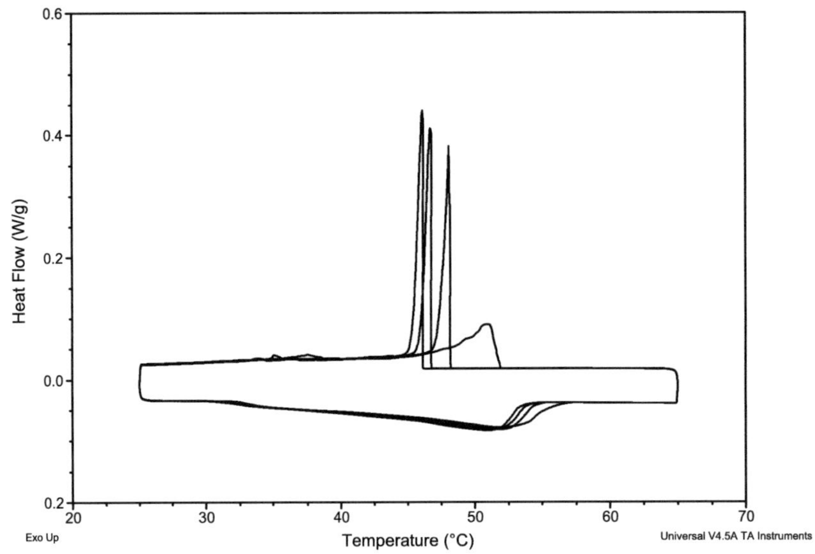

Fig. 4. DSC of two component lipids: SA and MeOA. Cycling of temperature enhances solids properties and uniformity of solids properties.

DSC of SA in MeOA (1/10). At 10% SA (wt/wt), the mixture with MeOA turned cloudy and a second phased forms. On cooling, a stable immiscible phase SA/MeOA (5/15) rapidly formed. Repeated cycling sharpened the phase transition on cooling but the very broad curve on heating remains quite similar.

In contrast, the very broad endothermic phase transition on heating occurred over a 20 °C temperature range. Mixing on heating took place by a different mechanism than separating out on cooling. Incorporating void volume into lipids is required for significant mixing to occur. Thus, the distribution of chemical composition and void volume during heating is necessarily localized. Since unit cell volume with different compositions have different mass, and unit cells with the same mass incorporating different void volumes will have a different unit cell volume, the rate of absorption of heat will not occur uniformly unit cell to unit cell. The unit cell volume, void volume and chemical composition must each be spatially uniform before the equal thermal properties at the molecular level can be spatially uniform.

Identifying fish oils by differences in thermal properties using DSC at very rapid heating and cooling rates has been reported [15]. Very rapid temperature ramping produced sharp phase transitions not evident in regular DSC experiments (as in Figure 1d). Rapid ramping can hide the asymmetry of fast cooling–slow heating kinetics, thus making both rates appear equal and the processes seem to be symmetrical.

Recently, modulated DSC (MDSC) procedures were developed [12]. Heat is added sinosoidally in place of linearly ramping temperature ($\Delta H_{mix} = 0$). MDSC can enable the thermodynamic and kinetic properties to be distinguished.

The temperature independent component (ΔS_{mix}) of the free energy of mixing (ΔG_{mix}) is accessible from constant temperature experiments. Thus the MDSC experiment was applied to 1/10 SA/MeOA (Figure 5). With a modulated heating rate and the sample held at a constant temperature for 100 minutes in each step (48 °C to 40 °C), changes were monitored. A very slight change in slope of the heat capacity (C_p) curves was observed for each temperature step until the sample reached 40 °C at which Cp increased by 23%. The thermal measurement was 5 - 10 °C lower than the phase transition temperature in the DSC experiment. Thus the DSC results included kinetic as well as thermodynamic components.

The MDSC result supports the conclusion that lipids do not necessarily transfer heat rapidly or uniformly. Thus some sites at the molecular level could be cooled to 40 °C even if the net temperature of the lipid was 48 °C. The change in Cp at 40 °C corresponds to the rapid conversion of a one phase-one unit cell volume into a two phase–two unit cell volume mixture in which each phase has a specific stoichiometry. In MDSC, solids properties form "quickly" in 100 minutes. The similar solids properties can be obtained from the same lipids in non-uniform temperatures in over 7000 minutes. Once formed, however, the solids properties last indefinitely. Latent heat in lipids may dissipate slowly because time is required for stoichiometry to be uniform enough for "relaxation" to occur. A simple mechanism to explain latent heat is that unit cells too large or too small to pack uniformly will diffuse into localized pockets of similar sized pockets. An equally viable explanation is that unit cell volumes containing variable amounts of packing inefficiency. Void volumes will migrate away from those which have less variability in packing volume. The unit cells which are more variable are most prone to absorb heat over a larger area; the areas which are most uniform in composition will heat and cool most uniformly. Non-uniformity in packing within a unit cell volume will most always correspond to non-uniform chemical composition within that unit volume.

The MDSC experiment corresponds to in effect an adiabatic constant temperature experiment. When the unit cell volumes are uniform, solids properties occur even when individual lipid molecules between unit cells may not be exactly uniformly packed. Even relatively small fluctuations in temperature may keep components mixed that at a constant temperature would in short order become immiscible.

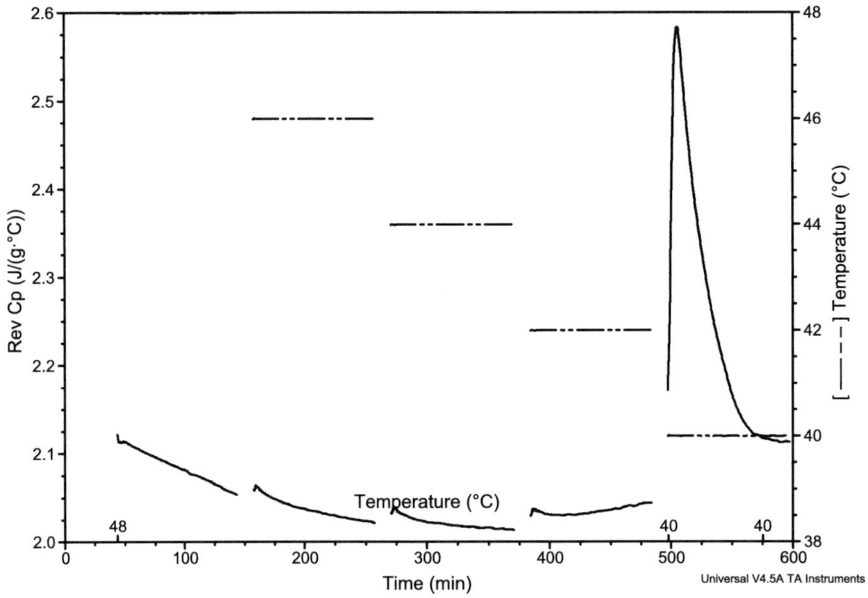

Fig. 5. Modulated DSC experiment in SA and MeOA demonstrates solids properties of lipid mixtures are thermodynamic properties. Kinetic properties of lipids can mask thermodynamic properties.

Although the precise chemical composition of and isolation procedures for natural lipids is variable, the molecular structure of DHA, seal oil, pig fat, and DHA-phosphotidylcholine (DHA-PC) has previously been characterized [2, 5, 6, 7, 9, 11]. Seal oil phase transition on cooling (42 °C) is easily distinguishable from the less unsaturated pig fat (51 °C). DHA phase transition (52 °C) is very different from DHA-PC (35 °C). The DSC of lipids (+ SA to form an immiscible phase) can be a rapid first pass tests for distinguishing whether two lipids are identical. This is evidence even though the SA portion in each has the identical size and shape, the 3-D packing around and within each unit cell volume depends upon the chemical composition of the non-SA lipids.

More important, however, is applying the thermal results to the molecular level packing of biochemically important lipids like DHA, lipids like the highly unsaturated DHA which dominates the composition of the photoreceptor, neurons, and synapses in the brain [3]. Ordered, close packing of the fatty acid chains in DHA neural lipids can facilitate the electrical functions (Crawford et al., 2008). DHA is a single chain lipid with six un-conjugated double bonds. SA + DHA had the DSC curve on cooling with the highest phase transition temperatures of the lipids analyzed. The shape of the DSC curve of DHA + SA was similar to that of MeOA + SA, except twice the level of SA was required to form an immiscible lipid phase and the phase transition temperature was higher.

The size and shape of a unit cell volume allows for only a specific number of molecules (each of which has its own size and shape). Especially large long molecules, inefficient packing always creates a large volume in which nothing large fits. The existence of stoichiometry in lipid unit cells is strong evidence that in fact unit cells are discrete sizes and shapes.

DHA molecular weight (328.5) is 111 % greater than for MeOA (296.5). Computational chemistry enabled comparing the packing in cubic unit cell volumes of immiscible phases containing (4/20) SA/DHA (volume = 14,484 A^3) with that of 2/20 SA/MeOA (volume = 13,128 A^3) (Figure 2a). The increase in mass was self consistent with the 110 % increase in volume, except the DHA volume contains four molecules of SA, not two as with MeOA. Thus with only one SA molecule per unit cell of DHA, a void volume equivalent to three molecules of SA would be present. Tight packing of the immiscible DHA phase at the molecular level can explain the high phase transition temperature of its DSC cooling curve. The thermodynamic data and the computational chemistry concur with the NMR study that previously reported that more highly unsaturated lipids pack tighter than less highly unsaturated lipids [13].

Interestingly, the molecular order within the unit cell parallels that of molecular order in lipid bilayer phases. Molecular level organization has previously been reported in lipid bilayers containing DHA [11]. They propose however molecular order in the bilayers is due to the presence of cholesterol. An alternative radically different explanation is that bilayer lipids already exist in unit cell volumes, and that cholesterol at the proper mole ratio fills up the void volume in the spacing of the lipids: in the presence of excess cholesterol, an immiscible phase forms. A similar mechanism can cause lipid bilayer formation. An unexpected conclusion of this research is that an ordered immiscible phase unit cell volume may routinely forms from an ordered miscible phase unit cell volume.

The miscibility/immiscibility phase separation in lipids is directly analogous to phase separation in ethyl acetate/water mixtures. Ethyl acetate freely dissolves in water up to a specific mole ratio; above that ratio, a second phase forms. The top layer is ethyl acetate saturated with water, the bottom layer is water saturated with ethyl acetate. As long as both phases are present, the further addition of ethyl acetate does not change the composition of either phase: only the volume fraction of each phase alters. The packing within the two distinct mole ratios of ethyl acetate to water results in a discrete phase difference. *There is no structural difference between the two layers because both layers contain exactly the same chemical components.* In the absence of a specific stoichiometry to the contrary, all lipids would be fully miscible. The simplicity of the experiments which result in lipid immiscibility is compelling evidence that the packing in the miscible phase and in the immiscible phase are not identical.

The immiscible phase in the case of SA/MeOA can be a soft solid, a gel, or even a liquid crystal. The immiscible phase is not a random event, but the direct consequence of a stoichiometry that exceeds the requirement of lipid miscibility. Moreover since it is the result of a thermodynamic process, once the immiscible phase forms, it stays around indefinitely.

A broad range of individual phase transition temperature and peak sharpness of DSC curves of in induced immiscible phase from only four structurally diverse lipids was found.

A very practical potential application of this technology is that by adding a small excess of SA (forming an immiscible phase) to a lipid, markers of biophysical characteristics of specific individual lipid compositions could be identified for quality control purposes or for distinguishing between natural and adulterated lipids.

Similar lipid phase transitions due to immiscibility most certainly occur routinely elsewhere. The difference between hard and soft bacon fat is primarily due to type of fat in the diet (i.e. saturated vs. unsaturated fat) [8]. Compositional difference between the two could be that soft bacon fat equals a miscible lipid phase and hard bacon equals an immiscible lipid phase. The primary difference between white and brown fat forming is the cell structure and tissue vascularization [16]. Brown fat can have systematically different physical properties from white fat in that white fat could have a different unit cell volume than brown fat. A diet rich in saturated and trans isomer fats is known to be a high risk factor for cardio-vascular disease [10]. These fats when present in the plasma membrane of the arterial endothelium could induce an accumulation of thicker, denser lipid in the membrane. This lipid phase immiscibility could explain the vasoconstriction causing the higher blood pressure required to force blood through smaller, less elastic capillaries. Trans fatty acids as well as saturated fats could similarly disrupt the packing of plasma membrane lipids. Exactly the same chemical components can be present below and above a critical triggering concentration ratio. In the immiscible phase, lipid mixtures packed more efficiently than precisely the same lipid components in a miscible phase: the fat in the newly formed phase would be more dense. All that changed chemically in forming a second phase would be a discrete change in the mole ratio of the new phase. The immiscible lipid phase would be thermodynamically stable.

Biodiesel mixtures of lipids are often initially perfectly clear. Days later, the same solutions turn cloudy. A simple explanation of cloudiness in biodiesel is that in some mixtures of biodiesel lipids, latent heat is released and some of the lipids pack more efficiently forming an immiscible phase. When latent heat is present, some units of volume with one mixture of lipid chemical structures retain more heat than per volume with a different ratio of lipid chemical structures. The molar volume over which chemical structure and thermal properties of lipids are integrated needs to be self-consistent. With spherical molecular volumes, summation of the global volume is larger than the volume of the spheres. A dam built of packed of soccer balls leaks because the volume of the dam is larger than the summation of the volumes of the soccer balls. The boundary between two discrete lipid phases is like a dam, slowing the mixing at the molecular level between two phases such that stoichiometry in each phase is discrete. The spherical model of lipid packing is "too leaky."

4. Conclusions

Structurally diverse lipids do not necessarily pack uniformly at the macroscopic or the molecular level. Since each of the mixtures of structurally diverse lipids had a finite capacity to incorporate long straight chain lipids [i.e. SA], macroscopic and/or molecular space had to have been available for the mixture of lipids to remain fully miscible. When this excess volume is filled [e.g. with SA], capacity for additional lipids of similar size/shape are precluded because the space has already been incorporated by the added lipid.

Additional SA does not perturb the miscible phase: in each of the lipid mixtures, Raman spectral frequencies are indistinguishable from of the same lipid phase before excess SA is added. The immiscible phase which forms unambiguously has more unsaturated lipid than saturated lipid. SA does not concentrate in an immiscible phase. Instead, it alters the packing of miscible phase such that the mixture is more dense. Adding additional SA does not alter the stoichiometry of the immiscible phase: it lower the mole fraction of the remaining miscible lipid phase. Unlike packing within a cubic unit cell volume, a spherical model of lipid packing neither predicts nor can explain a mechanism for this to occur.

Macroscopic stoichiometry occurs but it cannot explain any specific discrete molecular based stoichiometry. The smallest regularly shaped volume which adequately explains stoichiometry at the molecular level is the cubic unit cell volume. An immiscible phase perhaps may not be able to form without a new stoichiometry discretely different from the initial one.

DSC results demonstrate adding a small mole fraction of SA in structurally diverse lipids creates an ordered lipid phase. A spherical model of lipids predicts over time an ordered lipid state will diffuse into a uniform mixture. Instead, despite entropy, unit cells of similar size and shape form and then slowly pack uniformly, resulting in macroscopically observed lipid order that lasts indefinitely.

Stoichiometry in lipids is a normal consequence of molecular order at the unit cell level. Saturated lipids and trans-mono-unsaturated lipids are on average long straight rods; cis-mono-unsaturated lipids are at the molecular level are a flattened V shape; poly-cis-unsaturated lipids are a U shape. DHA is approximately an O shape. Mixtures of lipids of different shapes [and roughly the same molecular weight] appear to pack more efficiently than single component unsaturated fats alone. That more than one ratio of lipids can pack into a similar, if slightly smaller sized unit cell is the structural basis of immiscibility. The smallest volume in which the stoichiometry lipids can be uniform is a unit cell volume with one dimension being the molecular length of a single lipid molecule.

Since the physical properties of lipids correspond to the properties of aggregates of [e.g. 25] lipid molecule, mixtures of lipids of the same unit cell volume will always have physical properties similar to those of single component lipids to the extent that its unit cell volume is similar. Adding sufficient SA to a lipid alters the unit cell volume which alters its apparent density which in turn creates the macroscopically observed immiscible phase.

The stoichiometry between two immiscible phases will always be different.

5. References

[1] Aste, T. 2006. Volume fluctuations and geometrical constraints in granular packs. Physical Review Letters. 96, 018002.

[2] Broadhurst, C.L., Schmidt, W.F., Crawford, M.A., Wang, Y., Li R. 2004. 13C Nuclear Magnetic Resonance Spectra of Natural Undiluted Lipids: Docosahexaenoic-Rich Phospholipid and Triacylglycerol from Fish. J. Agric. Food Chem. 52, 4250-4255.

[3] Crawford M.A., Casperd, N.M., Sinclair, A.J. 1976. The long chain metabolites of linoleic and linolenic acids in liver and brain in herbivores and carnivores. Comp. Biochem. Physiol. 54B:395-401.

[4] Crawford M.A., Leigh, Broadhurst C., Galli, C., Ghebremeskel, K., Holmsen, H., Saugstad, L.F., Schmidt, W.F., Sinclair, A.J., Cunnane, S.C. 2008. The Role of Docosahexaenoic and Arachidonic Acids as Determinants of Evolution and Hominid Brain Development. In Fisheries for Global Welfare and Environment: K. Tsukamoto, T. Kawamura, T. Takeuchi, T. D. Beard, Jr. and M. J. Kaiser, eds., 5th World Fisheries Congress, pp. 57–76, Terrapub, Tokyo.

[5] Grahl-Nielson O. and O. Mjaavatten. 1991. Dietary influence on fatty acid composition of blubber fat of seals as determined by biopsy: a multivariate approach. Marine Biology. 110, 59-64.

[6] Gawrisch, K., Naddukkudy, V.E, Holte, L.L. 2003. The structure of DHA in Phospholipid membranes. Lipids. 38(4), 445-451.

[7] Huber, T, Rajamoorthi, K, Kurze V.F, Beyer, K, Brown M.F. 2002. Structure of docosahexanoic acid- containing phospholipid bilayers as studied by H2 NMR and molecular dynamics simulations. J. Am.Chem.Soc. 124(2), 298-309.

[8] Koch, D. E., Pearson, A. M., Magee, W. T., Hoefer J. A., Schweigert, B. S. 2008. Effect of Diet on the Fatty Acid Composition of Pork Fat. J. Anim. Sci. 27, 360-365.

[9] Maw, S.J, Fowler, V.R, Hamilton, M and Petchey, A.M. 2003. Physical characteristics of pig fat and their relation to fatty acid composition. Meat Science. 63, 185-190.

[10] Mozaffarian D., Katan, M..B., Ascherio, A. Stampfer, M.J. Willett W.C. 2006. Trans Fatty Acids and Cardiovascular Disease. N. Engl. J. Med. 354(15) 1601-13.

[11] Pitman, M.C, Suits, F., MacKerell, A.D., Feller, S.E. 2004. Molecular Level Organization of Saturated and Polyunsaturated Fatty Acids in a Phosphatidylcholine Bilayer Containing Cholesterol Biochemistry 43, 15318-15328.

[12] Rabel, S.R, Jona, J.A, Maurin, M.B. 1999. Applications of modulated differential scanning calorimetry in preformulation studies. J. Pharmaceutical and Biomedical Analysis. 21, 339-345.

[13] Schmidt, W.F, Barone, J.R, Francis, B, Reeves III, J.B. 2006. Stearic acid solubility and cubic phase volume. Chem.and Phys.of Lipids.142, 23-32.

[14] Schmidt, W.F, Mookherji, S.,Crawford, M.A. 2009. Unit cell volume and liquid-phase immiscibility in oleate-stearate lipid mixtures. Chem.and Phys.of Lipids. 158, 10-15.

[15] Schubring, R. Crystallization and melting behaviour of fish oil measured by DSC. 2009. J. Thermal analysis and Calorimetry. 95, 823-830.

[16] Seale, R., Bjork, B.,Yang, W., Kajimura, S., Chin, S., Kuang, S., Scime, A., Devarakonda, S., Conroe, H., Erdjument-Bromage, H., Tempst, P., Rudnicki, M.A., Beier, D.R., Spiegelman, B.M. 2008. PRDK16 controls a brown fat/skeletal muscle switch. Nature 454(21), 961-968.

[17] Seelig J and W Niederberger. 1974. Deuterium-labeled lipids as structural probes in liquid crystalline bilayers. Journal of American Chemical Society. 96(7), 2069-2072

[18] Uauy R., Hoffman D.R., Peirano P., Birch D.G., Birch E.E. 2001. Essential fatty acids in visual and brain development. Lipids. 36(9), 885-95.

[19] Yavin E., Himovichi E., Eilam R. 2009. Delayed cell migration in the developing rat brain following maternal Omega 3 alpha linolenic acid dietary deficiency. Neuroscience. 162(4):1011-22.

7

Stoichiometry of Polymer Complexes

A.Z. El-Sonbati, M.A. Diab and A.A. El-Bindary
Chemistry Department, Faculty of Science,
Mansoura University, Demiatta,
Egypt

1. Introduction

Polymer complexes have been attracting interest in many scientific and technological fields in recent years. Polymer complexes have found wide applications in bioinorganic industry (Fenger & Le Drian, 1998), wastewater treatment (Mizuta et al., 2000), pollution control (Orazzhanova et al., 2003), hydrometallurgy (Varvara et al., 2004), preconcentration (Ro et al., 2003), anionic polyelectrolyte hydrogels (Varghesa et al., 2001), cation-exchange resins (Ahmed et al., 2004) etc. Moreover, they recently showed potential applications in material science as catalytic, conductive, luminescent, magnetic, porous, chiral or non-linear optical materials (Janiak, 2003; James, 2003; Maspoch et al., 2004; Batten & Murray, 2003).

Although various extensive investigations on polymer complexes have been reported, most of these complexes are too complicated to be discussed quantitatively due to the non-uniformity of their structure. These compounds include not only "complexes of macromolecules" but also the structurally labile "metal complex". Before detailed information can be obtained about the properties of polymer complexes, in particular about the reactivity and the catalytic activity, their structure must be elucidated. A polymer complex possessing a uniform structure may be defined as follows:

- The structure within the coordination sphere is uniform, i.e. the species and the composition of the ligand and its configuration are identical in any complex unit existing in the polymer complex;
- The primary structure of the polymer ligand is known.
- If the structure within the coordination sphere is identical in a polymer and in a monomeric complex, their reactivity ought to be the same even though the complex is bound to a polymer chain. However, it is clear that the reactivity is sometimes strongly affected by the polymer ligand that exists outside the coordination sphere surrounding the metal complex. The effect of polymer ligands can be explained in terms of two factors:
- the steric effect, which is determined by the conformation and density of the polymer ligand chain;
- the special environment constituted by a polymer ligand domain.

Hence, it is possible to prepare polymer complexes having different use and applications by varying the polymer chain, the nature of the ligand and the metal ion.

A polymer complex is composed of synthetic polymer and metal ions, with the metal ions bound to the polymer ligand by a coordinate bond. A polymer ligand contains anchoring sites like nitrogen, oxygen or sulphur obtained either by polymerization of monomer possessing the coordinating site or by a chemical reaction between a polymer and a low molecular weight compound with coordinating ability. The synthesis results in an organic polymer with inorganic functions. The metal atoms attached to the polymer backbone are bound to exhibit a characteristic catalytic behavior, distinctly different from their low molecular weight analogues. Indeed, many synthetic polymer complexes have been found to possess high catalytic activity, in addition to semiconductivity, heat resistance and biomedical potentials.

This review will focus mainly on the stoichiometry and the characterization of polymer complexes structure by using elemental analyses, electronic spectra, magnetic susceptibilities, FT-IR, IR, ^{1}H-NMR, ESR and thermogravimetric analyses.

2. Classification of polymer metal complexes

The polymer complexes may be classified into three different groups according to the position occupied by the metal, which is decided by the methods of preparation:

1. Complexation of polymeric ligand with metal ions which could be divided into two categories:
   a. Pendant metal polymer complexes.
   b. Inter/intra-molecular bridged polymer complexes.
2. Complexation of multifunctional ligands with a metal.
3. Polymerization of metal containing monomers.

2.1 Complexation of polymeric ligand with metal ion

Only decades ago polychelats derived from polymeric ligands and transition metal ions attracted the attention of many investigators. Bamford, Jenkins and Johnson (Bamford et al., 1958) were the first who noticed and described that radical polymerization of vinyl monomers is accelerated by addition of an inorganic salt not participating in redox reactions. They showed that the rate of polymerization of acrylonitrile (AN) initiated by azobisisobutyronitrile (AIBN) in dimethyl formamide (DMF), increases when lithium chloride is dissolved in the reaction mixture. According to the kinetic measurements, the effect was ascribed to an increased propagation of the rate constant and explained by the complexation of the nitrile groups at the radicals with lithium chloride.

A number of authors (Tazuke & Okamura, 1966; Tazuke et al. 1966; Tazuke & Okamura, 1967) have studied radical polymerization of this type. From a kinetic point of view methyl methacrylate (MMA) and AN-metal salt ($AlCl_3$, $AlBr_3$, $ZnCl_2$, $GaCl_2$, etc) systems were most intensively investigated (Imoto et al., 1963; Bamford et al., 1966a & Zubov et al., 1968). The increased reactivity of the complexed monomer has been attributed to the delocalization of the electrons in the double and triple bonds of the acceptor monomer as a result of the complexation with the electron accepting metal halide (Fig. 1) (Lazuke et al., 1967).

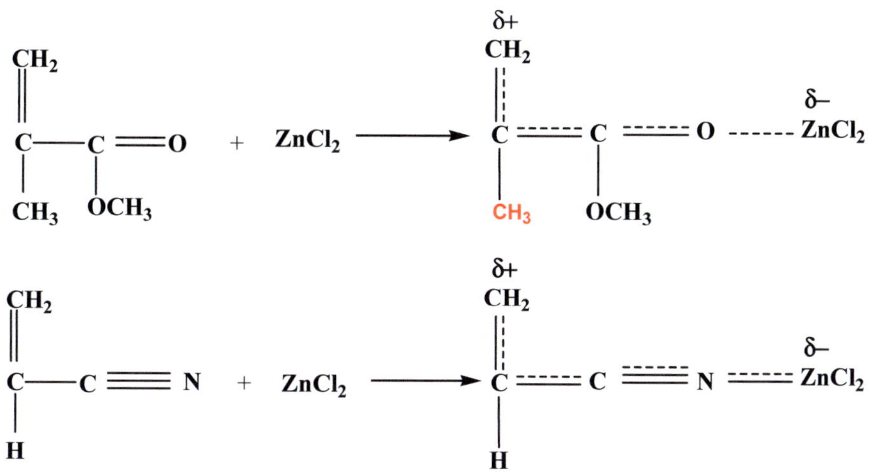

Fig. 1.

The new electrophilic acceptor monomer has an increased rate constant and an unchanged termination rate constant resulting in a more rapid rate of propagation and in the formation of a higher molecular weight polymer (Banford et al., 1966b). The kinetics of polymerization were extended to methyl acrylate (MA) with transition metal bromides (El-Sonbati et al., 1992). The presence of Cu(II), Ni(II) and Zn(II) bromides retards the rate of polymerization. This retardation effect of the polymerization of MA is attributable to the formation of addition products, which must be inactive in initiating the polymerization of MA and decrease the rate of polymerization in the order MA-$ZnBr_2$ < MA-$CuBr_2$ < MA-$NiBr_2$.

The enhanced reactivity of the complex monomer extends to copolymerization with olefinic or allylic monomer, which is poorly responsive to free radical initiated polymerization (Imoto et al., 1965; Serniuk & Thomas, 1965; Serniuk & Thomas, 1966). The free radical initiated copolymerization of such monomers which a metal halide complexed polar monomer results in an increased concentration of olefinic monomer in the polymer as compared with that obtained in the absence of the complexing agent, as well as an increase in the polymer molecular weight.

The reaction of polymer ligands with metal ions usually results in various coordination structures, which are divided into pendant and inter- and/or intra-molecular bridged complexes.

2.1.1 Pendant polymer complexes

The metal ion in a pendant metal complex is attached to the polymer ligand function, which is appended on the polymer chain. Based on the chelating abilities of the ligands, pendant complexes are classified as monodentate or polydentate polymer metal complexes.

a. Monodentate pendant polymer complexes

A metal ion or a metal complex has only one labile ligand, which is easily substituted by a polymeric ligand, and when other coordination sites are substitution inactive, the complex formed has a simple structure of monodentate type as shown in Fig. 2.

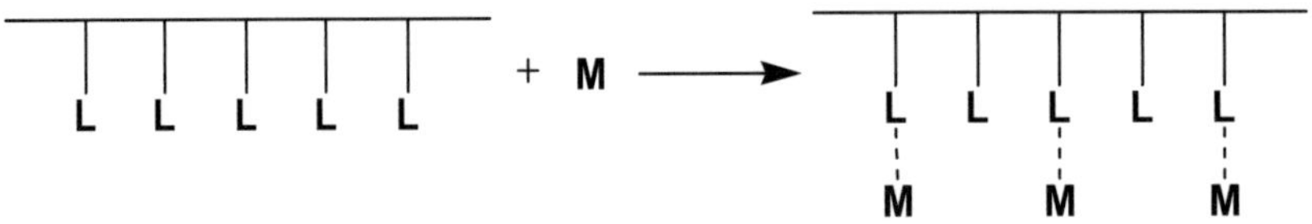

Fig. 2.

If the metal ion or metal complex has more than two labile ligands, it is often possible to realize a monodentate complex structure by selecting an appropriate reaction condition (Kaneko & Tsuchide, 1981). Important characteristics of this type of polymer complexes are:

i. The coordination is very clear.
ii. The effect of the polymer chain is clearly exhibited.
iii. The polymer complex is very often soluble in water or in organic solvents.

The reaction of poly(4-vinylpyridine)(PVP) with various metal chelates such as cis$[Co(en)_2Cl_2]Cl.H_2O$ (en = ethylendiamine), cis-α-$[Co(trien)Cl_2]Cl.H_2O$, (trien = triethylenetetramine) and cis-$[Co(en)_2PyCl]Cl_2$ (Py = pyridine) gives simple structures of monodentate type (Fig. 3) (Kurimura et al., 1971; Tsuchide et al., 1974).

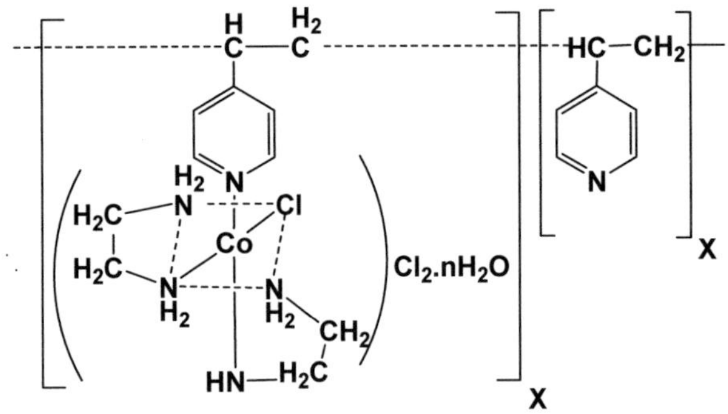

cis-$[Co(en)_2$ PVPCl] $Cl_2.nH_2O$

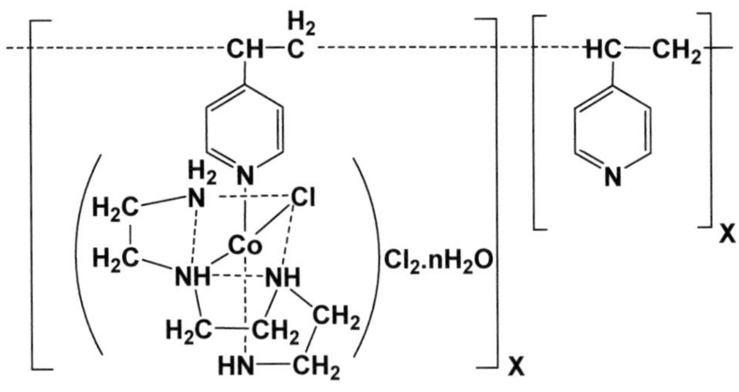

cis-$[Co(trien)_2PVPCl]Cl_2.nH_2O$

Fig. 3.

Soluble copper chloride complexes of poly(2-vinylpyridine) (P2VPy) were prepared (Lyons et al., 1988) in a methanol-water solution. Solubility was achieved with the proper solvent system due to the sterically hindered environment of the ligand, allowing only one pyridine moiety to complex each copper cation. Partial reduction of the cupric cation occurred during sample preparation, as observed by X-ray photoelectron spectroscopy (XPS) and magnetic susceptibility measurements.

b. Polydentate pendant polymer complexes

When the polymer pendant coordination group has a polydentate structure, the coordination structure of the polymer metal complex is very clear, and high stability can be expected as shown in Fig. 4.

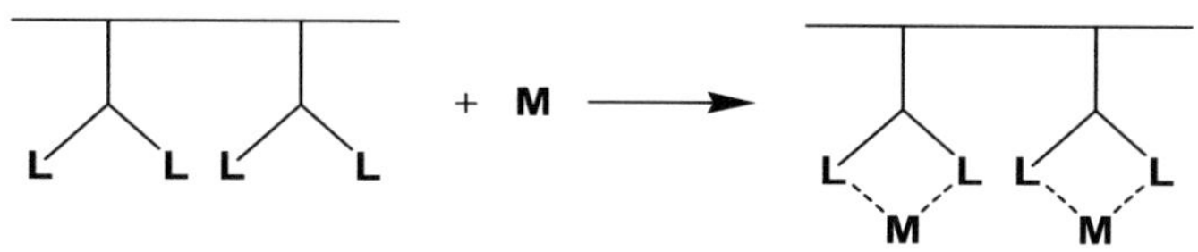

Fig. 4.

2.1.2 Inter-and/or intra-molecular bridging polymer complexes

The reaction of polymer ligands with metal ions very often results in inter-and/or interamolecular bridging (Fig. 5).

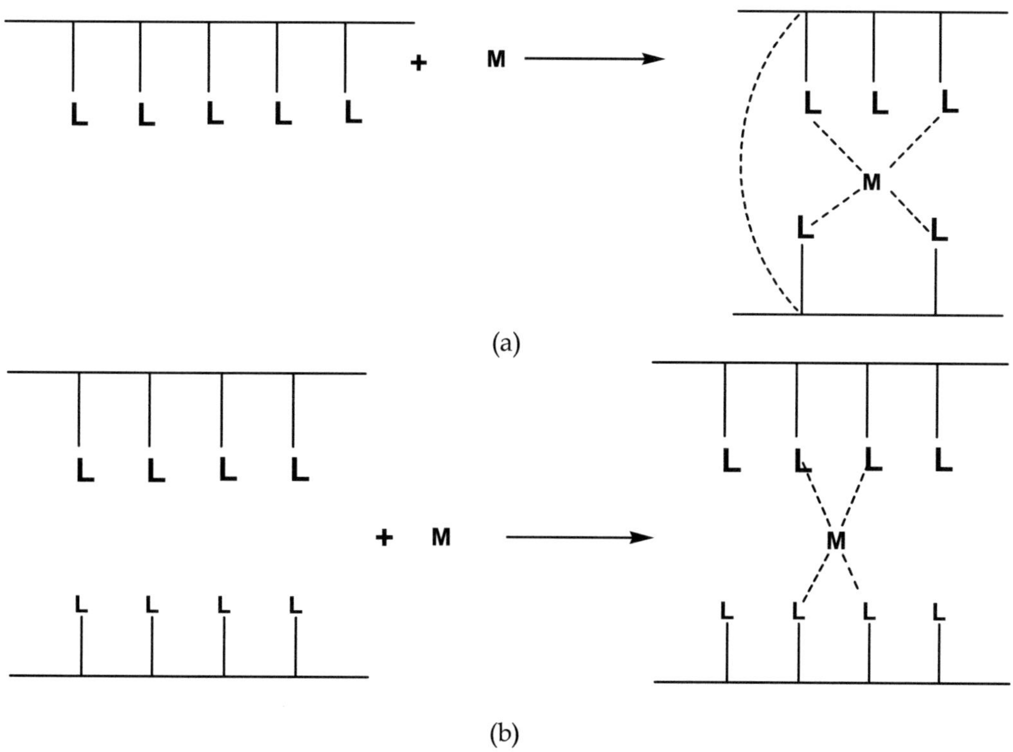

L : Coordinate atom (or) group, M = Metal ion, a : intra-polydentate, b : inter-polydentate

Fig. 5.

The coordination structure of the resulting polymer metal complex is not clear in this case, and the polymer complex is sometimes insoluble in water or in organic solvent. It is usually difficult to distinguish between the inter and intra-molecular bridging. The fact that it is not often easy to elucidate the polymer effect in studying the characteristics of the polymer complex. The simplest example of this type of polymer complex is the poly(vinyl alcohol)(PVA)-Cu(II) complex (Fig. 6) (Hojo & Shiria, 1972).

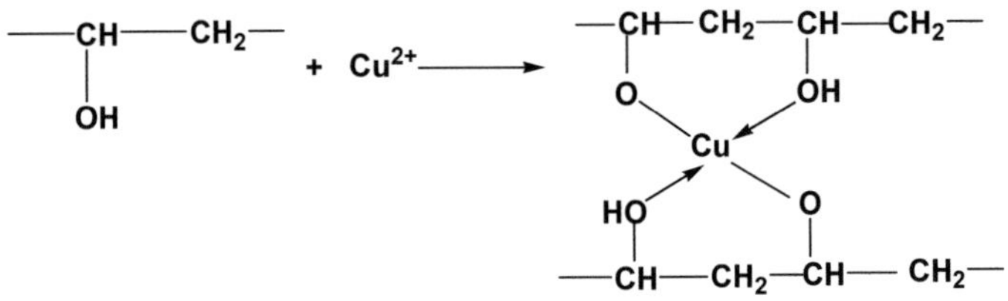

Fig. 6.

The coordination reaction is generally affected by the polymer ligand tacticity. The different coordination behavior of atactic poly (4-vinylpyridine)(PVP) and isotactic (2-vinylpyridine)(P2VP) with $M(II)Cl_2$, where M=Co, Ni, Cu or Zn, is reported (Agnew, 1976). Atactic PVP and $NiCl_2$ precipitated a mixture of a tetrahedral structure having stoichiometry $Ni(PVP)_2Cl_2$. Isotactic P2VP gave no precipitation with $NiCl_2$ in ethanol, showing no coordination in UV and visible spectra as shown in Fig. 7.

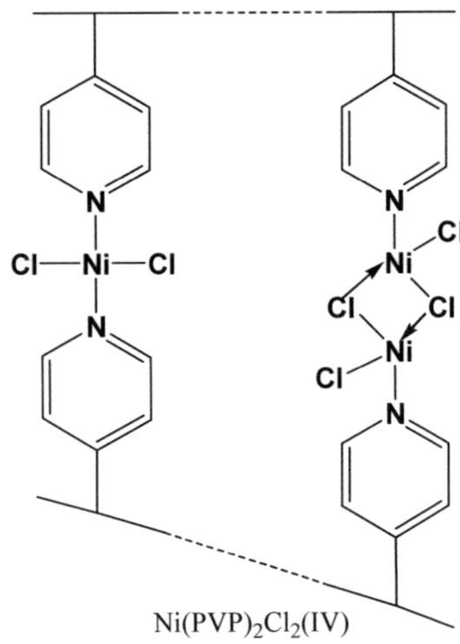

Fig. 7.

2.1.3 The chain linked through complexation of bifunctional ligands with metal ions

When bifunctional ligands form a complex with metal ions having more than two labile ligands, i.e. easily replaceable a polymer complex (Fig. 8) is formed through metal ion bridging.

This type of polymer metal complex has been synthesized as semiconducting organic materials (Katon, 1970), heat resistant organic polymer or polymer catalysts. Bridged ligands able to form polymer metal complexes of this type are classified as follows : (i) compounds having more than two coordinating groups, and (ii) simple compounds having more than two coordinating atoms, or simple ions which are able to function as bridged ligands. When the complex formation of ligands having four coordinating groups induces chemical reaction between the ligands, the resulting polymer complex sometimes has a network structure.

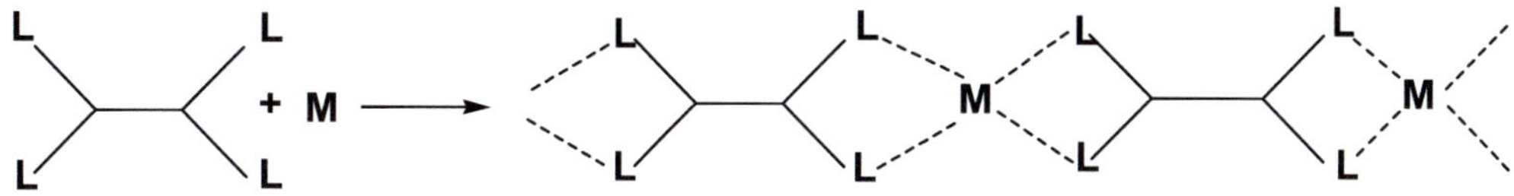

Fig. 8.

a. Linear coordinated polymer

i. Linked by a bifunctional ligand

Dithiooxamide (rubeanic acid) is a typical bifunctional ligand which forms a linear-type polymer metal complex with metal ions (Fig. 9) (Amon & Kane, 1950).

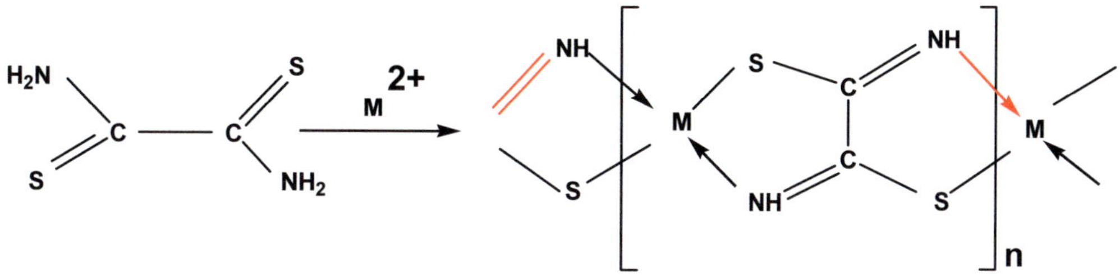

Fig. 9.

ii- Linked by simple compound or ion

A simple ion or compound can work as a bridging ligand giving a polymeric structure. A metal salt such as cupric chloride forms an associated structure (Fig. 10) in a very concentrated aqueous solution of hydrogen chloride (Wertz & Tyvoll, 1974) with the chloride ions occupying as bridging ligands both the axial and equatorial coordination sites of Cu^{2+}.

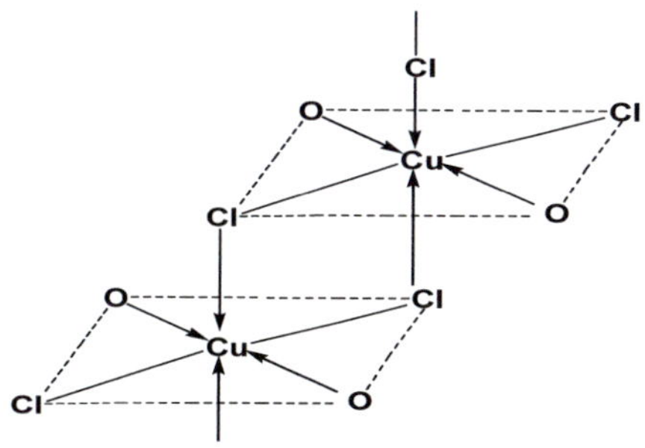

(V)

Fig. 10.

b. Network-coordinated polymers

The most usual method to prepare this type of complexes is use a "template reaction". This is a reaction between two functional groups of the ligand induced by their coordination to the metal ion, resulting in a chelated-type metal complex (Fig. 11).

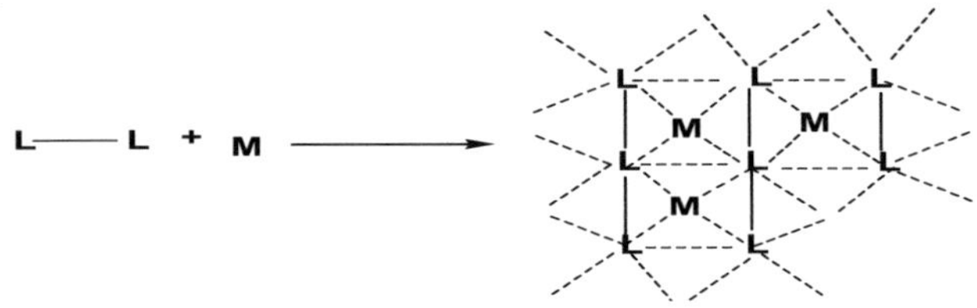

Fig. 11.

A typical example is poly(metal phthalocyanine) formed during the reaction of tetracyanobenzene with metal halides catalyzed by urea as shown in Fig. 12 (Epstein & Wildi, 1960).

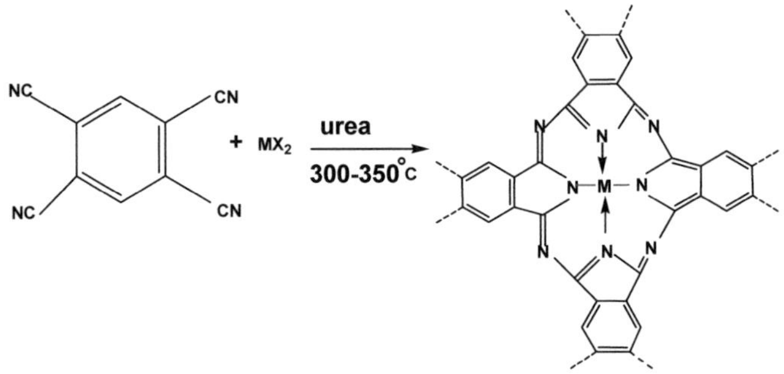

Fig. 12.

2.1.4 Formation through polymerization of metal complexes

Polymer containing the metal as part of a pendent or substituent group may be formed when complex possessing functionalized ligands undergo polymerization. The most widely studied are vinyl complexes and their derivatives, formed through radical polymerization of vinyl monomer containing transition metal ions. Vinyl compounds of metal complex are polymerized giving polymer metal complexes as shown in Fig. 13.

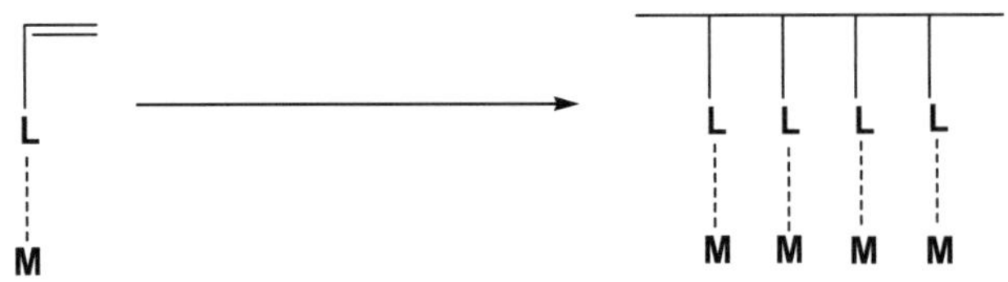

Fig. 13.

This type of polymer complex is characterized by its clear coordination structure. Nevertheless, the limitations of the vinyl compounds, and the metal complex tendency to hinder the vinyl polymerization, may constitute an obstacle in this type of polymerization.

Methacrylate monomer coordinated to Co(III) complex, e.g. methacrylato-pentaamine cobalt (III) perchlorate, was radically polymerized giving the polymer (VI) (Fig. 14) (Osada, 1975; Osada, 1976a; Osada, 1976b; Osada & Ishida, 1976).

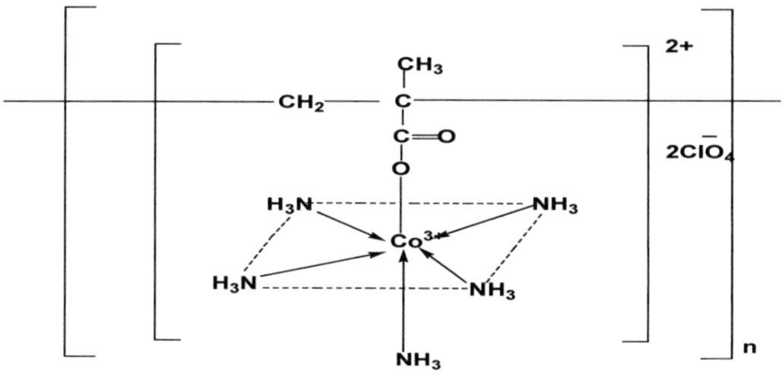

(VI)

Fig. 14.

The free radical initiated polymerization of polar monomers containing pendant nitrile and carbonyl groups, e.g. acrylonitrile and methyl methacrylate, in the presence of metal halides such as $ZnCl_2$ and $AlCl_3$ is characterized by an increased rate of polymerization. On the contrary, the formation of polymers with considerably higher molecular weight is likely in the absence of the metal halide (Bamford et al, 1957; Bovey, 1960; Arthur & Blouin, 1964).

The reaction of methyl methacrylate (MMA) with transition metal bromides gives examples of bidentated polymer complexes (El-Sonbati & Diab, 1988a) as shown in Fig. 15.

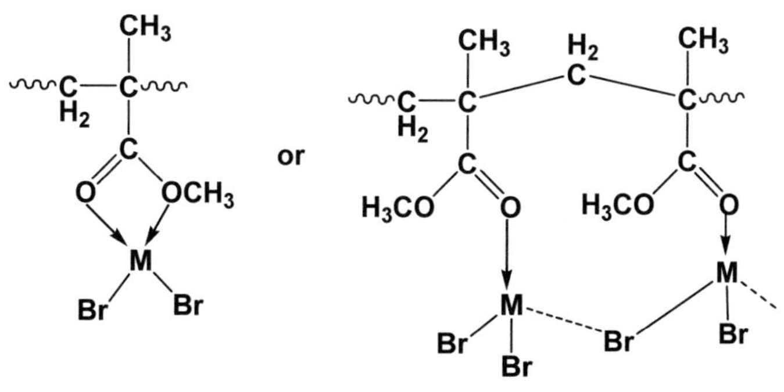

M = Cu(II), Co(II) and Ni(II)

Fig. 15.

This behavior is similar to the one suggested (Kabanov, 1969) for the polymerization of MMA in presence of inorganic salts such as $ZnCl_2$ and $AlBr_3$.

The polymerization of acrylonitrile (AN) in presence of Cu(I), Cu(II), Co(II), Ni(II) and Cd(II) bromides was studied (El-Sonbati & Diab, 1988b & 1988c). The IR spectrum of the formed AN-Cu(II) bromide polymer complex shows the absence of the C≡N band and the presence of two new bands corresponding to NH_2 and OH groups. These bands are not found with the other metal bromide polymer complexes (Fig. 16). It seem that Cu(II) is reduced to the stable Cu(I) during the polymerization of AN-Cu(II) bromide.

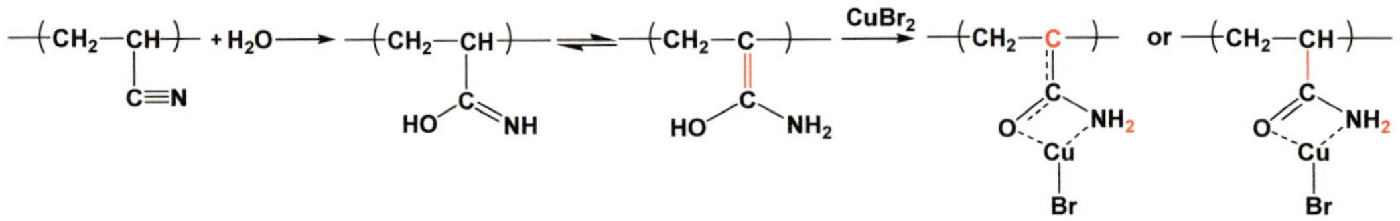

Fig. 16.

Poly(8-quinolyl acrylate)(P8-QA) and the polymers of the complexes of 8-quinolyl acrylate (8-QA) with some transition metal bromides and uranyl acetate have been prepared and characterized (El-Sonbati & Diab, 1988d). Dioxouranium(VI) acetate dehydrate reacts with 8-QA monomer in a 1:3 metal:ligand molar ratio. On the other hand, 8-QA reacts with Cu(II), Ni(II) and Co(II) bromides in such a way that the polychelates have 1:2, metal:ligand stoichiometry as shown in Fig. 17.

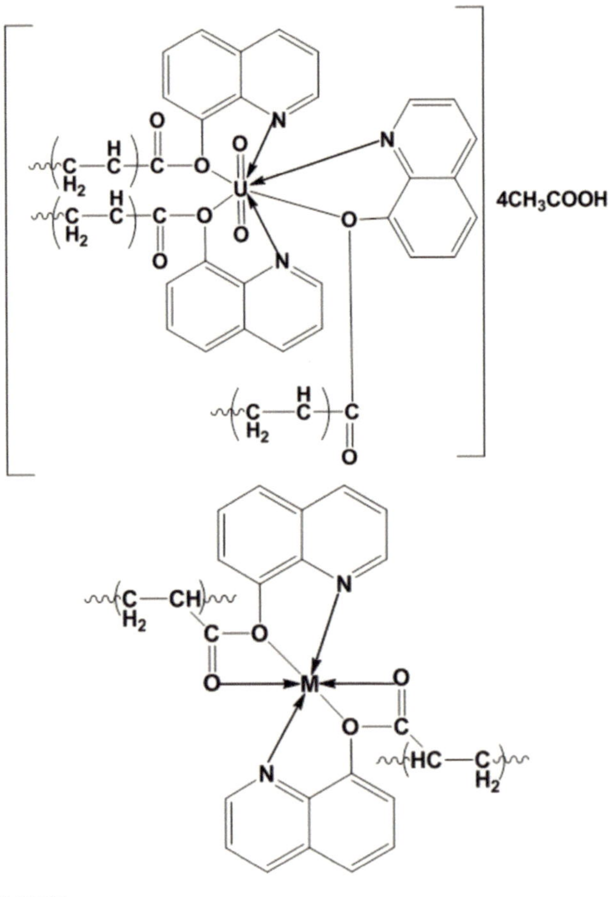

M = Cu(II), Co(II) and Ni(II)

Fig. 17.

Poly(acrylamido-4-aminoantipyrinyl)(PAA) homopolymer and polymer complexes of acrylamido-4-aminoantipyrinyl (AA) with some transition metal bromides and uranyl acetate have been prepared (El-Sonbat et al., 1989)). Dioxouranium(VI) acetate dehydrate reacts with AA in a 1:2 and with $CuBr_2$, $NiBr_2$ and $CoBr_2$ in 1:1 metal:ligand molar ratios and the polychelates of the types shown in Fig. 18.

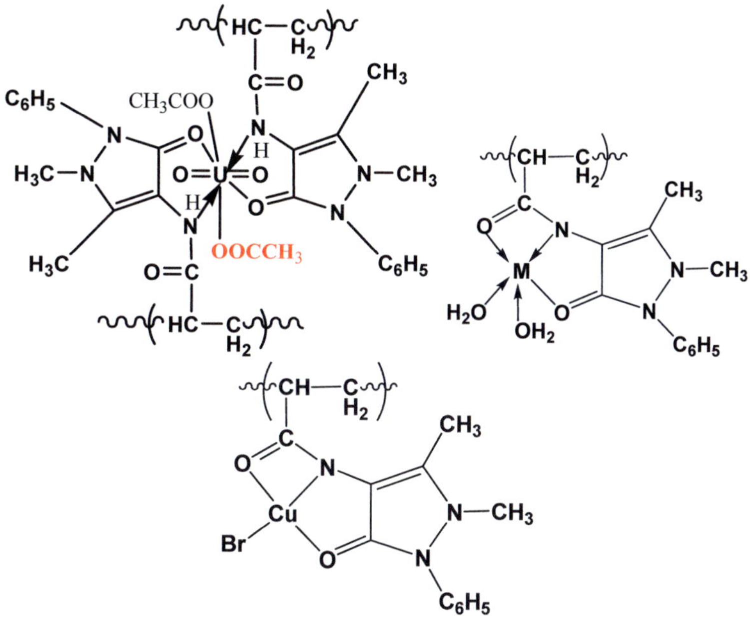

M = Co(II) and Ni(II)

Fig. 18.

Poly(2-acrylamidophenol)(PAP) homopolymer and polymer complexes of 2-acrylamidophenol (AP) with Cu(II), Ni(II), Co(II), Cd(II) chlorides and uranyl acetate were prepared and characterized (Diab et al., 1988). The phenolic C-O IR band has been shifted of ± 15 cm^{-1}, indicating that it is involved in the coordination of AP-$CuCl_2$ and AP-$CdCl_2$ polymer complexes (Fig. 19). There is a change in the position of NH band to lower frequency, indicating the recruitment of these groups in the coordination of AP-$CoCl_2$ and AP-$NiCl_2$ polymer complexes. The possible structures of AP-Cu(II), AP-Ni(II), AP-Co(II), AP-Cd(II) chlorides and uranyl acetate are the following:

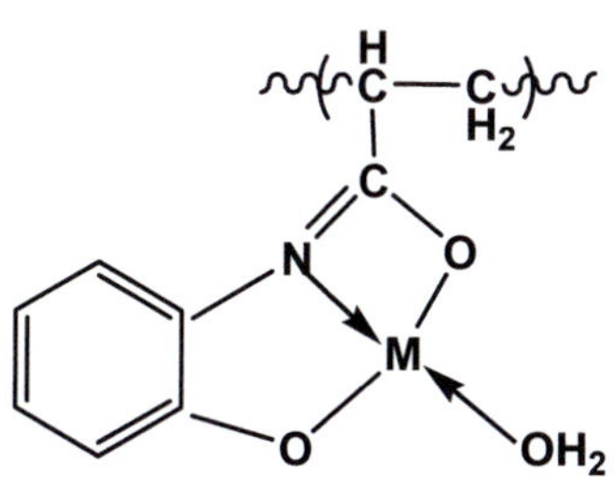

M = Cu(II) and Cd(II)

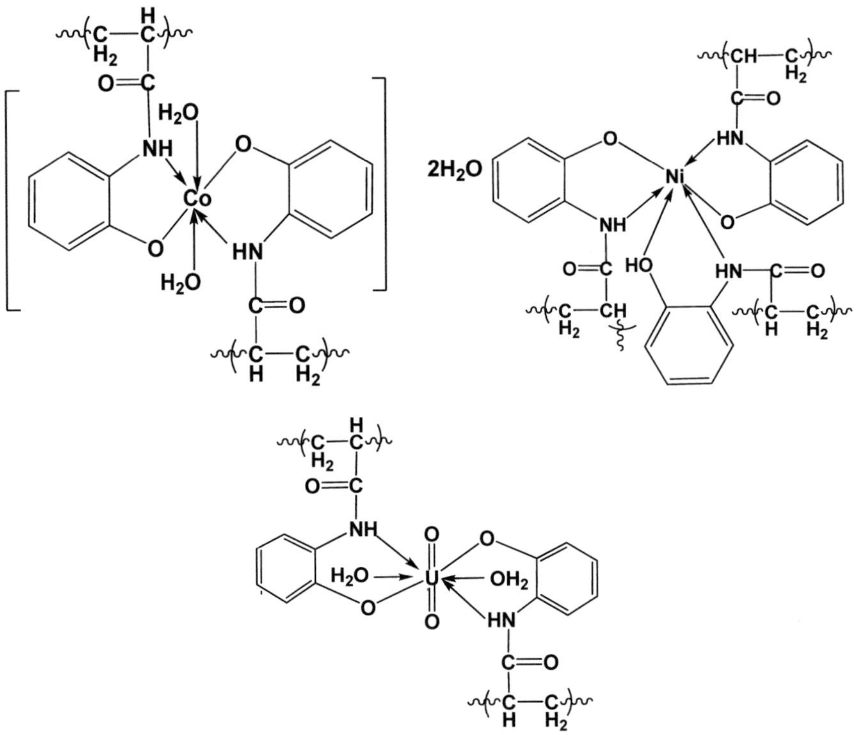

Fig. 19.

Poly(2-acrylamidopyridine)(PAP) homopolymer and polymer complexes of 2-acrylamidopyridine (AP) with some transition metal chlorides have been prepared and characterized (Diab et al., 1989a). IR spectrum of PAP homopolymer indicates two tautomeric forms are shown in Fig. 20.

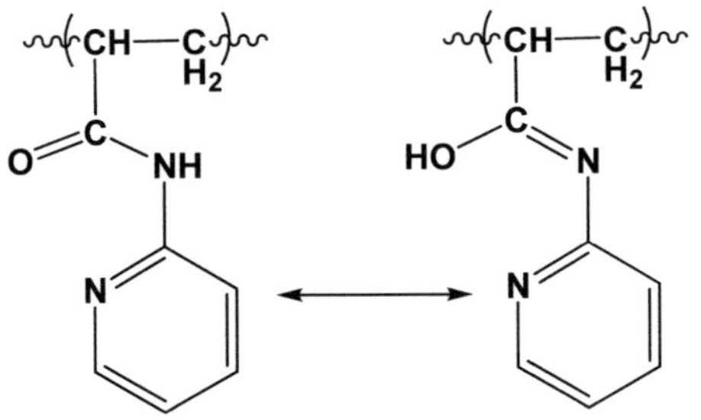

Fig. 20.

The IR spectrum of AP-$CuCl_2$ polymer complex shows a lowering of the OH stretching frequency by about 10-15 cm^{-1} indicating that the OH group is involved in the coordination (Fig. 21). An increase in the frequency of the pyridine nitrogen indicates that it takes part in the bond formation. Moreover, new bands appeared in the spectrum assigned to υ(M-O), υ(M-N) and υ(M-Cl). It may be deduced that the probable structure of AP-$CuCl_2$ polymer complex is:

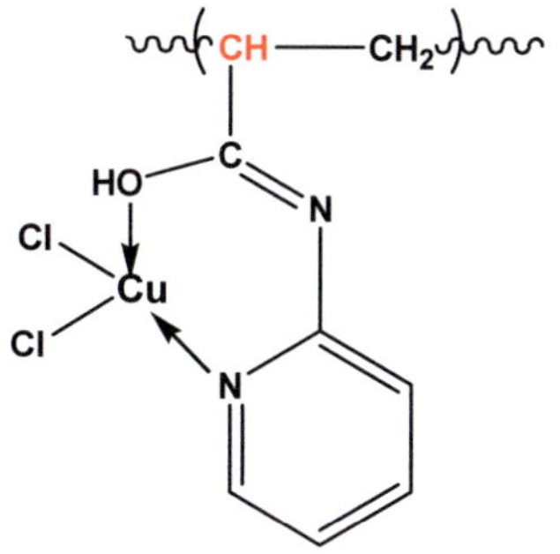

Fig. 21.

The IR spectra of AP-$CoCl_2$, AP-$NiCl_2$ and AP-$CdCl_2$ polymer complexes have the characteristic features of coordination between the nitrogen atom of the pyridine ring and the oxygen atom of the hydroxyl group. AP reacts with $NiCl_2$, $CoCl_2$ in a 2:1 ratio and with $CdCl_2$ in a 1:1 ratio. The possible structures of AP-$NiCl_2$, AP-$CoCl_2$ and AP-$CdCl_2$ polymer complexes (Fig. 22) are the following:

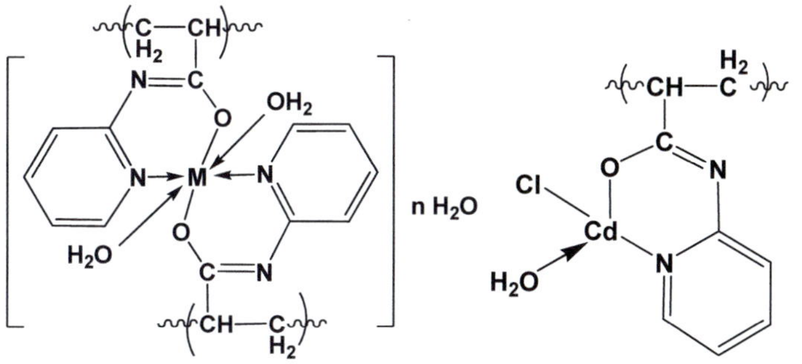

Fig. 22.

It was found that poly[bis(2,6-diaminopyridine sulphoxide)](PDPS) homopolymer and polymer complexes of bis(2,6-diaminopyridine sulphoxide)(DPS) with $CuCl_2$, $CuBr_2$ and CuI_2 were prepared and characterized (Diab et al., 1989b). The mode of complexation of the polymer complexes of PDPS with copper halides is derived as shown in Fig. 23.

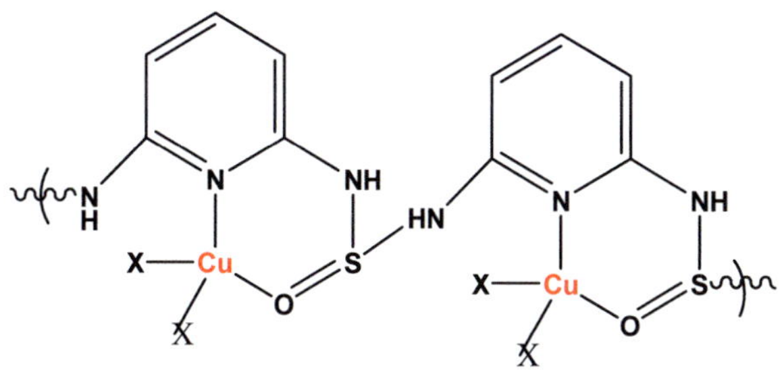

Fig. 23.

Poly(5-vinyl salicylaldehyde)(PVS) homopolymer and polymer complexes of 5-vinylsalicylaldehyde (VS) with $CuCl_2$, $CoCl_2$, $NiCl_2$ and uranyl acetate were synthesized and characterized (El-Hendawy, 1989). The IR spectrum of VS-$CuCl_2$ polymer complex shows a shift of υ(C=O) to a lower frequency by about 15 cm^{-1} and the υ(C-O) of the phenolic group is shifted to a higher frequency by about 25 cm^{-1} indicating that both groups are involved in the complexation. From the spectroscopic data, the magnetic moments and the elemental analysis, it is concluded that VS reacts with $CuCl_2$, $CoCl_2$ and $NiCl_2$ in the ratio 2:1. The possible structure of the polymer complexes VS-$CuCl_2$, VS-$CoCl_2$ and VS-$NiCl_2$ may be as shown in Fig. 24.

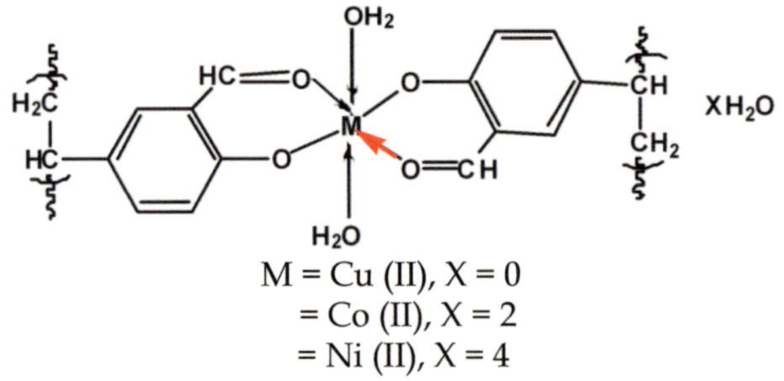

Fig. 24.

VS reacts with uranyl acetate in 1:2 metal:ligand stoichiometry (Fig. 25).

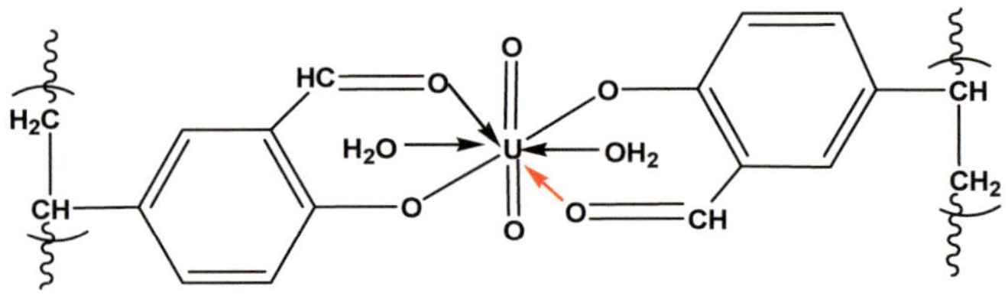

Fig. 25.

Polymer complexes of 2-acrylamidobenzoic acid (ABA) with transition metal chlorides and uranyl acetate were prepared and characterized (Diab et al., 1990a). ABA reacts with uranyl ions in a 2:1 molar ratio. The chelation occurs through one of the two oxygens of the carboxylate ion, which is represented as a tautomeric form as shown in Fig. 26.

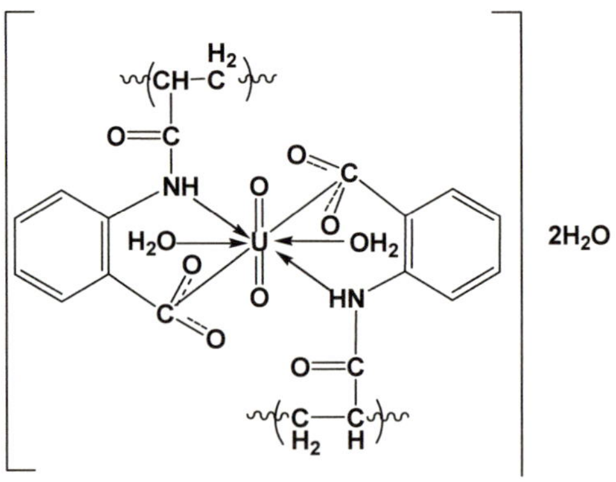

Fig. 26.

ABA reacts with Cu(II), Co(II), and Ni(II) in a 2:1 molar ratio of monomer unit: metal. The structure of the polychelates (Fig. 27) is of the type:

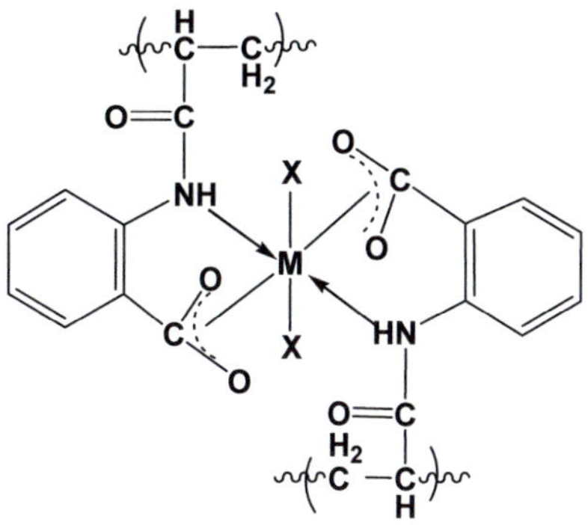

M = Co(II); X = H_2O
M = Cu(II) and Ni(II); X = 0

Fig. 27.

Poly(5-vinylsalicylidene anthranilic acid)(PVSA) homopolymer and polymer complexes of 5-vinylsalicylidene anthranilic acid (VSA) with some transition metal chlorides and uranyl acetate were prepared (Diab et al., 1990b). The IR spectrum of VSA-uranyl acetate polymer complex shows a change in the position of azomethine nitrogen and carboxylate ion groups indicating their involvement in coordination. Elemental analysis and IR spectrum reveal that VSA reacts with uranyl acetate, $NiCl_2$, $CuCl_2$ and $CoCl_2$ to form the structures shown in Fig. 28.

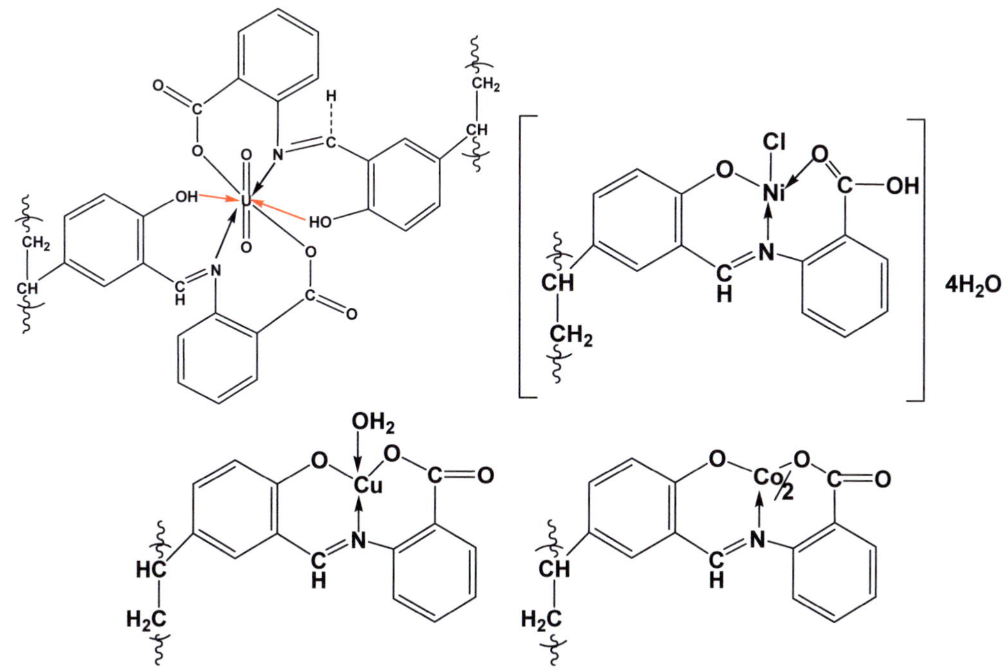

Fig. 28.

Poly(ethylene glycol)(PEG) reacts with Cu(II), Co(II), Ni(II) and Cd(II) chlorides to form polymer complexes in 2:1, ligand:metal molar ratios (Diab & El-Sonbati, 1990). The IR bands due to C-O are shifted to higher frequencies in the formed polymer complexes. This shift may be due to the increased covalence resulting from metal ion coordination. On the basis of the analytical data, electronic and IR spectral data, PEG reacts with $CuCl_2$, $CoCl_2$, $NiCl_2$ and $CdCl_2$ as shown in Fig. 29.

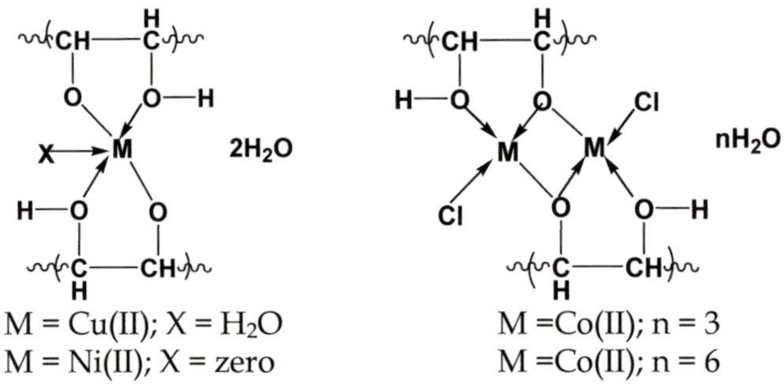

Fig. 29.

Polymer complexes of 5-vinylsalicylidene aniline (VSA) with Cu(II), Co(II), Ni(II), Cd(II) and UO_2(II). VSA reacts with uranyl nitrate in a 2:1 ratio and with uranyl acetate in a 1:1 ratio were found (El-Sonbati, 1992). A possible structure for the polymer complexes is shown in Fig. 30.

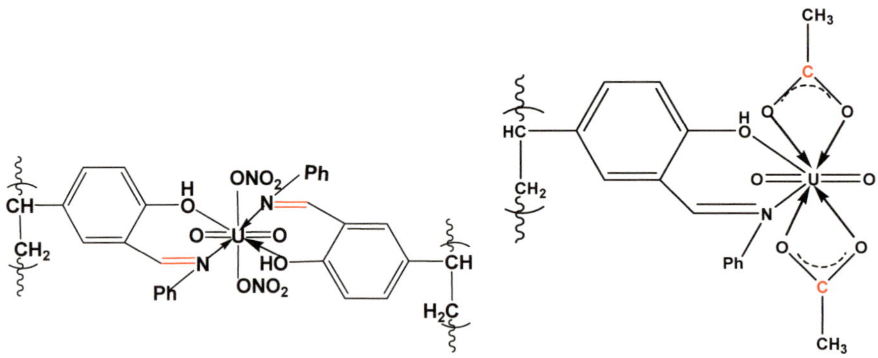

Fig. 30.

The IR, electronic spectra and elemental analyses data indicate that copper(II) salts react with VSA monomer in a 1:1 molar ratio (Fig. 31).

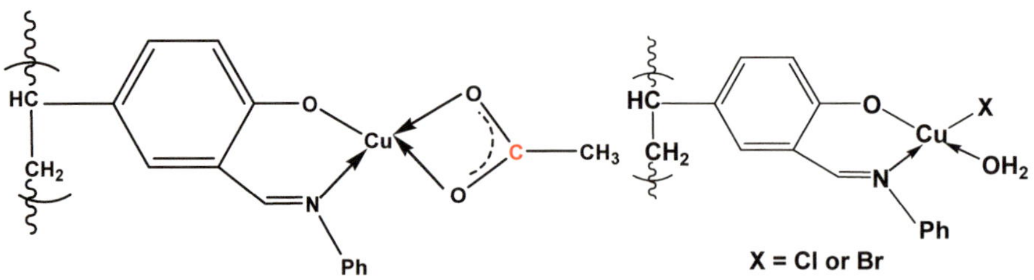

Fig. 31.

VSA reacts with Ni(II) and Co(II) in a 2:1 molar ratio and with Cd(II) in a 1:1 ratio (Fig. 32).

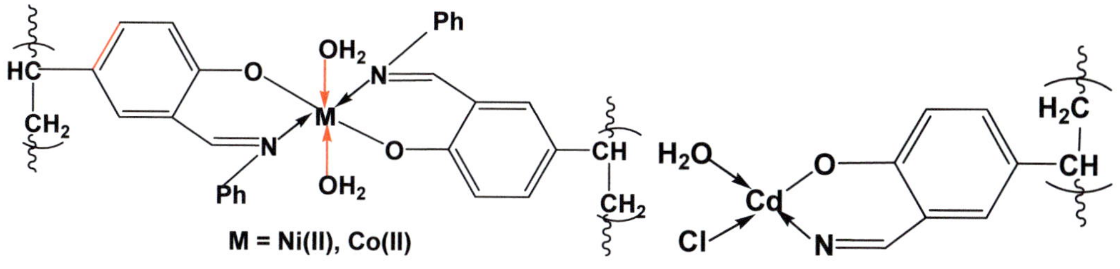

Fig. 32.

Homopolymer of 5-vinylsalicylidene-2-aminophenol (PVSA) and polymer complexes of 5-vinylsalicylidene-2-aminophenol (VSA) with transition metal acetate have been prepared and characterized (El-Sonbati, 1991a). The absence of the phenolic υ(O-H) in the copper(II), nickel(II), cadmium(II) and zinc(II) polymer complexes indicates the phenolic proton is lost upon metal ion complexation VSA appears to react with Cu(II), Ni(II), Cd(II) and Zn(II) acetate in a 1:1 ratio and with Co(II) and uranyl acetate in a 2:1 molar ratio. A possible structure for the polymer complexes is shown in Fig. 33.

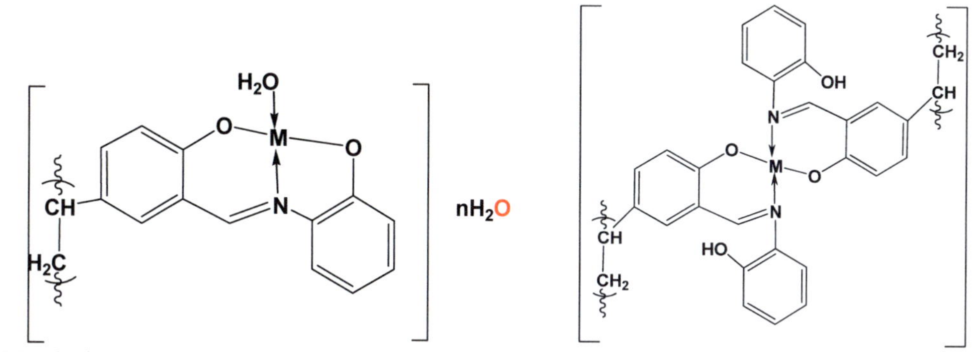

M =Cu(II); n = 2, M = Ni(II), Cd(II), Zn(II); n = 0 M = UO_2(II) or Co(II)

Fig. 33.

Polymer complexes derived from 5-vinylsalicylidene hydrazine-S-benzyl dithiocarbocarbazate (VSH) with $CuCl_2$, $NiCl_2$, $CdCl_2$ and uranyl acetate were prepared and characterized by elemental analyses, spectroscopic and magnetic measurements (El-Sonbati, 1991b). The IR spectra of VSH-$NiCl_2$ and VSH-$CdCl_2$ polymer complexes show the disappearance of the NH group and the appearance of new bands at 1625-1630 cm^{-1} which could be attributed to the stretching vibrational mode of the conjugated C=N-N=C group. There is a strong broad band at 3460-3350 cm^{-1} which is attributable to the associated water molecules. The absence of the phenolic υOH is an indication that the phenolic proton is lost upon complexation. Furthermore, it was found that there is a band around 1495 cm^{-1}, suggesting that the *o*-hydroxy group has entered into the band formation with metal ions. According to these results beside the electronic spectra and elemental analysis, the possible structure of the products of reaction of VSH with $NiCl_2$ and $CdCl_2$ as shown in Fig. 34.

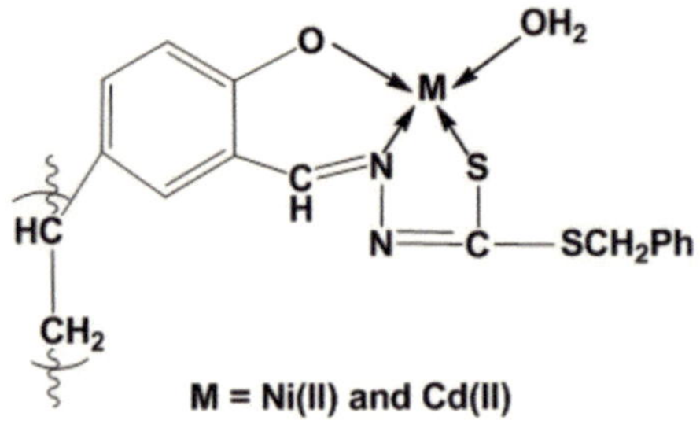

Fig. 34.

The IR spectrum of the VSH-$CuCl_2$ polymer complex shows the disappearance of the bands attributed to C=S and OH groups, suggesting that enolization occurred through the thioketonic group. The shift of the phenolic υ(C-O) to higher frequencies by about 15-20 cm^{-1} suggests the formation of an oxygen-bridge structure (Fig. 35). The structure appear to be of the following type:

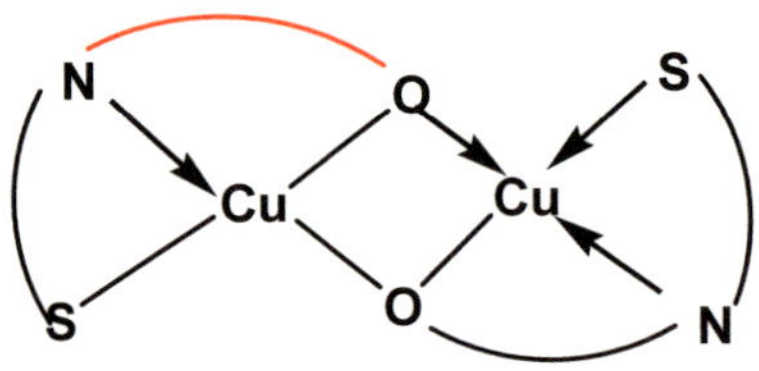

Fig. 35.

The stoichiometry between uranyl acetate and VSH are in agreement with a 1:2 molar ratio and the following type of structure is proposed (Fig. 36).

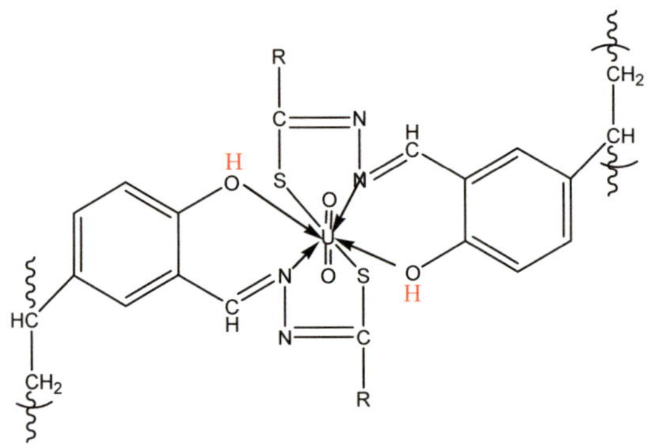

Fig. 36.

It was found that, 2-acrylamido-1,2-diaminobenzene (AAB) reacts with Cu(II), Ni(II), Zn(II) and UO_2(II) chlorides or acetate to give polymer complexes with different stoichiometry (El-Sonbati et.al., 1991), depending on the metal salt and the reaction conditions. The cobalt(II) polymer complexes may be classified into two groups. Those with the 1:1 composition are derived from ADB-Co(II) acetate and those with 1:2 stoichiometry are derived from ADB-Co(II) chloride. All these observations suggest the structures as shown in Fig. 37.

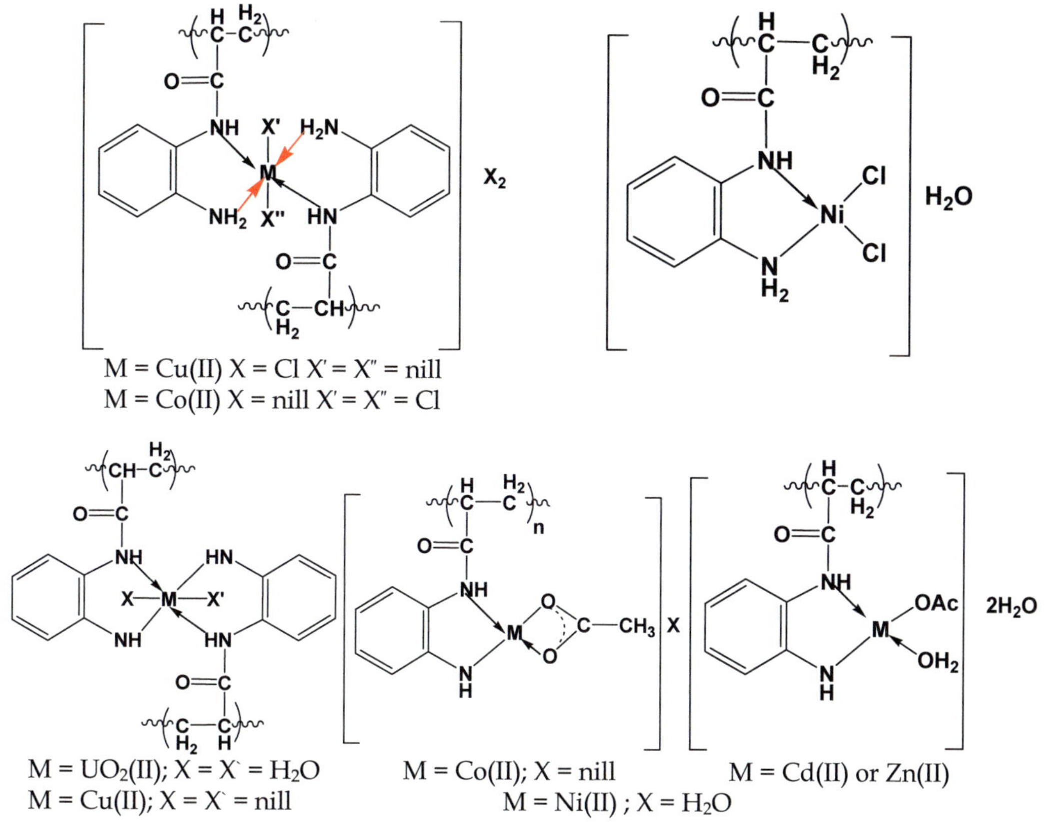

Fig. 37.

Polymer complexes of 5-vinylsalicylidene semicarbazone (VSSc) with Cu(II), Co(II), Ni(II), Cd(II), Zn(II) and UO_2(II) acetates were synthesized by mixing stoichiometric quantities (0.02 mol) of the VSSc in 30 ml DMF, the metal salt (0.01 mol) in 20 ml DMF and adding 0.1 w/v % 2,2`-azobisisobutyronitrile (AIBN) as initiator (El-Sonbati, 1991c). VSSc reacts with metal ions and uranyl acetate in a 2:1 molar ratio and a possible structure for the polymer complexes is shown in Fig. 38.

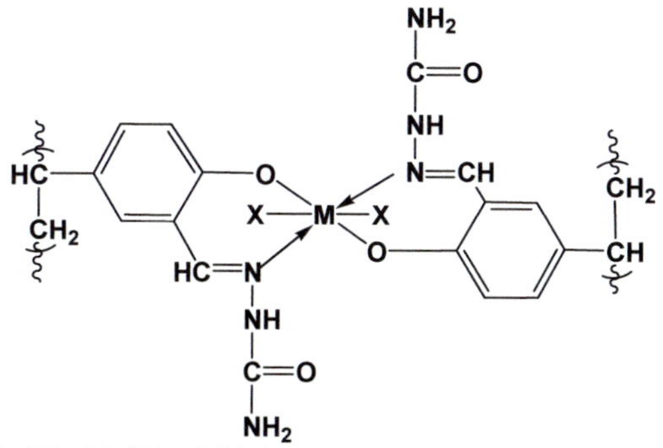

M = Cu(II), Co(II), Ni(II), Cd(II) or Zn(II); X = H_2O, M = UO_2(II); X = nill

Fig. 38.

Polymer complexes of 5-vinylsalicylidene-2-benzothiazoline ($VSBH_2$) with Cu(II), Ni(II), Co(II), Fe(II), Mn(II), Zn(II), Pd(II) and UO_2(II) were prepared and characterized (El-Sonbati & Hefni, 1993). Two IR bands of medium intensity at 1580 and 1530 cm^{-1} can be assigned to the thiazolines ring vibration. Therefore, $PVSBH_2$ homopolymer exists in benzothiazoline form as shown in Fig. 39.

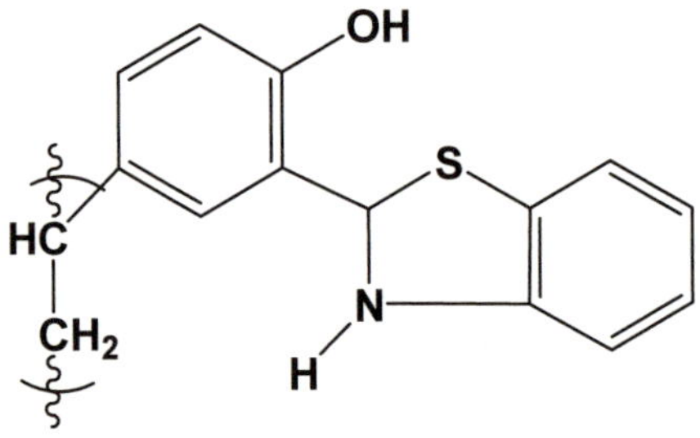

Fig. 39.

The electronic spectral data concluded that the five coordinate polymeric metal complexes of the general formula $[M(VSBH_2\text{-}2H).2H_2O]_n$ (M = Ni(II), Co(II), Mn(II) or Fe(II)) are dimetallic with octahedral geometry, while the remained ones are monomeric and present a square or tetrahedral structure (Fig. 40).

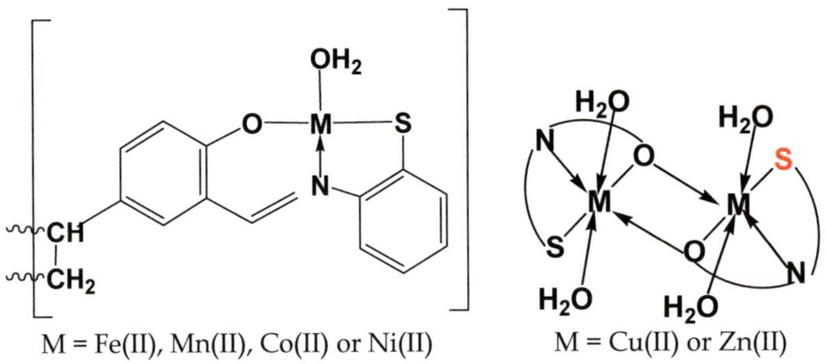

Fig. 40.

Polymer complexes derived from 5-vinylsalicylidene-2-aminomethylpyridine (VSAPH) with some transition metal salts were prepared and characterized (El-Bindary et al., 1993). All the IR and analytical data are commensurate with the structure shown in Fig. 41.

VSAPH may also act as a bidentate ligand, coordinating to the metal ion *via* the azomethine nitrogen and phenolic oxygen atoms. Loss in a proton from the latter group would allow formation of a six-membered chelate ring. The uranyl polymer complexes can be formulated as $[UO_2(VSAP)_2]$ and $[UO_2(VSAPH)(OAc)_2]$, indicating a probable coordination number of 6 for the uranium(VI) ion. The following structures are suggested (Fig. 42) for the polymer complexes:

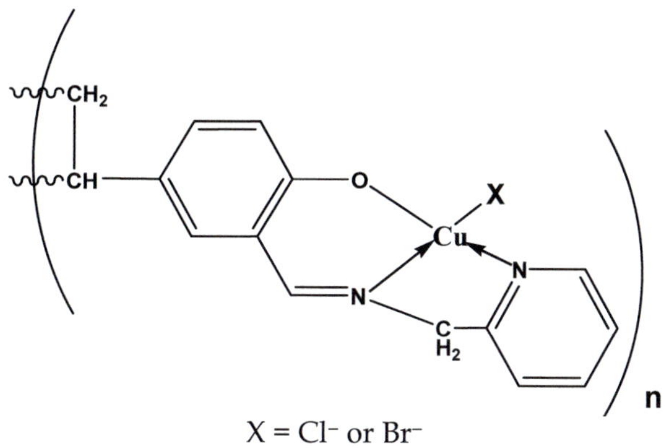

X = Cl^- or Br^-

Fig. 41.

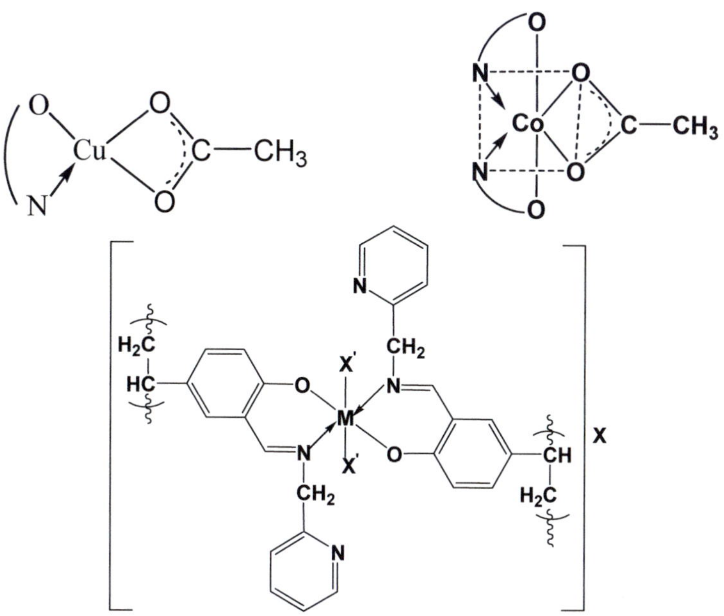

M = Co(II); X = Cl^- or Br^-; X' = H_2O; M = Ni(II); X = nil; X' = H_2O; M =Cd(II), Hg(II), UO_2(II);
X = X' = nill

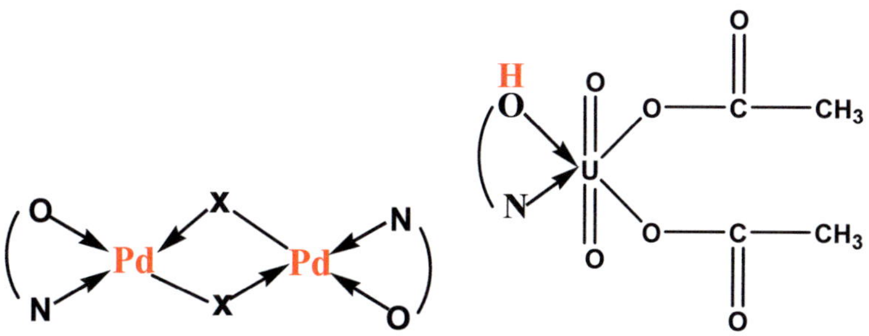

X = Cl^- or Br^-

Fig. 42.

Poly (cinnamaldehyde)-2-anthranilic acid (PCA) homopolymer and polymer complexes of cinnamaldehyde-2-anthranilic acid with Cu(II), Ni(II), Co(II), Zn(II), Cd(II) and Hg(II) has been synthesized and characterized (Fig. 43) (El- Sonbati et al., 1993a).

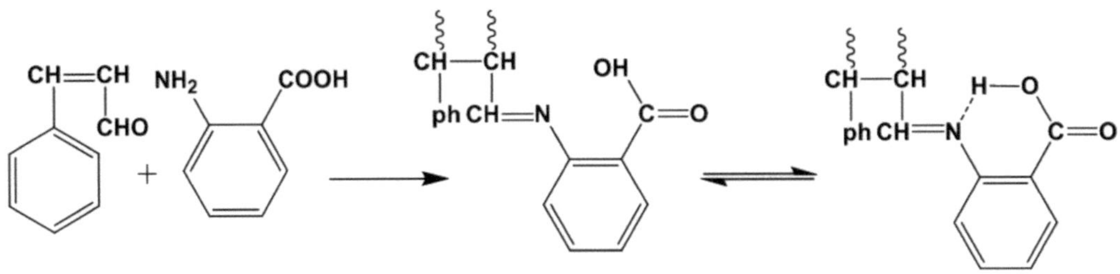

Fig. 43.

The analysis of the chelates show their formulae to be [M (PCA)- H)$_2$.2X], where M = Cu (II), Co(II); and M = Zn(II), Hg(II) and Cd(II) at X = nill, [M(PCA)-H]OAc.2X and [Ni(PCA)-H]XY] where M = Cu(II), Co(II), Ni(II) and X = H_2O, Y = Cl or Br. Their solubility varies in different common organic solvents. The 1:1 and 1:2 stoichiometries of the polymer complexes have been deduced from their elemental analyses. The presence of coordinated water was confirmed by TG data when a loss in weight corresponding to one water molecule was found for Ni(II) and two water molecules for Cu(II), Co(II) and Ni(II). No coordination water molecules were found in the case of Zn(II), Hg(II) and Cd(II) polymer complexes.

Polymer complexes of N,N`-*o*-phenylenediamine bis(cinnamaldehyde) (L) with Cu(II), Co(II), Ni^{II}, Zn^{II},UO_2^{II} and Pd^{II} were prepared and characterized (El-Sonbati et al., 1993b). A bidentate methine nitrogen atoms coordination of the ligand is assigned in the isolated complexes. The μ_{eff} values of cobalt(II) and nickel(II) polymer complexes are normal and indicate an octahedral stereochemistry around the metal ion, the moments for the cobalt and nickel complexes are in a range expected for six-coordination metal ions, with much orbital contribution. The electronic spectra are summarized in Table 1, together with the proposed assignments, ligand field parameters, magnetic susceptibilities and suggested geometries.

Mononuclear and binuclear complexes of poly(5-vinylsalicylidene-2-aminopyridine) (PVSA) were prepared by the reaction of the homopolymer with copper(II), cobalt(II), nickel(II), dioxouranium(VI) and palladium(II) salts (El-Sonbati et al., 1994a). Metal(II) acetates and palladium chloride were found to give mononuclear complexes, while cupric chloride gave a binuclear complex. The stereochemistry and the nature of the polymer complexes are markedly dependent upon the molar ratios of the reactants, the pH of the system and the nature of the anions involved. In all of the complexes the homopolymer was chelated to the metal ion through the nitrogen atom of the azomethine group and the oxygen atom of the phenolic group. The stoichiometric of the complexes indicate that the copper(II) complexes fall into two distinct categories. The reaction of metal acetate with the VSP monomer gives compounds with formulae which correspond to $[M(VSP\text{-}H)_2]_n$ while the reaction of $CuCl_2$ with VSP in the presence of an excess of ammonium hydroxide gives a compound with the formula $[Cu_2(VSP\text{-}H)_2Cl_2]_n$. The mononuclear and binuclear polymer complexes may be represented as shown in Fig. 44.

No	Species	Band position (cm^{-1})	Assignment	μ_{eff} (B.M)	Geometry
1	$[Co\ L_2Cl_2]$ 2X	8300 17350 19000 23450	$^4T_{1g} \rightarrow {}^4T_{2g}(F)\ \upsilon_1$ $^4T_{1g} \rightarrow {}^4A_{2g}(F)\ \upsilon_2$ $^4T_{1g} \rightarrow {}^4T_{1g}(P)\ \upsilon_3$	4.31	Octahedral
2	$[Co\ L_2Br_2]$ X	8050 16600 18700 23500	$^4T_{1g} \rightarrow {}^4T_{2g}(F)\ \upsilon_1$ $^4T_{1g} \rightarrow {}^4A_{2g}(F)\ \upsilon_2$ $^4T_{1g} \rightarrow {}^4T_{1g}(P)\ \upsilon_3$	4.05	Octahedral
3	$[Ni\ L_2Cl_2]$	10206 15272 22222	$^3A_{1g} \rightarrow {}^3T_{2g}(F)$ $^3A_{2g} \rightarrow {}^3T_{1g}(F)$ $^3A_{2g} \rightarrow {}^3T_{1g}(P)$	3.37	Octahedral
4	$[Ni\ L_2\ Br_2]$ X	10000 15625 24800	$^3A_{1g} \rightarrow {}^3T_{2g}(F)$ $^3A_{2g} \rightarrow {}^3T_{1g}(F)$ $^3A_{2g} \rightarrow {}^3T_{1g}(P)$	3.21	Octahedral
5 6	$[Cu\ L_2Cl_2]$ $[CuL_2\ Br_2]$ X	13900 - 16900 22200 - 24200	$^2E_g \rightarrow {}^2T_{2g}$ $^1A_g \rightarrow {}^1B_{1g}$	1.93 1.89	Octahedral
7 8 9	$[Pd\ LCl_2]$ $[Pd\ L_2]\ Cl_2$ $[Pd\ L]\ [PdCl_4]$	22200 - 24200 29000 - 31000	$^2E_g \rightarrow {}^2T_{2g}$ $^2A_g \rightarrow {}^1B_{1g}$	dia.	Square planner
11	$[UO_2\ L_2(NO_3)_2]$	21730	$E \rightarrow {}^2\Pi_4$	dia.	Octahedral

Polymer complexes (1-9) X = Cl or Br.

Table 1. Electronic spectral bands, assignments, ligand field parameters and proposed geometries for the polymer complexes.

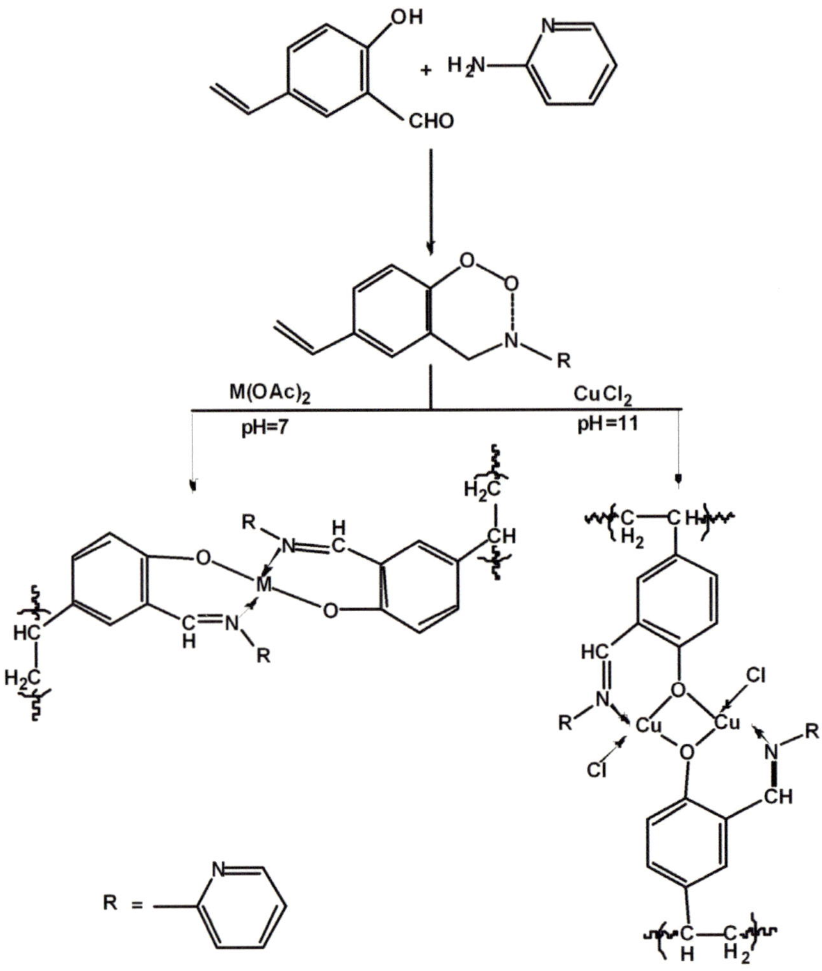

M = Cu(II), Fe(II), Co(II), Ni(II), Pd(II), Cd(II) and Zn (II)

Fig. 44.

Poly(5-vinylsalicylidene)-1,2-diaminobenzene (PVSB) homopolymer behaves as a monobasic tridentate chelating ligand and mixed ligand of PVSB and pyridine as a bidentate species. Polymer complexes of these ligands with Cu(II), Fe(II), Co(II), Ni(II), Pd(II), Cd(II) and Zn(II) were prepared and characterized (El-Sonbati & Hefni, 1994). In PVSB homopolymer, the principal IR bands of interest are two strong bands at 3365 and 3175 cm^{-1} attributed to the symmetric and asymmetric NH_2 stretching vibrations (Fig. 45). The frequencies of these bands are observed at a considerably lower wavenumber in the polymer complexes of the nitrogen atom of the amino group with metal ions. The absence of large systematic shifts of $\upsilon_{as}(NH_2)$, $\upsilon_s(NH_2)$ and $\delta(NH_2)$ bands in the spectra of mixed ligand polymer complexes, i.e. 2:1 species, implies that there is no interaction between the amino group nitrogen atom and the metal ions.

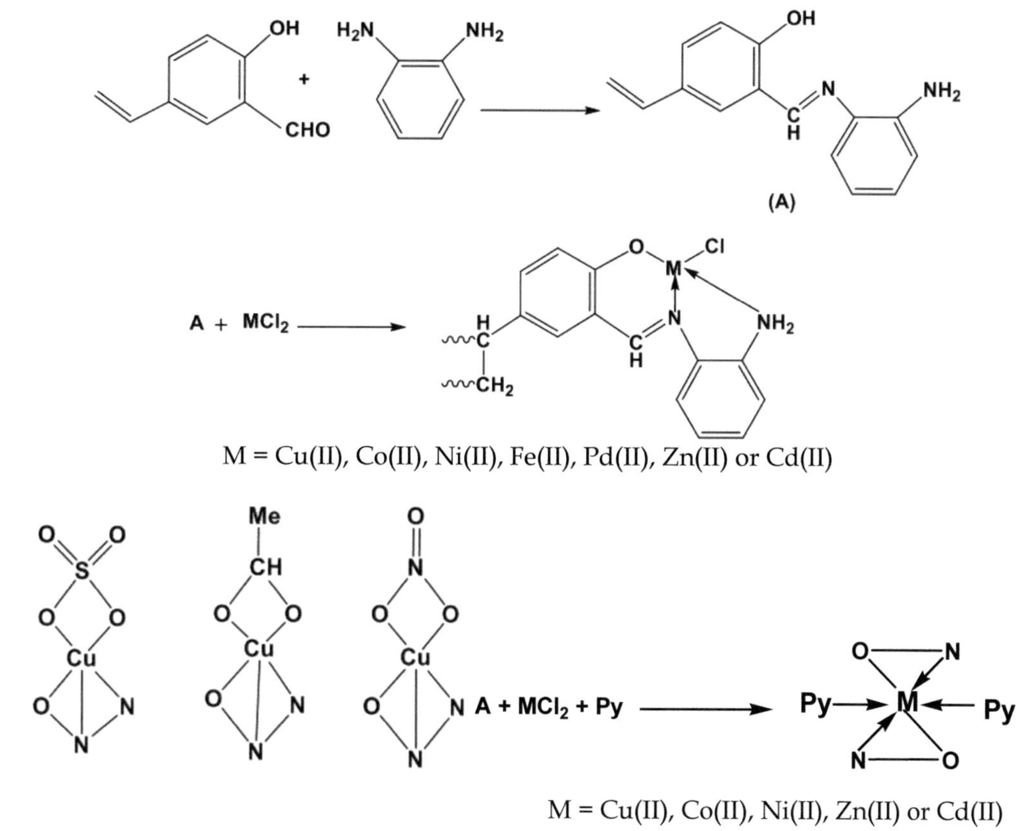

Fig. 45.

Polymer complexes of 2-acrylamido-1-phenyl-2-aminothiourea (APATH) with Rh(II) and Ru(II) ions in the presence and absence of N-heterocyclic bases as mixed ligand have been prepared and characterized through chemical analyses, thermal, electronic and infrared spectral studies (El-Sonbati et al., 1994b). The homopolymer shows three types of coordination behavior. In the mixed valence paramagnetic trinuclear polymer complexes $Rh_3(APATH)_2Cl_8$ (**1**) and $Ru_3(APATH)_2Cl_8$ (**2**), and in the mononuclear polymer compound $Ru(APATH)_2Cl_3$ (**3**) it acts as a neutral bidentate ligand coordinating through the thiocarbonyl sulphur and carbonyl oxygen atoms. In the mixed ligand paramagnetic polychelates, which are obtained from the reaction of APATH with $RuCl_3$. XH_2O in the presence of N-heterocyclic bases [B = H_2O, pyridine (Py)/or *o*-phenylendiamine (*o*-phen), DMF] consisting of polymer complexes $[Ru(APAT)_2(H_2O)Py]XCl$ (**7**) and $Ru(APAT)Cl_2$(*o*-phen.) H_2O (**8**) and in mononuclear compounds $Ru(APAT)_2Cl.DMF$ (**6**) and $Ru(APAT)_2Cl(H_2O)_2$ (**8**), it behaves as a monobasic bidentate ligand coordinating through the same donor atoms. In mononuclear compounds $[Ru(APAT)(APATH)Cl]2H_2O$ (**4**) and $[Ru(APAT)\ (APATH)Cl_2]2H_2O$ (**5**) it acts as a monobasic and neutral bidentate ligand coordinating only through the same donor atoms. Monometric distorted octahedral or trimeric chlorine-bridged, approximately octahedral structures are proposed for these polymer complexes. The polychelates are of 1:1, 1:2 and 3:2 (metal: poly-Schiff base) stoichiometry and exhibit five and six coordination (Fig. 46).

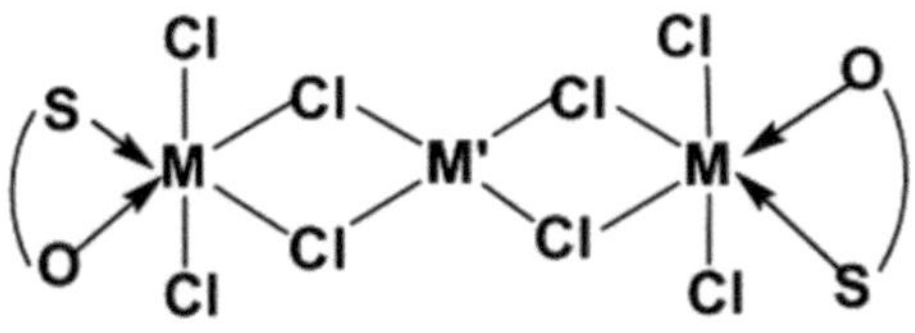

Fig. 46.

In the other hand, mononuclear and hetero bi-trinuclear polymer complexes of nickel(II), copper (II) and oxovanadium(VI) chloride with APATH monomer derived from amidation of acryloyl chloride with 2-amino-1-phenylthiourea have been prepared (El-Sonbati el al., 1995a). The elemental analyses show that these homonuclear polymer complexes have 2:1 and in bimetallic polymer complexes 2:1:1 (homopolymer: metal: metal), stoichiometry. These indicate that they fall into two distinct categories. The first is mononuclear, while the second is heterobinuclear. The following structures shown in Fig. 47 are suggested:

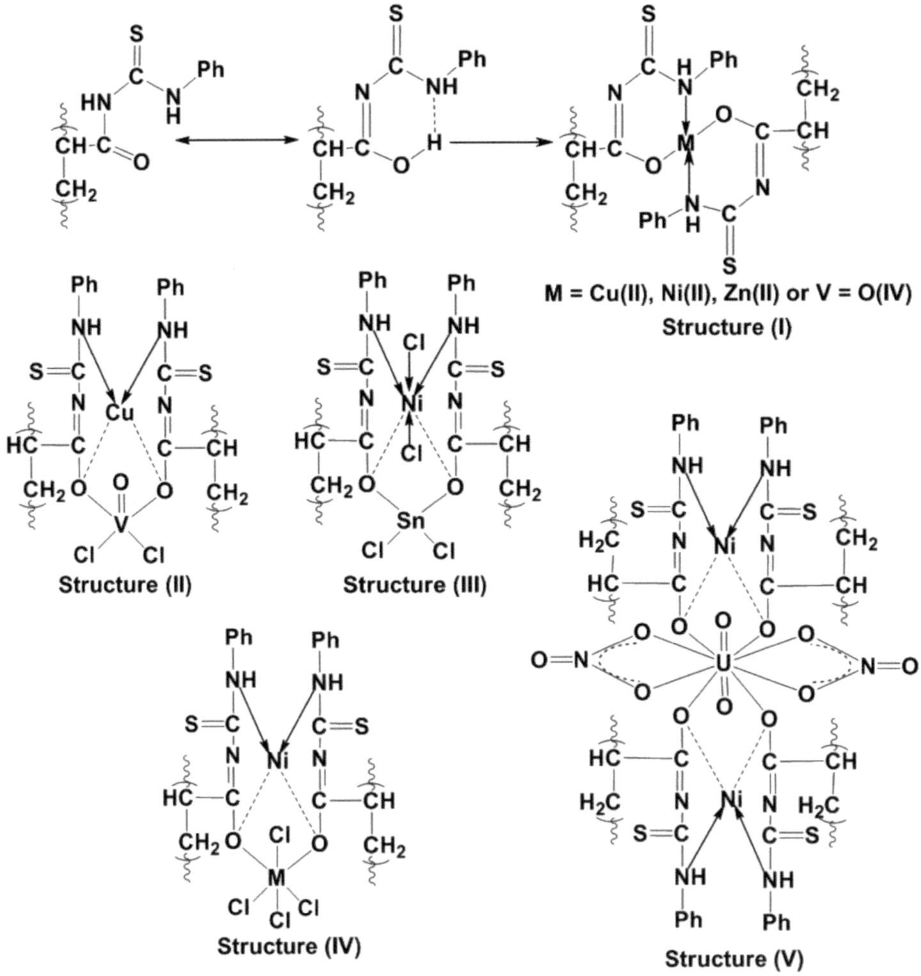

Fig. 47.

Poly[1-acrylamido-2(2-pyridyl)ethane)] (PAEPH) homopolymer and polymer complexes of 1-acrylamido-2(2-pyridyl) ethane AEPH with a number of bi and tetravalent transition metals have been prepared and characterized using spectral (^1H and ^{13}C-NMR, IR, UV-Vis) and thermal analysis, and magnetic measurements (El-Sonbati et al., 1995b). The stoiciometries of the polymer complexes have been deduced from their elemental analyses. These indicate that the metal-polymer complexes fall into two distinct categories, namely 1:1 and 1:2 (ligand: metal). PAEPH is mononucleating and hence requires one metal ion for coordination. The formation of the polymer complexes may be represented by the following reactions:

MX_2 + 2 AEPH ⟶ [M $(AEP)_2$] + 2HX (M = Pd, Pt or UO_2, X = Cl or CH_3COO)

$ZrCl_2$ + AEPH $\xrightarrow{\text{1:1 (6h or 9h)}}$ [Zr (AEP) Cl_3]$_n$ **A** or **C**

$ZrCl_2$ + AEPH $\xrightarrow{\text{1:2 (12h or 15h)}}$ [Zr $(AEP)_2$ Cl_2]$_n$ **B** or **D**

(Where AEP represents the anion of the corresponding monofunctional bidentate AEPH).

The reactions appear to proceed only up to a 1:2 molar ratio. Even on prolonged refluxing (~ 32 h) of 1:3 or 1:4 reaction mixture, replacement of a third chloride group by the homopolymer was not observed. This is probably due to steric factors. Plausible structures (Fig. 48) are given for the products (**A, C**) and (**B, D**) obtained from the reaction of 1:1 and 1:2 molar ratios, respectively.

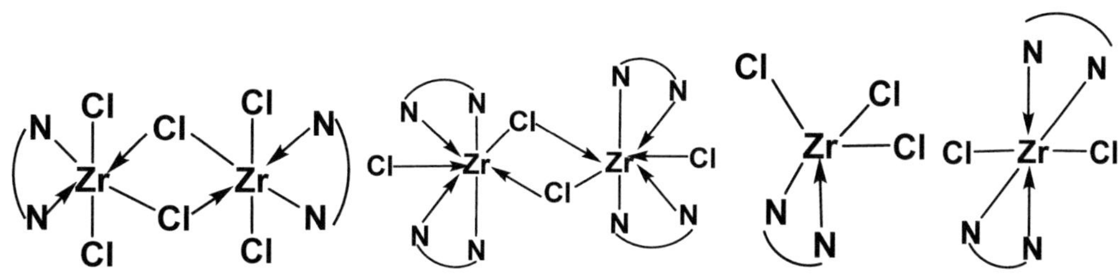

(A) **(B)** **(C)** **(D)**

Fig. 48.

The zirconium atoms appear to be hexa-(**A, B**) and hepta-(**B, C**) coordinated. In the polymer complexes of zirconyl isopropoxide, zirconium exhibits a coordination number of 5. The [$UO_2(AEP)(AcO)(OH_2)$] polymer complex spectrum exhibits characteristic bands for the monodentate acetate group at 1620 and 1395 cm^{-1} with $\Delta\upsilon$ = 235 cm^{-1}. The spectrum also exhibits three bands at 907, 790 and 275 cm^{-1} assigned to υ_3, υ_1 and υ_2 of the dioxouranium ion.

Trying to deepen the knowledge of this ligand, a studied polymer complexes of AEPH with copper(II), nickel(II), cobalt(II) and Zn(II) (El-Sonbati & El-Bindary, 1996). From IR and elemental analyses, the possible structures of the products of reaction of AEPH with transition metal ions shown in Fig. 49 are as follows:

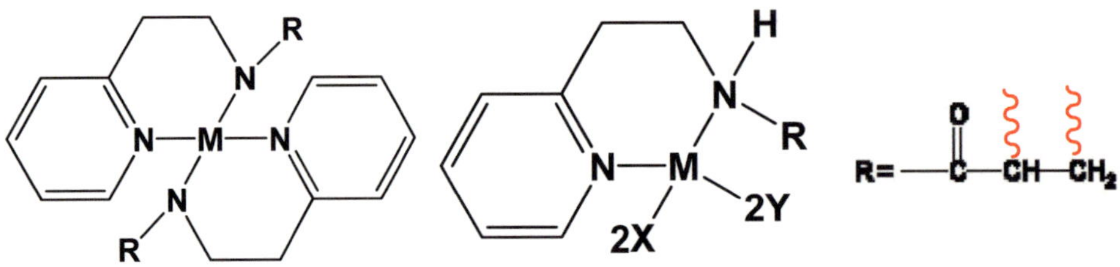

M = Cu(II) for $Cu(AEP)_2$
= Ni(II) for $Ni(AEP)_2$
= Zn(II) for $Zn(AEP)_2$

M = Cu(II), Ni(II) or Zn(II);
X = NO_3, Y = OH_2 for
$Cu(AEPH)(NO_3)_2(OH_2)_2$,
$Ni(AEPH)(NO_3)_2(OH_2)_2$ and
$Zn(AEPH)(NO_3)_2(OH_2)_2$;
M = Co(II); X = OAc; Y=OH_2 for Co(AEPH))$OAc)_2(OH_2)_2$
M = Zn(II); X = OAc;Y= nil for $Zn(AEPH)(OAc)_2$
M = Co(II); X = NO_3; Y= OH_2 for $Co(AEPH)(NO_3)_2(OH_2)_2$

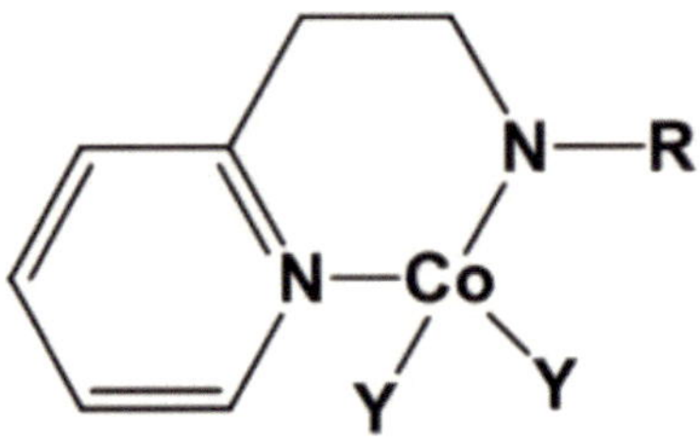

Y = OH_2 for $Co(AEP)(OH_2)_2$

Fig. 49.

Some binary and ternary novel polymer complexes dioxouranium(VI) with 5-vinylsalicylaldehyde (VSH) have been prepared and characterized by various physico-chemical techniques (El-Sonbati et al., 2002). Addition of ammonia to an ethanolic solution of uranyl nitrate give uranyl ammine complex which on treatment with VSA result in the formation of the imine complex (**C**). The reaction of the compound **C** with 1,2-diaminoethane and/or 1,2-diaminobenzene yield symmetrical tetradentate Schiff base complex of type (**1C**) as shown in Fig. 50.

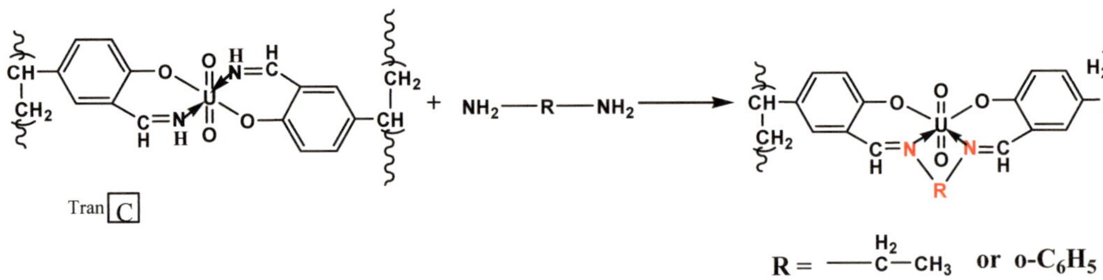

Fig. 50.

Reaction of $ZrCl_4$ with [Cu(VSR)] give heterobinuclear complexes Cu(VSED)$ZrCl_4$. [Cu(VSR)] has an additional lone pair of electron at each of the coordinated phenolic O^- and hence, it acts as a ligand and gets coordinated with $UO_2(CH_3COO)_2.2H_2O$. The Cu(II) band in the binuclear complex shows a shift from its value in mononuclear complex [Cu(VSR)] (Fig. 51). This lowering in the ligand field band of [Cu(VSR)] may be due to exchanges in the planarity of (VSR) and also to reduction in strength of Cu-O bond on the formation of second bond with metal(II) halides.

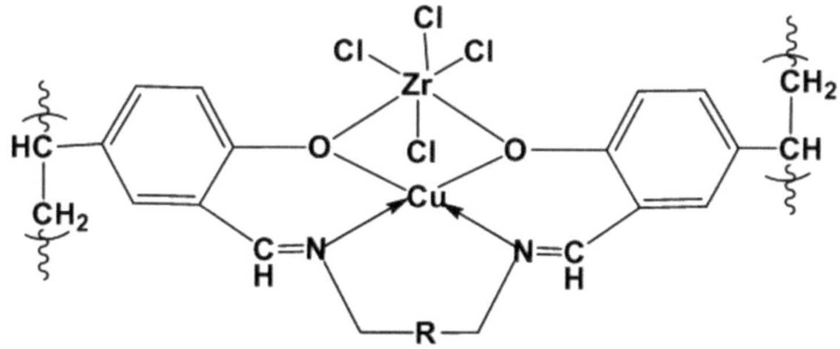

Fig. 51.

Novel seven, nine and ten-coordinated rare earth polymer complexes of N-acryloyl-1-phenyl-2-thiourea (APT) of the composition $[Ln(NO_3)_3(APT)_2]_n$ (Ln = La, Sm, Tb, Pr and Nd) and $[Ln(NCS)_3(APT)_x]_n$ (where Ln = La or Pr at X = 2 and Ln = Nd, Sm and Tb at X = 3) have been prepared and characterized on the basis of their chemical analyses, magnetic measurements, conductance, visible and IR spectral data (Mubarak & El-Sonbati, 2006). The data of elemental analysis indicate that the stoichiometric ratio for the reaction of monomer with various LnX_3 is 1:2 and 1:3 (Ln: monomer). The polymer complexes do not contain any water of coordination are all occupied by donor centers from the ligand groups. Therefore, the reaction between LnX_3 and ligand can be represented as follows:

$$LnX_3 + nAPT \rightarrow [Ln(NO_3)_3(APT)_2]_n$$

$$\rightarrow [Ln(NCS)_3(APT)_2]_n$$

$$\rightarrow [Ln(NCS)_3(APT)_3]_n$$

These data suggest that three nitrato and isothiocyanato ions are within the coordination sphere.

The build-up of polymer metallic supramolecules based on homopolymer 1-acrylamido-2-(2-pyridyl)ethane (AEPH) and ruthenium, rhodium, palladium as well as platinum complexes has been pursued with great interest (El-Sonbati et al., 2003a). AEPH is found to be a polyfunctional planar molecule with a delocalized π electronic system, with two nitrogen atoms which may act as basic centers and two labile N-H bands. The molecule may present in several tautomers and conformers. The equivalent conformers are the principle contributors to the molecular structure of this molecular in solution; they are in equilibrium and established by intramolecular hydrogen bonds. In the solid state reveals widely used intramolecular hydrogen bonding, which gives rise to six-membered ring (Fig. 52).

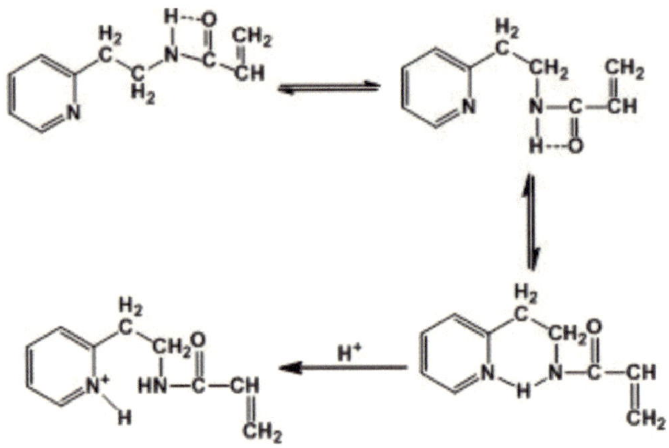

Fig. 52.

From the stoichiometries of all complexes, it is clear that the AEPH ligand function as bidentate N-N donors. Construction of molecular models suggest that the formation of a stable six-membered ring system with the central metal ions having N-N donor function taking one of the N-pyridyl ring and the N-imino (NH) of the monomer residue as bonding sites is the most probable proposition as shown in Fig. 53.

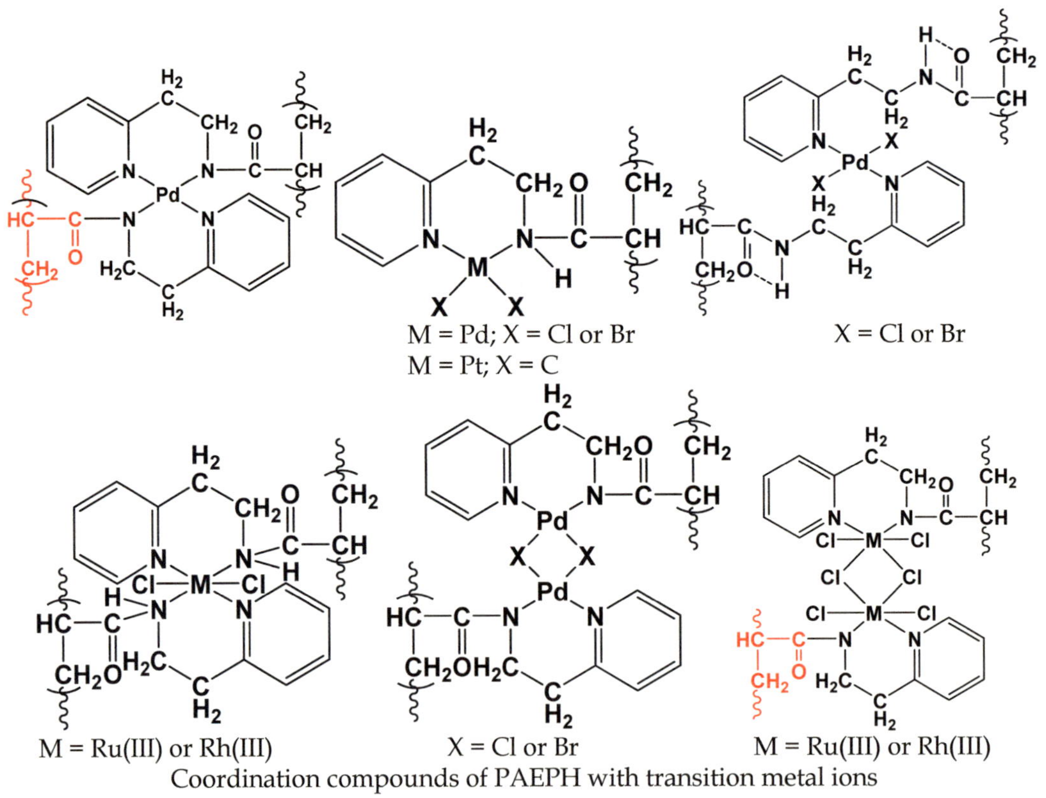

Coordination compounds of PAEPH with transition metal ions

Fig. 53.

Monomeric distorted octahedral or trimeric chlorine-bridged, approximately octahedral structures are proposed for these polymer complexes.

Mono, bis and tris-polymer complexes of ruthenium(III) and rhodium(III) chloride with 3-hydroxy-2-N-acrylamidopyridine (H_2L) monomer, derived from amidation of acryloyl chloride with 2-amino-3-hydroxypyridine have been proposed (El-Bindary et al., 2003). A few bimetallic mixed ligand polymer complexes have also been obtained by the reaction of rhodium(II) bidentate poly-chelate mixed ligand with palladium(II), platinum(II) or zirconium(IV) chlorides and uranyl acetate. The homopolymer shows three types of coordination behavior. The poly-chelates are of 1:1, 1:2 and 1:3 (metal:homopolymer) stoichiometry and exhibit six coordination.

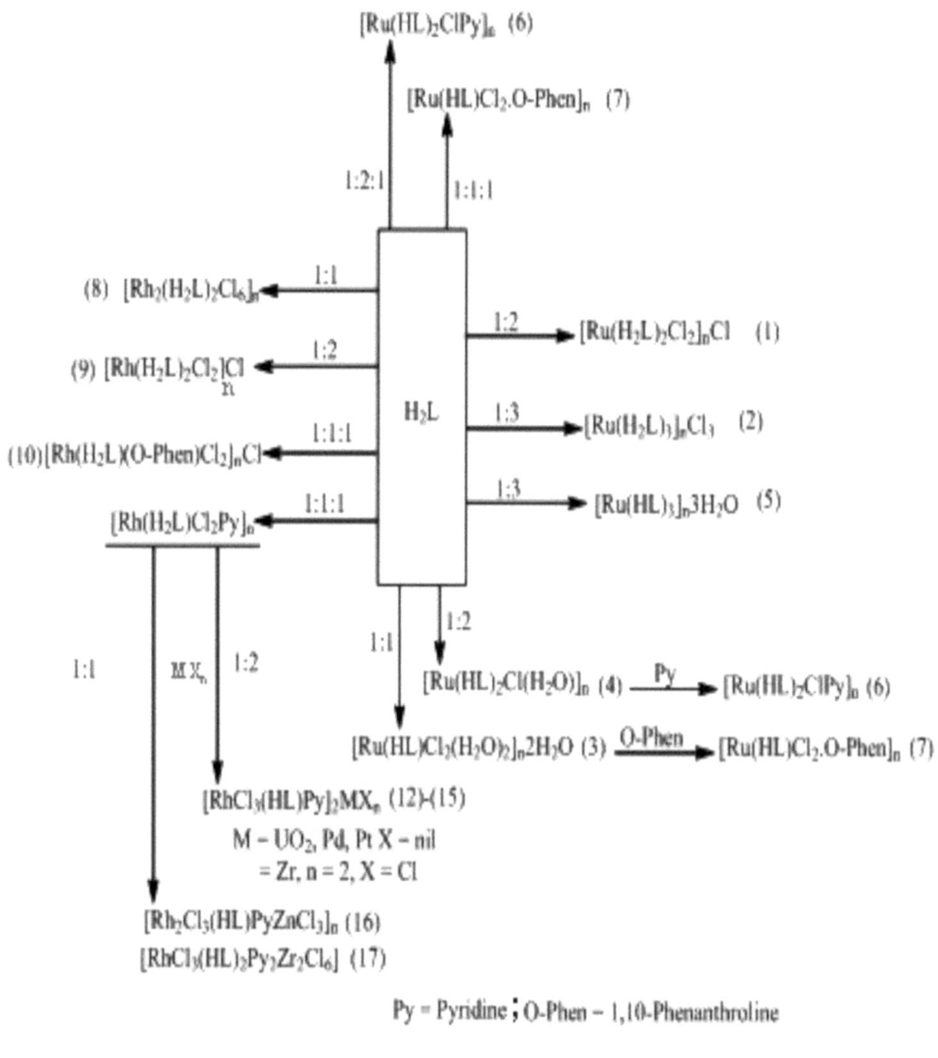

From the spectroscopic investigation of the rhodium complexes, it was concluded that the rhodium atom in each complex exists in an octahedral environments (Fig. 54).

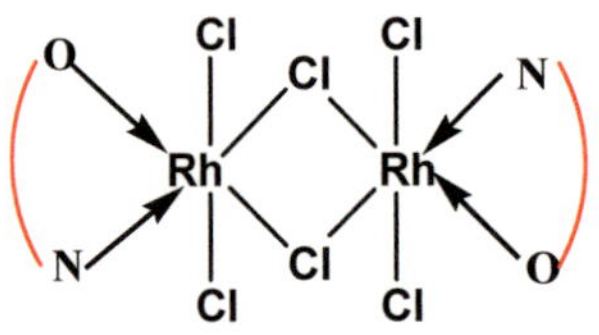

(8)

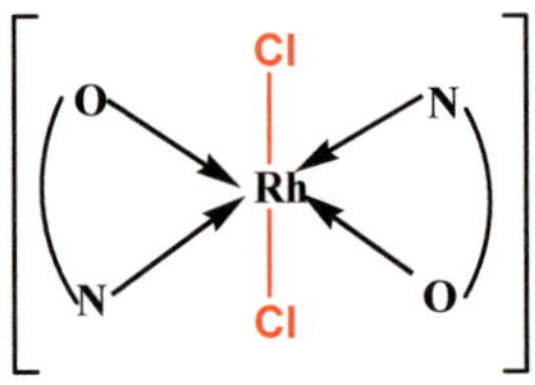

(9)

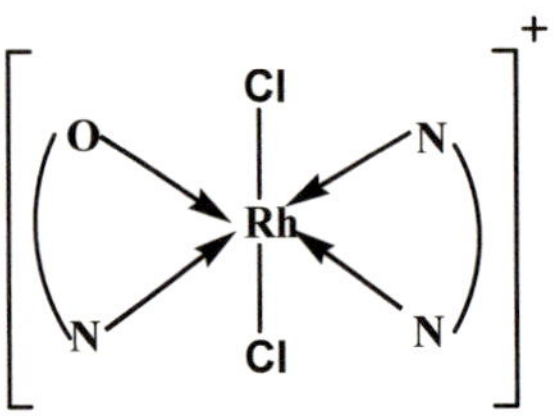

(10)

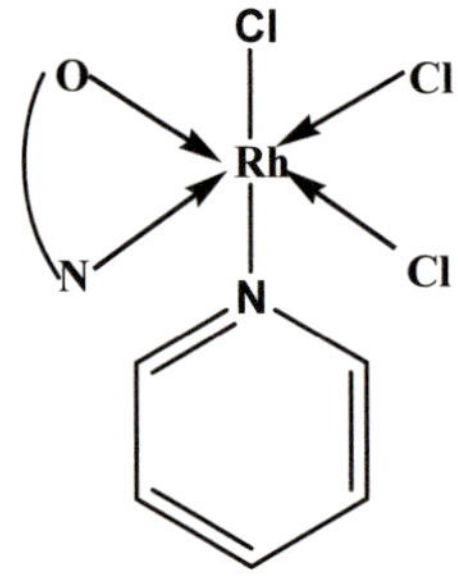

(11)

Fig. 54.

Plausible structures are given for the structures obtained from the reaction of 1:1 and 1:2 molar ratios (Fig. 55).

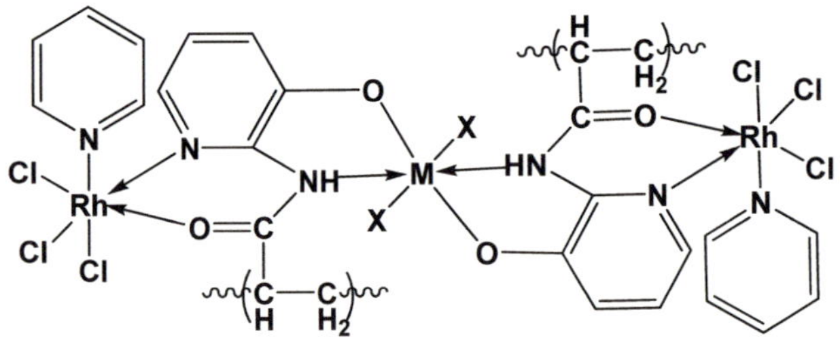

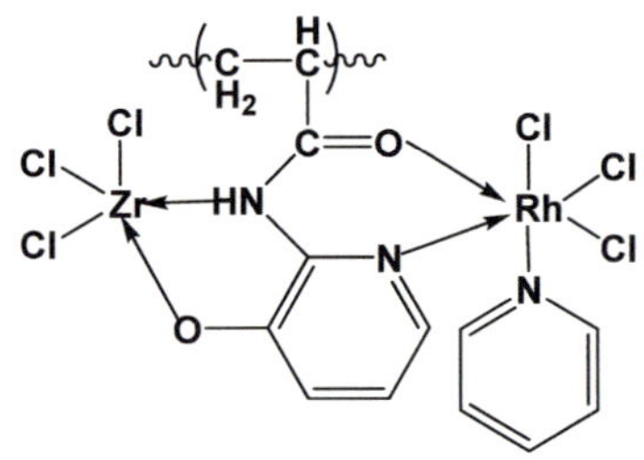

M = UO_2; Pt or Pd; X = nil

M = Zr; X = Cl.

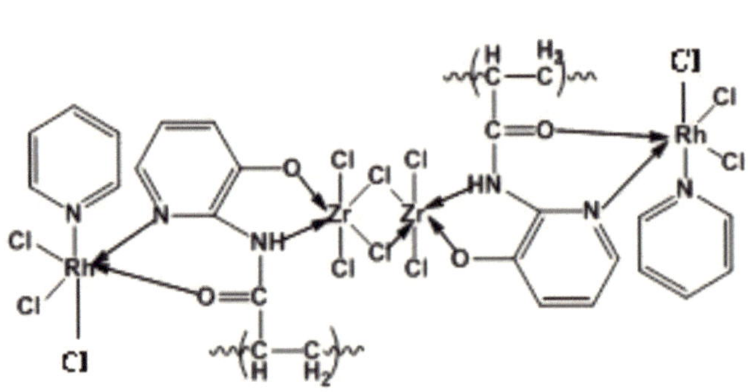

Fig. 55.

Two novel supramolecular complexes of types $UO_2(L)(H_2L)(OH_2)_2$ and $UO_2(HL_n)_2(OAc)_2$ (H_2L is a potential four-dentate ligand derived from hydrazine hydrate and malonylchloride and HLn is a potential bidentate ligand derived from coupling of allylazo-β-diketone have been synthesized and characterized by elemental analyses, conductance and spectral measurements (El-Sonbati et al., 2004a). Alcoholic solutions of uranyl acetate and malonic dihydrazide were refluxed for 8-9 h forms uranyldihydrazide complex as shown in Fig. 56.

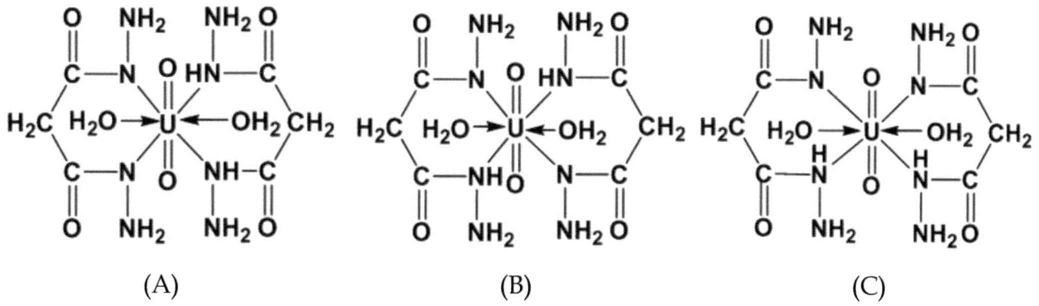

Fig. 56.

To the uranyl complex, an allyl-β-diketone was added using AIBN as initiator; the polymer complexes (Fig. 57) were characterized by IR spectroscopy:

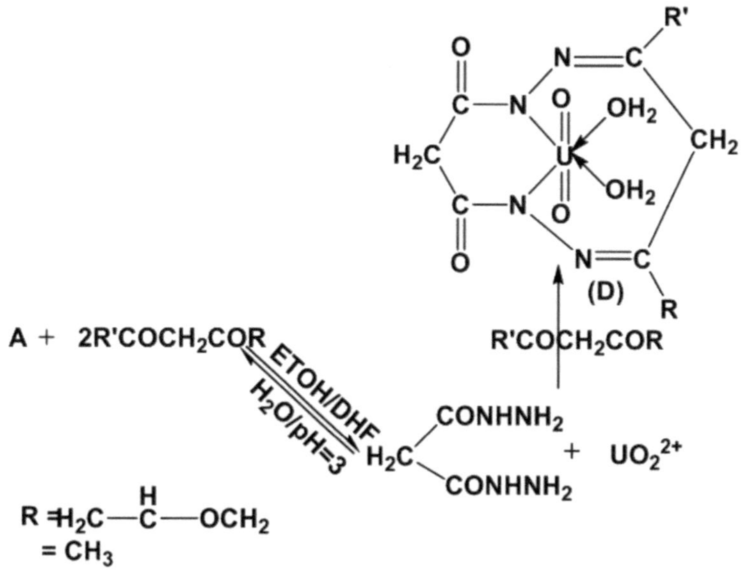

Fig. 57.

Polymer complexes of $[UO_2(HL_n)(OAc)_2]$ were prepared by refluxing a 0.5 M solution of the metal salt with the monomer using AIBN as initiator. The products of condensation reaction of allyl propenyl-2-(4-derivatives phenylazo) butan-3-one polymer complexes with malonyldihydrazide in ethanol/DMF in the presence of sodium acetate results in macrocyclic uranyl polymer complexes (Fig. 58).

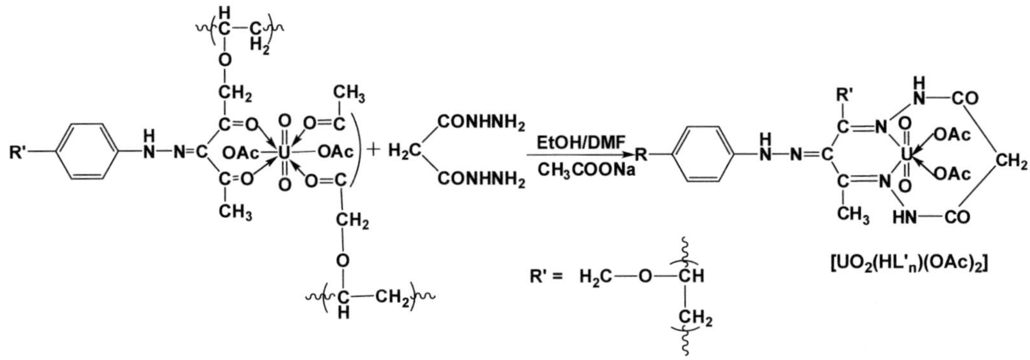

n =1(R = OCH_3), n =2(R=CH_3), n=3(R=H), n=4(R=Br), n=5(R=NO_2)

Fig. 58.

Copper(II) polymer complexes of emprical formula [Cu(ligands)$_2$X$_2$] (Fig. 59) (where X=Cl, Br, I, NO_3 and 1/2 SO_4) and [Cu(ligand)(CH_3COO)$_2$] have been prepared with poly(3-phenylacrylidine semicarbazone) (El-Sonbati et al., 2003b). It is propose that the uncomplexed polymer behaves as a bidentate coordinated ligand through the oxygen of the carbonyl and the nitrogen of azomethine.

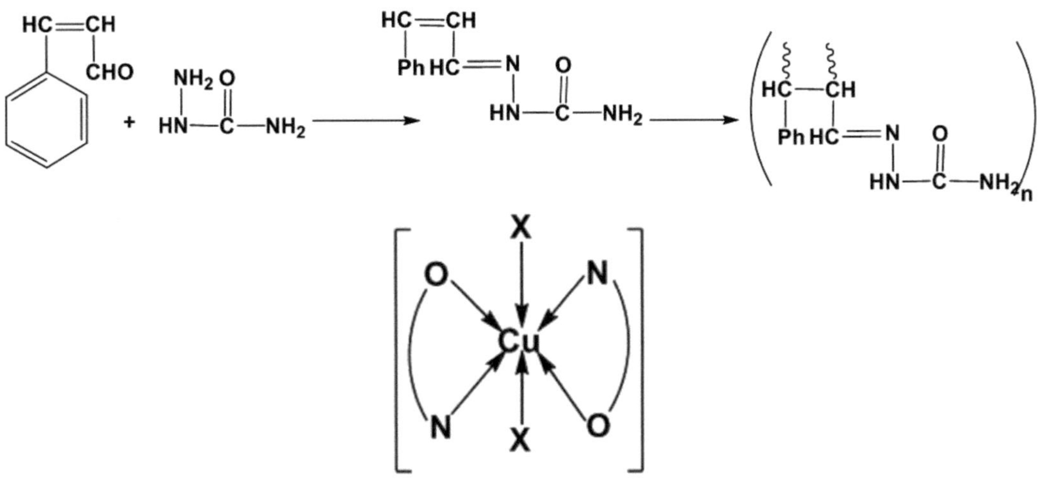

X = Cl, Br, I, NO_3

Fig. 59. Molecular structures proposed for poly(3-phenyl-acrylidine semicarbazone) and [Cu(ligand)$_2$X$_2$] complexes.

Poplymer complexes of N-(3-phenylacrylidene)-2-mercaptoaniline (HL_1) and cinnamaldehyde-2-aminophenol (HL_2) with Cu(II), Pd(II), Pt(II), UO_2(II), Rh(II), Ru(III), and Pd(IV) have been synthesized and characterized (Fig. 60) (El-Sonbati et al., 2003b). The electronic spectra of the derivatives of types [Ru(HL_n)Cl_3], have four bands in good agreement with the one-electron orbital schemes for trigonal bipyramidal d^5 complexes.

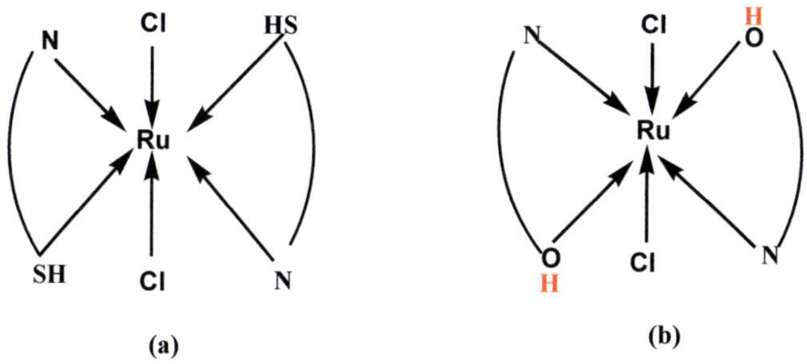

Molecular structures of (a) [Ru $(HL_1)_2Cl_2$] Cl, (b) [Ru $(HL_2)_2Cl_2$] Cl

Fig. 60.

Synthesis and characterization of ally propenyl-2-(4-derivatives phenylazo)butan-3-one (HL_n) are described as shown in Fig. 61 (Mubarak et al., 2006).

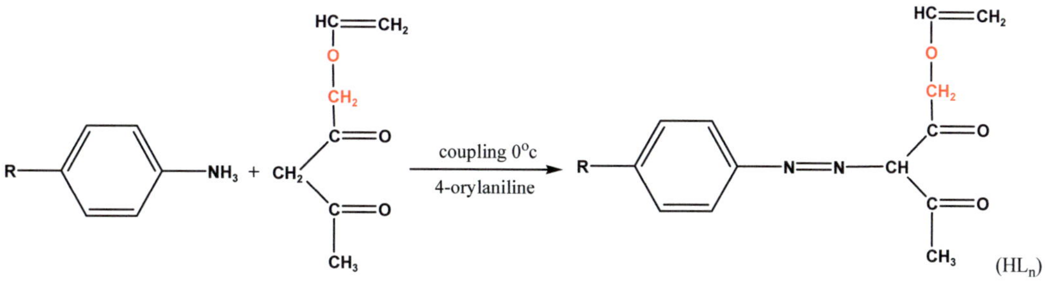

n = 1 R = OCH_3 (HL_1); n = 2 R = CH_3 (HL_2); n = 3 R = H (HL_3); n = 4 R = Br (HL_4); n = 5 R = NO_2 (HL_5)

Fig. 61.

The polymer complexes were prepared by mixing the appropriate uranyl acetate with two equivalents of HL_n/H_2L in DMF according to the following reaction scheme.

$$UO_2(CH_3COO)_2.2H_2O + HL_n \xrightarrow{DMF} [UO_2(HL_n)_2(OAc)_2]\ (n = 1\text{-}5) \quad (1)$$

$$UO_2(CH_3COO)_2.2H_2O + H_2L \xrightarrow{DMF} [UO_2(HL)_2(H_2O)_2] + 2CH_3COOH \quad (2)$$

The magnetic measurements of the dioxouranium(VI) polymer complexes are independent from field strength and temperature and the ground states of dioxouranium(VI) compounds contain no unpaired electrons. Allyl propenyl-2-(4-derivatives phenylazo) butan-3-one (HL_n) is a ligand whose reactivity towards metal ions varies as a function of the 4-substituents. The products, which are usually neutral, have two coplanar O,O metal-chelate rings in an O,O(O,O) trans geometry. Consequently, in the UO_2^{2+} case, the uranyl atom should be a six-coordinate octahedral with the oxygen atom in the apical position (Fig. 62).

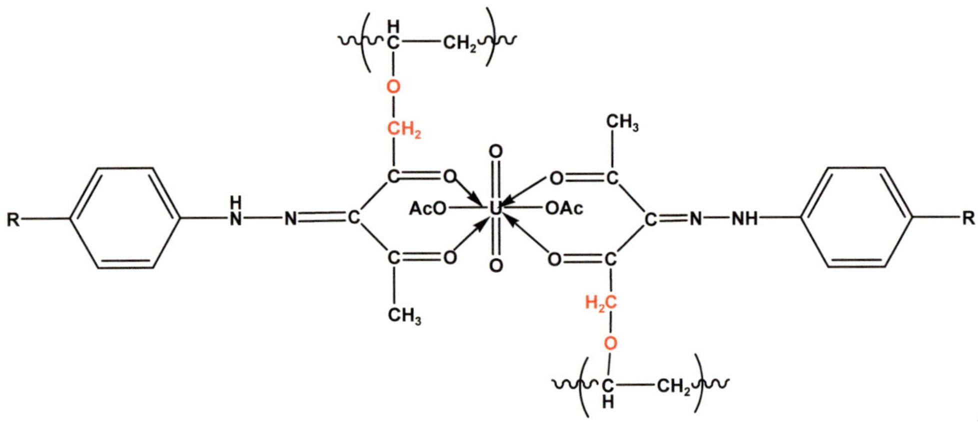

(n=1, R=OCH_3 (HL_1); n=2, R=CH_3 (HL_2); n=3, R=H (HL_3), n=4,R= Br (HL_4), and n=5, R=NO_2(HL_5)

Fig. 62. Molecular structure proposed for the VO $(L_n)_2$ complexes.

Novel supramolecular rare earth polymeric hydrazone complexes of 5-sulphadiazineazo-3-phenyl-2-thioxo-4-thiazolidinone (HL) of the composition $[(Ln)_2(HL)_3(NO_3)_6]_n$ where Ln = La(**1**), Y(**2**), Pr(**3**), Nd(**4**), Sm(**5**), Gd(**6**) and Ho(**7**) have been prepared and characterized on the basis of their chemical analyses, magnetic measurements, conductance, visible and IR spectral data (El-Sonbati et al., 2009). The IR spectrum of the ligand leads to assume the structure shown in Fig. 63.

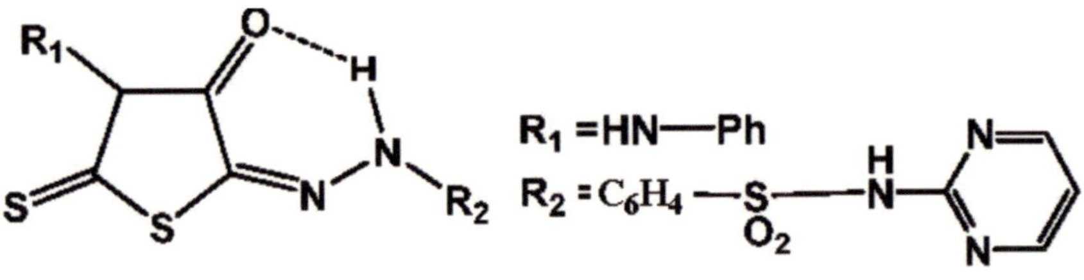

Fig. 63.

The spectral data show that all these act as tetradentate ligand. Electronic spectra indicate weak covalent character in the metal-ligand bond.

Polymer complexes of hydrazone sulphadrugs (HL_n) extended to novel five binuclear polymeric dioxouranium(VI) of azosulphadrugs (Fig. 64) (El-Sonbati et al., 2010a). The binding modes of the azosulphadrugs ligands towards uranyl(II) ions were critically assigned and addressed properly on the basis of their IR and their uranyl(II) complexes. 5-Sulphadiazinazo-3-phenyl-2-thioxo-4-thiozolidinone(HL_1) and 5-sulphamethineazo-3-phenyl-2-thioxo-4-thiozolidinone (HL_2) act as a tetradentate dibasic ligand, binding to the metal ion through nitrogen atom of diimide (N=N) group, nitrogen of azomethine pyridine atom (sulphadrugs moiety) and enolic OH group (sulphonyl oxygen) and through deprotonated hydrogen atom of phenolic oxygen atom (rhodanine). The sulphonamidic NH does not participate in bonding due to structure complication.

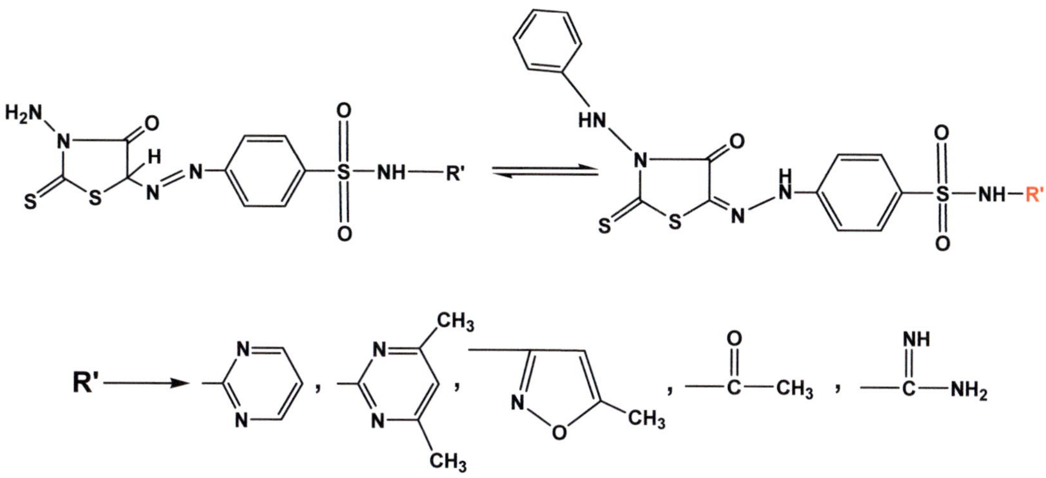

HL1 HL2 HL3 HL4 HL5

$HL_n + UO_2(NO_3)_2.2H_2O \rightarrow [(UO_2)_2(HL_n)(L_n)(NO_3)_2(OH_2)_2]_n + 2HNO_3$

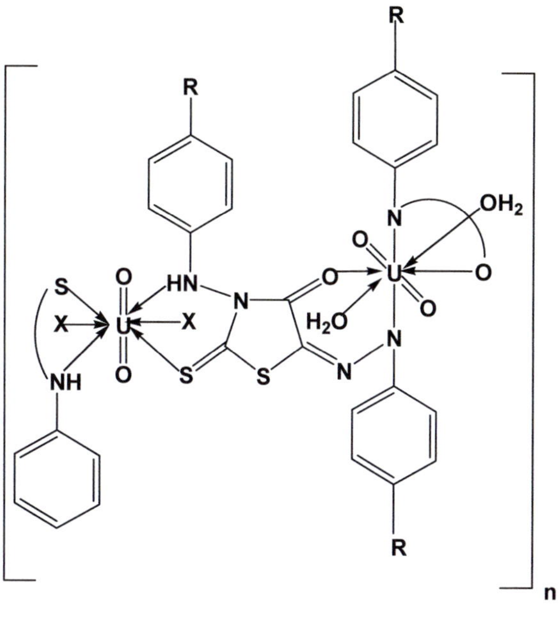

X = NO_3

Fig. 64. Geometrical formula of uranyl polymer complexes

Novel polymeric complexes with 5-sulphadiazineazo-3-phenyl-2-thioxo-4-thiazolidine (HL_1), 5-sulphamethazineazo-3-phenyl-2-thioxo-4- thiazolidine (HL_2) and 5-sulphamethoxazoleazo-3-phenyl-2-thioxo-4-thiazolidine (HL_3) and various anions were prepared (El-Sonbati et al., 2010b) according to the following scheme.

$2CuCl_2 + 3\ HL_n \rightarrow\ [(Cu)_2(HL_n)_3(Cl)_4]_n$

$2CuSO_4 + 3\ HL_n \rightarrow\ [(Cu)_2(HL_n)_3(SO_4)_2]_n$ where HL_n = tetradentate hydrazone, n = 1-3

The 2:3 stoichiometries of the polymeric complexes were calculated from their elemental analyses, and molar conductance reveal that three molecules of the ligand and four/two (Cl/SO_4) of the anions are coordinated to the two metal atoms in all complexes. The ligands coordinate to Cu(II) ion as an neutral and tetradentate *via* NH (hydrazone), oxygen of the carbonyl group (CO), nitrogen of the NH (3-phenylamine) and thion sulphur (CS) group.

A novel series of nickel(II) polymer complexes of 5-sulphadiazinazo-3-phenylamino-2-thio-4-thiozolidinone (HL_1), 5-sulphamethazine-3-phenylamino-2-thioxo-4-thiazolidinone (HL_2), 5-sulphamethoxazole-3-phenylamino-2-thioxo-4-thiazolidinone (HL_3), 5-sulpacetamide-3-phenyl-2-thioxo-4-thiozalidinone (HL_4) and 5-sulphaguanidine-3-phenylamino-2-thioxo-4-thiazolidinone (HL_5) were prepared and characterized (El-Sonbati et al., 2010c), IR spectra show that HL_n (n = 1-5) is coordinated to the metal ion in a neutral tetradentate manner with NSNO donor sites of NH (hydrazone`s), NH(3-phenylamine), carbonyl group and Ph-NH. The metal-to-ligand ratio of the nickel(II) polymer complexes was found to be 3:2, but all the Ni(II) polymer complexes have two additional bridged coordinated acetate molecules. So the Ni(II) ions appear to be five and hexa-coordinated acetate, and the geometry is octahedral for Ni(II) ion. The title $[Ni_3(HL_n)_2(\mu\text{-}OAc)_2(OAc)_4]_n$ consists of three Ni(II) atoms linked by interchain π-π interaction observed between aromatic rings of two (HL_n) which are further doubly bridged to two adjacent nickel atoms by acetate group. The geometrical structures of these complexes are found to be octahedral. The richness of electronic spectral in these is supporting evidence for the trinuclearity of the Ni(II) polymer complexes (Fig. 65).

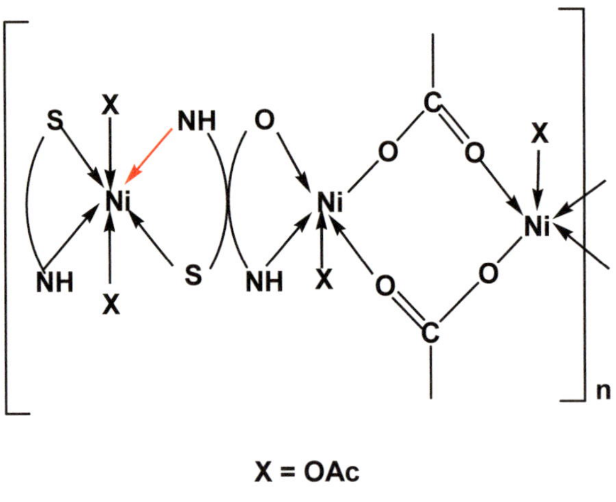

Fig. 65.

Polymer complexes of p-acrylamidyl sulphaguandine (HL) with Ni(II), Fe(II) and Pd(II) salts have been prepared (Fig. 66) (El-Sonbati et al., 2011a).

$NiX_2 + HL \rightarrow [Ni(HL)_2 X_2]_n$

where X = Cl^- (**1**), Br^- (**2**) I^- (**3**), NO_3^- (**4**) or SCN^- (**5**).

$FeSO_4 + HL \rightarrow [Fe(HL)(SO_4)(OH_2)_2]_n$ (**6**)

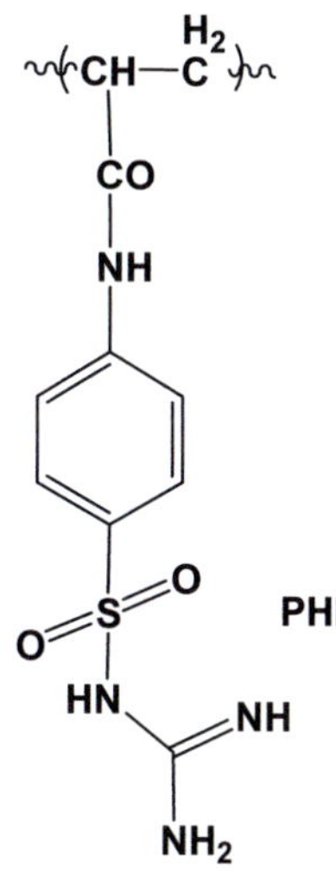

Fig. 66.

Nickel/iron mixed ligand polymer complexes were obtained by reacting pyridine (Py)/or ethylenediamine (en) with the calculated amount of trans-$[Ni(HL)_2Cl_2]$ (X = Cl^- or Br^-) as shown in Fig. 67.

$[Ni(HL)_2X_2]_n + Py \rightarrow [Ni(HL)_2(Py)_2]_nX_2$ where X = Cl^- (**7**), Br^- (**8**)

$[Fe(HL)(SO_4)(OH_2)]_n + en \rightarrow [Fe(HL)(en)(SO_4)(OH_2)]_n$ (**9**)

$PdX_2 + HL \rightarrow [Pd(LX)_2]_n$ where X = Cl^- (**10**), Br^- (**11**)

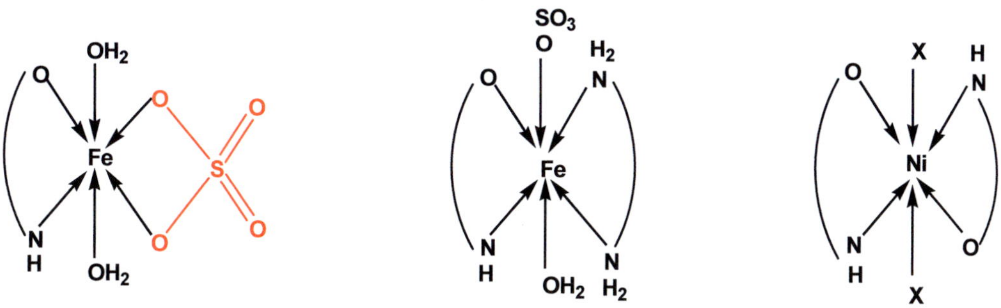

X = Cl (**1**), Br (**2**), I (**3**), ONO_2 (**4**), NCS (**5**), Py (**7,8**)

Fig. 67. Structure formulae of HL-metal polymer complexes

Novel polymer complexes of N-[3-(5-amino-1,2,4-triazolo)]acrylamide (ATA), formed by amidation of 3,5-diamino-1,2,4-triazole with acryloyl chloride were synthesized and characterized (Diab et al., 2011). Spectral studies reveal that the free ligand coordinates to the metal ion in a bidentate fashion through the oxygen of carbonyl group and a nitrogen azomethine of heterocyclic ring (Fig. 68). Elemental analyses of the polychelates indicate that the metal to ligand ratio was 1:1 and 1:2.

$$MCl_2 + ATA \xrightarrow{AIBN} P[M(ATA)Cl_2] \quad M = Cu(II) \text{ or } Cd(II)$$

$$MCl_2 + ATA \xrightarrow{AIBN} P[M(ATA)(OH_2)_2Cl_2] \quad M = Co(II) \text{ or } Ni(II)$$

$$UO_2(OAc)_2 + ATA \xrightarrow{AIBN} P[UO_2(ATA)(OAc)_2$$

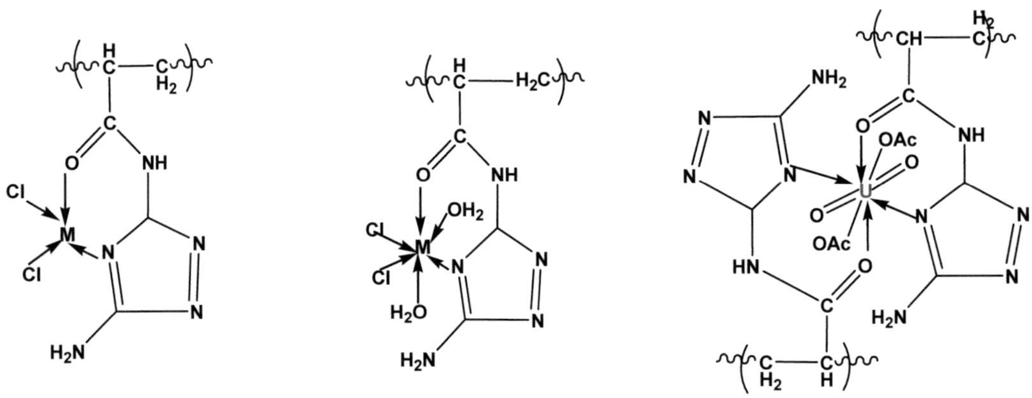

M = Cu(II) or Cd(II) M = Co(II) or Ni(II)

Fig. 68.

The amidation of acryloyl chloride with hydrazine hydrate in dry benzene forms acryloyl hydrazine (AH) monomer [(El-Bindary et al., 2011). Polymer complexes of AH with Cu(II), Ni(II), Co(II), Cd(II), UO_2(II) and Fe(III) salts have been prepared and characterized. AH has been shown to behave as a bidentate ligand via its nitrogen (NH_2 of the hydrazine group) and C-O/C=O (acryloyl) group in the polymer complexes, all of which exhibit supramolecular architectures assembled through weak interactions including hydrogen bonding and π-π staking. The elemental analyses, IR and electronic spectra data indicate that AN reacts with $CuCl_2$, $Cu(OAc)_2$, $FeCl_3$ and $CdCl_2$ in a 1:1 ratio (Structure I, III and V) and with $CoCl_2$ and $UO_2(OAc)_2$ in 2:1 molar ratios (Structure II and IV). The AH-$NiCl_2$ polymer complex is a mixture of both structure I and II. The magnetic and spectral data indicate a square planar geometry for Cu^{2+} complexes and an octahedral geometry for Co(II) and UO_2(II) complexes (Fig. 69). The ESR spectral data of the Cu(II) complexes showed that the metal-ligand bonds have considerable covalent character.

Oxovandium(IV) polymer complexes of formulation $\{[(VO)L]_2\}_n$(1) and $[(VO)LB]_n$ (2-4), where H_2L is tridentate and dianionic ligand, 3-allyl-2-thioxo-1,3-triazolidine-4,5-dione-5[*o*-hydroxylphenyl] and B is planar heterocyclic and aliphatic bases, bipyridyl (bipy); pyridine (py) and ethylenediamine (en) have been prepared and characterized (El-Sonbati et al., 2011b).

$$VOSO_4.5H_2O + H_2L \rightarrow \{[VOL]_2\}_n + H_2SO_4$$

$$VOSO_4.5H_2O + H_2L + B \rightarrow [VOLB]_n + H_2SO_4$$

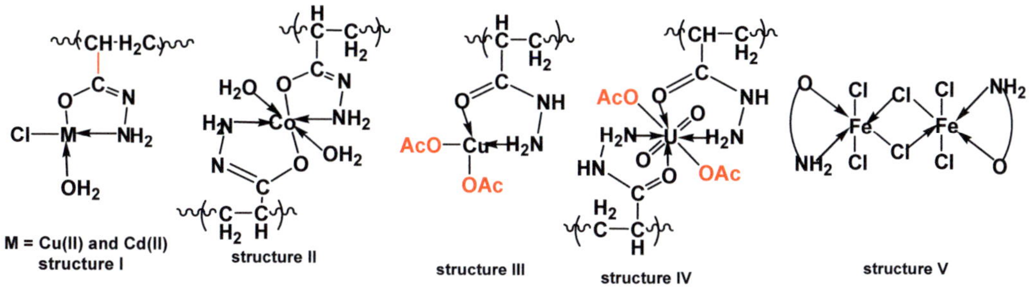

Fig. 69. Proposed structures of polymer complexes

The molecular structrure shows the presence of a vanadyl group in six-coordinate VNO_3/VN_2O_3 coordination geometry. The N,N-donor heterocyclic and aliphatic base displays an N-donor site *trans* to the vanadyl oxo-group. In all polymeric complexes (**1-4**) the ligand coordinates through oxygen of phenolic/enolic and azodye nitrogen. Formation of the polymer complexes has been done on the basis of their elemental analytical data, molar conductance values and magnetic susceptibilty data. All the complexes show 1:1$\{[VOL]_2\}_n$/1:1:1$[VOLB]_n$ metal:ligand/metal:ligand:base stoichiometry (Fig. 70).

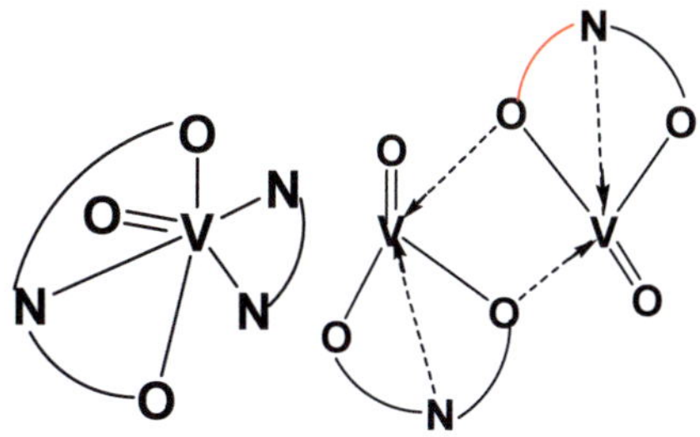

Fig. 70. Ternary structure of $[VOLB]_n$ (**2-4**) and the bases (B) used Tentative structure of polymer complex $\{[VOL]_2\}_n$ (**1**)

Recently, a novel ligand of N-[2-(6-aminopyridino)] acrylamide (APA) was prepared via amidation of 2,6-diaminopyridine with acryloyl chloride in dry benzene as solvent (El-Sonbati et al., 2011c). Metal-polymer complexes are reported and characterized. The formation of these polymer complexes proceeds according to the following equations:

$MCl_2 + APA \rightarrow [M(APA)Cl.OH_2]_n$ M = Cu(II) or Cd(II)

$MCl_2 + APA \rightarrow [M(APA)(OH_2)_3Cl]_n$ M = Co(II) or Ni(II)

$UO_2(OAc)_2 + APA \rightarrow [UO_2(APA)_2(OH_2)_2]_n$

The proposed strucrure for the polychelates is shown in Fig. 71.

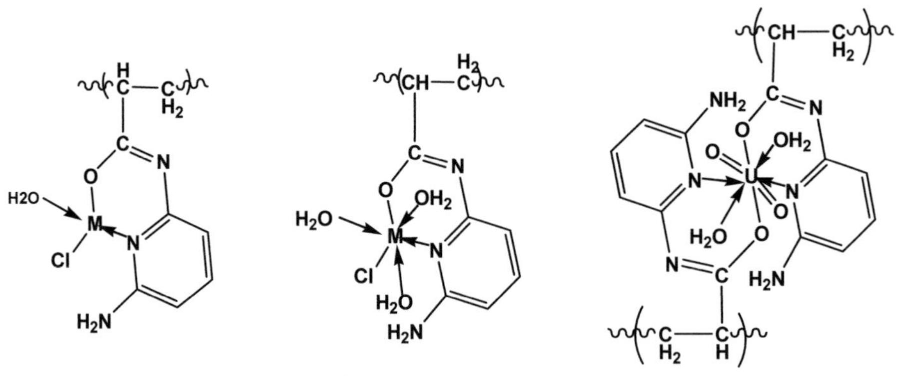

M = Cu(II) or CdII) M = Co(II) or Ni(II)

Fig. 71. Proposed structure of the polymer complexes

3. Conclusions

The coordination polymer research field of study is a vast and one of the fastest growing areas of chemistry in recent times, with important work being done on a large variety of different aspects. Polymer complexes are an important class of new materials due to the coupling of the chemical, optical and electronic properties of the metal moiety to those of the polymer. This review, however, provides a uniquely broad overview of the stoichiometry of polymer complexes by using elemental analyses, FT-IR and IR spectra. The geometry of the polymer complexes was evaluated by electronic spectra (UV.-Vis.) and magnetic moment measurements.

4. Acknowledgement

The authors are grateful to Dr. M.M. El-Halawany, Department of Mathematics and Physics Sciences, Faculty of Engineering, Mansoura University for his patience and neat diligent drawing all the structures of the review.

5. References

Agnew, N.H. (1976). *Transition metal complexes of poly(vinylpyridines)*, J. Polym. Sci., Polym. Chem. Ed. 14, 2819-2830.

Ahmed, M., Malik, M.A., Pervez, S. & Raffiq, M. (2004). *Effect of porosity on sulfonation of macroporous styrene-divinylbenzene beads*, Eur. Polym. J. 40, 1609-1613.

Amon, W.F. & Kane, K.W. (1950). *Macrocyclic beryllium chelates and their polymers*, US Pat. 2, 505, 85 - 88.

Arthur, J.C.Jr. & Blouin, F.A. (1964). *Radiochemical yield of graft polymerization reactions of cellulose*, J. Appl. Polym. Sci. 8 (6), 2813-2824.

Bamford, C.H., Jenkins, A.D. & Johnston, R.J.(1957).*Studies in polymerization XII. Salt effects on the Polymerization of acrylonitrile in non-aqueous solution*, Proc. Royal Soc. (London) A 241, 364-375.

Bamford, C.H., Jenkins, A.D. &. Johnston, R.J. (1958). *Kinetic effects of salts on vinyl polymerization in non- aqueous systems*, J. Polym. Sci. 28 (120), 355-366.

Bamford, C.H., Brumby, S. & Wayne, R.P. (1966a). *Effect of zinc chloride on the velocity coefficients in the polymerization of methyl methacrylate*, Nature 209, 292-294.

Bamford, C.H., Brumby. S & Wayne, R.P. (1966b). *Photolysis of nitrosyl chloride by ultraviolet radiation*, Nature 209, 292-295.

Batten, S.R. & Murray, K.S. (2003). *Structure and magnetism of coordination polymers containing dicyanamide and tricyanomethanide*, Coord. Chem. Rev. 246 (1-2), 103-130.

Bovey, F.A. (1960). *Polymer NSR spectroscopy. V. The effect of zinc chloride on the free radical polymerization of methyl methacrylate*, J. Polym. Sci. 47(149), 480-481.

Diab, M.A., El-Sonbati, A.Z., El-Sanabari, A.A. & Taha, F.I. (1988). *Polymer complexes: Part VI-Thermal stability of poly(2-acrylamidophenol) homopolymer and complexes of poly(2-acrylamidophenol) with some transition metal salts* , Polym. Deg. & Stab. 23, 83-90.

Diab, M.A., El-Sonbati, A.Z., El-Sanabari, A.A. & Taha, F.I. (1989a). *Polymer complexes: Part VIII-Thermal stability of poly(2-acrylamidopyridine) homopolymer and polymer complexes of 2-acrylamidopyridine with some transition metal chlorides*, Polym. Deg. & Stab. 24, 51-58.

Diab, M.A., El-Sonbati, A.Z. & Ghoniem, M.M. (1989b). *Polymer complexes. IX. Thermal stability of poly[bis(2,6-diaminopyridine sulphoxide)] and polymer complexes of bis (2,6-diaminopyridine sulphoxide) with copper halides*, Acta Polymerica 40 (8), 545-547.

Diab, M.A., El-Sonbati, A.Z., El-Sanabari, A.A. & Taha, F.I. (1990a). *Polymer complexes. XIII. Thermal stability Of poly(2-acrylamidobenzoic acid) homopolymer and polymer complexes of 2-acrylamidobenzoic acid with transition metals*, Acta Polymerica 41(1), 45-48.

Diab, M.A., El-Sonbati, A.Z. Hilali, A.S., Killa, H.M. & Ghoniem, M.M. (1990b). *Polymer complexes: Part XIV. Thermal stability of poly(5-vinyl salicylidene anthranilic acid) homopolymer and polymer complexes of 5-vinyl salicylidene anthranilic acid with some transition metal salts*, Polym. Deg. & Stab. 29, 165-173.

Diab, M.A. & El-Sonbati, A.Z. (1990). Polymer complexes: Part XV. *Thermal stability of poly(ethylene glycol) homopolymer and polymer complexes of poly(ethylene glycol) with some transition metal chlorides*, Polym. Deg. & Stab. 29, 271-277.

Diab, M.A., M.E., El-Sonbati, A.Z., & Attallah, M.E. (2012). *Polymer complexes. LV. Spectroscopic and thermal studies on supramolecular complexation of transition elements with N-[3-(5-amino-1,2,4-triazolo) acrylamide*, J. Coord. Chem. 65, 539-549.

El-Bindary, A.A.., El-Sonbati,. A.Z., Diab, M.A., El-Ela,. M.A, & Mazrouh, S.A. (1993). *Polymer complexes. XXII. Metal chelates of poly[(5-vinylsalicylidene)-2-aminomethylpyridine]*, Synth. React. Inorg. Met.-Org. Chem., 23 (6), 875-888.

El-Bindary, A.A., El-Shihri, A.S. & El-Sonbati, A.Z. (2003). *Polymer complexes. XLI. Supramolecular assemblies comprised a novel structural models of mixed metal polymer complexes*, Desig. Mono. & Polym. 6 (3), 283- 298.

El-Bindary, A.A., El-Sonbati, A.Z., Diab, M.A., & Attallah, M.E. (2012). *Polymer complexes. LVI. Supramolecular architectures consolidated by hydrogen bonding and π-π interaction*, Spectrochim. Acta, Part A 79, 1057-1062.

El-Hendawy, A.M., El-Sonbati, A.Z. & Diab, M.A. (1989). *Polymer complexes. XI. Thermal stability of poly(5-vinyl salicyldehyde) with some transition metal salts*, Acta Polymerica 40 (11), 710-713.

El-Sonbati, A.Z. & Diab, M.A. (1988a). *Polymer complexes. I. Stability of methyl methacrylate-transition metal bromide polymer complexes*, Acta Polymerica 39 (3), 124-127.

El-Sonbati, A.Z. & Diab, M.A. (1988b). *Polymer complexes. II. Polymerization of acrylonitrile in presence of some transition metal bromide*, Acta Polymerica 39 (10), 558-562.

El-Sonbati, A.Z. & Diab, M.A. (1988c). *Polymer complexes. III. Stability and degradation of acrylonitrile- transition metal bromide polymer complexes*, Acta Polymerica 39 (11), 651-653.

El-Sonbati, A.Z. & Diab, M.A. (1988d). *Polymer complexes. IV. Thermal stability of poly(8-quinolyl acrylate) and the polymers of the complexes of 8-quinolyl acrylate with some transition metal salts*, Polym. Deg. & Stab. 22, 295-302.

El-Sonbati, A.Z., El-Dissouky, A. & Diab, M.A. (1989). *Polymer complexes. V. Thermal stability of poly(acrylamido-4-aminoantipyrinyl) homopolymer and polymer complexes of acrylamido-4-aminopyrinyl with some transition metal salts*, Acta Polymerica 40 (2), 112-116.

El-Sonbati, A.Z. (1991a). *Polymer complexes. XVII. Thermal stability of poly(5-vinyl salicylidene)-2- aminophenol homopolymer and polymer complexes of 5-vinyl salicylidene-2-aminophenol with transition metal acetate*, Transition Met. Chem. 16, 45-47.

El-Sonbati, A.Z. (1991b). *Polymer complexes.XVIII. polychelates from poly(5-vinyl salicylidene hydrazine-S-benzyl dithiocarbozate) with some transition metal salts*, Synth. React. Inorg. Met.-Org. Chem. 21 (2), 203- 216.

El-Sonbati, A.Z., Diab, M.A., Kotb, M.F. & Killa, H.M. (1991). *Polymer complexes. XIX. Structural chemistry of poly(2-acrylamido-1,2-diaminobenzene) complexes*, Bull. Soc. Chim. Fr. 128, 623-627.

El-Sonbati, A.Z. (1991c). *Polymer complexes. XX. Stability studies in relation to IR data and structural chemistry of polychelate from poly(5-vinyl salicylidene) semicarbazone with some transition metal acetates*, Synth. React. Inorg. Met.-Org. 21 (6&7), 977-990.

El-Sonbati, A.Z., Killa, H.M., Kotb, M.F. & Diab, M.A. (1992). *Polymer complexes. XII. Polymerization of methyl acrylate in the presence of some transition metal salts*, Polym. Deg. & Stab. 35, 255-260.

El-Sonbati, A.Z. (1992). *Polymer complexes. Part XVI. Structural chemistry of poly(5-vinyl salicylidene) aniline complexes* Transition Met. Chem. 17, 19-22.

El-Sonbati, A.Z. & Hefni, M.A. (1993). *Polymerization complexes. Part XXI. Stereochemical changes of metal chelates of poly(5-vinyl salicylidene-2-benzothiazoline)*, Monat. fur Chemie 124, 419-424.

El-Sonbati, A.Z., El-Bindary, A.A., Diab, M.A., El-Ela, M.M. & Mazrouh, S.A. (1993a). *Polymer complexes. XXIV. Physico-chemical studies on coordination and stability in relation to IR data for poly(cinnamaldehyde-2-anthranilic acid) complexes of d-block elements*, Polym. Deg. & Stab. 42, 1-11.

El-Sonbati, A.Z., El-Bindary, A.A., Diab, M.A. & Mazrouh, S.A.. (1993b). *Polymer complexes. XXIII. Synthesis and physico-chemical studies on transition metal complexes of symmetric novel poly(N,N`-o- phenylenediamine)bis(cinnamaldehyde)*, Monat. fur Chemie 124, 793-801.

El-Sonbati, A.Z., El-Bindary, A.A., Diab, M.A., El-Ela, M.A. & Mazrouh, S.A. (1994a). *Polymer complexes: 25. complexing ability of poly(5-vinyl salicylidene-2-aminopyridine) towards different metal(II) salts*, Polymer 35 (3), 647-652.

El-Sonbati, A.Z. & Hefni, M.A. (1994). *Polymer complexes. Part XXVI. Novel mixed ligand poly(5-vinyl salicylidene)-1,2-diaminobenzene complexes,* Polym. Deg. & Stab. 43, 33-42.

El-Sonbati, A.Z., Hassanein, A.M., Mohamed, M.T. & Abd El-Moiz, A.B. (1994b). *Polymer complexes. Part XXVII. Novel mixed-valence-ligand poly(2-acrylamido-1-phenyl-2-aminothiourea) complexes,* Polym. Deg. & Stab. 46, 31-40.

El-Sonbati, A.Z., Abd El-Moiz, A.B. & Hassanein, A.M. (1995a). *Polymer complexes. XXVIII. Novel mixed-metal poly(2-acrylamido-1-phenyl-2-aminothiourea) complexes,* Polym. Deg. & Stab. 48, 35-44.

El-Sonbati, A.Z., Abd El-Moiz, A.B. & Hassanein, A.M. (1995b). *Polymer complexes. XXIX. Novel polymer complexes prepared from poly[1-acrylamido-2(2-pyridyl)] ethane,* Polym. Deg. & Stab. 48, 45-53.

El-Sonbati, A.Z. & El-Bindary, A.A. (1996). *Polymer complexes. XXX. Novel polymer complexes prepared in the present investigation from poly[1-acrylamido-2(2-pyridyl)-ethane],* New Polymeric Mater. 5 (1), 51-60.

El-Sonbati, A.Z., El-Bindary, A.A. & Rashed, I.G.A. (2002). *Polymer complexes. XXXVII. Novel models and structural of symmetrical poly-Schiff base on heterobinuclear complexes of dioxouranium(VI),* Spectrochim. Acta, Part A 58, 1411-1424.

El-Sonbati, A.Z., El-Bindary, A.A. & Diab, M.A. (2003a). *Polymer complexes. XXXX. Supramolecular assembly on coordination models of mixed-valence-ligand poly[1-acrylamido-2(2-pyridyl)ethane] complexes,* Spectrochim. Acta, Part A 59, 443-454.

El-Sonbati, A.Z., Al-Shihri, A.S. & El-Bindary, A.A. (2003b). *Polymer complexes. XLIII. EPR spectra and stereochemical versatility of novel copper(II) polymer complexes,* J. Inorg. & Organomet. Polym. 13 (2), 99- 108.

El-Sonbati, A.Z., El-Bindary, A.A., Issa, R.M. & Kera, H.M. (2004a). *Polymer complexes. XLII. Supramolecular assemblies comprised of macrocyclic polymer complexes,* Desig. Mon. & Polym. 7 (5), 445-459.

El-Sonbati, A.Z., Al-Shihri, A.S. & El-Bindary, A.A. (2004b). *Polymer complexes. XLV. Spectral studies on metal-ligand bonding in novel poly-Schiff base complexes,* J. Inorg. & Organomet. Polym. 14 (1), 53-71.

El-Sonbati, A.Z., Al-Sarawy, A.A. & Moqbal, A.M. (2009). *Polymer complexes. XLIX. Supramolecular modeling of bonding in novel rare earth polymeric rhodanine drug complexes,* Spectrochim. Acta, Part A 74, 463- 468.

El-Sonbati, A.Z., Diab, M.A., El-Shehawy, M.S. & Moqbal, M. (2010a). *Polymer complexes. XLV. Novel supramolecular coordination modes of structure and bonding in polymeric hydrazone sulphadrugs uranyl complexes,* Spectrochim. Acta, Part A 75, 394-405.

El-Sonbati, A.Z., Diab, M.A., El-Halawany, M.M. & Salam, N.E. (2010b). *Polymer complexes. XLXI. Supramolecular spectral studies on metal-ligand bonding of novel rhodanine sulphadrugs hydrazone,* Mat. Chem. & Phys. 123, 439-449.

El-Sonbati, A.Z., Diab, M.A., El-Halawany, M.M. & Salam, N.E. (2010c). *Polymer complexes. XLXII. Interplay of coordination π-π stacking and hydrogen bonding in supramolecular assembly of [sulpha drug derivatives- N,S:N,O] complexes,* Spectrochim. Acta, Part A 77, 755-766.

El-Sonbati, A.Z., Belal, A.A.M., Diab, M.A. & Mohamed, R.H. (2011a). *Polymer complexes. LIV. Structural and spectral studies of supramolecular coordination polymers built from Ni(II), Fe(II) and Pd(II) with sulphadrug,* J. Mol. Str. 990, 26-31.

El-Sonbati, A.Z., Diab, M.A. & Bulboula, M.Z. (2011b). *Polymer complexes. LXIII. Structures of supramolecular assemblies of vanadium chelating groups Spectrochim.* Acta, Part A 78, 1119-1125.

El-Sonbati, A.Z., Diab, M.A. & Mohamed, R.H. (2011c). *Polymer complexes. LIX. Supramolecular structural, spectral and thermal analysis of N-[2-(6-aminopyridino)] acrylamide polymer complexes,* Polym. Int. 60, 1467-1474.

Epstein, A. & Wildi, B.S. (1960). Electrical properties of poly-copper phthalocyanine, J. Chem. Phys. 32 (2), 324- 329.

Fenger, I. & Le Drian, C. (1998). *Reusable polymer-supported palladium catalysts: An alternative to tetrakis(triphenylphine) palladium in the suzuki cross-coupling reaction,* Tetrahedron Lett. 39, 4287-4290.

Hojo, N. & Shiria, H. (1972). *Kinetics of ligand exchange reaction of Cu(II)-amine complex with poly(vinyl alcohol) in aqueous solution,* Nippon Kagatu Kaishi, 1316-1320.

Imoto, M., Otsu, T. & Shimizu, S. (1963). *Vinyl polymerization. LXVI. The effect of zinc chloride on the radical polymerization of vinyl monomers,* Die Makromol. Chemie 65 (1), 174-179.

Imoto, M., Otsu, T., Yamada, B. & Shimizu, A. (1965). *Further results on the effect of zinc chloride in the copolymerization of methyl methacrylate or acrylonitrile with some butenes or allylic compounds,* Die Makromol. Chemie 82, 277-280.

James, S.L. (2003). *Metal-organic frameworks,* Chem. Soc. Rev. 32, 276-288.

Janiak, C. (2003). *Engineering coordination polymers towards applications,* Dalton Trans. 2781-2804.

Kabanov, V.A. (1969). *Effect of formation of complexes on radical polymerization processes.*IUPAC International Symposium on Macromolecular Chemistry, Budapest, 435-462.

Kaneko, M. & Tsuchide, E. (1981). *Formation, characterization and catalytic activities of polymer-metal complexes,* J. Polym. Sci., Macromol. Rev. 16 (1), 397-522.

Katon, J.E. (1970). "*Organic semiconducting polymers*", Marcel Dekker, New York.

Kurimura, Y., Tsuchide, E. & Kaneko, M. (1971). *Preparations and properties of some water-soluble cobalt(III)- poly-4-vinylpyridine complexes,* J. Polym. Sci., Part A-1: Polym. Chem. 9 (12), 3511-3519.

Lazuke, S., Tsugi, K., Yanezawa, T. & Okamura, S. (1967). *Reactivity of coordinated ligands as studied by molecular orbital calculation. I. Radical polymerizability of zinc complexes of vinyl compounds,* J. Phys. Chem. 71 (9), 2957-2968.

Lyons, A.M., Vasile, M.J., Pearce, E.M. & Wasjczok, J.V. (1988). *Copper chloride complexes with poly(2-vinylpyridine): preparation and redox properties,* Macromolecules 21 (11), 3125-3134.

Maspoch, D., Ruiz-Molina, D. & Veciana, J. (2004). *Magnetic nanoporous coordination polymers,* J.Mater. Chem. 14, 2713-2723.

Mizuta, T., Onishi, M. & Miyoshi, K. (2000). *Photolytic ring-opening polymerization of phosphorous-bridged [1]. Ferrocenophane coordinating to an organometallic fragment,* Organometallics 19 (24), 5005-5009.

Mubarak, A.T. & El-Sonbati, A.Z. (2006). *Novel ligation of some rare earth metal supramolecular polymer complexes*, Polym. Bull. 57, 683-690.

Mubarak, A.T., El-Sonbati, A.Z., El-Bindary, A.A., Issa, R.M. & Kera, H.M. (2006). *Polymer complexes: supramolecular modeling for determination and identification the band length in novel polymer complexes from their infrared spectra*, J. Appl. Organomet. Chem. 20, 819-829.

Osada, Y. (1975). *Microtacticity of the polymers obtained by radical polymerization of methacrylic acid coordinated to Co(II) complexes*, Die Makromol. Chemie 176 (6), 1893-1896.

Osada, Y. (1976a). *Radical polymerization reactivities of methacrylic acid coordinated to cobalt(III) complexes*, Die Makromol. Chemie 177 (5), 1259-1271.

Osada, Y. (1976b). *Configurational effects of metal complexes attached to methacrylic acid in the process of radical polymerization*, Die Makromol. Chemie 177 (5), 1273-1282.

Osada, Y. & Ishida, K. (1976). *Alternative copolymer with-(ABA)-sequences from the radical copolymerization of methacrylic acid coordinated to Co(III) complex with sodium styrene-4-sulfonate*, Die Makromol. Chemie, 177 (7), 2209-2213.

Orazzhanova, L.K., Yashkarova, H.G., Issue, L.A. & Kudaibergenov, S.E. (2003). *Binary and ternary polymer- strontium complexes and the capture of radioactive strontium-90 from the polluted soil of the semipalalinsk nuclear test site*, J. Appl. Polym. Sci. 87 (5), 759-764.

Ro, K.W., Chang, W.J., Kim, H., Koo, Y.M. & Hahn, J.H. (2003). *Capilary electrochromatography and preconcentration of neutral compounds on poly(dimethylsiloxane) microchips*, Electrophoresis 24 (18), 3253-3259.

Serniuk, S.E. & Thomas, R.M. (1965). *Copolymerization of polar with nonpolar monomers in the presence of a Friedal-Crafts and a free radical initiator.* (to Essa Research & Engineering Co.), US Pat. 3, 183-217.

Serniuk, S.E. & Thomas, R.M. (1966). *Copolymerization with monomer complexes.* (to Esso Research & Engineering Co.), US Pat. 3, 278, 503.

Tazuka, S. & Okamura, S. (1966). *Effect of metal salts on polymerization. Part 1. Polymerization of vinylpyridine initiated with cupric acetate*, J. Polym. Sci. 4 (1), 141-157.

Tazuka, S., Sato, N. & Shimizu, S. (1966). *Effects of metal salts on polymerization. Part II. Polymerization of vinylpyridine complexed with the group IIb metal salts*, J. Polym. Sci., Part A-1: Polym. Chem. Ed. 4 (10), 2461-2478.

Tazuka, S., Okamura, S. (1967). *Effects of metal salts on polymerization. Part III. Radical polymerizabilities and infrared spectra of vinylpyridines complexed with zinc and cadmium salts*, J. Polym. Sci., Part A-1: Polym.Chem. Ed. 5 (5), 1083-1099.

Tsuchide, E., Nishide, H. & Takeshita, M.. (1974). *Steric and electrostatic factors on the formation and the structure of polymeric cobalt(III) complexes*, Die Makromol. Chemie 175 (8) 2293-2306.

Varghese, S., Lele, A.K., Sirnivas, D. & Mashellear, R.A. (2001). *Role of hydrophobicity on structure of polymer- metal complexes*, J. Phys. Chem. B 105 (23), 5368-5373.

Varvara, S., Muresane, L., Popescu, I.C. & Maurin, G. (2004). *Copper electrodeposition from sulfate electrolytes in the presence of hydroxyethylated-2-butyne-1, 4-diol*, Hydrometallurgy 75, 147-156.

Wertz, D.L. & Tyroll, L. (1974). *The coordination of Cu(II) in a nearly saturated solution of* $CuCl_2$ *in hydrochloric acid,* J. Inorg. & Nucl. Chem. 36 (12), 3713-3717.

Zubov, V.P., Lachinov, N.B., Golubov, V.B., Kilikova, V.F., Kabanov, V.A., Polak, L.S. & Kargin, V.A. (1968). *The influence of complexing agents on the polymerization of vinyl and allyl monomers,* J. Polym. Sci., Part C 23 (1), 147-155.

8

Dermatological Application of PAMAM – Vitamin Bioconjugates and Host-Guest Complexes – Vitamin C Case Study

Stanisław Wołowiec[1], Marek Laskowski[1], Barbara Laskowska[1], Agnieszka Magoń[2], Bogdan Mysliwiec[2] and Marek Pyda[2]
[1]*Department of Cosmetology, University of Information Technology and Management,*
[2]*Faculty of Chemistry, Rzeszów University of Technology, Rzeszów*
Poland

1. Introduction

Stoichiometry of reaction describes the quantitative relationships among substances as they participate in chemical reactions. Furthermore the term stoichiometry is used to describe the quantitative relationship among elements in compounds. This is also valid in the quantitative description of so-called weak complexes formed between molecules through non-covalent and non-ionic interactions. They generally arise from hydrogen bonding or Van der Waals interactions and are very common in biological chemistry, like in the case of enzyme-substrate, enzyme-inhibitor, or enzyme-coenzyme complexes. In less specific systems, stoichiometry may be referred to the number of small molecules interacting with one macromolecule to form complex structure. Depending on the interaction type between the components of the complex they are often desribed as host (macromolecule, H) - guest (small molecule, g) complexes. The host-guest complexes can sometimes be isolated as compounds of defined strochiometry, however their dissolution always leads to establishing an equilibrium between complexes and free guest, according to the scheme:

$$Hg_n \Leftrightarrow Hg_{n-1} + g \Leftrightarrow Hg_{n-2} + 2g \Leftrightarrow Hg_{n-3} + 3g \ldots\ldots\ldots \Leftrightarrow H + ng \qquad (1)$$

described by overall formation constant:

$$K = [Hg_n]/[H][g]^n \qquad (2)$$

This weak interaction between H and g leads to the formation of multiple complexes Hg_n, with n = 1, 2, 3, …. n, depending on g concentration, which is in excess compared to H one. Its larger amount is necessary to determine n_{max}, i.e. the maximum amount of guest molecules which are able to interact with one host macromolecule. Thus the n_{max} is often referred to as host-guest complex stoichiometry or host capacity in relation to specific guest.

Commonly employed molecular complex is the one used in iodometric titration, where the equivalent point is determined by the deeply blue color of starch (macromolecular host) and iodine (guest) complex disappearance with the iodine completely consumed by thiosulfate (Rundle & Frank, 1943).

Starch is a glucose polymer containing mainly α(1-4) glycosidic bonds with an amylose moiety forming polyiodide complexes with maximum absorbance at 620 nm. Being starch a polydisperse polymer, the equilibrium constant for the blue iodine complex formation is actually the averaged value (Saenger, 1984).

More adequate formation constants can be determined for monodisperse macromolecules, such as dendritic polymers. The dendrimer chemistry developed very fast over the last two decades, and it has been the subject of many reviews due to dendrimers numerous applications, such as: nanomaterials for molecular electronics, photonics, sensors (Astruc et al., 2010, Lo & Burn, 2007) and nanomedicine (D'Emanuele & Attwood, 2005, Caruthers et al., 2007). Polyethyleneimine (PEI), polyester (PES) and polyamidoamine (PAMAM) dendrimers invented in Frechet's and Tomalia's group macromolecules own a signifficant position among dendrimeric molecules (Frechet et al., 1995, Tomalia , 2005a and b).

2. Polyamidoamine dendrimers (PAMAM)

2.1 General characteristics of PAMAM dendrimers

The dendritic molecules are globular shaped monodisperse objects. The polyamidoamine dendrimers (PAMAM) were synthesized in Tomalia's group (Tomalia et al., 2003, Tomalia, 2005). The PAMAM dendrimers of full generation posses several surface amine groups which make them perfectly soluble in water. They can be obtained by alternate addition of methyl acrylate to amine (in our study ethylenediamine has been used as starting diamine core) resulting in doubling the surface methyl propionate groups, followed by condensation of ester groups with diamine (ethylenediamine being the best choice). The latter step introduces further amine function on surface. Thus the full generation (Gn) PAMAM dendrimers posses: 8, 16, 32, and 64 surface amine groups in G1, G2, G3, and G4, respectively. The synthetic pattern is shown in Scheme 1. The hydrodynamic diameters of full generation PAMAM dendrimers are: 1.5, 2.2, 2.9, 3.6, and 4.5 nm for G0, G1, G2, G3, and G4, respectively. The surface structure of full generation dendrimers can be widely modified by surface amine groups conversion, resulting in change in their solubility and permeability properties (Jevprasesphant et al., 2003, Imae et al., 2000). The PAMAM dendrimers are molecules with inner cavities, which are able to absorb small molecules to form host-guest complexes. During the synthesis of PAMAM dendrimers in methanol, the final removal of this solvent from the dendrimer spherical macromolecule requires prolonged vacuum evaporation. PAMAM dendrimers ability to encapsulate hydrophobic guests was extensively used as a strategy for promoting water insoluble drugs transportation into tissues and cells (vide infra).

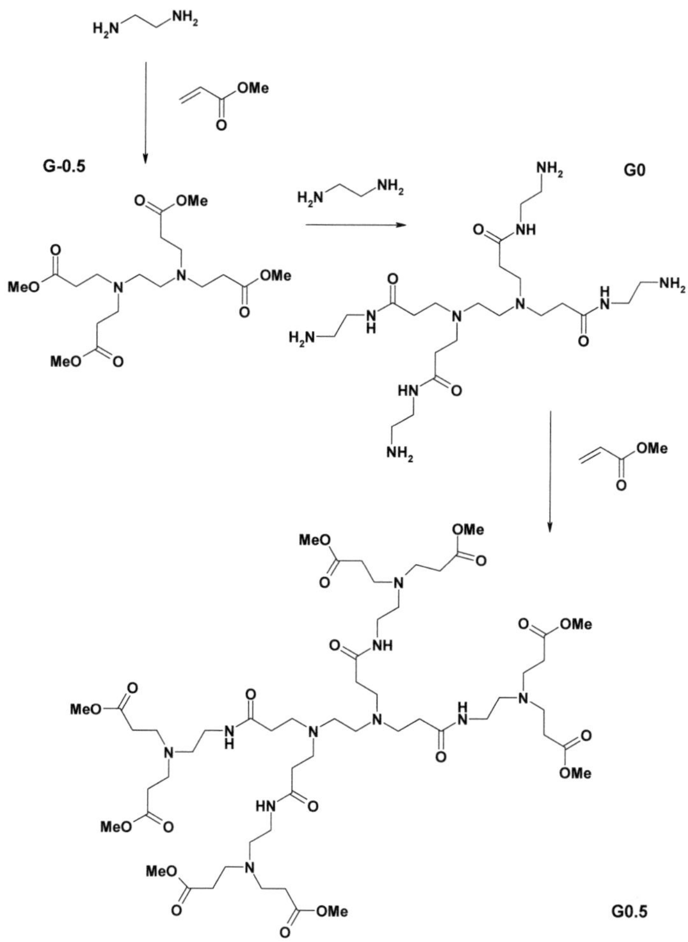

Scheme 1. The scheme of synthesis of PAMAM dendrimers on ethylenediamine (en) core. Addition of methyl acrylate to en results in formation of -0.5 half-generation PAMAM dendrimer (G-0.5) with four methyl ester groups on surface. The condensation of G-0.5 with four en equivalents leads to full-generation PAMAM dendrimer (G0). Further addition of methyl acrylate gives G0.5 PAMAM dendrimer, which upon next condensation with eight en equivalents results in obtaining full generation PAMAM dendrimer G1 (not shown). Repeated sequence of addition/condensation protocol leads to G1.5, G2, G2,5, G3 and so on.

2.2 Medical applications of PAMAM dendrimers

PAMAM dendrimers are relatively low toxic (Jain et al., 2010, Mukherjee et al., 2010, Kolhatkar et al., 2007, Hans & Lowman, 2002). Therefore they are extensively studied as drug carriers. There are two strategies commonly applied: 1) diffusion of prodrug covalently bound to the dendrimer, and 2) diffusion of drug encapsulated in the dendrimer. Thus, the PAMAM dendrimers act as solubilizers for anti-inflamatory drugs *ketoprofen* (Yiyun et al., 2005), *ibuprofen* (Milhem et al., 2000) and *indomethacin* (Chauhan et al., 2003) and promote their prolonged release both *in vitro* and *in vivo* (Na et al., 2006, Kolhe et al., 2003). Similar concept was used to increase solubility and uptake flux of several anticancer drugs, like *methoxyestradiol* (Wang et al., 2011), *adriamycin* and *methotrexate* (Kojima et al., 2000), a plant alkaloid *camptothecin* (Cheng et al., 2008), *doxorubicidin* (Papagiannaros et al., 2005), and *dimethoxycurcumin* (Markatou et al. 2007). Moreover, *nifedipine* - a calcium channel blocking agent (Devarakonda et al., 2004, 2005), a loop diuretic *furosemide* (Devarakonda et al., 2007, antipsychotic drug *risperidone* (Prieto et al., 2011), a hypolipidemic drug (Kulhari et al., 2011), antibiotic *quinolones* (Cheng et al., 2007), antibacterial *sulfamethoxazole* (Ma et al., 2007), as well as ophtalmic drugs *pilocarpine nitrate* and *tropicamide* (Vandamme & Brobeck, 2005) were also supported by PAMAM dendrimers as carrier. Surprisingly PAMAM – drug complexes were proven to be effectively transdermal increasing the flux of *5-fluorouracil* - a drug for treatment of psoriasis, premalignant and malignant skin conditions (Venuganti & Perumal, 2008, Bhadra et al., 2003) of dermatologically important vitamins, like *nicotinic acid* Cheng & Xu, 2005) and *riboflavin* (Filipowicz & Wołowiec, 2011) as well as of *psoralene* – the photosensitizer used for treatment of psoriasis (Borowska et al., 2010).

A more advanced strategy is based on a covalent bonding of the prodrug, bioconjugates being extremely promising for site-directed therapy. Thus, the PAMAM bioconjugates with drugs synthesized and tested *in vitro* so far are the one with *methotrexate* and *folate* (Patri et al., 2005, Chandrasekar et al., 2009), *ibuprofen* (Kolhe et al., 2006, Kurtoglu et al., 2010), *methylprednisolone* (Khandare et al., 2005), *adriamycin* (Kono et al., 2008), *triamcinolone* (Ma et al., 2009), *propranolol* (D'Emanuele et al., 2004), *5-aminosalicylic acid* (Wiwattanapatapee et al., 2003), and especially important for skin treatment *phosphorylcholine* (Jia et al., 2011), *cholic acid* (Zhang et al., 2011), *biotin* (Yang et al., 2009), and *riboflavin* (Thomas et al., 2010). Similar studies are currently being performed in our laboratory to clarify the skin penetration of vitamins supported by PAMAM dendrimers. In some cases PAMAM dendrimers act as solubilizers and enhance the skin load, while in other cases the vitamin flux decreases. Here we present the latest results on vitamin C permeation in the presence of PAMAM dendrimers.

3. PAMAM dendrimers as carriers for vitamin C

Ascorbic acid (vitamin C) is an essential nutrient protecting living tissues from oxidation processes by free radicals and reactive oxygen derived species. It is also an important co-factor in collagen synthesis, hence present in most cosmetic products. The bioavailability of topically applied vitamin C is very high compared with other dermatologically important vitamins and depends on the specific delivery system, like o/w, w/o emulsions and hydrogels (Rozman et al., 2009) and liposomes, niosomes or solid lipid nanoparticles as dispergents (Kaur et al., 2007) as well as microemulsions (Kogan and Garbi, 2006). Due to its instability vitamin C is usually present in cosmetics as ester derivatives which are thermally and oxidatively more stable. Besides they also promote diffusion through epidermis. Though ascorbic palmitate is generally used, recently some other esters (Shibayama et al., 2008, Kumano et al., 1998, Tai et al., 2004) and even tandem retinyl ascorbate (Abdulmayed and Herda, 2004) were synthesized and their skin bioavailability tested.

The permeation rate through whole mouse skin was estimated as 3.43 (± 0.74) $\mu g/cm^2/h$ (Lee and Tojo, 1998) assuming that the least permeable barrier of *stratum corneum* was a matrix of intercellular lipid due to its low water content. This also demonstrated that the rapid permeation of vitamin C when released from delivering formulation is not necessarily a cosmetic target. Macromolecular carriers can be used for controlling the transdermal diffusion rate of cosmetic ingredients; polyamidoamine (PAMAM) dendrimers, widely used as transdermal carriers for drugs have been shown to be amongst the best candidates (Svenson, 2009). For water-insoluble vitamins, like A and E, they can serve as solubilizers, while for water soluble vitamins, like ascorbic acid (**1**), they might allow to increase the skin load. In such a case the PAMAM dendrimers could be used as valuable additives for cosmetic creams.

Here we present the results on simple host-guest chemistry between PAMAM dendrimers and **1** in solution and in neat dendrimers **G2,5**, **G3**, **G3,5**, and **G4** studied by the ^{1}H NMR and differential scanning calorimetry (DSC) methods in order to establish the proper stochiometry of host-guest complexes available for cream formulation. The preliminary *in vitro* studies on diffusion of **1** absorbed in PAMAM dendrimers through artificial model membrane (polyvinydifluoride, PVDF) and pig ear skin (PES) were also performed.

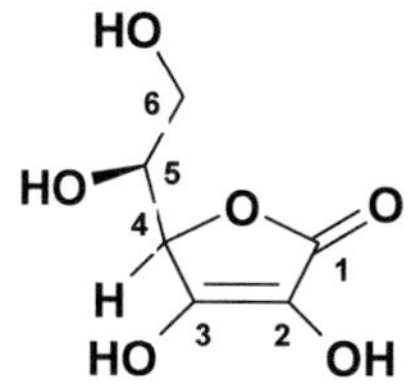

1

3.1 Materials and methods

3.1.1 Reagents

Ascorbic acid (vitamin C, **1**, MW = 176.12 g/mol, m.p. = 190 - 194°C with decomposition) was used as received. All solvents and reagents were of reagent grade purity (Aldrich) and used without further purification.

3.1.2 Syntheses of PAMAM dendrimers

PAMAM dendrimers of generation 2, 2,5, 3, 3,5, and 4 (**G2**, **G2,5**, **G3**, **G3,5**, and **G4**, respectively) on ethylenediamine core were synthesized according to the published method by alternate addition of methyl acrylate to **Gn** and condensation of ethylenediamine with **Gn,5** [Tomalia et al., 2003]. The dendrimers were characterized by the ^{1}H and ^{13}C NMR spectra in deuterium oxide and in methanol-d_4 using standard 1-D and 2-D COSY, HMBC, and HSQC methods with 500 MHz Bruker UltraShield spectrometer to confirm their purity.

3.1.3 Solubilization of 1 in methanol containing host dendrimers

The solubility of **1** in methanol-d_4, estimated by reference chloroform addition into the saturated solution is 0.36 mol dm^{-3}. ^{1}H and ^{13}C resonances assignement has been performed based on 1-D and 2-D NMR experiments.

^1H NMR (chemical shift [ppm], intensity, multiplicity, assignment): 4.88 ([1H], d, H^4); 3.90 ([1H], d of t, H^5); 3.68 ([2H], d, H^6); ^{13}C NMR: 172.1 (C^1); 153.4 (C^3); 118.5 (C^2); 75.5 (C^4); 69.2 (C^5); 62.2 (C^6).

The solubilization of **1** in presence of dendrimers was studied by straight addition of solid **1** into 700 μL of **G3**, **G4**, **G2,5** or **G3,5** solutions at variable concentration in methanol-d_4 after added a measured amount of chloroform as quantitative reference. The H^4 doublet of **(1)** shifted from 4.88 to 4.73 ppm upon dissolving in solution containing **G3** or **G4** dendrimers. Partial precipitation of the complex occurred when added amount of **1** added reached **1**:**G3** and **1**:**G4** ratio equal to 3:1. The analysis of separated solid indicated that the composition of water-soluble solid complex was 3:1, independently on dendrimers concentration. Solubilization of **1** in methanol-d_4 in presence of **G2,5** or **G3,5** showed no complexes precipitation within studied range of dendrimer concentration (up to 0.003 mol·dm^{-3}); the solubility of **1** depending linearly on it.

Linear regression of **1** versus **G2,5** and **G3,5** concentrations are shown in Figure 1 and 2, respectively. The proton resonances in the ^1H NMR spectrum of **1** in solutions containing **G2,5** or **G3,5** were not shifted compared with **1** in pure methanol-d_4.

3.1.4 Differential scanning calorimetric studies on PAMAM-1 stoichiometry

Glass transition temperature T_g was examined using heat-flux differential scanning calorimeter DSC, Q1000™ from TA Instruments, Inc., equipped with a mechanical refrigerator from temperatures 183.15 K (-90°C) to 393.15 K (120°C) (dry nitrogen gas with a flow rate of 50 cm^3·min^{-1} was purged through the DSC cell in the instrument and cooling was accomplished with a refrigerated cooling system). Samples of neat **G2,5**, **G3**, **G3,5**, and **G4** dendrimers were examined as well as host-guest complexes prepared by dissolving **Gn** or **Gn,5** in methanol followed by addition of measured amount of **1** and extensive vacuum evaporation. The oily samples of **1** and **Gn** or **Gn,5** exhibited a higher T_g value than the neat dendrimers (Table 1) within **1**:**PAMAM** ratio 6:1 for **G2,5** and 3:1 for other generations of PAMAM dendrimer. The original T_g of pure dendrimers was recovered once exceeded these molar ratios, with a subsequent lost of the sample homogeneity.

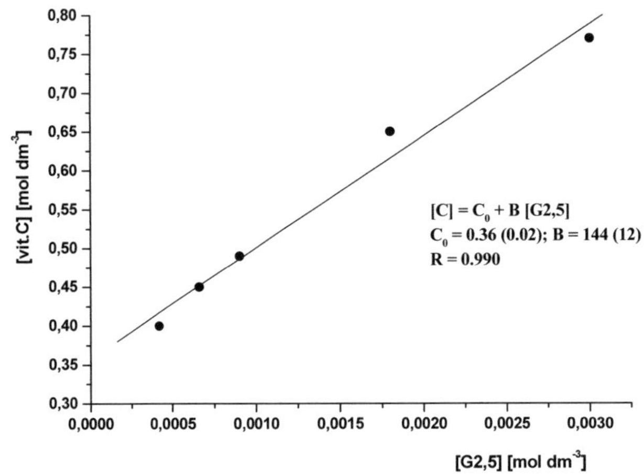

Fig. 1. The dependence of solubility of 1 in methanol containing variable concentration of G2.5.

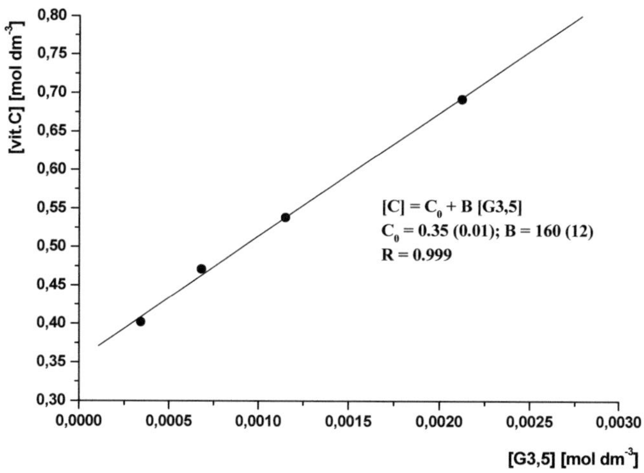

Fig. 2. The dependence of solubility of 1 in methanol containing variable concentration of G3.5.

1 : Gn ratio	G2,5	G3	G3,5	G4
0:1	229	253	224	248
1:1	243	265	240	263
2:1	243	268	251	269
3:1	247	267	255	259
4:1	246	257	224	249
5:1	244	254		248
6:1	250			
7:1	225			

Table 1. Glass transition temperatures [K] for Gn dendrimers and mixtures of Gn and 1.

3.1.5 *In vitro* permeation of Gn-1 and Gn,5-1 complexes

Permeation of **Gn-1** and **Gn,5-1** complexes was studied using Franz diffusion assembly (Thermo Scientific (UK) model DC 600 equipped with 6 cm^3 acceptor compartments). The o/w emulsion was used as donor. The emulsion was prepared using cetearyl alcohol (1.5 g), Brij 72 (1.2 g), Brij 58 (0.3 g) as emulsifiers, vaseline (5.0 g), stearine (0.5 g), glycerin (1.5 g) and water (40.0 g). The samples containing **Gn-1** complexes were prepared on 1 g scale by dissolving **1** (*ca* 5 mg) and **Gn** (*ca* 50 mg) in 1 g of the emulsion. Preliminary samples were obtained by dissolving the host-guest complexes **Gn-1** (prepared by mixing **1** and **Gn** in methanol followed by vacuum evaporation) in emulsion on the same scale. No difference in the permeation studies were noticed related to the protocols. For the analysis ca 250 mg samples were mounted over commercial polyvinydifluoride membrane (PVDF, 0.125 mm thickness) or prepared pig ear skin membrane (PES, 0.55 mm thickness), with 0.067 M phosphate buffer pH = 7.4 : ethanol 7:3 v/v. as receptor medium. The progress of diffusion was monitored spectrophotometrically at 264 nm using the extinction coefficient calculated for the solution of **1** in receptor solution ($1.1{\cdot}10^4$, Figure 3). The receiving solution was stirred magnetically with 1000 rpm at 32°C. 10 ml aliquots of receptor solution were taken at 0.5 hour or longer time intervals and the receiver compartment was filled with 6 ml portion of a new receptor solution. The experiments were carried on until at least 10% of initial amount of **1** was received in receptor solution. The results were analyzed calculating the flux in [$\mu mol \cdot hour^{-1} \cdot cm^{-2}$]. The active area of membrane determined by size of the ring in Franz cell was 0.176 cm^2. The cumulated amount of **1** received as a function of diffusion time was crucial to determine the diffusion properties of **Gn-1** complexes. The time of 10% diffused **1** ($\tau_{0.1}$) was used as quantitative parameter to compare diffusion efficency. Permeation experiments were repeated 7 times. The mean standard deviation and workup of data were performed as previously (Filipowicz and Wołowiec, 2011).

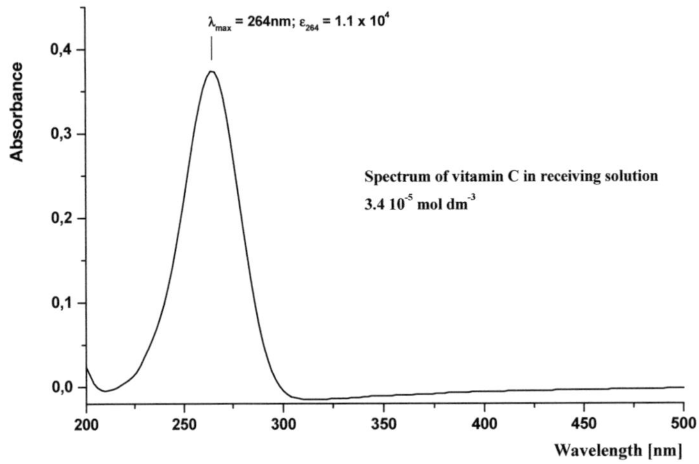

Fig. 3. The UV-Vis spectrum of **1** in receptor solution.

3.2 Results and discussion

3.2.1 Solubilization of 1 in presence of dendrimers studied by the ^{1}H NMR

Ascorbic acid (**1**) is well soluble in water, while its solubility in methanol-d_4, determined by ^{1}H NMR spectroscopy is 0.35 $mol \cdot dm^{-3}$. It increases when bound to PAMAM dendrimers **G2**, **G3**, **G4**, **G2,5** and **G3,5**, respectively. When **1** is dissolved in methanol-d_4, the doublet resonance of H^4 shifts considerably from 4.80 into 4.62 ppm when **1**:**G4** ratio is 1:1. The species formed between **1** and **G3** or **G4** dendrimers become insoluble when the **1**:**Gn** ratio reaches 3:1 and 6:1 for **1**:**G3** and **1**:**G4**, respectively. The isolated complexes are readily water soluble. Presumably their stoichiometry does not correspond to the dendrimers ability to absorb small molecules of ascorbic acid, rather than to the limit of their solubility in methanol.

Opposite to **G3** or **G4** the **G2,5** and **G3,5** dendrimers which have similar sizes and molecular weights act as effective solubilizers of **1** in methanol. They are able to solubilize *ca* 144-160 molecules of **1** per molecule of dendrimer, almost independently on the host size. When methanol is evaporated from such a samples, the separation of **1** from dendrimer is observed resulting in formation of non-homogeneous mixture. In order to establish the stoichiometry of neat host-guest complexes another method was used.

3.2.2 Differential scanning calorimetric studies of neat complexes of 1 with dendrimers

Recently we have used DSC method to evaluate the stoichiometry of host-guest complexes between PAMAM dendrimers and *8-methoxypsoralene* (Borowska et al., 2010). Water insoluble host formed oily host-guest complexes which revealed higher temperature of glass transition (T_g) than PAMAM dendrimers. When the guest amount was increased above the host maximum capacity, the separation of PAMAM dendrimers and guest took place, followed by T_g returning to its original value. Similar phenomenon was observed in all cases studied here. However, the results on T_g were slightly surprising, because the limit of encapsulation for dendrimers **G3**, **G3,5** and **G4** was 3 molecules of **1** per macromolecule, i.e. lower in comparison with **G2,5**, for which 6 molecules of **1** per molecule of **G2,5**, showed increased value of T_g. However it confirms the ^{1}H NMR results on solubilization in methanol, which also showed that **G2,5** interacts with more molecules of guest than larger hosts. This might be due to different types of interaction between host and **1**. Vitamin C, unlike hydrophobic *8-methoxypsoralene* is able to form ion-pair complex, this interaction prevailing in case of full-generation dendrimers **G3** and **G4**. The ion-pairs decompose when solvent is removed from solution upon preparation of neat samples. Besides, the larger dendrimers are used, the more dense are the cavities of host and self organization of vitamin C crystals prevails over weak intramolecular interaction within host-guest complex. Furthermore we noticed that homogeneous samples of host-guest complexes formed between PAMAM dendrimers and **1** can be obtained in every case when the stoichiometry is maintained as 3:1. These complexes were then used to perform transdermal permeability experiments on skin-model membranes (see below).

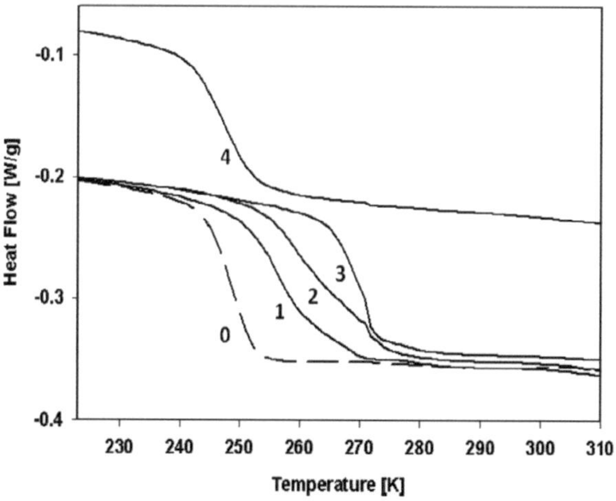

Fig. 4. The DSC curves for **1** : **G4** mixtures at molar ratio (from bottom to top): 0:1; 1:1; 2:1; 3:1; 4:1.

3.2.3 Permeation studies

The permeation experiments of **1** through PVDF and PES membranes using **1** dispersed in o/w emulsion indicated a typical change in the flux of **1**; after 0.5 hr induction time, the flux rapidly grew finally stabilizing within 1.5 hour of experiment.

Addition of PAMAM dendrimers of **G2**, **G2,5**, **G3**, **G3,5**, and **G4** only slightly influenced the rate of diffusion through PVDS membrane. The experiments were conducted until ca 50% of **1** was transferred through PVDS and the time of 10% transfer, $\tau_{0.1}$. was used as reference in all the experiments. Addition of smaller size dendrimers **G2, G2,5, G3** caused elongation of $\tau_{0.1}$, presumably due to host-guest complexes diffusion or diffusion of **1** preliminarily released from them in emulsion. The larger size dendrimers **G3,5**, and **G4** had no such impact (Figure 5a). Generally the diffusion of **1** through PVDF was fast, with 10% of **1** transferred within ca 1 hour. Unlikely, the diffusion through much thicker PES membrane occurred slower being strongly affected by the added dendrimer (Figure 5b). This influence could be clearly demonstrated by comparison of $\tau_{0.1}$ (Figure 6 and Table 2). The slowest diffusion was found in case of **1-G2,5** composition. The diffusion rate was diminished by a factor of 4 if compared with **1** itself. **G3** considerably decreased the rate by a factor of 3.7, while other dendrimers, larger **G3,5** and **G4** and smaller **G2**, showed lower impact. The results obtained for diffusion experiments through PES confirm the PVDF ones, nevetheless remarkable differentiation of diffusion efficiency was found in case of PES.

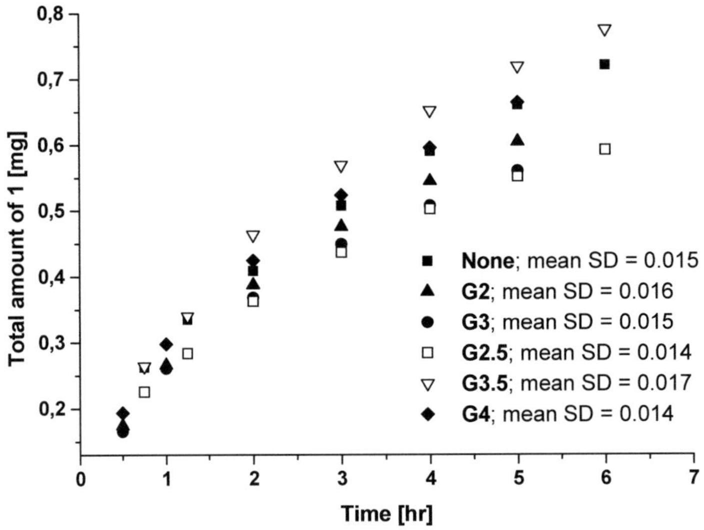

Fig. 5a. The cumulated amount of **1** diffused through PVDF membrane vs time. The load of **1** was 2.8 (± 0.2) mg in every case.

Comparing the supposed stoichiometry of host-guest complexes based on DSC measurements as well as remarkable solubilization of **1** in methanol containing **G2,5** and **G3,5** we can assume that these dendrimers form the most stable host-guest complexes, with **1** encapsulated within macromolecule, while **G3** and **G4** encapsulate **1** weakly to give the 3:1 **1**: **Gn** complexes. Moreover, **1** interacts with **G2**, **G3** and **G4** surface amine groups with this interaction prevailing on encapsulation. When **1** is released from ionic complexes with **Gn**, it diffuses similarly like from emulsion. When the whole host-guest complex diffuse, the rate is considerably lower. This phenomenon is quite opposite to what was observed for the systems in which PAMAM dendrimers were used as solubilizers of water-insoluble *psoralene* or *riboflavin* (Borowska et al, 2010, Filipowicz and Wołowiec, 2011); in these cases the transdermal diffusion of these compounds was enhanced. Both of these behaviors are useful for controlling transdermal diffusion of dermatologically important agents. Finally the emulsion containing vitamin and dendrimeic carrier can be easily prepared by addition of pre-formed host-guest complex in ethanol and addition of oily complex to the prepared emulsion. Such prepared creams may carry both water-soluble and water-insoluble vitamins, as well as some vitamin derivatives bonded covalently, like retinal, pyridoxal or biotin. These bioconjugates are currently under investigation in our laboratory.

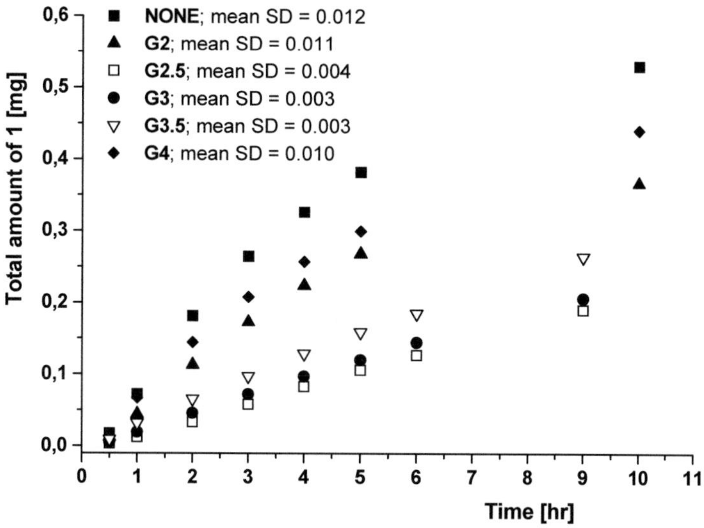

Fig. 5b. The cumulated amount of **1** diffused through PES membrane vs time. The load of **1** was 2.8 (± 0.2) mg in every case.

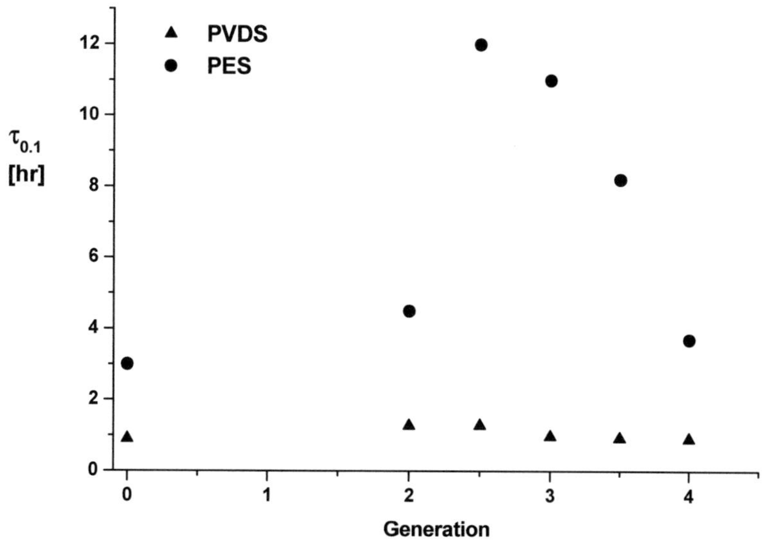

Fig. 6. The dependence of $\tau_{0.1}$ in experiments of transdermal diffusion through PVDS and PES membranes in function of PAMAM dendrimer generation.

Sample (o/w)	$\tau_{0.1}$ [hr]	
	PVDS	PES
1	0.9 (±0.12)	3.0 (±0.21)
1-G2	1.3 (±0.15)	4.5 (±0.26)
1-G2.5	1.3 (±0.15)	12.0 (±0.29)
1-G3	1.0 (±0.13)	11.0 (±0.28)
1-G3.5	0.9 (±0.12)	8.2 (±0.20)
1-G4	0.9 (±0.12)	3.7 (±0.22)

Table 2. The time of 10% transfer of **1** ($\tau_{0.1}$) from emulsions containing dendrimers.

4. Conclusions

1. PAMAM dendrimers influence the solubility of ascorbic acid (**1**) in methanol. The solubility of ionic complexes between **1** and full-generation PAMAM dendrimers in methanol is lower in comparison with **1** itself. 3:1 stoichiometry adducts between vitamin **1** : **G3** and **1** : **G4**, can be isolated from methanolic solutions as homogeneous, solvent-free oily complexes.
2. Half-generation PAMAM dendrimers: **G2,5** and **G3,5** solubilize **1** in methanol due to non-specific interaction up to *ca* 150 molecules of **1** per molecule of dendrimer.
3. The ionic interactions, encapsultation, and surface absorption of **1** by PAMAM dendrimers result in host-guest complexes formation. Based upon DSC measurements the stoiochiometry of the homogeneous, oily complexes was determined as 6:1 (for **1** : **G2,5**) and 3:1 (for **1** : **G3**, **1** : **G3,5** and **1** : **G4**).
4. When 10% of **1** per dendrimer compositions are placed in o/w emulsions, the permeation profile of **1** through the polyvinyldifluoride (PVDF) and pig ear skin (PES) membranes depends on the presence and size of dendrimer used as vitamin carrier in the emulsion. Transdermal diffusion through PES is considerably slowed down by dendrimers according to the order:

$$G2,5 \cong G3 > G3,5 >> G2 \cong G4 > \text{none}$$

5. Finally, the **G2,5** and **G3** dendrimers can be applied as transdermal carriers to control vitamin C release kinetics from emulsions or hydrogels. Vitamin C retardation is surprisingly in contrast with previously studied water insoluble 8-methoxypsoralene or riboflavin which showed a promotion of the diffusion process.

5. Acknowledgment

The work was supported by the Grant no N N302 432839, obtained from Ministry of Higher Education and Research, Poland.

6. References

Abdulmajed, K., Herda, C.M., 2004. Topical delivery of retinyl ascorbate co-drug. 1. Synthesis, penetration into and penetration across human skin. *International Journal of Pharmaceutics*, Vol. 280, pp. 113-124.

Astruc, D., Boisselier, E., Ornelas, C. (2010) Dendrimers Designed for Functions: From Physical, Photophysical, and Supramolecular Properties to Applications in Sensing, Catalysis, Molecular Electronics, Photonics, and Nanomedicine. *Chemical Reviews,* Vol. 110, No. 4, pp. 1857-1959.

Bhadra, D., Bhadra, S., Jain, S., Jain, N.K. (2003) A PEGylated dendritic nanoparticulate carrier of fluorouracil. *International Journal of Pharmaceutics* Vol. 257, pp. 111–124.

Borowska, K., Laskowska, B., Magoń, A., Myśliwiec, B., Pyda, M., Wołowiec, S. (2010) PAMAM dendrimers as solubilizers and hosts for 8-methoxypsoralene enabling transdermal diffusion of the guest. International Journal of Pharmaceutics, Vol. 398, pp. 185-189.

Caruthers, S.D., Wickline, S.A., Lanza, G.M. (2007) Nanotechnological applications in medicine. *Current Opinion in Biotechnology,* Vol. 18, pp. 26–30.

Chandrasekar, D., Sistla, R., Ahmad, F.J., Khar, R.K., Diwan, P.V. (2007) The development of folate-PAMAM dendrimer conjugates for targeted delivery of anti-arthritic drugs and their pharmacokinetics and biodistribution in arthritic rats. *Biomaterials,* Vol. 28, pp. 504–512.

Chauhan, A.S, Sridevi, S., Chalasani, K.B, Jain, A.K., Jain, S.K., Jain, N.K., Diwan, P.V. (2003) Dendrimer-mediated transdermal delivery: enhanced bioavailability of indomethacin. *Journal of Controlled Release,* Vol. 90, pp. 335–343.

Cheng, Y., Qu, H., Ma, M., Zhenhua Xu, Z, Xu, P, Fang, Y., Xu, T. (2007) Polyamidoamine (PAMAM) dendrimers as biocompatible carriers of quinolone antimicrobials: An in vitro study. *European Journal of Medicinal Chemistry,* Vol. 42, pp. 1032-1038

Cheng, Y., Li, M., Xu, T. (2008) Potential of poly(amidoamine) dendrimers as drug carriers of camptothecin based on encapsulation studies. *European Journal of Medicinal Chemistry* Vol. 43, pp. 1791-1795.

D'Emanuele, A., Attwood, D. (2005) Dendrimer–drug interactions. *Advanced Drug Delivery Reviews* , Vol. 57, pp. 2147– 2162.

D'Emanuele, A., Jevprasesphant, R., Penny, J., Attwood, D. (2004) The use of a dendrimer-propranolol prodrug to bypass efflux transporters and enhance oral bioavailability. *Journal of Controlled Release,* Vol. 95, pp. 447– 453.

Devarakonda, B. Hill, R.A., de Villiers, M.M. (2004) The effect of PAMAM dendrimer generation size and surface functional group on the aqueous solubility of nifedipine. *International Journal of Pharmaceutics* , Vol. 284, pp. 133–140.

Devarakonda, B., Li, N., de Villiers, M.M. (2005) Effect of Polyamidoamine (PAMAM) Dendrimers on the In Vitro Release of Water-Insoluble Nifedipine From Aqueous Rels. *AAPS PharmSciTech,* Vol. 6, No. 3, pp. E504-E512.

Devarakonda, B.,, Daniel P. Otto, D.P., Judefeind, A., Hill, R.A., de Villiers, M.M. (2007) Effect of pH on the solubility and release of furosemide from polyamidoamine (PAMAM) dendrimer complexes. *International Journal of Pharmaceutics,* Vol. 345, pp. 142–153.

Filipowicz, A., Wołowiec, S. (2011) Solubility and *in vitro* transdermal diffusion of riboflavin assisted by PAMAM dendrimers. *International Journal of Pharmaceutics,* Vol. 408, pp. 152-156.

Fréchet, J.M., Henni, M., Gitsov, I., Aoshima, S., Leduc, M.R., Grubbs, R. B.(1995) Self-Condensing Vinyl Polymerization: An Approach to Dendritic Materials. *Science* Vol. 269, pp.1080-1083.

Hans, M.L., Lowman, A.M. (2002) Biodegradable nanoparticles for drug delivery and targeting. *Current Opinion in Solid State and Materials Science*, Vol.6, pp. 319–327.

Imae, T., Ito, M., Aoi, K., Tsutsumiuchi, K., Noda, H., Okada, M. (2000) Formation of organized adsorption layers by amphiphilic dendrimers. *Colloids and Surfaces A: Physicochemical and Engineering Aspects*, Vol. 175, pp. 225-234.

Jain K., Kesharwani, P., Gupta, U., Jain, N.K. (2010). Dendrimer toxicity: Let's meet the challenge. *International Journal of Pharmaceutics*, Vol. 394, pp. 122–142

Jevprasesphant, R., Penny, J., Jalal, R., Atwood, D., McKeon, N.B., D'Emanuele, A. (2003) The influence of surface modification on the cytotoxicity of PAMAM dendrimers. *International Journal of Pharmaceutics*, Vol. 252, pp. 263-266.

Jia, L., Xu, J.-P., Wang, H. Ji, J. (2011) Polyamidoamine dendrimers surface-engineered with biomimetic phosphorylcholine as potential drug delivery carriers. *Colloids and Surfaces B: Biointerfaces*, Vol. 84, pp. 49–54.

Kaur, I., Kapila, M., Agrawal, R. (2007) Role of novel delivery systems in developing topical anitoxidants as therapeutics to combat photoageing. *Aging Research Reviews,*Vol. 6, pp. 271-288.

Khandare, J., Kolhe, P., Pillai, O., Kannan, S., Lieh-Lai, M., Kannan, R.M. (2005) Synthesis, Cellular Transport, and Activity of Polyamidoamine Dendrimer-Methylprednisolone Conjugates. *Bioconjugate Chemistry*, Vol. 16, pp. 330-337.

Kogan, A., Garbi, N., 2006. Microemulsions as transdermal drug delivery vehicles. *Advances in Colloid Interface Science*, Vol. 123-126, pp. 369-385.

Kojima, C., Kono, K., Maruyama, K., Takagishi, T. (2000) Synthesis of Polyamidoamine Dendrimers Having Poly(ethyleneglycol) Grafts and Their Ability To Encapsulate Anticancer Drugs. *Bioconjugate Chemistry,* Vol. 11, pp. 910-917.

Kolhatkar, R.B., Kitchens, K.M., Swaan, P.W., Ghandehari, H. (2007) Surface Acetylation of Polyamidoamine (PAMAM) Dendrimers Decreases Cytotoxicity while Maintaining Membrane Permeability. *Bioconjugate Chemistry* Vol. 18, pp. 2054–2060

Kolhe, P., Khandare, J., Pillai, O., Kannan, S., Lieh-Lai, M., Kannan, R.M. (2006) Preparation, cellular transport, and activity of polyamidoamine-based dendritic nanodevices with a high drug payload. *Biomaterials*, Vol. 27, pp. 660–669.

Kolhe, P., Misra, E., Kannan, R.M., Kannan, S., Lieh-Lai, M. (2003) Drug complexation, in vitro release and cellular entry of dendrimers and hyperbranched polymers. *International Journal of Pharmaceutics*, Vol. 259, pp. 143-160.

Kono, K, Kojami, C., Hayashi, N., Nishisaka, E., Kiura, K., Watarai, S., Harada, A. (2008) Preparation and cytotoxic activity of poly(ethylene glycol)-modified poly(amidoamine) dendrimers bearing adriamycin. *Biomaterials*, Vol. 29, pp. 1664-1675.

Kulhari, H., Pooja, D., Prajapati, S.K., Chauhan, A.S.. (2011) Performance evaluation of PAMAM dendrimer based simvastatin formulations. *International Journal of Pharmaceutics,* Vol. 405, pp. 203–209.

Kumano, Y., Sakamoto, T., Egawa, M., Iwai, I., Tanaka, M., Yamamoto, I., 1998. In vitro and In Vivo Prolonged Activieties of Novel Vitamin C Derivative, 2-0-α-D-Glucopyranosyl-L-Ascorbic Acid (AA-2G), in Cosmetic Fields. *Journal of Nutritional Science and Vitaminology*, Vol. 44, pp. 345-359.

Kurtoglu, Y.E., Mishra, M.K., Kannan, S., Kannan, R.M. (2010) Drug release characteristics of PAMAM dendrimer–drug conjugates with different linkers. *International Journal of Pharmaceutics*, Vol. 384, pp. 189–194.

Lee, Ae-Ri C., Tojo, K. (1998) Characterization of Skin Permetation of Vitamin C: Theoretical Analysis of Penetration Profiles and Differential Scanning Calorimetry Study. *Chemical and Pharmaceutical Bulletin*, Vol. 46, pp. 174-177.

Lo, S.-C., Burn, P.L. (2007) Development of Dendrimers: Macromolecules for Use in Organic Light-Emitting Diodes and Solar Wells. *Chemical Reviews*, Vol. 107, No. 4, pp. 1097-1116.

Ma, M., Cheng, Y., Xu, Z., Xu, P., Qu, H., Fang, Y., Xu, T., Wen, L.. (2007) Evaluation of polyamidoamine (PAMAM) dendrimersas drug carriers of anti-bacterial drugs using sulfamethoxazole (SMZ) as a model drug. *European Journal of Medicinal Chemistry*, Vol. 42, pp. 93-98.

Ma, K., Hu, M.-Z., Qi, Y., Zou, J.-H., Qiu, L.-Y., Jin, Y., Ying, X.-Y., Sun, H.-Y. (2009) PAMAM–Triamcinolone acetonide conjugate as a nucleus-targeting gene carrier for enhanced transfer activity. *Biomaterials*, Vol. 30, pp. 6109–6118.

Markatou, E., Gionis, V. Chryssikos, G.D., Hatziantoniou, S.,Georgopoulos, A., Demetzos, C. (2007) Molecular interactions between dimethoxycurcumin and Pamam dendrimer carriers. *International Journal of Pharmaceutics*, Vol. 339, pp. 231–236.

Milhem, O.M., Myles, C., McKeown, N.B., Attwood, D., D'Emanuele, A. (2000) Polyamidoamine Starburst® dendrimers as solubility enhancers. *International Journal of Pharmaceutics*, Vol. 197, pp. 239–241.

Mukherjee, S.P., Davoren, M., Byrne, H.J. (2010) In vitro mammalian cytotoxicological study of PAMAM dendrimers - Towards quantitative structure activity relationships. *Toxicology in Vitro*, Vol. 24, pp. 169–177.

Na, M., Yiyun, C., Tongwen, X, Yang, D., Xiaomin, W., Zhenwei, L., Zhichao, C., Guanyi, H., Yunyu, S., Longping, W. (2006) Dendrimers as potential drug carriers. Part II. Prolonged delivery of ketoprofen by in vitro and in vivo studies. *European Journal of Medicinal Chemistry*, Vol. 41, pp. 670–674.

Papagiannaros, A., Dimas, K., Papaioannou, G.Th., Demetzos, C. (2005) Doxorubicin-PAMAM dendrimer complex attached to liposomes: Cytotoxic studies against human cancer cell lines. *International Journal of Pharmaceutics*, Vol. 302, pp. 29–38.

Patri, A.K., Kukowska-Latallo, Jamek.F.,. Baker Jr., J.R. (2005) Targeted drug delivery with dendrimers: Comparison of the release kinetics of covalently conjugated drug and non-covalent drug inclusion complex. *Advanced Drug Delivery Reviews*, Vol. 57, pp. 2203– 2214.

Prieto, M.J, Temprana, E.F., del Río Zabala, N.E., Marotta, C.H., del Valle Alonso, S. (2011) Optimization and in vitro toxicity evaluation of G4 PAMAM dendrimer-risperidone complexes. *European Journal of Medicinal Chemistry*, Vol. 46, pp. 845-850

Rozman, B., Gasperlin, M., Tinois-Tessoneaud, E., Pirot, F., Falson, F. (2009) Simultaneous absorption of vitamins C and E from topical microemulsions using reconstructed human epidermis as a skin model. *European Journal of Pharmaceutics and Biopharmaceutics*, Vo. 72, pp. 69-75.

Rundle, R.E., Frank C. Edwards, F.C. (1943) The Configuration of Starch in the Starch-Iodine Complex. IV. An X-Ray Diffraction Investigation of Butanol-Precipitated Amylose. *Journal of the American Chemical Society*, Vol. 65,. No. 11, pp 2200–2203.

Saenger, W. (1984) The structure of the blue starch-iodine complex. *Naturwissenschaften*, Vol. 71, No.1, pp. 31-36.

Shibayama, H., Hisama, M., Matsuda, S., Ohtsuki, M., 2008. Permeation and Metabolism of a Novel Ascorbic Acid Derivative, Disodium Isostearyl 2-O- L -Ascorbyl Phosphate, in Human Living Skin Equivalent Models. *Skin Pharmacology and Physiology*, Vol. 21, pp. 235-243.

Svenson, S. (2009) Dendrimers as versatile platform in drug delivery applications. *European Journal of Pharmacutics and Biopharmaceutics*, Vol. 71, pp. 445-462.

Tai, A., Goto, S., Ishiguro, Y., Suzuki, K., Nitowa, T., Yamamoto, I., 2004. Permeation and metabolizm of a serie sof novel lipophilic ascorbic acid derivatives, 6-*O*-acyl-2-*O*--α-D-Glucopyranosyl-L-ascorbic acid with a branched-acyl chain, in human living skin equivalent model. *Bioorgorganic and Medicinal Chemistry Letters*, Vol. 14, pp. 623-627.

Thomas, T.P., Choi, S.K., Li, M-H., Kotlyar, Jamek., Baker Jr., J.R. (2010) Design of riboflavin-presenting PAMAM dendrimers as a new nanoplatform for cancer-targeted delivery. *Bioorganic & Medicinal Chemistry Letters*, Vol. 20, pp. 5191–5194.

Tomalia, D.A. (2005b) Birth of a New Macromolecular Architecture: Dendrimers as Quantized Building Blocks for Nanoscale Synthetic Organic Chemistry. *Aldrichimica Acta*, Vol. 37, No.2, pp. 39-57.

Tomalia, D.A., Huang, B., Swanson, D.R., Brothers II, H.M., Klimash, J.W. (2003) Structure control within poly(amidoamine) dendrimers: size, shape and region-chemical mimicry of globular proteins. *Tetrahedron*, Vol. 59, pp. 3799-3813.

Tomalia, D.A. (2005a) Birth of a new macromolecular architecture - dendrimers asquantized building blocks for nanoscale synthetic polymer chemistry, *Progress in Polymer Science*, Vol. 30, pp. 294–324.

Vandamme, Th.F., Brobeck, L. (2005) Poly(amidoamine) dendrimers as ophthalmic vehicles for ocular delivery of pilocarpine nitrate and tropicamide. *Journal of Controlled Release*, Vol. 102, pp. 23–38.

Venuganti, V.V.K., Perumal, O.P. (2008) Effect of poly(amidoamine) (PAMAM) dendrimer on skin permeation of 5-fluorouracil. *International Journal of Pharmaceutics* Vol. 361, pp. 230–238.

Wang, Y., Guo, R., Cao, X., Shen, M., Shi, X. (2011) Encapsulation of 2-methoxyestradiol within multifunctional poly(amidoamine) dendrimers for targeted cancer therapy. *Biomaterials*, Vol. 32, pp. 3322-3329.

Wiwattanapatapee, R, Lomlim, L., Saramunee, K. (2003) Dendrimers conjugates for colonic delivery of 5-aminosalicylic Acid. *Journal of Controlled Release*, Vol. 88, pp. 1–9.

Yang, W., Cheng, Y., Xu, T., Wang, X., Wen, L.-p. (2009) Targeting cancer cells with biotinedendrimer conjugates. *European Journal of Medicinal Chemistry*, Vol. 44, pp. 862-868.

Yiyun, C. Tongwen, X., Rongqiang, F. (2005) Polyamidoamine dendrimers used as solubility enhancers of ketoprofen, *European Journal of Medicinal Chemistry*, Vol. 40, pp. 1390–1393.

Zhang, K., Yu, A., Wang, D., Yang, W., Li, J., Zhang, X, Wang, Y. (2011) Solvent-controlled self-assembly of amphiphilic cholic acid-modified PAMAM dendrimers. *Materials Letters*, Vol. 65, pp. 293–295.

Part 4

The Role of Stoichiometry in the Determination of Protein Interactions

9

Stoichiometry of Signalling Complexes in Immune Cells: Regulation by the Numbers

Elad Noy, Barak Reicher and Mira Barda-Saad
The Mina and Everard Goodman Faculty of Life Sciences, Bar-Ilan University, Ramat-Gan Israel

1. Introduction

Host protection against pathogens and tumor cells is mediated mainly via white blood cells or leukocytes. As an inappropriate immune response can result in damage to the host and/or failure in pathogen clearance, the activation and function of leukocytes are tightly regulated processes. Regulation of immune cells is carried out by complex networks of receptors and cellular mediators. While the progress of the signal cascade is necessary for leukocyte activation and the development of an immune response, improper signaling and cellular activation are associated with various pathologies. The study of such networks constitutes a cornerstone of immunological research and has great implications for the understanding of the immune system and for the development of immunotherapies for cancer, infectious diseases, as well as autoimmunity.

In this chapter, we will describe the importance of the stoichiometry of signalling complexes in the regulation of leukocyte activation and function. We will focus on techniques used to analyze the formation, composition, and stoichiometry of multiprotein complexes, and we will also review current information and implications of stoichiometry on immune-cell activation and regulation.

1.1 Leukocytes and their regulation

Protection against infectious diseases is mediated by the immune system, which includes both humoral and cellular responses that enable the protective function or resistance against pathogens (Viret & Janeway, 1999). While humoral immunity is mediated by secreted proteins, peptides and small molecules and participates in host protection, responses of immune cells are cardinal for most immunological functions.

Immune cells, or leukocytes (white blood cells) are divided into two main cell types based on their nuclear shape; these include mononuclear cells (including monocytes, macrophages, dendritic cells and lymphocytes) and polymorphonuclear cells, also termed "granulocytes" (including neutrophils, eosinophils, and basophils). In general, each of these cell types plays a role in a different aspect of the immune response (Risso, 2000). Some of the leukocytes such as macrophages, neutrophils and dendritic cells, also termed "phagocytes", are responsible for the phagocytosis of pathogens. Others, as the granulocytes, secrete bactericidal agents, while one type of lymphocytes (B lymphocytes- described below) produce and secrete target-specific antibodies. The leukocytes are also responsible for the destruction of virus infected cells, as well as for the identification and eradication of cancerous cells (Doherty, 1996; Jager et al., 2001).

The leukocytes belong to two arms: either to the innate or to the adaptive immune system. Cells of the innate immune system constitute the first responders to pathogens and cancerous cells. Phagocytes are responsible for pathogen removal as they engulf, ingest and digest these invaders. Cells belonging to the mononuclear phagocyte family, such as macrophages and dendritic cells, process ingested particles, releasing peptide fragments and displaying them on their cell surface. The presentation of these peptide chains, or antigens, in the context of immune cell recognition, constitutes the corner stone of the activation of the adaptive arm of the immune system (Davis & Bjorkman, 1988). The cells that display foreign antigen complexes on their surfaces are termed "antigen presenting cells" (APCs) and include, among others, macrophages and dendritic cells.

The lymphocytes are divided into three cell types: Natural killer cells (NK), T lymphocytes (also termed T cells) and B lymphocytes (also termed B cells). While NK cells play a major role in the innate immune response, T and B cells play a major role in the adaptive immune response. In contrast to NK cells, which do not express receptors for specific antigens, T and B cells express a stochastically generated receptor, the T-cell antigen receptor (TCR) or the B-cell receptor (BCR), capable of interacting with a single specific antigen. The large repertoire of different lymphocyte clones expressing different receptors allows the recognition of virtually all antigens (Davis & Bjorkman, 1988). T cells are involved in cell-mediated immunity, whereas B cells are primarily responsible for humoral immunity (secretion of antibodies) (Davis & Bjorkman, 1988).

Antigen presentation is mediated via the Major Histocompatibility Complex molecules (MHC). Class I MHC is expressed by all nucleated cells while Class II MHC is expressed only by dedicated APCs mentioned above, and B lymphocytes.

Class I MHC molecules, in addition to their role in antigen presentation, act as NK inhibiting ligands. Disruption of MHC Class I expression, occurring in certain virus infected cells and in tumor cells, while facilitating escape from recognition by T cells, reduces NK inhibitory signaling, thereby enhancing cytotoxic NK activity (Chini & Leibson, 2001; Wu & Lanier, 2003).

In response to pathogens, a type of T cells, called T helper cells, produce cytokines that direct the immune response, while another type, called cytotoxic T cells, produce also cytotoxic granules, similarly to NK cells, which induce the death of pathogen infected cells (Chini & Leibson, 2001; Wu & Lanier, 2003).

Cytokines are proteins that act as messengers between cells. In the immune system, cytokines facilitate communication among immune cells and between immune cells and other host cells. Cytokines are responsible for inducing immune cell proliferation and for enhancing, suppressing and terminating immune responses (Weber & Iacono, 1997).

Given their role in the coordination of the immune response, the development of long term immunity, and their role in the recognition and elimination of cancerous and virally infected cells, T lymphocytes are the subject of a vast amount of studies. Deciphering the processes governing T cell activation constitutes a focal point of immunological research (Smith-Garvin et al., 2009; Wucherpfennig et al., 2010).

T cell activation begins with the binding of the TCR complex to peptide bound MHC (Dembic et al., 1986; Saito & Germain, 1987). Along with this engagement, T cell specific co-receptors called either CD4 (present on T helper cells) or CD8 (present on T cytotoxic cells) recognize and bind to MHC class II or MHC class I, respectively (Viret & Janeway, 1999) (Fig. 1). During these binding processes, the TCR and co-receptor molecules undergo clustering, allowing the protein kinase, Lck, bound to the intercellular portion of either CD4 or CD8, to phosphorylate tyrosine sites on cytoplasmic proteins of the TCR complex (Rudolph et al., 2006). These tyrosine motifs belong to a family called ITAMs (immunoreceptor tyrosine based activation motifs) (Love & Hayes, 2010; Reth, 1989). Upon phosphorylation, these tyrosine residues on the TCR ζ chain associate with the SH2 (Src Homology 2) domains of the kinase ZAP-70 (zeta chain-associated protein of 70 kDa) (Chan et al., 1992). As ZAP-70 is recruited to the complex, it undergoes phosphorylation by Lck, and is thereby itself activated (Barber et al., 1989; Samelson et al., 1986; Samelson et al., 1990; Veillette et al., 1988). ZAP-70 then phosphorylates the downstream T cell signalling molecules, LAT (linker for the activation of T cells) (Zhang et al., 1998) and SLP-76 (SH2 domain-containing leukocyte protein of 76 kDa) (Bubeck Wardenburg et al., 1996; Samelson, 2002). Phosphorylated LAT complexes with SLP-76 via the adaptor proteins Gads and Grb2 and acts as a scaffold for the recruitment of additional signalling proteins, promoting downstream activation events (Liu et al., 1999; Sommers et al., 2004). PLC-γ (Phosphoinositide phospholipase C γ) recruited to phosphorylated SLP-76, catalyzes the breakdown of the membranal phospholipid Phosphatidylinositol 4,5-bisphosphate (PIP2) into the secondary messengers, diacylglycerol (DAG) and inositol-1,4,5-trisphosphate (IP3) (Beach et al., 2007; Ebinu et al., 1998). DAG activates PKCθ (Protein kinase C θ), and through it, activates the cellular transcription factors NF-κB (nuclear factor κB) and AP-1 (activator protein 1) (Melowic et al., 2007; Smith-Garvin et al., 2009), while IP3 induces the opening of calcium channels, further facilitating T cell activation (Imboden & Stobo, 1985). Increased cellular calcium levels induce the release of the nuclear factor, NFAT (Nuclear factor of activated T-cells), from the calcium binding protein, Calcineurin (Hogan et al., 2003). These transcription factors promote the expression of proteins necessary for T cell activation and for its effector functions, including the production and secretion of cytokines governing immune responses (Smith-Garvin et al., 2009).

Phosphorylated SLP-76 is also a key player in the activation of the cellular actin polymerization machinery, facilitating the reorganization of the cytoskeleton necessary for enhancing the T-cell/APC interface and enabling T cell effector functions (Jordan et al., 2006; Reicher & Barda-Saad, 2010). By recruiting the adaptor protein Nck (non-catalytic region of tyrosine kinase adaptor protein) and VAV1, an activator of Rho family GTPases, SLP-76 mediates between TCR proximate activation events and actin polymerization and reorganization (Koretzky et al., 2006). Nck, in turn, recruits the actin nucleation factor, WASp (Wiskott–Aldrich Syndrome Protein) (Zeng et al., 2003). With the recruitment of WASp by Nck, and activation of actin nucleation and polymerization machinery by VAV1 activated GTPases, the cytoskeleton undergoes remodelling, enabling enhanced cell spreading and the reorientation of cellular polarity (Billadeau et al., 2007). In cytotoxic T cells, cellular polarity allows for the direction of cytotoxic granules at the intended target cell (Reicher & Barda-Saad, 2010; Smith-Garvin et al., 2009).

B cells share many points of similarity with T cells, in aspects of antigen-induced cellular activation, subsequent signalling complex formation, and cytoskeletal remodelling. In analogy to T cells, B cell activation is triggered by ligation of the BCR to its cognate antigen (Fig. 1). The BCR is comprised of a membrane-bound immunoglobulin (mIg) component with a short cytoplasmic domain that has no direct interaction with downstream signalling molecules. Therefore, the mIg associates with two additional immunoglobulin chains, Igα/β, which contain ITAMs (Pierce, 2009; Tolar et al., 2005). Antigen binding by the BCR initiates rapid phosphorylation of the ITAMs within the Igα/β chains by Src family kinases e.g. Lyn, and leads to the recruitment of intracellular signalling molecules and adapters, including Syk (Spleen tyrosine kinase), Blnk (B cell linker), VAV and PLCγ2. These molecules interact to form a multi protein signalling complex known as the signalosome (Batista et al., 2010). Similar to T cells, the membrane recruited signalling molecules induce calcium influx (mediated by PLCγ2) and the subsequent activation of transcription factors such as NF-κB. Eventually, antigen binding by the BCR leads to B-cell proliferation, differentiation, and antibody production and secretion. Actin cytoskeleton reorganization is pivotal for the activation and function of B-cells, as it facilitates BCR clustering and organization, and B cell spreading (Fleire et al., 2006; Treanor et al., 2010; Weber et al., 2008). In this context, signalling molecules such as VAV may also facilitate actin polymerization in B-cells (Weber et al., 2008), by functioning as activators of Rho GTPases. However, the exact molecular mechanisms underlying actin reorganization in B-cells are not completely understood, and are under extensive investigation.

Deciphering of the underlying mechanisms of lymphocyte activation is of great importance to the understanding of the direct activity of T cells in anti-tumoral and anti-viral immunity, as well as its function as a key regulator of immune responses and autoimmunity. The regulation and function of numerous cellular processes are dependent on protein-protein interactions. In the immune system, protein-protein interactions are the main mechanisms leading the regulation of lymphocyte activation, and indeed, rule the initiation and termination of the immune response by various cells of the immune system. Understanding the molecular mechanisms underlying these multi-protein complexes requires the characterization of their composition and stoichiometry.

Below, we describe major techniques for exploring protein-protein interactions regulating immune cell activation and function, with the focus on technologies used for determining the stoichiometric ratios of protein complexes.

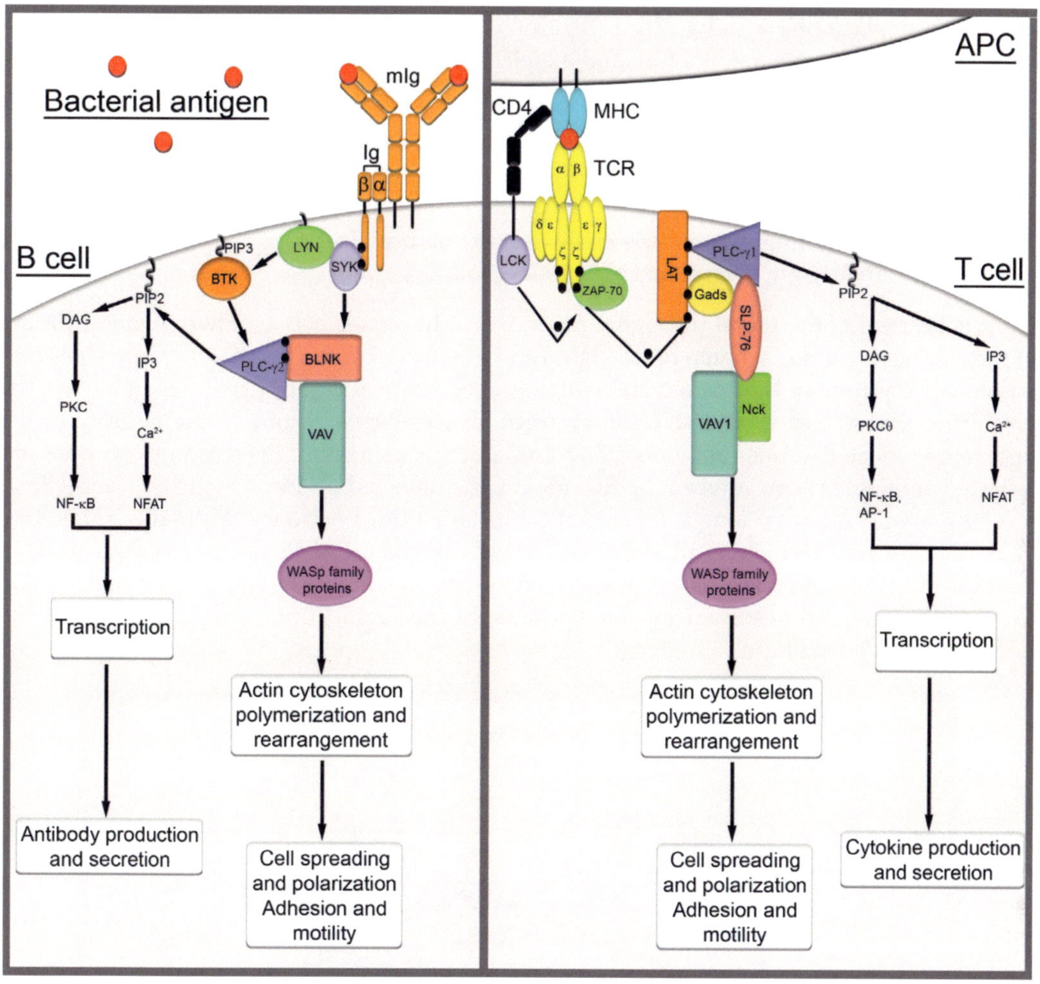

Fig. 1. B and T cell signalling cascades.

The above scheme describes key events downstream of TCR (right panel) or BCR (left panel) activation that are mentioned in the current review. The black spots represent phosphorylation sites.

2. Methods used in researching the stoichiometry of leukocyte regulatory complexes

As protein/protein interactions regulate and control a multitude of cellular functions, various methods for investigating protein-protein binding were developed. Here we review leading methods used for the investigation of inter protein binding and to determine the stoichiometry of these interactions.

2.1 Surface Plasmon Resonance (SPR)

Surface Plasmon Resonance-based sensing makes use of the photonic excitation of electrons into surface plasmons - delocalized electrons that oscillate at the interface between a molecule adsorbed onto a metal film and a dielectric medium (Ritchie, 1957).

The interaction between photons, electrons in the metal film, and the adsorbent allow the investigation of inter-molecular interactions. Binding of molecules, such as proteins or small molecular ligands, to proteins immobilized to the metal film changes the interaction of the projected light photons and the electrons in the metal, causing a shift in the intensity of reflected light, and thus allows the investigation of protein-protein binding, as detailed below (McDonnell, 2001; Rich & Myszka, 2000).

Light is beamed at the metal through a prism. As light passes between two media differing in their refractive indices, some of the light can be reflected at the point of the inter-medium interface. Projection of light at a certain angle, called "critical angle" (itself dependent on the proportion of the two refractive indices), or at larger angles, results in the entirety of the light to be reflected, a phenomenon called total internal reflection. Even though photons are reflected at the interface between the two media, the reflected photons create an electric field reaching about one wavelength beyond the inter-medium boundary (Pattnaik, 2005). This field, called evanescent wave, allows photons reaching the metal surface at a certain angle to excite surface plasmons at the opposite side of the metal sheet (Fig. 2) (Pattnaik, 2005). Exciting photons are absorbed by the electrons of the metal film, leading to a detectable reduction in reflected light (Fig. 2).

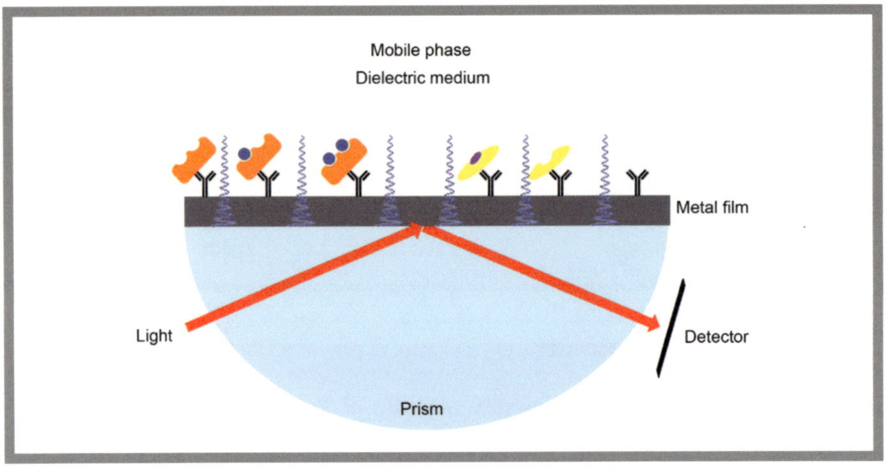

Fig. 2. Illustration of the principles underlying Surface Plasmon Resonance (SPR) technology.

Light reflected at the intermedium boundary can cause surface plasmon resonance on a metal film, reducing the intensity of the reflected light. The induction of surface plasmon is highly dependent on the angle of light incident, as the evanescent waves responsible for SPR propagate into the other side of the metal film, and the angle at which incident light can induce surface plasmon is dependent on the conditions proximate to the metal film. Proteins are adsorbed to the metal film either by direct immobilization or with the use of antibodies.

As proteins adsorbed to the metal film bind ligands (either other proteins or small molecules), the angle of maximal SPR changes, enabling the monitoring of the binding.

The angle at which photons are capable of exciting plasmon is dependent on the refractive indices of the metal and the adjacent. As proteins are adsorbed, the refractive index at the boundary changes, thus affecting the degree at which light can excite surface plasmons. By plotting the intensity of reflected light as a function of incidence angle and finding the angle at which light reflection is minimal, it is possible to find the angle of maximal surface plasmon induction. Comparison of the difference between angles of maximal surface plasmon induction before and after protein adsorption allows the calculation of the difference in refractive index of the medium, from which the mass of the protein adsorbate is easily calculable (due to the high identity between the reflective indices of all proteins) (Pattnaik, 2005).

In the SPR based inter-protein interaction assays, a protein is first immobilized on one side of the metal film, via binding to different bait molecules attached to the metal film such as streptavidin or carboxymethyl groups. During the experiment, changes in the intensity of reflected light, occurring due to the excitation of surface plasmon, are detected with a charge-coupled device (CCD). As ligand proteins in the mobile phase bind to the immobilized proteins, the refractive index at the inter-medium boundary changes, affecting light reflection, from which various aspects of the protein-protein binding can be deciphered. By measuring protein adsorption and dissociation from the immobilized proteins bound to the metal film, the equilibrium constant (Kd), the association and dissociation constants (ka and kd, respectively) and the stoichiometry governing the protein complex formation can be calculated (McDonnell, 2001; Pattnaik, 2005).

Biacore is the oldest and most commonly commercially available SPR system.

2.2 Isothermal Titration Calorimetry (ITC)

Inter-protein interactions results in the formation and termination of non-covalent bonds such as van der Waals interactions, hydrogen bonds and hydrophobic interactions. Isothermal titration calorimetry takes advantage of the thermodynamic outcomes of such reactions to measure molecular interactions. By recording heat changes due to binding enthalpy, isothermal titration calorimetry allows the monitoring of molecular interactions. Measurement of the heat change occurring during the reaction allows for the determination of the thermodynamic variables of the molecular interaction: changes in enthalpy, entropy and free energy (ΔH, ΔS and ΔG, respectively), binding constants (Ka), heat capacity (Δ Cp) and the reaction stoichiometry (n) (Ladbury, 2007).

The ITC apparatus is composed of two identical cells, or chambers, housed in an isothermal jacket. One chamber contains a solution of one of the components participating in the reaction, while the second chamber is filled with buffer (or water) and serves as a control (Fig. 3). The jacket is cooled, thus requiring energy investment to maintain the temperature of the chambers. Temperature detectors (thermopile/thermocouple circuits) allow heaters to keep the temperature of each chamber fixed (Ladbury, 2007; Liang, 2008; Roselin et al., 2009).

At the beginning of the experiment, the two chambers are at the same temperature. The reacting component is injected into the sample chamber, resulting in enthalpic change; in the case of an exothermic reaction, less heat per time will be needed to maintain the sample chamber at a temperature equal to that of the reference chamber, while an endothermic reaction will require more heat to maintain the equilibrium between the two chambers. As titrant aliquots are injected into the sample chamber, changes in power required to maintain the sample chamber at the same temperature of the reference chamber are recorded (Fig. 3). In addition to heat changes due to the reaction between the two macro-molecules, dilution of the reactant adds its own enthalpy. In order to compensate for dilution heat, the reactants are independently added to the buffer, with heat changes recorded and subtracted from raw ITC data.

Using data from multiple titrations, a titration plot is drawn, with the relation between energy released or used during the reaction plotted against the reactants' molar ratio. From the curve, the reaction enthalpy, binding constant and stoichiometry are calculated in a single experiment, using non-linear regression. Using these variables, the other thermodynamic constants can be calculated with the use of basic thermodynamic relations (Ladbury, 2007).

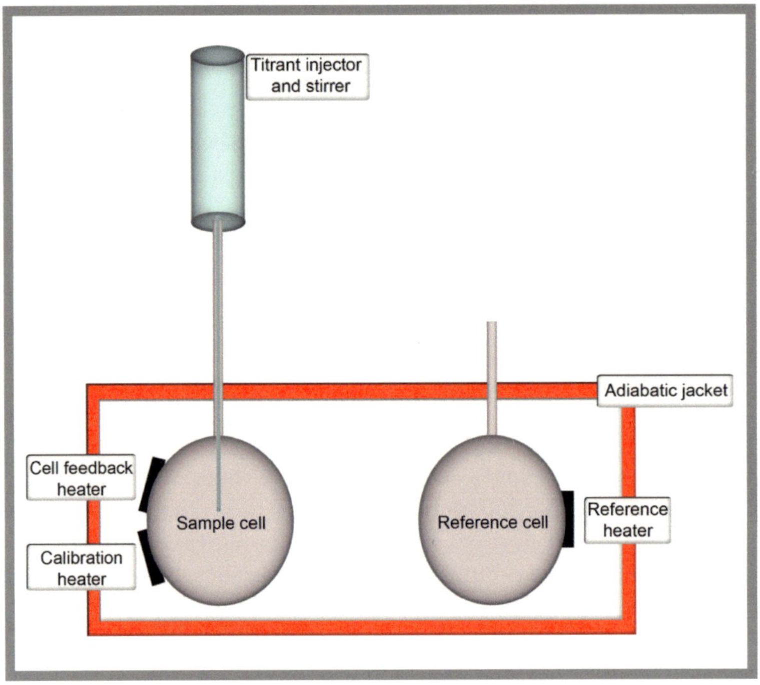

Fig. 3. Illustration of the principles of Isothermal Titration Calorimetry (ITC).

The sample cell is filled with one of the reactants, and the injector is filled with the other. The reference cell is filled either with distilled water or buffer. Continuous power is applied to the reference heater, while the cell feedback heater keeps the temperature of the sample cell equal to that of the reference cell. As titrant is injected into the sample cell, heat is either taken up or evolves. This causes the power required by the cell feedback heater to keep the temperature of the cells equal to either increase or decrease, respectively. These changes are monitored to produce ITC data.

While both ITC and SPR are powerful methods for the real-time in-vitro analysis of protein-protein interactions, ITC is preferable to SPR in the study of stoichiometry ratios of units of protein complexes, as it offers greater resolution and does not require prior immobilization of one of the proteins (Jecklin et al., 2009).

2.3 Analytical Ultracentrifugation (AUC)

Making use of the analysis of the sedimentation of macromolecules under centrifugal forces, analytical ultracentrifugation allows the observation of the shape, size, and stoichiometry of complexes, as well as association constants, molecular mass and intermolecular interactions. Analytical Ultracentrifugation was first developed by Nobel Prize laureate Theodor Svedberg in 1925, but costly instrumentation and arduous data acquisition and processing limited its usage. With the development of computerized data management and new types of detectors, the increased usability and versatility of AUC occurred starting in the 1990s (Cole et al., 2008).

Analytical Ultracentrifugation aims to differentiate and characterize macromolecules based on their behaviour under acceleration. Prior to centrifugation, the distribution of the macromolecules in the solution is dependent on inter molecular forces and on entropy, with the effect of gravity being negligible. During centrifugation, molecules in the solution are redistributed, as centrifugal forces compete with diffusion (Fig. 4).

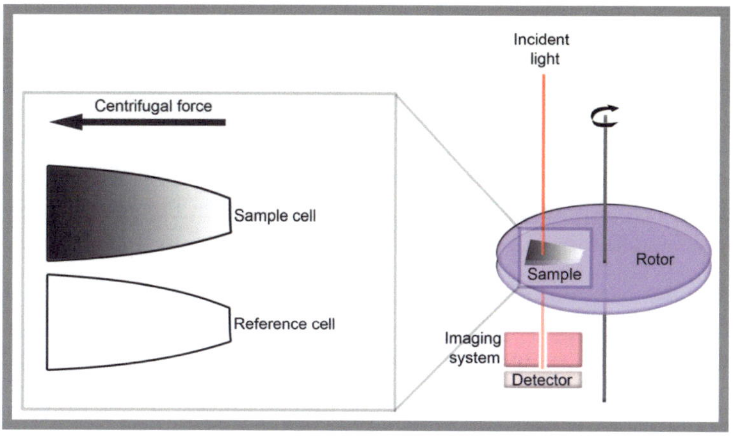

Fig. 4. Illustration of the principle technology of Analytical Ultracentrifugation (AUC).

Under centrifugation, protein complexes are redistributed according to their mass and hydromantic properties. In sedimentation velocity experiments, an optical detector is used to measure the radial concentration of proteins during sedimentation. In sedimentation equilibrium, the sedimentation gradient is monitored not during its formation but at the end of the process, when the centrifugal force is at equilibrium with diffusion. Sample cell readings are compared to those of a reference cell.

Concentration distribution under centrifugation is described by the Lamm equation:

$$\frac{\partial c}{\partial t} = D\left[\frac{\partial^2 c}{\partial r^2} + \frac{1}{r}\frac{\partial c}{\partial r}\right] - s\omega^2\left[r\frac{\partial c}{\partial r} + 2c\right] \quad (1)$$

The solution concentration at time t and position r is represented by c. D is the diffusion coefficient; s represents the sedimentation coefficient; and ω is the angular speed of the rotor.

In sedimentation equilibrium experiments, the equilibrium state of molecule distribution under acceleration is monitored. The sedimentation equilibrium is the state where sedimentation due to centrifugation (simulating gravity) equals diffusion-driven transport. By examining the rate at which the solution reaches the new equilibrium it is possible to observe intermolecular interactions and define the shape, the size, and the stoichiometry of the complexes. On the other hand, in sedimentation equilibrium experiments, the concentration distribution at equilibrium is examined, allowing the determination of molecular mass, association constants and complex stoichiometry. In sedimentation equilibrium experiments, the hydrodynamic properties of the investigated molecules do not influence the results, which are dependent only on thermodynamic properties, simplifying data analysis (Balbo et al., 2005; Schuck, 2010b; Zhao et al., 2011).

However, the advantages of sedimentation velocity measurements, namely, shorter run time (hours instead of days), higher precision, wider versatility and the collection of multiple data points, combined with the robust data processing offered by modern analysis programs, make it the most commonly used AUC technique.

During centrifugation, molecules are radially redistributed. Measurements of radial concentration distribution, also called "scans", are acquired at various time intervals (minutes in sedimentation velocity experiment, hours in sedimentation equilibrium experiments) (Demeler, 2010). Detection of proteins in analytical ultracentrifugation experiments is performed via optical detectors. Absorbance detection is the most commonly used method, making use of the strong excitation peaks of proteins (and nucleic acids, when relevant) in the UV range. It does require the use of non-absorbing buffer, preventing its use in cases where the sedimentation experiment is performed in the presence of UV absorbing additives, such as nucleotides or certain reducing agents, such as dithiothreitol.

Interference optics uses differences in refractive indices between the centrifuged sample and a reference. In addition to being unaffected by UV absorption of medium components, interference optics offers greater precision than absorbance-based detection, and has a higher dynamic range, a characteristic advantageous for the measurement of highly concentrated solutions. Data density is also higher than that gained from absorbance optics. A disadvantage of interference optics is that all the components dissolved in the medium affect its interference pattern; thus, the reference buffer components must match in content and concentration to the buffer used for the sample. Use of interference optics also requires the use of measurement cell windows that do not affect the refraction pattern. The sample should also be devoid of components with absorbance at the wavelength of the laser used in this system (commonly 675nm). Another option is the use of fluorescence detection; this method allows greater sensitivity and selectivity compared to absorbance optics, but requires the prior labelling of the proteins. This requirement negates a major advantage of AUC, namely, the ability to use untagged proteins (Cole et al., 2008; Demeler, 2010).

Data analysis is performed using dedicated programs such as SEDANAL, SEDFIT/SEDPHAT, BPFIT and ULTRASCAN. In sedimentation velocity experiments, the analytical programs are commonly used to interpret the data by computationally fitting it to the Lamm equation, an approach called discrete Lamm equation modelling (DLEM) (Brown et al., 2009; Schuck, 2009, 2010a).

2.4 Analytical Native Antibody-based Mobility-Shift (NAMOS) assay

Gel electrophoresis is a common process utilized in multiple protein research methods. Unlike the widely used sodium dodecyl sulfate polyacrylamide gel electrophoresis (SDS-PAGE) and other gel electrophoresis assays preformed under denaturing conditions, blue native polyacrylamide gel electrophoresis (BN-PAGE) allows the separation of proteins according to their sizes in a native, non-denaturing environment (Schagger & von Jagow, 1991; Schamel & Reth, 2000; Swamy et al., 2006). The negatively charged Coomassie blue reagent binds nonspecifically to all proteins, bestowing its negative charge uniformly, thus allowing the proteins to migrate through the polyacrylamide gel during electrophoresis. Unlike electrophoresis performed in the presence of denaturing agents, the BN-PAGE assay allows the conservation of multi-protein complexes (Schagger & von Jagow, 1991; Schamel & Reth, 2000; Swamy et al., 2006). The native antibody-based mobility-shift (NAMOS) assay, developed and used to investigate the stoichiometry of the TCR complex, uses antibodies specific to various components of the TCR protein complex (Swamy et al., 2006). Samples of the complex are incubated in the presence of various antibodies at different concentrations prior to electrophoresis. Antibody binding to the complex increases its overall mass and size, thereby slowing down its passage through the gel. Furthermore, antibody binding to the complex is dependent on the availability of sites recognized by the antibody (epitopes) and the complex/antibody ratio. In the absence of antibodies, all the protein complex molecules migrate in the gel according to the original size of the complex, forming a single band. As antibody binding slows down the movement of the protein complex, bound complexes will form additional bands, corresponding to the increased size of the complex that includes bound antibody. As complexes are treated with increasing concentration of antibodies, the band corresponding to the unbound complex begins to disappear while the band or bands corresponding to bound complexes increase in intensity. If two antibodies are able to bind to the complex, as antibody concentration is increased, the band corresponding to the binding of one antibody begins to disappear as well, with the band corresponding to the protein bound to two antibodies increasing in strength. Additional binding sites will result in bands corresponding to higher molecular weight. It is thus possible to learn from the resulting band pattern the number of complex sites recognizable by the antibodies, and thereby deduce complex stoichiometry (Swamy et al., 2006).

The NAMOS assay allows the investigation of the stoichiometry of complexes in a relatively simple manner, requires only small amounts of protein complexes (femtograms to nanograms), and does not require their prior purification. On the other hand, the NAMOS assay is highly dependent on the ability of the antibodies to reach and bind to all relevant binding sites, as well as on the properties of the antibodies used. Some antibodies form aggregates, creating an unintelligible "ladder" pattern instead of bands, and are thus unusable for this assay. Bivalent antibodies may bind two complex molecules at the same time, creating an additional band interfering with correct stoichiometry analysis. This problem may be mitigated with the use of monovalent antigen binding fragments (Fab fragments) derived from the whole antibodies. Epitopes of the target can also be sterically inaccessible, thereby causing an underestimation of the complex stoichiometry. If the inaccessibility is caused by the proximity of the epitopes, with one antibody sterically interfering with the binding of an antibody to the adjacent epitope, use of Fabs may also negate this problem, as they are considerably smaller than full sized antibodies (Swamy et al., 2006).

Based on an understanding of the most common analytical techniques, we will now review major studies that contributed to the understanding of the stoichiometry of regulatory protein complexes in immune cells.

3. Current understanding of stoichiometry of the complexes involved in immune cell regulation

With the development and application of new technologies allowing the investigation of protein-protein contacts, studies conducted to understand the key mechanisms of immune cell regulation have shed light on the stoichiometric ratios in fundamental immune regulatory complexes.

The stoichiometry of the BCR was initially investigated by quantifying radioactivity of protein complexes incorporating 35S-labeled methionine. As the number of methionine residues in each of the BCR proteins is known, it was possible to calculate the molar ratios between different subunits of the receptor complex. A 1:1 stoichiometry was found between the immunoglobulin and the Igα/β heterodimer required for signal transduction (Swamy et al., 2006).

This finding was later confirmed in a study utilizing quantitative fluorescence resonance energy transfer (FRET) analysis to characterize the distances between the different chains of the BCR, its conformation during cell rest and during activation, and the clustering of multiple BCRs during antigen binding. In that experiment, FRET between BCR complex proteins genetically tagged with the fluorescent protein, monomeric YFP (mYFP), and Cy3-labeled antibodies specific to either the immunoglobulin or to the Igβ chain, indicated a 1:1 stoichiometry between the immunoglobulin and the Igα/β heterodimer (Tolar et al., 2005).

Knowledge of the stoichiometric ratio between the Ig-α/β heterodimer and the immunoglobulin was later used in the development of the NAMOS assay, validating its use in the investigation of the TCR complex stoichiometry (Swamy et al., 2007).

In the past, stoichiometry of the TCR complex was determined using classical methods, making use of 35S-labeled methionine incorporation into the proteins, followed by the purification of the radiolabeled protein complexes, as described above for the BCR. The subunits were detected by phosphoimaging and quantified by densitometry. The results indicated that a TCRα-TCRβ heterodimer binds a single CD3δ-CD3ε heterodimer, a single CD3γ-CD3ε heterodimer and a CD3ζ-CD3ζ homodimer. Thus, the overall stoichiometry of the TCR complex was found to be 1:1:1:1:2:2 (for αTCR, βTCR, CD3γ, CD3δ, CD3ε, and CD3ζ, respectively) (Rudolph et al., 2006; Wucherpfennig et al., 2010) These findings corroborated the stoichiometry proposed in a previous study (Blumberg et al., 1990), and are supported by other results, as well (Call et al., 2004). However, other works suggested that a second αβ heterodimer was incorporated into the complex, suggesting an $(\alpha\beta)_2\gamma\varepsilon\delta\varepsilon\zeta\zeta$ stoichiometry (Exley et al., 1995; Fernandez-Miguel et al., 1999; San Jose et al., 1998). Finally, an αβ $(\gamma\varepsilon)_2\delta\varepsilon\zeta\zeta$ configuration was also suggested (Rubin et al., 2002).

A later study utilized the NAMOS technique to study the stoichiometry of the TCR-CD3 complex (Swamy et al., 2007). The assay was first validated using the BCR complex, whose stoichiometry (two heavy chains, two light chains and a single Ig-α/β heterodimer) is well characterized (Reth et al., 2000; Schamel, 2001; Schamel & Reth, 2000). Purified BCRs were incubated with increasing concentrations of antibodies specific to various subunits of the complex. The protein complexes incubated with antibodies were then subjected to electrophoresis. Antibody binding to protein complexes slows their movement through the electrophoresis gel. With increasing concentration of antibodies specific to the Ig-α/β heterodimer, the band corresponding to BCR not bound to antibodies began to disappear, and a single band at a higher molecular weight appeared. However, increasing the concentration of antibodies specific to the heavy chain caused two bands to appear along with the disappearance of the original band, with the first band corresponding to the binding of one heavy chain specific antibody appearing at lower antibody concentration, and a second one, corresponding to the binding of two antibodies specific to the BCR heavy chain appearing at higher antibody concentrations, along with the disappearance of the band corresponding to the binding of a singular antibody. Use of antibodies specific to the BCR light chain yielded the same pattern. From this, a 2:2:1 heavy chain, light chain, Ig-α/β heterodimer was suggested, in accordance with previous findings (Reth et al., 2000; Schamel, 2001; Schamel & Reth, 2000; Tolar et al., 2005).

The NAMOS assay was then used to explore the stoichiometry of the TCR-CD3 complex. Use of antibodies specific for either TCRα or TCRβ each resulted in the appearance of a single band, indicating a single TCRα and TCRβ subunit in the complex. Use of antibodies specific to CD3ζ chain yielded the appearance of two bands, indicating the presence of two CD3ζ chains in the complex (Swamy et al., 2007). It should be noted that even at high concentrations of CD3ζ specific antibodies, the band corresponding to a complex bound to a single antibody did not disappear completely, possibly due to the small size of the CD3ζ subunit, resulting in steric interference with the simultaneous binding of two antibodies at once to the spatially proximate CD3ζ monomers. Next, antibodies specific to CD3ε were used. The band pattern included, aside from the original band of complexes not bound to antibodies, the appearance of three bands, interpreted as the TCR-CD3 complex bound to either one antibody, two antibodies, or the binding of one antibody to two TCR-CD3 complexes. In order to avoid this complicated pattern, monovalent CD3ε binding antibody fragments were used, yielding a band pattern consistent with the presence of two CD3ε in the complex. Complexes incubated with antibodies specific for CD3γ yielded an electrophoresis pattern consistent with the binding of a single antibody per complex. Finally, use of CD3δ specific antibodies did not result in an intelligible band pattern, as these antibodies tend to form aggregates, resulting in a smear. Therefore, it was impossible to directly observe CD3δ stoichiometry in the TCR-CD3 complex from these results. However, given that the presence of two CD3ε and one CD3γ, and that previous studies showed that CD3ε forms heterodimers with CD3γ and with CD3δ (Alarcon et al., 2003) an overall stoichiometry of the TCR-CD3 complex as αβγεδεζζ was suggested (Swamy et al., 2008; 2007).

A later study used electron microscopy to characterize the structure of the TCR-CD3 complex. It revealed that the actual three dimensional structure of the complex is larger than expected given a composition of αβγεδεζζ. Due to this discrepancy, the authors suggested the possible existence of a second αβ heterodimer in the complex, sterically inaccessible to antibodies, which would explain its lack of detection with the use of the NAMOS assay and in previous studies. This study therefore contradicts the model of αβγεδεζζ stoichiometry, reviving the suggestion of $(\alpha\beta)_2\gamma\varepsilon\delta\varepsilon\zeta\zeta$ complex stoichiometry (Arechaga et al., 2010). Further research is therefore necessary to clarify the issue of the stoichiometry of the TCR-CD3 complex.

At the initiation of the T cell activation, recognition of the peptide bound MHC by the TCR is accompanied by binding of the appropriate co-receptor (CD4/8) to the MHC protein, bringing together the co-receptor bound protein kinase, Lck, with its target ITAMs in the TCR complex, and allowing ZAP-70 to be recruited to the TCR complex. The stoichiometric ratios between the clustered TCR molecules and the Lck-bound co-receptors, also governed by the dynamics of lipid rafts, remain the subject of further studies.

ZAP-70, with its recruitment to the TCR complex, phosphorylates LAT, thereby enabling its recruitment to cellular membrane and allowing the recruitment of additional signalling proteins to the activation site. LAT constitutes a major adaptor protein, forming a complex of multiple proteins taking part in T cell activation.

Grb2 is an adaptor protein that recruits SOS1 to LAT, thereby allowing SOS1 to perform as a guanine exchange factor, activating GTPases of the Ras family (Koretzky, 1997; Samelson, 2002; Zhu et al., 2003). Alternatively, Grb2 molecules bind Cbl, an E3 ubiquitin-protein ligase capable of chemically attaching ubiquitin monomers to proteins involved in the cellular activation process, modifying their functionality and regulating their degradation (Samelson, 2002). Binding of these two proteins is facilitated by the Grb2 SH3 domain, capable of recognizing their proline rich domains. SPR was used for determining the binding affinity of the signalling adaptor molecule, Grb2, to the epidermal growth factor receptor (EGFR) and to SOS1 and the stoichiometry of the complex. Grb2 uses the same binding motifs for interacting with either EGFR or, in T cells, with LAT (Lowenstein et al., 1992; Weber et al., 1998). Therefore, these findings are also relevant for the Grb2-SOS1 binding-mediated regulation of Ras activity during the activation of T cells. Using the BIAcore SPR system, the binding of Grb2 to the epidermal growth factor receptor was determined to be of 1:1 stoichiometry, while the binding stoichiometry of Grb2 to SOS1 was 2:1 (respectively) (Lemmon et al., 1994). A later study utilized SV ultracentrifugation to measure the binding of Grb2 to SOS1 and to LAT. It was found that two Grb2 molecules are able to bind to a single SH3 ligand (either SOS1 or Cbl). ITC was used to examine Grb2 binding with either the N terminal domain or the C terminal domains of SOS1. It was determined that the binding stoichiometry Grb2 to either protein fragment was 1:1, while binding of Grb2 to SOS1 proteins containing both proline rich Grb2 binding domains was found to be 2:1 (Houtman et al., 2006). These results were in disagreement with those of a previous study that described a 1:1 stoichiometry between Grb2 and SOS1 (Chook et al., 1996); the cause of this discrepancy may be due to the usage of gel filtration analysis and of SE ultracentrifugation, which are of relatively lower resolution compared to the SV ultracentrifugation method; the techniques used may be less suitable to differentiate between 2:1 and 1:1 Grb2:SOS1 sedimenting species, along with the use of the full length SOS1 in the older study (Houtman et al., 2006). Stoichiometric analysis of the binding of Grb2-SOS1 complexes to LAT molecules was performed with the use of SV ultracentrifugation. While a 1:2:1 LAT–Grb2–SOS1 complex was observed, detection of peaks signifying of sedimentation of larger complexes indicates that Grb2-SOS1 complexes can bind additional LAT molecules, facilitating the clustering and oligomerization of LAT. The presence of these rapidly sedimenting species is indeed highly dependent on the concentration of LAT, Grb2 and SOS1, indicating that they are formed by clustering of LAT in the presence of Grb2-SOS1 complexes. This mechanism serves to oligomerize LAT molecules subsequent to TCR activation. LAT clustering serves as a mechanism enhancing T cell activation, and may play a critical role in T cell activation under weakly stimulating conditions, occurring *in-vivo*. Indeed, transfection of Jurkat E6.1 T cell line with truncated SOS1 proteins, containing only the C-terminal proline-rich, Grb2- binding domain, reduced T cell activation in comparison to mock transfected cells and to cells transfected with the SOS1 containing both proline rich Grb2 binding domains. This effect was more pronounced with the use of low concentration of anti-CD3 activating antibody (Houtman et al., 2006). The function of Grb2-SOS complexes in LAT clustering was later verified with the use of ITC technology (Houtman et al., 2007).

To analyze the interaction between SLP-76, a scaffold protein and a key player in T cell activation, and Gads, an adaptor protein responsible for the recruitment of SLP-76 upon cellular activation events downstream to TCR engagement, ITC was used. To this end, an 18mer oligopeptide of SLP-76, and the Gads C-SH3 domain to which it binds were titrated. Calorimetric analysis showed that the stoichiometry of this inter-protein interaction responsible for T cell activation is 1:1 (Seet et al., 2007).

Characterization of the stoichiometric ratios between LAT and SLP-76 and PLCγ was also performed. Using ITC, these proteins were found to exhibit a 1:1 binding ratio (Houtman et al., 2004). The interactions of SLP-76 with its binding partners VAV1 and Nck was studied by our group. Study of these interactions and their stoichiometry was preformed with the use of SV ultracentrifugation and ITC technologies (Barda-Saad et al., 2010)

First, ITC was used to measure the affinity, specificity and stoichiometry of the binding of Nck and VAV to SLP-76. To that end, short (17mers) phosphopeptides bearing the sequences of phosphorylated SLP-76 binding domains were prepared. Our results indicated that VAV1 and Nck both bind at the pY113 and pY128 sites. We then used longer peptides (49mers), containing both pY113 and pY128, both pY113 and pY145, both pY128 and pY145, or pY113, pY128 and pY145. Binding stoichiometry of VAV1 to the pY113-pY128 doubly phosphorylated peptide was surprisingly 1:1, while VAV1 was able to bind to both the pY113 and the pY128 containing peptides. Although Nck binding to the pY113-pY145 or to pY113-pY145 peptides was of a 1:1 stoichiometry, Nck engaged in low affinity binding to pY145, in contrast to VAV1. Surprisingly, binding of either Nck or VAV1 to the pY113-pY128-pY145 triply phosphorylated peptide was of 2:1 stoichiometry.

In order to further study the SLP76-Nck-VAV1 complex, we utilized ultracentrifugation. We performed SV analytical ultracentrifugation, using full sized Nck protein, the SH3–SH2–SH3 domains of VAV1 (which are responsible for its inter-protein interactions), and SLP-76 peptides containing different combinations of binding sites. The VAV1 truncated protein was tagged with a site specific label (VAV-FAM), and SLP-76 peptides were labelled with rhodamine TAMRA. We examined the formation of complexes of different SLP-76 derived peptides, Nck and truncated VAV1, by monitoring the effects of different combinations of SLP-76 derived peptides, in the presence of either Nck, VAV1, or both, on the sedimentation velocity. The AUC results corroborated the results of the ITC experiments, suggesting that the stoichiometry of the complex SLP76-Nck-VAV1 was 1:2:2, respectively (Barda-Saad et al., 2010).

The activity of WASp, an actin nucleation-promoting factor, is required for reorganization of the actin cytoskeleton and therefore is crucial for T cell activity (Jordan et al., 2006; Reicher & Barda-Saad, 2010). WASp is recruited to the site of TCR activation by Nck, and is activated by VAV1. WASp, by activating the Arp2/3 complex, promotes the branching of actin filaments and the development of cytoskeletal networks (Machesky et al., 1999; Rohatgi et al., 1999). The C-terminal domain of WASp, called VCA, binds to the Arp2/3 complex. The VCA domain is divided into three regions, with the C and A regions contributing most to the association energy of the Arp2/3 complex (Marchand et al., 2001), driving a conformational change in Arp2/3 and facilitating its activity (Chereau et al., 2005; Dayel & Mullins, 2004; Rodal et al., 2005); the V region binds an actin monomer, delivering it to the Arp2/3 complex upon Arp2/3-WASp binding (Dayel & Mullins, 2004; Machesky & Insall, 1998; Marchand et al., 2001; Rohatgi et al., 1999). The increased activity of dimerized VCA domains suggests that more than one WASp molecule is able to bind to the Arp2/3 complex (Padrick et al., 2008; Padrick et al., 2011). To study the binding stoichiometry of Arp2/3 and WASp, the WASp VCA domain was tagged with Alexafluor-488 (Padrick et al., 2011). Its binding stoichiometry with Arp2/3 was then investigated using SV AUC. Experiments were performed in the presence of excess VCA molecules. The co-sedimentation pattern of Arp2/3 and the tagged WASp VCA domain indicated a 2:1 VCA:Arp2/3 binding stoichiometry. While Arp2/3 was shown to bind two VCA molecules simultaneously, it is possible that it can accommodate only one VCA molecule bound to an actin monomer at the same time. To address this issue, VCA bound to actin was used. Analysis of SV ultracentrifugation results indicated that two VCA-actin molecules were able to simultaneously bind to the Arp2/3 complex. Mass spectroscopic analysis of these species yielded an apparent mass of 333 kDa, consistent with the molecular mass predicated for one Arp2/3, two VCA and two actin molecules (Padrick et al., 2011). Together with the increased activity of VCA dimers (Padrick et al., 2008), these findings suggest that VCA:Arp2/3 complexes of 2:1 stoichiometry are likely to be the main mechanism for WASp activation of Arp2/3. WASp proteins are bound to scaffolding proteins, limiting their orientation. Since simultaneous binding of two WASp molecules may bias the orientation of the Arp2/3 complex, this new insight suggests that the 2:1 binding stoichiometry may limit the directions in which Arp2/3 may promote actin filament branching. This mechanism may guide the creation of actin networks towards the cellular membrane, facilitating cell spreading required for its immune functions (Padrick et al., 2011).

4. Conclusion

The study of the stoichiometry of the protein complexes governing immune-cell activity constitutes an important element in understanding the processes controlling the immune system. Methods used for the investigation of the stoichiometric ratios between these proteins yield new insights regarding the mechanism and the function of immune signalling complexes. As illustrated, the binding stoichiometry of Grb2 and SOS1 to LAT serves as a mechanism of LAT oligomerization responsible for a lower cellular activation threshold, thus facilitating T-cell activation under physiological conditions (Houtman et al., 2006). The study of the stoichiometry of WASp binding to the actin nucleating factor Arp2/3 suggests a mechanism that is responsible for the directionality of actin-filament branching, guiding actin polymerization, and thus assisting in the cell spreading necessary for the function of immune cell (Padrick et al., 2011).

While the new, innovative technologies and techniques have greatly assisted in the ongoing effort to decipher the mechanisms controlling the activation of immune cells, especially those regulating T-cell activity, much remains to be discovered in the field of interactions and stoichiometric ratios between immune regulatory proteins.

5. Acknowledgment

We thank Dr. Alex Braiman for critical reading of the review. MBS thanks the following agencies for their research support: The Israel Science Foundation for grants no.1659/08, 971/08, 1503/08 and 491/10, the Ministries of Health & Science for grant no. 3-4114 and 3-6540, the Israel Cancer Association through the Estate of the late Alexander Smidoda, and the Taubenblatt Family Foundation for the Bio-medicine excellence grant.

6. References

Alarcon, B.; Gil, D.; Delgado, P. & Schamel, W. W. (2003). Initiation of TCR signaling: regulation within CD3 dimers. *Immunol Rev*, 191, pp. 38-46.

Arechaga, I.; Swamy, M.; Abia, D.; Schamel, W. A.; Alarcon, B. & Valpuesta, J. M. (2010). Structural characterization of the TCR complex by electron microscopy. *Int Immunol*, 22, pp. 897-903.

Balbo, A.; Minor, K. H.; Velikovsky, C. A.; Mariuzza, R. A.; Peterson, C. B. & Schuck, P. (2005). Studying multiprotein complexes by multisignal sedimentation velocity analytical ultracentrifugation. *Proc Natl Acad Sci U S A*, 102, pp. 81-86.

Barber, E. K.; Dasgupta, J. D.; Schlossman, S. F.; Trevillyan, J. M. & Rudd, C. E. (1989). The CD4 and CD8 antigens are coupled to a protein-tyrosine kinase (p56lck) that phosphorylates the CD3 complex. *Proc Natl Acad Sci U S A*, 86, pp. 3277-3281.

Barda-Saad, M.; Shirasu, N.; Pauker, M. H.; Hassan, N.; Perl, O.; Balbo, A.; Yamaguchi, H.; Houtman, J. C.; Appella, E.; Schuck, P. & Samelson, L. E. (2010). Cooperative interactions at the SLP-76 complex are critical for actin polymerization. *EMBO J*, 29, pp. 2315-2328.

Batista, F. D.; Treanor, B. & Harwood, N. E. (2010). Visualizing a role for the actin cytoskeleton in the regulation of B-cell activation. *Immunol Rev*, 237, pp. 191-204.

Beach, D.; Gonen, R.; Bogin, Y.; Reischl, I. G. & Yablonski, D. (2007). Dual role of SLP-76 in mediating T cell receptor-induced activation of phospholipase C-gamma1. *J Biol Chem*, 282, pp. 2937-2946.

Billadeau, D. D.; Nolz, J. C. & Gomez, T. S. (2007). Regulation of T-cell activation by the cytoskeleton. *Nat Rev Immunol*, 7, pp. 131-143.

Blumberg, R. S.; Ley, S.; Sancho, J.; Lonberg, N.; Lacy, E.; McDermott, F.; Schad, V.; Greenstein, J. L. & Terhorst, C. (1990). Structure of the T-cell antigen receptor: evidence for two CD3 epsilon subunits in the T-cell receptor-CD3 complex. *Proc Natl Acad Sci U S A*, 87, pp. 7220-7224.

Brown, P. H.; Balbo, A. & Schuck, P. (2009). On the analysis of sedimentation velocity in the study of protein complexes. *Eur Biophys J*, 38, pp. 1079-1099.

Bubeck Wardenburg, J.; Fu, C.; Jackman, J. K.; Flotow, H.; Wilkinson, S. E.; Williams, D. H.; Johnson, R.; Kong, G.; Chan, A. C. & Findell, P. R. (1996). Phosphorylation of SLP-76 by the ZAP-70 protein-tyrosine kinase is required for T-cell receptor function. *J Biol Chem*, 271, pp. 19641-19644.

Call, M. E.; Pyrdol, J. & Wucherpfennig, K. W. (2004). Stoichiometry of the T-cell receptor-CD3 complex and key intermediates assembled in the endoplasmic reticulum. *EMBO J*, 23, pp. 2348-2357.

Chan, A. C.; Iwashima, M.; Turck, C. W. & Weiss, A. (1992). ZAP-70: a 70 kd protein-tyrosine kinase that associates with the TCR zeta chain. *Cell*, 71, pp. 649-662.

Chereau, D.; Kerff, F.; Graceffa, P.; Grabarek, Z.; Langsetmo, K. & Dominguez, R. (2005). Actin-bound structures of Wiskott-Aldrich syndrome protein (WASP)-homology domain 2 and the implications for filament assembly. *Proc Natl Acad Sci U S A*, 102, pp. 16644-16649.

Chini, C. C. & Leibson, P. J. (2001). Signal transduction during natural killer cell activation. *Curr Protoc Immunol*, Chapter 11, pp. Unit 11 19B.

Chook, Y. M.; Gish, G. D.; Kay, C. M.; Pai, E. F. & Pawson, T. (1996). The Grb2-mSos1 complex binds phosphopeptides with higher affinity than Grb2. *J Biol Chem*, 271, pp. 30472-30478.

Cole, J. L.; Lary, J. W.; T, P. M. & Laue, T. M. (2008). Analytical ultracentrifugation: sedimentation velocity and sedimentation equilibrium. *Methods Cell Biol*, 84, pp. 143-179.

Davis, M. M. & Bjorkman, P. J. (1988). T-cell antigen receptor genes and T-cell recognition. *Nature*, 334, pp. 395-402.

Dayel, M. J. & Mullins, R. D. (2004). Activation of Arp2/3 complex: addition of the first subunit of the new filament by a WASP protein triggers rapid ATP hydrolysis on Arp2. *PLoS Biol*, 2, pp. E91.

Dembic, Z.; Haas, W.; Weiss, S.; McCubrey, J.; Kiefer, H.; von Boehmer, H. & Steinmetz, M. (1986). Transfer of specificity by murine alpha and beta T-cell receptor genes. *Nature*, 320, pp. 232-238.

Demeler, B. (2010). Methods for the design and analysis of sedimentation velocity and sedimentation equilibrium experiments with proteins. *Curr Protoc Protein Sci*, Chapter 7, pp. Unit 7 13.

Doherty, P. C. (1996). Cytotoxic T cell effector and memory function in viral immunity. *Curr Top Microbiol Immunol*, 206, pp. 1-14.

Ebinu, J. O.; Bottorff, D. A.; Chan, E. Y.; Stang, S. L.; Dunn, R. J. & Stone, J. C. (1998). RasGRP, a Ras guanyl nucleotide- releasing protein with calcium- and diacylglycerol-binding motifs. *Science*, 280, pp. 1082-1086.

Exley, M.; Wileman, T.; Mueller, B. & Terhorst, C. (1995). Evidence for multivalent structure of T-cell antigen receptor complex. *Mol Immunol*, 32, pp. 829-839.

Fernandez-Miguel, G.; Alarcon, B.; Iglesias, A.; Bluethmann, H.; Alvarez-Mon, M.; Sanz, E. & de la Hera, A. (1999). Multivalent structure of an alphabetaT cell receptor. *Proc Natl Acad Sci U S A*, 96, pp. 1547-1552.

Fleire, S. J.; Goldman, J. P.; Carrasco, Y. R.; Weber, M.; Bray, D. & Batista, F. D. (2006). B cell ligand discrimination through a spreading and contraction response. *Science*, 312, pp. 738-741.

Hogan, P. G.; Chen, L.; Nardone, J. & Rao, A. (2003). Transcriptional regulation by calcium, calcineurin, and NFAT. *Genes Dev*, 17, pp. 2205-2232.

Houtman, J. C.; Brown, P. H.; Bowden, B.; Yamaguchi, H.; Appella, E.; Samelson, L. E. & Schuck, P. (2007). Studying multisite binary and ternary protein interactions by global analysis of isothermal titration calorimetry data in SEDPHAT: application to adaptor protein complexes in cell signaling. *Protein Sci*, 16, pp. 30-42.

Houtman, J. C.; Higashimoto, Y.; Dimasi, N.; Cho, S.; Yamaguchi, H.; Bowden, B.; Regan, C.; Malchiodi, E. L.; Mariuzza, R.; Schuck, P.; Appella, E. & Samelson, L. E. (2004). Binding specificity of multiprotein signaling complexes is determined by both cooperative interactions and affinity preferences. *Biochemistry*, 43, pp. 4170-4178.

Houtman, J. C.; Yamaguchi, H.; Barda-Saad, M.; Braiman, A.; Bowden, B.; Appella, E.; Schuck, P. & Samelson, L. E. (2006). Oligomerization of signaling complexes by the multipoint binding of GRB2 to both LAT and SOS1. *Nat Struct Mol Biol*, 13, pp. 798-805.

Imboden, J. B. & Stobo, J. D. (1985). Transmembrane signalling by the T cell antigen receptor. Perturbation of the T3-antigen receptor complex generates inositol phosphates and releases calcium ions from intracellular stores. *J Exp Med*, 161, pp. 446-456.

Jager, D.; Jager, E. & Knuth, A. (2001). Immune responses to tumour antigens: implications for antigen specific immunotherapy of cancer. *J Clin Pathol*, 54, pp. 669-674.

Jecklin, M. C.; Schauer, S.; Dumelin, C. E. & Zenobi, R. (2009). Label-free determination of protein-ligand binding constants using mass spectrometry and validation using surface plasmon resonance and isothermal titration calorimetry. *J Mol Recognit*, 22, pp. 319-329.

Jordan, M. S.; Sadler, J.; Austin, J. E.; Finkelstein, L. D.; Singer, A. L.; Schwartzberg, P. L. & Koretzky, G. A. (2006). Functional hierarchy of the N-terminal tyrosines of SLP-76. *J Immunol*, 176, pp. 2430-2438.

Koretzky, G. A. (1997). The role of Grb2-associated proteins in T-cell activation. *Immunol Today*, 18, pp. 401-406.

Koretzky, G. A.; Abtahian, F. & Silverman, M. A. (2006). SLP76 and SLP65: complex regulation of signalling in lymphocytes and beyond. *Nat Rev Immunol*, 6, pp. 67-78.

Ladbury, J. E. (2007). Measurement of the formation of complexes in tyrosine kinase-mediated signal transduction. *Acta Crystallogr D Biol Crystallogr*, 63, pp. 26-31.

Lemmon, M. A.; Ladbury, J. E.; Mandiyan, V.; Zhou, M. & Schlessinger, J. (1994). Independent binding of peptide ligands to the SH2 and SH3 domains of Grb2. *J Biol Chem*, 269, pp. 31653-31658.

Liang, Y. (2008). Applications of isothermal titration calorimetry in protein science. *Acta Biochim Biophys Sin (Shanghai)*, 40, pp. 565-576.

Liu, S. K.; Fang, N.; Koretzky, G. A. & McGlade, C. J. (1999). The hematopoietic-specific adaptor protein gads functions in T-cell signaling via interactions with the SLP-76 and LAT adaptors. *Curr Biol*, 9, pp. 67-75.

Love, P. E. & Hayes, S. M. (2010). ITAM-mediated signaling by the T-cell antigen receptor. *Cold Spring Harb Perspect Biol*, 2, pp. a002485.

Lowenstein, E. J.; Daly, R. J.; Batzer, A. G.; Li, W.; Margolis, B.; Lammers, R.; Ullrich, A.; Skolnik, E. Y.; Bar-Sagi, D. & Schlessinger, J. (1992). The SH2 and SH3 domain-containing protein GRB2 links receptor tyrosine kinases to ras signaling. *Cell*, 70, pp. 431-442.

Machesky, L. M. & Insall, R. H. (1998). Scar1 and the related Wiskott-Aldrich syndrome protein, WASP, regulate the actin cytoskeleton through the Arp2/3 complex. *Curr Biol*, 8, pp. 1347-1356.

Machesky, L. M.; Mullins, R. D.; Higgs, H. N.; Kaiser, D. A.; Blanchoin, L.; May, R. C.; Hall, M. E. & Pollard, T. D. (1999). Scar, a WASp-related protein, activates nucleation of actin filaments by the Arp2/3 complex. *Proc Natl Acad Sci U S A*, 96, pp. 3739-3744.

Marchand, J. B.; Kaiser, D. A.; Pollard, T. D. & Higgs, H. N. (2001). Interaction of WASP/Scar proteins with actin and vertebrate Arp2/3 complex. *Nat Cell Biol*, 3, pp. 76-82.

McDonnell, J. M. (2001). Surface plasmon resonance: towards an understanding of the mechanisms of biological molecular recognition. *Curr Opin Chem Biol*, 5, pp. 572-577.

Melowic, H. R.; Stahelin, R. V.; Blatner, N. R.; Tian, W.; Hayashi, K.; Altman, A. & Cho, W. (2007). Mechanism of diacylglycerol-induced membrane targeting and activation of protein kinase Ctheta. *J Biol Chem*, 282, pp. 21467-21476.

Padrick, S. B.; Cheng, H. C.; Ismail, A. M.; Panchal, S. C.; Doolittle, L. K.; Kim, S.; Skehan, B. M.; Umetani, J.; Brautigam, C. A.; Leong, J. M. & Rosen, M. K. (2008). Hierarchical regulation of WASP/WAVE proteins. *Mol Cell*, 32, pp. 426-438.

Padrick, S. B.; Doolittle, L. K.; Brautigam, C. A.; King, D. S. & Rosen, M. K. (2011). Arp2/3 complex is bound and activated by two WASP proteins. *Proc Natl Acad Sci U S A*.

Pattnaik, P. (2005). Surface plasmon resonance: applications in understanding receptor-ligand interaction. *Appl Biochem Biotechnol*, 126, pp. 79-92.

Pierce, S. K. (2009). Understanding B cell activation: from single molecule tracking, through Tolls, to stalking memory in malaria. *Immunol Res*, 43, pp. 85-97.

Reicher, B. & Barda-Saad, M. (2010). Multiple pathways leading from the T-cell antigen receptor to the actin cytoskeleton network. *FEBS Lett*, 584, pp. 4858-4864.

Reth, M. (1989). Antigen receptor tail clue. *Nature*, 338, pp. 383-384.

Reth, M.; Wienands, J. & Schamel, W. W. (2000). An unsolved problem of the clonal selection theory and the model of an oligomeric B-cell antigen receptor. *Immunol Rev*, 176, pp. 10-18.

Rich, R. L. & Myszka, D. G. (2000). Advances in surface plasmon resonance biosensor analysis. *Curr Opin Biotechnol*, 11, pp. 54-61.

Risso, A. (2000). Leukocyte antimicrobial peptides: multifunctional effector molecules of innate immunity. *J Leukoc Biol*, 68, pp. 785-792.

Ritchie, R. H. (1957). Plasma Losses by Fast Electrons in Thin Films. *Physical Review*, 106, pp. 874-881.

Rodal, A. A.; Sokolova, O.; Robins, D. B.; Daugherty, K. M.; Hippenmeyer, S.; Riezman, H.; Grigorieff, N. & Goode, B. L. (2005). Conformational changes in the Arp2/3 complex leading to actin nucleation. *Nat Struct Mol Biol*, 12, pp. 26-31.

Rohatgi, R.; Ma, L.; Miki, H.; Lopez, M.; Kirchhausen, T.; Takenawa, T. & Kirschner, M. W. (1999). The interaction between N-WASP and the Arp2/3 complex links Cdc42-dependent signals to actin assembly. *Cell*, 97, pp. 221-231.

Roselin, L. S.; Lin, M. S.; Lin, P. H.; Chang, Y. & Chen, W. Y. (2009). Recent trends and some applications of isothermal titration calorimetry in biotechnology. *Biotechnol J*, 5, pp. 85-98.

Rubin, B.; Alibaud, L.; Hucheng-Champagne, A.; Arnaud, J.; Toribio, M. L. & Constans, J. (2002). Some hints concerning the shape of T-cell receptor structures. *Scand J Immunol*, 55, pp. 111-118.

Rudolph, M. G.; Stanfield, R. L. & Wilson, I. A. (2006). How TCRs bind MHCs, peptides, and coreceptors. *Annu Rev Immunol*, 24, pp. 419-466.

Saito, T. & Germain, R. N. (1987). Predictable acquisition of a new MHC recognition specificity following expression of a transfected T-cell receptor beta-chain gene. *Nature*, 329, pp. 256-259.

Samelson, L. E. (2002). Signal transduction mediated by the T cell antigen receptor: the role of adapter proteins. *Annu Rev Immunol*, 20, pp. 371-394.

Samelson, L. E.; Patel, M. D.; Weissman, A. M.; Harford, J. B. & Klausner, R. D. (1986). Antigen activation of murine T cells induces tyrosine phosphorylation of a polypeptide associated with the T cell antigen receptor. *Cell*, 46, pp. 1083-1090.

Samelson, L. E.; Phillips, A. F.; Luong, E. T. & Klausner, R. D. (1990). Association of the fyn protein-tyrosine kinase with the T-cell antigen receptor. *Proc Natl Acad Sci U S A*, 87, pp. 4358-4362.

San Jose, E.; Sahuquillo, A. G.; Bragado, R. & Alarcon, B. (1998). Assembly of the TCR/CD3 complex: CD3 epsilon/delta and CD3 epsilon/gamma dimers associate indistinctly with both TCR alpha and TCR beta chains. Evidence for a double TCR heterodimer model. *Eur J Immunol*, 28, pp. 12-21.

Schagger, H. & von Jagow, G. (1991). Blue native electrophoresis for isolation of membrane protein complexes in enzymatically active form. *Anal Biochem*, 199, pp. 223-231.

Schamel, W. W. (2001). Biotinylation of protein complexes may lead to aggregation as well as to loss of subunits as revealed by Blue Native PAGE. *J Immunol Methods*, 252, pp. 171-174.

Schamel, W. W. & Reth, M. (2000). Monomeric and oligomeric complexes of the B cell antigen receptor. *Immunity*, 13, pp. 5-14.

Schuck, P. (2009). On computational approaches for size-and-shape distributions from sedimentation velocity analytical ultracentrifugation. *Eur Biophys J*, 39, pp. 1261-1275.

Schuck, P. (2010a). Diffusion of the reaction boundary of rapidly interacting macromolecules in sedimentation velocity. *Biophys J*, 98, pp. 2741-2751.

Schuck, P. (2010b). Sedimentation patterns of rapidly reversible protein interactions. *Biophys J*, 98, pp. 2005-2013.

Seet, B. T.; Berry, D. M.; Maltzman, J. S.; Shabason, J.; Raina, M.; Koretzky, G. A.; McGlade, C. J. & Pawson, T. (2007). Efficient T-cell receptor signaling requires a high-affinity interaction between the Gads C-SH3 domain and the SLP-76 RxxK motif. *EMBO J*, 26, pp. 678-689.

Smith-Garvin, J. E.; Koretzky, G. A. & Jordan, M. S. (2009). T cell activation. *Annu Rev Immunol*, 27, pp. 591-619.

Sommers, C. L.; Samelson, L. E. & Love, P. E. (2004). LAT: a T lymphocyte adapter protein that couples the antigen receptor to downstream signaling pathways. *Bioessays*, 26, pp. 61-67.

Swamy, M.; Dopfer, E. P.; Molnar, E.; Alarcon, B. & Schamel, W. W. (2008). The 450 kDa TCR Complex has a Stoichiometry of alphabetagammaepsilondeltaepsilonzetazeta. *Scand J Immunol*, 67, pp. 418-420; author reply 421.

Swamy, M.; Kulathu, Y.; Ernst, S.; Reth, M. & Schamel, W. W. (2006). Two dimensional Blue Native-/SDS-PAGE analysis of SLP family adaptor protein complexes. *Immunol Lett*, 104, pp. 131-137.

Swamy, M.; Minguet, S.; Siegers, G. M.; Alarcon, B. & Schamel, W. W. (2007). A native antibody-based mobility-shift technique (NAMOS-assay) to determine the stoichiometry of multiprotein complexes. *J Immunol Methods*, 324, pp. 74-83.

Tolar, P.; Sohn, H. W. & Pierce, S. K. (2005). The initiation of antigen-induced B cell antigen receptor signaling viewed in living cells by fluorescence resonance energy transfer. *Nat Immunol*, 6, pp. 1168-1176.

Treanor, B.; Depoil, D.; Gonzalez-Granja, A.; Barral, P.; Weber, M.; Dushek, O.; Bruckbauer, A. & Batista, F. D. (2010). The membrane skeleton controls diffusion dynamics and signaling through the B cell receptor. *Immunity*, 32, pp. 187-199.

Veillette, A.; Bookman, M. A.; Horak, E. M. & Bolen, J. B. (1988). The CD4 and CD8 T cell surface antigens are associated with the internal membrane tyrosine-protein kinase p56lck. *Cell*, 55, pp. 301-308.

Viret, C. & Janeway, C. A., Jr. (1999). MHC and T cell development. *Rev Immunogenet*, 1, pp. 91-104.

Weber, J. R.; Orstavik, S.; Torgersen, K. M.; Danbolt, N. C.; Berg, S. F.; Ryan, J. C.; Tasken, K.; Imboden, J. B. & Vaage, J. T. (1998). Molecular cloning of the cDNA encoding pp36, a tyrosine-phosphorylated adaptor protein selectively expressed by T cells and natural killer cells. *J Exp Med*, 187, pp. 1157-1161.

Weber, M.; Treanor, B.; Depoil, D.; Shinohara, H.; Harwood, N. E.; Hikida, M.; Kurosaki, T. & Batista, F. D. (2008). Phospholipase C-gamma2 and Vav cooperate within signaling microclusters to propagate B cell spreading in response to membrane-bound antigen. *J Exp Med*, 205, pp. 853-868.

Weber, R. L. & Iacono, V. J. (1997). The cytokines: a review of interleukins. *Periodontal Clin Investig*, 19, pp. 17-22.

Wu, J. & Lanier, L. L. (2003). Natural killer cells and cancer. *Adv Cancer Res*, 90, pp. 127-156.

Wucherpfennig, K. W.; Gagnon, E.; Call, M. J.; Huseby, E. S. & Call, M. E. (2010). Structural biology of the T-cell receptor: insights into receptor assembly, ligand recognition, and initiation of signaling. *Cold Spring Harb Perspect Biol*, 2, pp. a005140.

Zeng, R.; Cannon, J. L.; Abraham, R. T.; Way, M.; Billadeau, D. D.; Bubeck-Wardenberg, J. & Burkhardt, J. K. (2003). SLP-76 coordinates Nck-dependent Wiskott-Aldrich syndrome protein recruitment with Vav-1/Cdc42-dependent Wiskott-Aldrich syndrome protein activation at the T cell-APC contact site. *J Immunol*, 171, pp. 1360-1368.

Zhang, W.; Sloan-Lancaster, J.; Kitchen, J.; Trible, R. P. & Samelson, L. E. (1998). LAT: the ZAP-70 tyrosine kinase substrate that links T cell receptor to cellular activation. *Cell*, 92, pp. 83-92.

Zhao, H.; Balbo, A.; Brown, P. H. & Schuck, P. (2011). The boundary structure in the analysis of reversibly interacting systems by sedimentation velocity. *Methods*, 54, pp. 16-30.

Zhu, M.; Janssen, E. & Zhang, W. (2003). Minimal requirement of tyrosine residues of linker for activation of T cells in TCR signaling and thymocyte development. *J Immunol*, 170, pp. 325-333.

10

Determination of the Binding Site-Size of the Protein-DNA Complex by Use of the Electrophoretic Mobility Shift Assay

Cheng-Yang Huang
Department of Biomedical Sciences, Chung Shan Medical University,
Department of Medical Research, Chung Shan Medical University Hospital,
Taichung City,
Taiwan

1. Introduction

In this chapter we describe how to perform an electrophoretic mobility shift assay (EMSA), also known as the band shift or gel retardation assay, to determine the binding site-size of the DNA binding protein using a series of DNA polymers. The binding site-size information of the DNA binding protein is a prerequisite for formulating any model of the proteins' function in DNA replication. EMSA is simple and quick, and if needed, the use of radioactive DNA make it highly sensitive and allow us to "see" the formation of distinct complexes of the DNA binding protein. The expectation of EMSA is that, once the length of the nucleotides is sufficient for the binding of protein, the protein-DNA complex remains intact and migrates as distinct band during gel electrophoresis. In addition, once the length of the nucleotides is sufficient for the binding of two or more proteins, the protein-DNA complexes migrate as distinct bands, usually referred to as a super shift: the higher the oligomeric protein-DNA complex, the lower the electrophoretic mobility. This technique can be used for both highly sequence-specific (e.g., transcription factor) (1,2) and non-specific proteins (e.g., single-stranded DNA binding protein) (3-7).

2. Some general considerations

1. Although EMSA was originally used in the detection of DNA-binding proteins in the crude cell extracts, it is thought that cell extracts contain many other DNA-binding proteins (and their regulatory proteins), and some small molecules (such as ATP and DNA metabolites), that are also able to interact with the DNA and the target protein; these molecules may cause some unpredictable effects on the reaction. Therefore, it is highly recommended to use purified protein(s) for EMSA.
2. When the studied protein has low DNA-binding activity, needs other loading factors, or binds to DNA in a strong sequence-specific way, a relatively high concentration of protein (in μM range) may be required to facilitate protein-DNA complex formation.
3. Protein binding to DNA usually needs to be in the "suitable" condition for optimal complex formation and stabilization. The conditions for the DNA binding process may

vary significantly in terms of pH, ionic strength, and necessary factors (such as metal ions or ATP).

4. When the protein-DNA interaction is highly cooperative, a particular care must be taken for determining its binding site-size by use of EMSA. If only one protein-DNA complex is visible when the DNA length is further increased (for example, to dT60 or more), it is likely inappropriate to determine its binding site-size using EMSA.

3. Experimental systems

1. Polyacrylamide gels. Differences in the size, aggregation state and pI of protein-DNA complexes will affect the choice of conditions used for EMSA. Generally, the lower percent of polyacrylamide gel will be considered for the bigger protein. Polyacrylamide gels, usually in 6-12% w/v, are made using an acrylamide to bisacrylamide weight ratio of 19:1 and TBE as the buffer in the gel and for electrophoresis.
2. Electrophoresis buffers. The process of electrophoretic separation may destabilize protein-DNA complexes, and thus the ionic strength, pH and composition of electrophoresis buffers should be adjusted to fit the need of the protein-DNA complex formation. If the binding condition for the formation of the protein-DNA complex is known, the electrophoresis buffer can be kept similar to the binding buffer. The most common buffer used in both polyacrylamide and agarose gels is TBE buffer. However, some metal-containing or metal-binding proteins should be analyzed in a buffer without EDTA. Sometimes the use of low ionic strength electrophoresis buffers at the same pH value can improve the stability of the protein-DNA complexes and the resolutions between bands; TE (10 mM Tris–HCl, 0.1 mM EDTA) or HE (10 mM HEPES, 0.1 mM EDTA) might be used in this case.
3. Sample buffers. Protein-DNA complexes are loaded on the polyacrylamide gel usually in the presence of 5-10% glycerol or sucrose. This can be included in the binding buffer or added before the protein-DNA complexes loading to the gel. Bromophenol blue and/or xylene cyanol (0.02% w/v) is usually used as an electrophoresis marker.
4. Visualization of gels. After electrophoresis, the gels are placed on filter paper, dried under vacuum at 80 °C, and then visualized by either autoradiography (exposed to X-ray film) or using a phosphorimager (exposed to the phosphor storage plate). Phosphorimaging is much more sensitive and the dynamic range is much greater than that of X-ray film. For phosphorimaging, the phosphor storage plate is scanned, and the data are digitized for quantitative analysis.

4. Determination of the binding site-size of the protein-DNA complex by use of the electrophoretic mobility shift assay: Single-stranded DNA binding protein (SSB)

Step 1. Use of a purified protein

As mentioned above, cell extracts contain many other proteins and some small molecules, able to interact with the target DNA and protein, which may cause some unpredictable effects on the DNA-binding reaction. Therefore, it is highly recommended to use purified protein(s) for EMSA. More and more proteins have become available in a pure form now, especially by using recombinant technology. The overexpression of DNA-binding proteins or their domains is essential for their purification, characterization and structure determination. The bacterial host *E. coli* is the first choice of expression system; it is simple to use and inexpensive to culture. For example, the gene encoding the single-stranded DNA binding protein (SSB) from *Pseudomonas aeruginosa* PAO1 can be PCR-amplified from the genomic DNA (3), inserted into the pET21b vector, and the gene can be expressed in transformed *E. coli* cell by using the inducer isopropyl thiogalactoside (IPTG). *P. aeruginosa* SSB can be then purified from the soluble supernatant by Ni^{2+}-affinity chromatography (HiTrap HP; GE Healthcare Bio-Sciences, Piscataway, NJ, USA). Protein purity can be determined by Coomassie-stained SDS-PAGE.

Step 2. Preparation of protein-DNA complexes

Binding mode is not always the same for several DNA-binding proteins. For example, differences in the binding condition, such as the ionic strength, pH and some small molecules included in the reaction mixture, can affect the binding mode of SSB (8). These factors also influence the stability of the SSB-DNA complexes in the binding reaction. For determination of the binding site-size of SSB using EMSA, various lengths of ssDNA oligonucleotides or other series of ssDNA homopolymers will be needed; radiolabeling can be carried out with [γ^{32}P]ATP (6000 Ci/mmol; PerkinElmer Life Sciences) and T4 polynucleotide kinase (Promega, Madison, WI, USA). The SSB-DNA complexes will be formed with different protein concentrations, usually at range of 10^{-9}–10^{-7} M. For *P. aeruginosa* PAO1 SSB, 0, 19, 37, 77, 155, 310, 630, 1250, 2500, and 5000 nM protein was used for the complexes formation, respectively. *P. aeruginosa* PAO1 SSB was incubated for 30 min at 25°C with 1.7 nM radioactive DNA substrates (dT15, 20, 25, 30, 35, 40, 45, 50, 55, 60, 65, 70, 75, and 80) in a total volume of 10 µL in 20 mM Tris-HCl pH 8.0 and 100 mM NaCl. The composition of the binding buffer may be adjusted to fit the need of study or the nature of the protein of interest.

Step 3. Fractionation of the SSB-DNA complexes using EMSA

Polyacrylamide or agarose gels can be used to fractionate mixture of protein-DNA complexes prior to further analysis. For *P. aeruginosa* PAO1 SSB, the complexes were formed in a total volume of 10 µL (see above), and aliquots (5 µL) were removed from each reaction solution and added to 2 µL of gel-loading solution (0.25% bromophenol blue and 40% sucrose). The resulting samples can be resolved on a native 8% polyacrylamide gel at 4 °C in TBE buffer for 1 h at 100 V and visualized by autoradiography or phosphorimaging.

Step 4. Determination of the binding site-size of protein-DNA complexes

After fractionating and phosphorimaging, complexed and free DNA bands can be visualized and quantified, and the binding site-size of DNA-protein complex can be determined. For example, various lengths of radioactive ssDNA oligonucleotides d(T5)n were complexed with SSB and with different protein concentrations. If the DNA space (length) is enough, the second or third studying protein will bind to the same complex where one protein of interest has been already pre-bound. Therefore, we can calculate the length of DNA required for the second joining protein (Figure 1). For example, SSB from *Klebsiella pneumoniae* binds to short ssDNAs (dT30–50) to form a complex in which a single protein is bound to the ssDNA (Figure 2), and two proteins could bind to dT55–75 (Figure 3). The presence of an extra 5 nt in dT55, as compared with dT50, provides enough interaction space for the binding of a second SSB protein, which occupies around 27 nt ssDNA (55/2=27.5). Furthermore, three SSB proteins could bind to dT80–85 (Figure 4), which occupies around 26 nt ssDNA per SSB protein (80/3=26.7). Thus, combining together the EMSA results with the number of the SSB-DNA (dT30–85) complexes, it can be found that the binding-site size of SSB from *Klebsiella pneumoniae* is 27 ± 1 nt, as determined using EMSA under this binding condition (Figure 5).

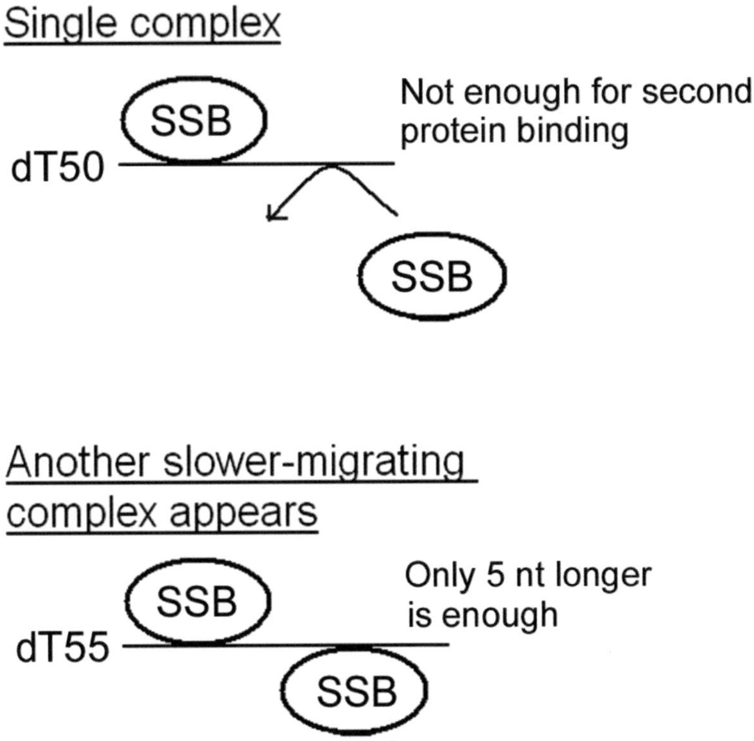

Fig. 1. Schematic model for the supershift of the SSB binding to the ssDNA. If the DNA provides enough interaction space for the binding of a second protein, we can observe another slower-migrating complex from EMSA when the protein concentration is increased.

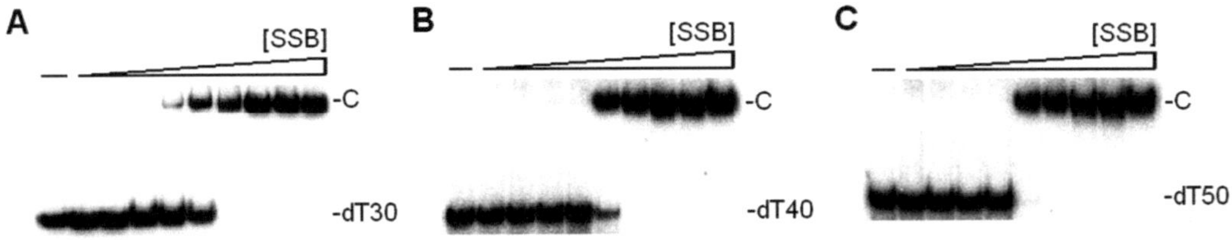

Fig. 2. Binding of *Klebsiella pneumoniae* SSB to dT30–50. The reaction solutions contained DNA substrate dT30, dT40, or dT50 and the SSB (0–5.0 μM). SSB (0, 19, 37, 77, 155, 310, 630, 1250, 2500, and 5000 nM) was incubated for 30 min at 25 °C with 1.7 nM of (A) dT30, (B) dT40, or (C) dT50 in a total volume of 10 μL in 20 mM HEPES pH 7.0 and 500 mM NaCl. Aliquots (5 μL) were removed from each reaction solution and added to 2 μL of gel-loading solution (0.25% bromophenol blue and 40% sucrose). The resulting samples were resolved on a native 8% polyacrylamide gel at 4 °C in TBE buffer (89 mM Tris borate and 1 mM EDTA) for 1 h at 100 V and visualized by autoradiography. This SSB binding to dT30–50 forms a single complex.

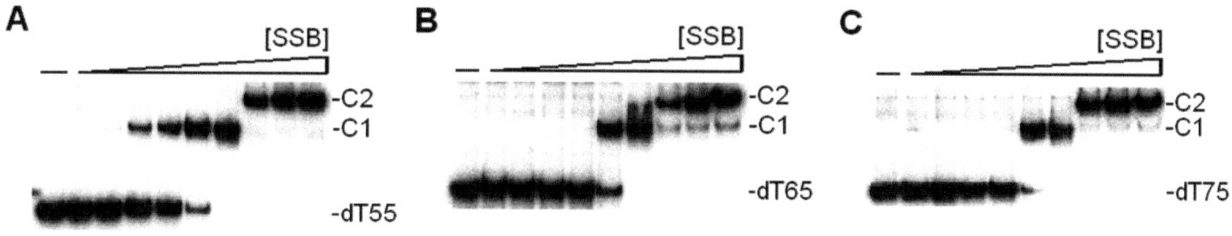

Fig. 3. Binding of *Klebsiella pneumoniae* SSB to dT55–75. The reaction solutions contained DNA substrate dT55, dT65, or dT75 and the SSB (0–5.0 μM). SSB (0, 19, 37, 77, 155, 310, 630, 1250, 2500, and 5000 nM) was incubated for 30 min at 25 °C with 1.7 nM of (A) dT55, (B) dT65, or (C) dT75 in a total volume of 10 μL in 20 mM HEPES pH 7.0 and 500 mM NaCl. Aliquots (5 μL) were removed from each reaction solution and added to 2 μL of gel-loading solution (0.25% bromophenol blue and 40% sucrose). The resulting samples were resolved on a native 8% polyacrylamide gel at 4 °C in TBE buffer (89 mM Tris borate and 1 mM EDTA) for 1 h at 100 V and visualized by autoradiography. This SSB binding to dT55–75 forms two different complexes.

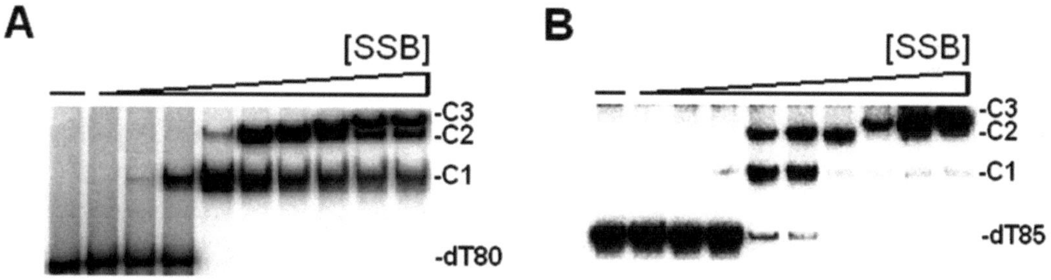

Fig. 4. Binding of *Klebsiella pneumoniae* SSB to dT80–85. The reaction solutions contained DNA substrate dT80 or dT85 and the SSB (0–5.0 μM). SSB (0, 19, 37, 77, 155, 310, 630, 1250, 2500, and 5000 nM) was incubated for 30 min at 25 °C with 1.7 nM of (A) dT80 or (B) dT85 in a total volume of 10 μL in 20 mM HEPES pH 7.0 and 500 mM NaCl. Aliquots (5 μL) were removed from each reaction solution and added to 2 μL of gel-loading solution (0.25% bromophenol blue and 40% sucrose). The resulting samples were resolved on a native 8% polyacrylamide gel at 4 °C in TBE buffer (89 mM Tris borate and 1 mM EDTA) for 1 h at 100 V and visualized by autoradiography. This SSB binding to either dT80 or dT85 forms three different complexes.

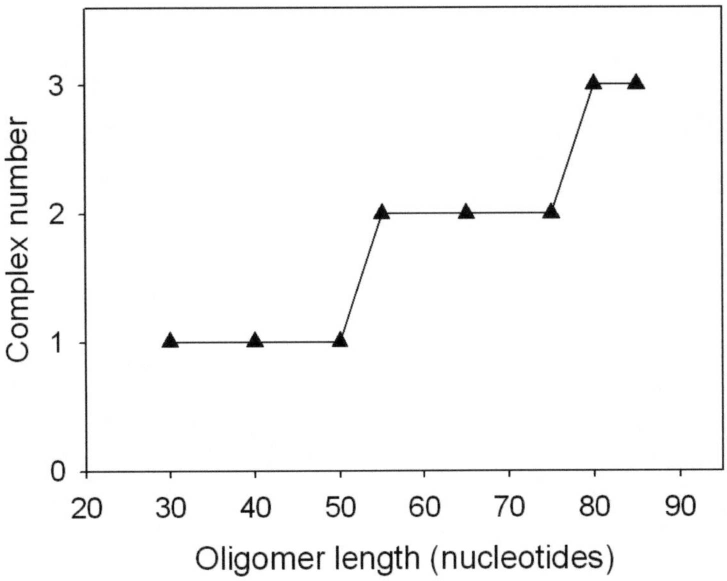

Fig. 5. Complex number of *Klebsiella pneumoniae* SSB as a function of the length of the ssDNA determined using EMSA. The binding site-size of other DNA-binding protein may also be determined using a similar protocol.

Step 5. Estimation of the apparent dissociation constants

In addition to the binding site-size, EMSA can also be used to estimate the apparent dissociation constants for the protein-DNA complexes when the protein concentration is known accurately and the used DNA is at low concentrations. If the DNA concentration is much lower than the apparent dissociation constant, its value will be equal to the protein concentration needed to have 50% of protein-DNA complex formed. The radio-intensity of free DNA and each protein-DNA complex, with increasing amounts of the protein, can be scanned and quantified by using phosphorimaging. For example, using *Salmonella enterica* serovar Typhimurium LT2 SSB (4), the apparent dissociation constant for the SSB-ssDNA complex 1 (K_{d1}) was estimated from the protein concentration that binds 50% of the input DNA; the apparent dissociation constant for the SSB-ssDNA complex 2 (K_{d2}) was estimated from the protein concentration that forms 50% of the complex 2, and K_{dn} could be also calculated in a similar manner if multiple complexes are formed.

Step 6. Analysis of oligomeric state by gel filtration chromatography

We have previously described how to determine the binding-site size of DNA-binding protein like SSB. Information about the oligomeric state of protein of interest may also be important for analysis of its binding mode. Assuming that the protein has a shape and partial specific volume similar to the standard proteins, the native molecular mass of the protein can be estimated and compared with its predicted mass in monomer from the amino acid sequence. For example, the native molecular mass for *S. enterica* serovar Typhimurium LT2 SSB is approximately 4.1 times the molecular mass of a *St*SSB monomer, and thus *S. enterica* serovar Typhimurium LT2 SSB in solution is a tetramer.

5. Conclusion

Development of more targeted drugs or antibiotics against many pathogenic bacteria has been hampered due to the lack of knowledge of DNA replication and the overall molecular biology of the organisms. For example, *K. pneumoniae* used here is a ubiquitous opportunistic pathogen that colonizes at the mucosal surfaces in humans and causes severe diseases; many clinical strains of *K. pneumoniae* are highly resistant to antibiotics. Since SSB is required for DNA replication, blocking the activity of SSB would be detrimental to bacterial survival. A characteristic of any protein-nucleic acid complex is its "site size", i.e. the average number of nucleotide residues occluded by the bound protein. Here we describe how to determine the binding-site size of DNA-binding protein using EMSA in different binding conditions. The information obtained through the use of this methodology may be very helpful in studying the binding mode(s) of DNA-binding protein. However, a particular care must be taken when the DNA-binding protein of interest binds to DNA with high cooperativity, as like PriB. If only one protein-DNA complex is visible when the length of the DNA is further increased (for example, to dT60 or more), it is likely inappropriate to determine its binding site-size using EMSA.

6. Acknowledgement

This work was supported by a grant from the National Research Program for Genome Medicine (NSC 100-3112-B-040-001 to C.Y. Huang).

7. Experimental protocol

Determination of the binding site-size of SSB (or other DNA-binding protein)

Equipment and reagents

- 30% acrylamide/bis- acrylamide stock solution
- Binding buffer: 20 mM Tris-HCl, pH 8.0, 100 mM NaCl. The composition of the binding buffer may be adjusted to fit the particular study or the nature of the studied protein
- Various lengths of ssDNA homopolymers. The duplex DNA can be used for other DNA-binding protein
- [γ^{32}P]ATP solution at 10mCi/mL, specific activity 3000 Ci/mmol
- T4 polynucleotide kinase
- Purified SSB protein
- Loading buffer: 0.25% bromophenol blue and 40% sucrose
- TBE buffer (89 mM Tris borate and 1 mM EDTA)
- Vertical electrophoresis system and a power pack

Experimental method

1. Phosphorylate the ssDNA homopolymers of varying length in 10 μL of T4 polynucleotide kinase buffer (70 mM Tris-HCl, pH 7.6, 10 mM $MgCl_2$, 5 mM dithiothreitol) supplemented with 1 μL of [γ^{32}P]ATP and 1 μL of T4 polynucleotide kinase. Incubate at 37 °C for 1 h.
2. Dilute radiolabeled DNA substrates to suitable concentration (for example, 1-10 nM; for determination of the apparent dissociation constant) using binding buffer.

3. Incubate radiolabeled DNA substrates with different concentrations of protein, respectively, for 30 min at 25 °C, in a total volume of 10 μL in binding buffer.
4. Remove aliquots (5 μL) from each reaction solution and add it to 2 μL of loading buffer and load on a native 8% polyacrylamide gel at 4°C in TBE buffer for 1–2 h at 100 V, depending on the length of DNA.
5. Dry the gel under vacuum and autoradiograph.
6. Summarize the number of DNA-protein complexes formation for each length of DNA used.
7. Evaluate DNA length required for two and three complexes formation.
8. Calculate the length (the binding site-size) needed for one protein binding.

8. References

[1] Tsai, K. L., Sun, Y. J., Huang, C. Y., Yang, J. Y., Hung, M. C., and Hsiao, C. D. (2007) *Nucleic Acids Res* 35, 6984-6994
[2] Tsai, K. L., Huang, C. Y., Chang, C. H., Sun, Y. J., Chuang, W. J., and Hsiao, C. D. (2006) *J Biol Chem* 281, 17400-17409
[3] Jan, H. C., Lee, Y. L., and Huang, C. Y. (2011) *Protein J* 30, 20-26
[4] Huang, Y. H., Lee, Y. L., and Huang, C. Y. (2011) *Protein J* 30, 102-108
[5] Hsieh, H. C., and Huang, C. Y. (2011) *Biochem Biophys Res Commun* 404, 546-551
[6] Huang, C. Y., Hsu, C. H., Sun, Y. J., Wu, H. N., and Hsiao, C. D. (2006) *Nucleic Acids Res* 34, 3878-3886
[7] Liu, J. H., Chang, T. W., Huang, C. Y., Chen, S. U., Wu, H. N., Chang, M. C., and Hsiao, C. D. (2004) *J Biol Chem* 279, 50465-50471
[8] Lohman, T. M., and Ferrari, M. E. (1994) *Annu Rev Biochem* 63, 527-570

11

Stoichiometry of Protein Interactions in Bacteriophage Tail Assembly

Fumio Arisaka
Tokyo Institute of Technology, Graduate School of Bioscience and Biotechnology
Department of Life Science
Japan

1. Introduction

The concept of self-assembly of supramolecules from subunit proteins originated from the study of tobacco mosaic virus, TMV, by Fraenkel-Conrat & Williams in 1955. They succeeded in reassembly of viable TMV from the isolated coat protein and detergent-extracted RNA. Since then, disassembly and reassembly or self-assembly have been investigated in various systems including simple plant viruses and bacteriophages. Disassembly and reassembly, however, was only successful for simple single-stranded RNA viruses and phage, and have never been successful for other phages including single-stranded DNA phage such as phiX174. The reason is that in the case of bacteriophages even such simple phage has so-called scaffolding proteins which are not present in the mature phage. Larger and more complicated phage such as phage T4 has virion proteins which undergo "processing" or cleavage at the N-terminal region during assembly. Also, most of the virion has extremely stable capsid which can be dissociated only under denaturing conditions. Thus, phage assembly has been studied using "assembly-naïve" proteins (King, 1968). "Assembly naïve" means that the proteins have never experienced assembly. In *in vitro* complementation, "assembly-naive" proteins in the lysates of mutant phage-infected cells were mixed to let them assemble to form viable virions. Overexpression system can be used to produce "assembly-naive" proteins in place of the phage-infected lysate. Constituent subunit proteins of supramolecules including viruses, muscle myosin/actin, bacterial flagella etc. or oligomeric proteins have the intrinsic properties to assemble spontaneously.

Bacteriophage or phage is a virus that infects bacterium. Bacteriophage has some distinct features as compared with animal or plant viruses. First, they all inject DNA into the host cell leaving the protein capsids outside. Secondly, more than 95% of bacteriophage have tails (Ackerman, 2009). Tails are thought to be evolved in order to inject DNA efficiently through bacterial cell membrane which is fortified by outer membrane and peptideglycan layer in the case of Gram-negative bacteria or thick peptidoglycan layer containing teichoic acids in the case of Gram-positive bacteria. Bacteriophage which have tails are collectively called *Caudovirares* consisting of three sub-families, *Myoviridae* which have a long, contractile tail, *Podoviridae* which have a short non-contractile tail and *Siphoviridae* which have long, non-contractile tail.

Bacteriophage T4 is a *Myoviridae* which infects *Escherichia coli*, a Gram-negative bacterium. The virion consists of a head which packages viral genomic DNA, a contractile tail sheath and six tail fibers, LTF, which are the sensor to detect the receptor of the host cell (Figure 1). The head protects the viral DNA from external perturbation including nuclease activity. Tail is an intricate and complex molecular machine which protects DNA from accidental ejection, but also functions as facilitating efficient injection of the DNA in the head into the cytosol of *E. coli* when it encounters the host. Phage T4 is known to have extremely high efficiency of infection, almost 100%, which means that once the virion recognizes and is adsorbed to the outer membrane, it successfully inject its DNA. Phage adsorption, or receptor recognition, takes place in two steps and the first step is the binding of the tip of LTFs to the glucose residue of the core oligosaccharide LPS (Prehm, 1976). This binding is reversible. The signal of the binding is then transmitted to the baseplate by unknown mechanism, through gp9 (gp: gene product) which is the socket of LTFs and induces the conformational change of the baseplate from "hexgon" to "star" (Crowthe et a., 1977). Six short tail fibers, STF, concomitantly spring out downward and the tip of the STFs now bind to the heptose part of the LPS core oligosaccharide tightly. The conformational change of the baseplate triggers the tail sheath contraction. Recently, the C-terminal domain structure of gp37 which constitutes the distal half fibers has been determined by Bartual et al. (2010), which revealed that gp37 turns back at residue number 950 to form elongated six-stranded anti-parallel beta-strand needle.

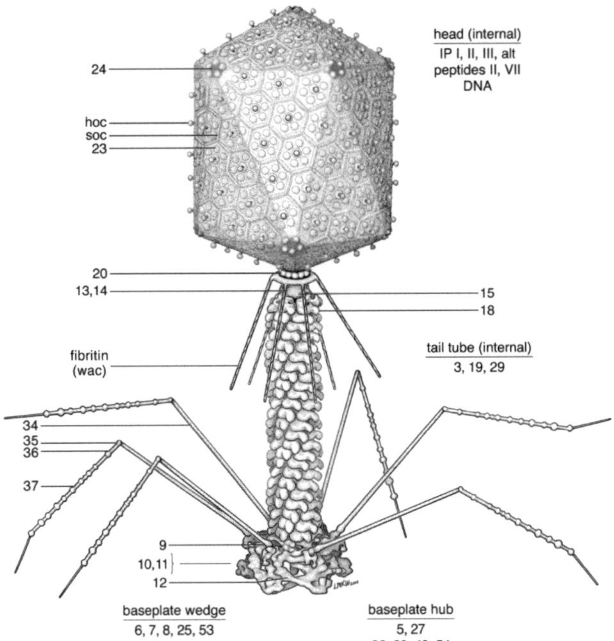

Fig. 1. Bacteriophage T4 (Courtesy of F. E. Eiserling)

Head, tail and six tail fibers are independently assembled. The head first binds a tail and then six tail fibers bind to form a viable phage. For the attachment of the tail fibers to the baseplate through gp9, a baseplate protein, "whisker" protein facilitates the attachment by transiently binding tail fibers at the kink position to properly orient the tail fibers. Gp63 also plays a role in facilitating the attachment.

The assembly pathway of the tail of phage T4 has been worked out by a pioneering work by Kikuchi and King (1975a, 1975b, 1975c) (Figure 2). Recently, Yap et al. (2010a) reexamined and confirmed their assembly pathway. Also, they presented experimental results which strongly support the notion that the strictly ordered wedge assembly is based on the conformational change of the subunit proteins upon binding to the precursor complex.

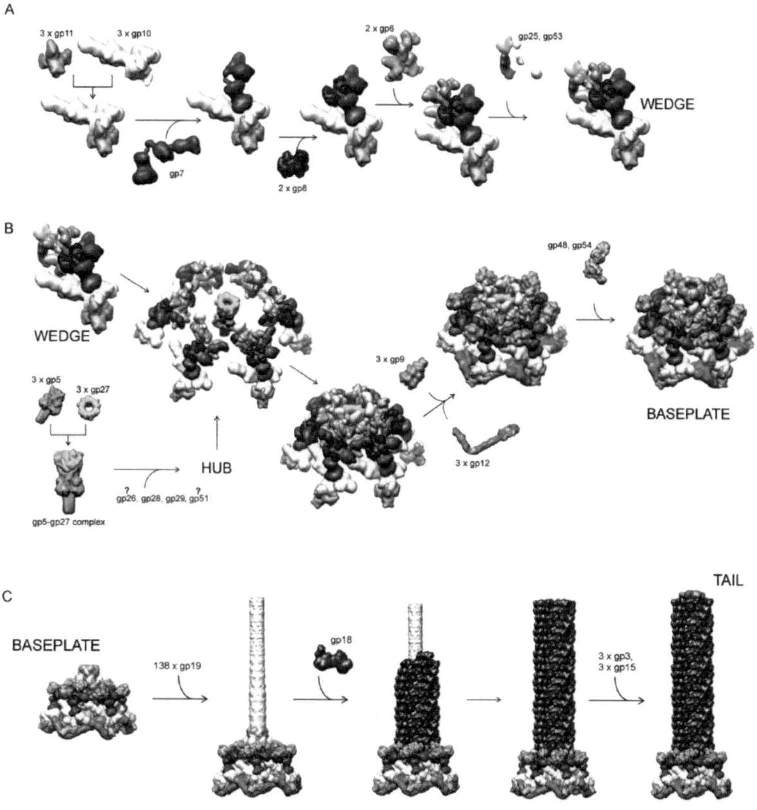

Fig. 2. Assembly of the tail of bacteriophage T4 (P. Leiman et al., 2010)

Structure of the tail in atomic level has been determined by the efforts of Michael G. Rossmann's group at Purdue in collaboration with Vadim V. Mesyanzhinov's, Mark van Raaij's and our group. These results are reviewed by Petr Leiman et al. in the special issue for T4 and T4-related phages of the Virology Journal (Leiman et al., 2010).

Thus, the stoichiometry of most of the tail proteins in phage T4 has been eventually determined by X-ray crystallography, but in this review focus will be made on the methodology of stoichiometry determination in solution before high resolution structures of the components were determined. Also, we would like to emphasize the importance of study of solution interactions. Occasionally, the oligomeric states of subunits are different from what is expected from the X-ray structure (See 3.3 Hub).

2. Methodology

In any interacting systems, stoichiometry and the binding constant are the two most important physical parameters to be determined. If the binding is too tight or irreversible under the normal conditions, the binding constant is difficult to determine, but the stoichiometry is readily determined by measuring the molecular weight of the complex if that of each constituent subunit molecule is known and they are not too different in molecular weight.

2.1 SDS-PAGE

Molecular weights of the constituent subunit proteins can be empirically estimated by SDS-PAGE. It can be also used to estimate the weight ratio of the constituent proteins, keeping in mind that the intensity of the staining by Coomassie brilliant Blue may depend on the amino acid composition to some extent.

2.2 Size-exclusion chromatography

Size exclusion chromatography (SEC, also called gel filtration chromatography) can be used for both analytical and preparative purposes. For molecular weight determination, it takes advantage of the elution volume of the solute which is a linear function of the logarithm of molecular weights. Various gel materials of different pore sizes are available and one could choose the appropriate gels and apply molecular markers. Elution volumes depend on the Stokes radius of the solute and not on the molecular weights. In our research, SEC was therefore only used for preliminary experiments.

2.3 Analytical ultracentrifugation

There are two modes in analytical ultracentrifugation; sedimentation velocity (SV) and sedimentation equilibrium (SE). Both SV and SE give absolute molecular weight (Mw) in solution independent of its molecular shape. They also give quantitative information concerning molecular interactions. SV is particularly sensitive in detecting minor components as low as 1% of the total concentration, but SE is more accurate in determining Mw. If the solute is not homogeneous, SE will give the weight average Mw. Due to the recent advancements particularly in SV analysis, including c(s) analysis (Schuck, 1998), SV has been extensively used in the present study, but when necessary, SE was also carried out. Both SV and SE can deal with quantitative analyses of protein interactions.

Experiments were carried out in Beckman-Coulter Optima XL-I equipped with either 4-hole An60Ti or 8-hole An50Ti rotors at 20°C. For SV experiments, normal double sector cells were used and 400 μl of the sample solution and 430 μl of dialysate or equilibrium buffer for SEC were applied in the sample and reference sector, respectively. Dialysate or the buffer solution used for the last step of purification were used as a reference solution in all experiments. All data were acquired without time intervals between successive scans. The sedimentation coefficient distribution function, c(s), was obtained by using the SEDFIT program (Schuck, 2000). Molecular mass distribution, c(M), was obtained by converting c(s) into c(M), on the assumption that the frictional ratio f/f_0 was common to all the molecular species (as implemented in the SEDFIT program).

For SE experiments, double sector cells or standard six channel centerpieces and quartz windows were used. 110 μl of each sample and 120 μl of the corresponding dialysate or buffer were loaded. When double sector cells were used, 120 μl and 140 μl of the sample and reference solutions were loaded. Loading concentrations of the samples as absorbance at 280 nm were 0.2, 0.3 and 0.5 and the measurements were made at 20 °C. Rotor speeds were decided by using calculator function of SEDFIT. Scans were recorded every 2 h and the equilibrium of the system was judged by the superimposition of the last three scans. Totally nine datasets were globally fitted to a single species model to determine the weight average molecular weight by non-lin software implemented in the Beckman-Coulter software package. The partial specific volumes based on the amino acid composition of the proteins, the solvent viscosity and solvent density were calculated by Sednterp program (Laue et al., 1992).

2.4 Electron microscopy

With regard to stoichiometry, electron microscopy (EM) has been used to identify the symmetry of oligomeric complexes. If some oligomer has a six-fold symmetry, it is likely that the oligomer is hexamer or the multi-mer of 6 as in the case of gp3 and gp15.

Purified sample with approximately 0.1 mg/ml concentration was loaded on a thin carbon film (supported on top of copper mesh grids) made hydrophilic by glow discharge in a partial vacuum. The sample was washed with five drops of double-distilled water, negatively stained twice with 2% uranyl acetate solution for 30 s each time, blotted, and air dried and subjected to observation.

3. Stoichiometry and protein interactions in the tail of phage T4

Tail consists of two parts, i.e. a baseplate and a long co-cylinder consisting of a tube and a contractile tail sheath. The baseplate consists of a hub and six wedges surrounding the former. Several other gene products bind to the precursor to complete the baseplate which is then ready to initiate tube and sheath polymerization, which is terminated by gp3 and gp15. Neck made of gp13 and 14 which connects a head and a tail is not a part of the tail, but stoichiometry determination of that part will be included in this section.

3.1 Wedge

There are seven gene products in the wedge, i.e. gp11, gp10, gp7, gp8, gp6, gp53 and gp25. The association state and sedimentation coefficient of each gene product are listed in Table 1. Gp11 and gp10 are trimer; gp7 is monomer; gp8 and gp6 are dimer, whereas gp53 and gp25 are monomer in solution. Except for gp11 which can bind to gp10 at any stage of wedge assembly, incorporations of all other gene products are strictly ordered. "Strictly ordered" means that if any of the six gene products is missing, intermediate complex up to that point is formed, but all other gene products that are to be incorporated later will remain unassociated. In order to look at interactions between all the combinations of gene products and assembly pathway, Yap et al. devised a novel method in which each gene was expressed separately in *E. coli*, cells were mixed and then lysed and the association products were analyzed. The results are listed in Table 2 (Yap et al., 2010b).

All the interactions in the strictly ordered assembly pathway were confirmed. Sedimentation velocity experiments indicated that there are not very strong, but significant interactions among gp6, gp53, and gp25, which does not comfort to the strictly ordered pathway. Since the interactions were not strong, it was not possible to isolate the complexes by size exclusion chromatography. It is noted that the interaction between gp6 and gp53 was much stronger when gp6 had been associated with the prior wedge intermediate up to gp8. Gp6 in that complex then could not directly bind gp25, but was bound after the binding of gp53. The results strongly suggested that the strict sequential assembly is based on the 'induced-fit' mechanism, where the binding of each subunit induced a conformational change in the complex to create a binding site for the next subunit entry.

Gene product (gp)	a.a. residue number	Stoichiometry in solution	Stoichiometry in the tail	Sedimentation coefficient	Comments, PDB
gp11	219	3	18	4.2S(trimer)	1EL6
gp10	602	3	18	7.8S(trimer)	2FKK
gp7	1032	1	6	5.7S(monomer)	
gp8	334	2	12	5.0S(dimer)	1N7Z
gp6	660	2	12	6.0S(dimer)	3H2T
gp53	196	1	6	2.1S(monomer)	
gp25	132	1	6	1.8S(monomer)	
gp5	575	3	3	ND	1K28, SE*)
gp27	391	1	3	ND	1K28, SE
gp29	590	ND	3	ND	
gp26	208	ND	ND	ND	
gp28	177	ND	ND	ND	
gp9	288	3	18	ND	1S2E
gp12	527	3	18	ND	1H6W, 1OCY, SE
gp48	364	ND	6	ND	
gp54	320	ND	6	ND	
gp18	659	1	138	4.2S(monomer)	3FOA
gp19	163	1	138	ND	
gp3	176	6	6	7.76S(hexamer)	
gp15	272	6	6	6.20S(hexamer)	
gp57A	79	3 or 6	-	ND	molecular chaperone
gp51	249	ND	ND	ND	catalytic

ND: not determined *) SE: sedimentation equilibrium has been done.

Table 1. Tail proteins and complexes

Gp10-gp11 complex constitutes the six tail pins at the corners of the dome-shaped baseplate hexagon. Plishker et al. (1988) overexpressed genes 11, 10, 7, and 8, mixed these gene products in various combinations and the formed complexes were then analyzed by native gel electrophoresis. They confirmed the strictly ordered sequential pathway which was proposed by Kikuchi and King (1975), but did not reach the correct stoichiometry.

Protein/protein complex	gp11	gp7	gp8	gp6	gp53	gp25
gp10	++	++	-	-	-	-
gp7	-		-	-	-	-
gp8	-			-	-	-
gp6	-				+	+
gp53	-					+
gp10-gp7	++		++	-	-	-
gp10-gp7-gp8	++			++	-	-
gp10-gp7-gp8-gp6	++				++	-
gp10-gp7-gp8-gp6-gp53	++					++

++: strong interaction, +: weak interaction, -: no interaction

Table 2. Interactions among wedge proteins

In 2000, Zhao et al. co-expressed gp11 and gp10, isolated the complex and demonstrated by SDS-PAGE, Edman degradation of the complex, and sedimentation equilibrium (SE) that gp10 and gp11 formed a 3:3 stoichiometry complex (Zhao et al., 2000). From the results of Edman degradation and SDS-PAGE, the molar ratio of gp10 and gp11 was determined to be approximately 1. On the other hand, the molecular weight of the purified gp10-gp11 complex was determined by sedimentation equilibrium to be 284,000 which is close to the expected value of 269,840, assuming that the stoichiometry is 3:3. Furthermore, comparison of the results in the presence and absence of reducing reagent, 2-mercaptoethanol (2-ME), in SDS-PAGE revealed that two molecules of gp10 in the complex formed a disulfide bond, while the third gp10 molecule did not participate in the disulfide bond formation.

Yap et al. (2010a) utilized their novel method to isolate all the possible intermediate complexes with and without gp11, which is an exception due to the fact that gp11 can bind to gp10 at any step of the assembly pathway (2010b) . The stoichiometry of intermediate complexes are summarized in Table 3. At present, stoichiometry of gp53 and gp25 is still unkown, although it is clear that they are monomer in solution. Regarding the binding affinities of these association steps of the wedge, their bindings are so tight that once bound they are almost irreversible and the binding constants have not been determined.

Yap et al. also found that when the wedge intermediate $(gp10)_3(gp7)_1(gp8)_2(gp6)_2$ complex binds gp53, it spontaneously forms a baseplate-like structure in a "star" conformation in the absence of gp25. The biological significance of the baseplate-like structure needs further investigation.

3.2 Hub

The main components of the hub are gp5 and gp27. Gp5 is the "tail lysozyme" which is a structural component of the baseplate and possesses the lysozyme activity. In 1980, it was reported by Kao & McClain (1980) that the lysozyme activity for the so-called "lysis from without" is gp5. Nakagawa et al (1985) later confirmed the results, isolated gp5 from the tail and identified the lysozyme activity to be N-acetyl muramidase which is the same as that of T4 lysozyme of gp e (gp: gene product). The nucleotide sequence of gene 5 was determined by Mosig et al. (1989).

Complex	Stoichiometry	$s_{20,w}$ (f/f_0)
gp10-gp7	3:1	10.2 S (1.52)
gp10-gp7-gp8	3:1:2	12.1 S (1.53)
gp10-gp7-gp8-gp6	3:1:2:2	14.5 S (1.64)
gp10-gp7-gp8-gp6-gp53	3:1:2:2:x	15.0 S (1.51); 43.7 S (1.53)
gp10-gp7-gp8-gp6-gp53-gp25	3:1:2:2:x:x	15.3 S (1.49); 42.0 S (1.44)
gp11-gp10	3:3	9.7 S
gp11-gp10-gp7	3:3:1	11.9 S (1.59)
gp11-gp10-gp7-gp8	3:3:1:2	13.4 S (1.56)
gp11-gp10-gp7-gp8-gp6	3:3:1:2:2	15.3 S
gp11-gp10-gp7-gp8-gp6-gp53	3:3:1:2:2:x	ND
gp11-gp10-gp7-gp8-gp6-gp53-gp25	3:3:1:2:2:x:x	16.0 S (1.67); 40.6 S (1.59)

x: stoichiometry not determined, f/f_0: frictional ratio

Table 3. Sedimentation coefficient and frictional ratio of wedge intermediate complex

Kanamaru et al. (1999) have cloned and overexpressed gene 5, and isolated gp5. They proved that it was cleaved at Ser351 and Ala352 during assembly and that the C-terminal domain remained associated to the rest of gp5 until the phage infected the host bacterium. The cleavage between Ser351 and Ala352 gave rise to gp5* and gp5C. Trimeric nature of gp5 in solution was determined by sedimentation equilibrium which revealed that the molecular weight in solution was 194,400 which was close to 189,300 about three times the molecular weight of monomer pre-gp5-his, 63,100, estimated from the amino acid sequence. Trimeric nature of gp27 in the "tail lysozyme complex" was inferred from the interaction study of gp27 and gp5 (Sarkar et al., 2006). The measured molecular weight of gp27-gp5 complex was 319,000 which is close to the expected value of 322,818, indicating that most of the solute remained as a whole complex, $(gp27)_3(gp5^*)_3(gp5C)_3$. Measurement of molecular weight at 20°C, after heat treatment at 37°C for half an hour, showed that the complex dissociated into $(gp27)_1(gp5^*)_1$ hetero-dimer and $(gp5C)_3$ trimer at pH 8.6, but when the pH was lowered down to 6.0, the hetero-dimer dissociated into monomers, whereas $(gp5C)_3$ stayed as a stable trimer. This result was considered relevant to the infection process, as the low pH in periplasm makes gp5* free so that it can cleave peptidoglycan layer to make a local hole through which tail tube can penetrate and reach the inner membrane and probably helps forming a pore in the inner membrane for DNA injection.

The X-ray crystal structure of the tail lysozyme complex was determined by Kanamaru, Leiman et al. (2001). They confirmed the stoichiometry of $(gp27)_3(gp5)_3$ and also localized the complex beneath the baseplate by superimposing the high resolution structure into the low resolution electron density of the 3D-reconstituted baseplate from cryo-electron micrographs. Later, Kanamaru et al. (2006) designed a series of mutant gp5 in which amino acid replacements were made at residue 351 to prevent from cleavage. They found that the amino acid replacements caused a various degrees of cleavage suppression. They have crystallized one of the gp5 mutants, S351L, in complex with gp27, and determined the structure around the cleavage site, which was not possible in the previous study. Interestingly, the mutant phage did not lose the phenotype although it showed some cold sensitive phenotype.

The localization and stoichiometry of gp29, which is the ruler molecule (Abuladze et al., 1994), has not been worked out yet. Gp29 has been difficult to isolate. It is assumed that it first forms a spherical-shape oligomeric complex, binding to the upper central part of the hub. The current model states that, as the tail tube polymerizes, it elongates itself and when it is completely extended, gp3 binds to the tip of gp29 and gp19, the tube protein to stop the polymerization. The tail length determination is the first system where the mechanism was explained by the ruler molecule or tape measure protein.

Neither the localization nor the number of molecules of gp26 and gp28 per a baseplate has been determined. It has been reported that when gene 27 is expressed together with gp28, gp27 is found in the membrane fraction (Nieradko and Koszalka, 1999). Gp51, which is essential for the assembly of the baseplate, has been reported to function catalytically, but how gp51 works as a catalyst is not known (Snustad, 1968).

Kikuchi & King's model (1975a) stated that 6 wedges surrounded a hub to form a baseplate intermediate complex. On the other hand, Yap et al. (2010a) found that upon binding of gp53 to the intermediate complex, a baseplate-like structure in a "star" conformation took place. The significance of this observation has to wait for further study, but the observation should be related to the association property of the wedge complex.

KVP40 is a T4-related vibrio phage which has a broad host range. Nemoto et al. (2008) have cloned, overexpressed, purified, and biophysically characterized two proteins encoded in the KVP40 genome, namely, gp5 and ORF334. Homology-based comparison between KVP40 and phage T4, was used to estimate the two KVP40 proteins functions. KVP40 gp5 shared significant homology with T4 gp5 in the N- and C-terminal domains, but lacked the internal lysozyme domain. Like T4 gp5, KVP40 gp5 was found to form a homotrimer in solution. In contrast, KVP40 ORF334 shared no significant homology with any known proteins from T4-related phages. KVP40 ORF334 was found to form a heterohexamer with KVP40 gp5 in solution in a fashion nearly identical to the interaction between the T4 gp5 and gp27 proteins. Electron microscope image analysis of the KVP40 gp5-ORF334 complex indicated that it had a very similar size to the T4 gp5-gp27 structure. On the basis of biophysical characterization, along with positional genome information, ORF334 was concluded to be the ortholog of T4 gp27, playing the role of a linker between gp5 and the phage baseplate.

3.3 Other baseplate proteins

After the baseplate precursor structure is formed, gp9, which is the socket molecule for the long tail fibers, binds to the upper six corners of the baseplate, and gp12, which constitutes the short tail fibers, binds beneath the baseplate. Gp9 is the first among tail proteins whose crystal structure was determined by X-ray crystallography (Kostychenko et al., 1999). Gp9 is a trimer both in solution and in the baseplate, showing two domains which are connected by a flexible linker. This linker makes it possible for the tail fiber to assume two different orientations. The N-terminal domain of gp9 which binds the tail fibers tightly can point to a direction away from the tail sheath, but at lower pH, they take retracted configuration or bind along the tail sheath. Gp12 is also a trimeric protein. It is a trimer in solution at 37°C, but the trimer reversibly associates into 18-mer (trimer x 6) at 20°C, based on sedimentation equilibrium (Yamazaki & Arisaka, unpublished results). Hexamerization of the trimer is strongly dependent on the salt concentration and in the presence of 1 M KCl, gp12 is trimeric 20°C. In retrospect, the hexamer might have been the "garland" as Kostychenco et al. have called it (Kostychenko et al., 2003), where trimeric gp12 form an outer most ring of the baseplate. Under the baseplate, the N-terminal gp12 tightly binds to the domain IV of gp10 and the C-terminal gp12 binds to the N-terminal domain of the neighboring trimeric gp12. When the baseplate changes its conformation from "hexagon" to "star", the C-terminus of gp12 detaches from the N-terminus of the neighbouring gp12 and springs out downward and tightly binds to the heptose part of LPS.

Following gp9 and gp12 binding to the baseplate, gp48 and gp54 bind to the upper center part of the baseplate in this order to complete the baseplate formation and now ready for tail tube, gp19, polymerization (Berget and Warner, 1975). The stoichiometry of gp48 and gp54 in solution is not known, but six molecules each are present in the baseplate.

3.4 Phage-encoded molecular chaperone, gp57A

Folding of short tail fibers requires the presence of phage-encoded molecular chaperone, gp57A. Gp57A is also required for the folding of proximal and distal half fibers, gp34 and gp37. Analytical ultracentrifugation (AUC), differential scanning microcalorimetry (DSC), and stopped-flow circular dichroism (CD) were used to establish the association scheme of gp57A (Ali et al., 2003). It is an oligomeric α-helix protein with 79 amino acids. Analysis of the sedimentation velocity data by direct boundary modelling with Lamm equation solutions together with a more detailed boundary analysis incorporating association schemes, led us to conclude that at least three oligomeric species of gp57A are in reversible and fast association equilibrium, and that a 3mer-6mer-12mer model describes the data best. On the other hand, DSC revealed a highly reversible two-step transition of dissociation/denaturation, both of which were accompanied by a decrease in CD at 222 nm. The melting curve analysis revealed that it is consistent with a 6mer-3mer-1mer model. The refolding/association kinetics of gp57A, measured by stopped-flow CD, was consistent with the interpretation that the bimolecular reaction from trimer to hexamer is preceded by a fast α-helix formation in the dead-time. Trimer or hexamer is likely the functional oligomeric state of gp57A.

3.5 Tail tube and sheath

The 138 subunits of both tail tube, gp19, and sheath, gp18, assemble on the baseplate to form 23 hexameric rings which are terminated by gp3 and gp15, respectively (Zhao et al., 2003). The number of the rings were determined by 3D-image reconstruction of the tail from electron micrographs (Kostychenko et al., 2005). Previously, the number of rings were reported to be 24 (Amos and Klug, 1975), but that was due to the difficulty of counting rings at the baseplate attachment site with the available resolution at that time. Higher resolution of the recent studies made it clear that the number is 23. X-ray crystal structure of C-terminal deleted mutant gp18M (1-510 a.a.res.) has been solved by Aksyuk et al. (2009) to 3.5 A resolution. The high resolution structure and the fold of gp18 confirmed our previous results that the protease-resistant domain is between residue 82 and 316 and that the C-terminus is close to the N-terminus based on both chemical modification and mutation analysis (Takeda et al., 1990; Arisaka et al. 1990;Takeda et al., 2004).

Tube and sheath make identical helices and each gp19 tube subunit spatially corresponds to gp18 sheath subunit. Each ring is 40.6 A and is rotated by 17.2^{o} in a right-handed manner relative to the previous ring. The sheath surrounds the tail tube and the tube has the same helical parameter as the tail sheath. Tails can be isolated from head^{-} mutant (23^{-}) infected cells. When the isolated tails are exposed to low ionic strength buffer, the tail sheath are readily dissociated from the tube-baseplate complex into monomers. If the monomeric sheath protein is mixed with the tube-baseplate and 0.1 M KCl is added, the monomeric protein self-assembles onto the tube-baseplate to form the extended tail sheath. The sheath assembly is very cooperative; in the reassembled solution, only complete sheath and tube-baseplates are present and incomplete sheath are rarely seen under electron microscopy of negatively stained specimens. Sedimentation velocity experiment confirmed the cooperativity, where only tube-baseplate, 70S, and the complete tail, 120S, are observed (Arisaka et al., 1979). The sheath is not dissociated once the head is attached, but the stabilization mechanism is not known. The whisker, gpwac, is not responsible for the stabilization, because wac^{-} phage has a stable sheath.

4. Neck proteins, gp13 and gp14

Once packaging of DNA into the head of bacteriophage T4 is completed, a neck is formed at the portal vertex of the head to be ready for the tail attachment. The main components of the neck are gp13 and gp14, which consist of 309 and 256 amino acid residues, respectively. In order to elucidate the structure and subunit arrangement in the neck, overexpression systems of gene 13 and gene 14 were constructed and purified to homogeneity (Akhter, T., 2007). Far-UV circular dichroism (CD) spectra of gp13 and gp14 indicated that gp13 is rich in α-helices whereas gp14 is rich in β-sheets. Sedimentation velocity analysis of gp13 and gp14 revealed that both proteins are present as monomers in solution. The frictional ratios (f/f_0) of the two proteins indicated that gp14 has a more elongated shape than gp13. Although isolated gp13 and gp14 do not interact with each other when mixed under physiological conditions, they form a hetero-oligomer complex with the stoichiometry of 10:5 after treatment with ammonium sulfate. Electron microscopy of this complex has shown that it forms a ring-like structure of 15 nm in diameter.

5. Conclusions and perspectives

Investigations on the assembly of bacteriophage have been facilitated by the isolation of conditional lethal mutants such as temperature sensitive and amber mutants in the early 1960s (Epstein et al., 1964). The former mutants can grow at 30°C, but not 42°C. The latter cannot grow on the wild type *E. coli*, but grow on the amber suppressor strains of *E. coli*. The phenotype of amber mutants can be examined by using wild type bacterium as a host and when necessary the mutants can grow on the permissive strains. The assembly pathway of the phage has been investigated by sucrose density gradient, SDG, of the lysate in combination with in vitro complementation (Kikuchi & King, 1975a, b, c; Coombs & Arisaka).

A number of head proteins such as the major capsid protein, gp23, and minor capsid protein, gp24, undergo processing and lose 65 and about 20 residues, respectively, before DNA packaging, but no tail proteins except for gp5, tail lysozyme, are cleaved during assembly.

Assembly of the wedge part is strictly ordered, which means that in the absence of a particular gene product, gene products up to that point form an intermediate and the other gene products stay free in the cytosol. Assembly of other parts of the phage are not so strict , but also ordered to various degrees. Ordered assembly pathway is common to all the viral assembly and necessary presumably to avoid undesired interaction of the incomplete parts for the ultimate complete assembly of virion which is viable. The ordered assembly of the wedge was originally demonstrated by Kikuchi and King in 1975,, and it was later confirmed by in vivo pulse-chase analysis by Ferguson and Coombs (2000) and by recent solution study by Yap et al. (2010). Meanwhile, high resolution structures of many of the gene products have been determined, which was recently reviewed by Petr Leiman et al. (2010).

There are totally 22 genes which are essential for the formation of the tail. Among them, gp57A is a phage-encoded molecular chaperone for long and short tail fibers and gp51 is known to function catalytically. Neither of them are present in the final virion. Amon the 20 gene products which constitutes parts of the virion, complete structure of gp11, gp8, gp5, gp27, gp9, and partial structures gp10, gp6, gp12, gp18 have been determined by X-ray crystallography. Structures of the remaining ten gene products, gp7, gp53, gp25, gp29, gp26, gp28, gp48, gp54, gp19, gp3 and gp15 remain to be determined.

The final product of the assembly, a bacteriophage virion, is a robust and stable structure. On the other hand, some of the intermediate structures during assembly are unstable and easily dissociable. These reversible interactions are facilitated and stabilized by irreversible interactions in the later stages. For example, tail sheath protein interactions involved in forming the extended sheath are relatively weak, but stabilized when the head is attached to the tail.

How the phage-encoded molecular chaperone, gp57A, functions is not known. The hypothesis that the ruler molecule or tape measure protein, gp29, determines the length of the tail by stopping the polymerization of the tail tube protein upon full extension of the originally spherical molecule has not been proved.

Further structure determination of the tail proteins and study on their interactions are necessary for the full understanding of the mechanism of assembly and infection.

6. Acknowledgment

The author would like to give sincere thanks to M. G. Rossmann and V. V. Mesyanzhinov and our collaborators, especially S. Kanamaru, P. Leiman, and V. Kostychenko, for their long-standing collaboration. This study was supported by a Human Frontier Science Program _HFSP_ to Michael G. Rossmann, Vadim V. Mesyanzhinov, and F.A.; Grant-in-Aid for Scientific Research on Priority _B_ from the Ministry of Education, Culture, Sports, Science and Technology; and Grant-in-Aid for Scientific Research _C_ from Japan Society for the Promotion of Science to F. A.

7. References

Abuladze, N.K., Gingery, M., Tsai, J. and Eiserling, F.A. (1994) Tail length determination in bacteriophage T4. *Virology* Vol. 199, pp. 301–310

Ackerman, H.-W. (2009). Phage classification and characterization. *Methods Mol.Bio.,* Vol.510, pp.127-140

Akhter T., Zhao L., Kohda A., Mio K., Kanamaru S., Arisaka F. (2007) The neck of bacteriophage T4 is a ring-like structure formed by a hetero-oligomer of gp13 and gp14 Biochim Biophys Acta. 1774(8):1036-43

Aksyuk A. A., Leiman P. G., Kurochkina L. P., Shneider M. M., Kostyuchenko V.A., Mesyanzhinov V. V., Rossmann M. G. (2009) The tail sheath structure of bacteriophage T4: a molecular machine for infecting bacteria. EMBO J. Vol. 28, pp.821-829.

Ali S.A., Iwabuchi N., Matsui T., Hirota K., Kidokoro S.-I., Arai M., Kuwajima K., Schuck P., and Arisaka F. (2003) Reversible and Fast Association Equilibria of a Molecular Chaperone, gp57A, of Bacteriophage T4, *Biophys. J.* Vol.85, pp.1-13

Amos, L. A. and Klug, A. (1975) Three-dimensional image reconstruction of the contractile tail of the T4 bacteriophage, J. Mol. Biol. Vol.99, pp.51-73

Arisaka F., Takeda S., Funane K., and Ishii, S.-I. (1990) Structural Studies of the Contractile Tail Sheath Protein of Bacteriophage T4 II. Structural Analyses of the Tail Sheath Protein, gp18, by Limited Proteolysis, Immunoblotting and Immuno-electron Microscopy. Biochemistry 29:5057-5062

Arisaka, F., Tschopp, J., van Driel, R., and Engel, J. (1979) Reassembly of the Bacteriophage T4 Tail from the Core-Baseplate and the Monomeric Sheath Protein P18: A Cooperative Association Process, J. Mol. Biol. Vol. 132, pp. 369-386

Bartual, S.G., Otero J.M., Garcia-Doval C., Llamas-Saiz A.L., Kahn R., Fox GC, van Raaij MJ.(2010) Structure of the bacteriophage T4 long tail fiber receptor-binding tip, *Proc Natl Acad Sci U S A.* Vol.107 No.4,pp.20287-92

Berget, P. B., and Warner, H. R. (1975) Identification of P48 and P54 as components of bacteriophage T4 baseplate, *J. Virol.* Vol.16, pp.1669-1677

Coombs, D.H., Arisaka, F. (1994) T4 Tail Morphogenesis, in "Molecular Biology of Bacteriophage T4" (ed. by Jim Karam), pp.259-281 American Society for Microbiology, Washinton, DC

Crowther, R.A., Lenk, E.V., Kikuchi, Y., and King, J. (1977) Molecular reorganization in the hexagon to star transition of the baseplate of bacteriophage T4. *J. Mol. Biol.* Vol. 116, pp.489-523

Epstein, R. H., Bolle, A., Steinberg, C., Kellenberger, E., Boy de la Tour, E., Chevalley, R., Edgar, R., Susman, M., Denhart, C., and Lielausis, I. (1964) Physiological studies of conditional lethal mutants of bacteriophage T4D. Cold Spring Harbor Symp. Quant. Biol. Vol.28, pp.375-392

Ferguson PL, Coombs DH. (2000) Pulse-chase analysis of the in vivo assembly of the bacteriophage T4 tail. J Mol Biol. 297(1):99-117.

Fraenkel-Conrat, H., and Williams, R. C. (1955) Proc Natl Acad Sci U S A. Vol. 41, pp. 690 - 698

Kanamaru, S., Gassner, N. C., Ye, N., Takeda, S., and Arisaka, F. (1999)The C-Terminal Fragment of the Precursor Tail Lysozyme of Bacteriophage T4 Stays as a Structural Component of the Baseplate after Cleavage *J. Bacteriol.* Vol. 181, No. 9, pp.2739-2744

Kanamaru S., Leiman P. G., Kostychenco V. A., Chipman P. R., Mesyanzhinov V. V., Arisaka, F., and Rossmann, M.G. (2002) Structure of the cell-puncturing device of bacteriophage T4. *Nature* Vol. 415, pp. 553-557

Kanamaru, S., Ishiwata, Y., Suzuki, T. Rossmann, M. G., Arisaka, F. (2005) Control of Bacteriophage T4 Tail Lysozyme Activity During the Infection Process *J. Mol. Biol.* Vol. 346, pp.1013–1020

Kao, S. H. and W.H. McClain, W. H. (1980) Baseplate protein of bacteriophage T4 with both structural and lytic functions. *J. Virol.* Vol. 34, pp95-103

Kikuchi, Y. and King, J. (1975) Genetic control of bacteriophage T4 baseplate morphogenesis I. Sequential assembly of the major precursor, in vivo and in vitro. *J. Mol. Biol.* 99: 645-672

Kikuchi, Y. and King, J. (1975) Genetic control of bacteriophage T4 baseplate morphogenesis II. Mutants unable to form the central part of the baseplate. *J. Mol. Biol.* 99:673-694

Kikuchi, Y. and King, J. (1975) Genetic control of bacteriophage T4 baseplate morphogenesis III. *J. Mol. Biol.* 99:695-716

King, J. (1968) Assembly of the tail of bacteriophage T4, J. Mol. Biol. Vol. 32, pp.231-262

Kostyuchenko, V. A., Navruzbekov, G. A., Kurochkina, L. P., Strelkov, S. V., Mesyanzhinov, V. V., and Rossmann, M. G. (1999) The structure of bacteriophage T4 gene product 9: the trigger for tail contraction. *Structure Fold Des.*Vol. 7, pp.1213-1222

Kostychenko V.A., Leiman P.G., Chipman, P.R., Kanamaru, S., van Raaij, M.J., and Arisaka, F., Mesyanzhinov, V.V., Rossmann, M.G. (2003) Three-dimensional structure of bacteriophage T4 baseplate. Nat. Struct. Biol. Vol.10, pp.688-693

Kostyuchenko V.A., Chipman P.R., Leiman P.G., Arisaka F., Mesyanzhinov, V.V. Rossmann M.G. (2005) The tail structure of bacteriophage T4 and its mechanism of contraction. Nat Struct Mol Biol. Vol.12, pp.810-813

Laue, T. M., Shah, B.D., T. M. Ridgeway, T. M., and S. L. Pelletier, S. L., (1992) Computer-aided interpretation of analytical sedimentation data for proteins, p.90–125. *In* S. E. Harding, A. J. Rowe, and J. C. Horton (ed.), *Analytical ultracentrifugation in biochemistry and polymer science.* Royal Society of Chemistry, Cambridge, United Kingdom.

Leiman, P., Fumio Arisaka, Mark J. van Raaij, Victor A. Kostychenko, Anastasia A. Aksyuk, Shuji Kanamaru, Michel G. Rossmann (2010) *Virology J.* Vol. 7, pp.355-382

Mosig, G., Lin, G. W., Franklin, J., and Fan, W. H. Functional relationship and structural determination of two bacteriophageT4 lysozymes: a soluble (gene e) and a baseplate-associated (gene 5) protein. *New Biol.* 1:171-179 (1989)

Nemoto M., Mio K., Kanamaru S., Arisaka F.: ORF334 in Vibrio phage KVP40 plays the role of gp27 in T4 phage to form a hetero-hexameric complex. J. Bacteriol. 190(10): 3606-3612 (2008)

Nakagawa, H., Arisaka, F., and Ishii, S.-I. (1985) Isolation and characterization of the bacteriophage T4 tail-associated lysozyme. *J. Virol.* Vol. 54, pp.460-466

Nieradko, J. and Koszałka, P. (1999) Evidence of interactions between gp27 and gp28 constitutes the central part of bacteriophage T4 baseplate. *Acta Microbiol. Pol.* Vol. 48, pp. 233-242

Plishker, M. F. , Rangwala, S. H., Berget, P. B. (1988) Isolation of bacteriophage T4 baseplate protein P7 and P8 and in vitro formation of the P10/P7/P8 assembly imtermediate. *J. Virol.* Vol. 62, No. 2, pp. 400-406.

Prehm, P., Jann, B., Jann, K., Schmidt, G., and Stirm, S. (1976) On a bacteriophage T3 and T4 receptor region within the cell wall lipopolysacchride of E.coli B. *J. Mol. Biol.* Vol. 101, pp.277-281

Sarkar, S. K., Takeda, Y., Kanamaru, S., Arisaka, F. (2006) Association and dissociation of the cell puncturing complex of bacteriophage T4 is controlled by both pH and temperature *Biochim. Biophys. Acta* Vol.1764, pp.1487–1492

Schuck, P. (1998) Sedimentation analysis of noninteracting and self-associating solutes using numerical solutions to the Lamm equation. *Biophys. J.* Vol. 75, pp.1503-1512

Schuck P. (2000) Size distribution analysis of macromolecules by sedimentation velocity ultracentrifugation and Lamm equation modeling. *Biophys. J.* 78:1606-1619.

Snustad, D. P. (1968) Dominance interactions in Escherichia coli cells mixedly infected with T4D wild-type and amber mutants and their possible implications as to type of gene-product function: catalytic vs. Stoichiometric. *Virology* Vol. 35, pp.550-563

Takeda S., Arisaka F., Ishii S.-I., and Kyogoku Y. (1990) Structural Studies of the Contractile Tail Sheath Protein of Bacteriophage T4 I. A Conformational Change of the Tail Sheath Upon Contraction As Probed by Differential Chemical Modification. Biochemistry 29:5050-5056

Takeda S., Suzuki M., Yamada T., Kageyama M., and Arisaka F. (2004) Mapping of functional sites on the primary structure of the contractile tail sheath protein of bacteriophage T4 by mutation analysis. Biochim. Biophys. Acta 1699(1-2): 163-171

Yap, M.L., Mio, K., Leiman, P.G., Kanamaru, S., and Arisaka, F. (2010a) The Baseplate Wedges of Bacteriophage T4 Spontaneously Assemble into Hubless Baseplate-like Structure In Vitro. *J. Mol. Biol.* 395:349-360

Yap, M. L., Mio, K., Ali, S., Minton, A., Kanamaru, S., Arisaka, F. (2010b) Sequential Assembly of the Wedge of the Baseplate of Phage T4 in the Presence and Absence of gp11 as Monitored by Analytical Ultracentrifugation. *Macromol. Biosci.* Vol. 10, pp. 808-813

Zhao L., Takeda S., Leiman, P. G., Arisaka F. (2000) Stoichiometry and inter-subunit interaction of the wedge initiation complex, gp10-gp11, of bacteriophage T4. *Biochim. Biophys. Acta.* Vol.1479, No.1-2, pp.286-92.

Zhao L., Kanamaru S., Chaidirek C., Arisaka F. (2003) P15 and P3, the Tail Completion Proteins of Bacteriophage T4, Both Form Hexameric Rings, *J. Bacteriol.* Vol. 185, pp. 1693-1700 (2003)

Part 5

Experimental Techniques for the Evaluation of Stoichiometry

12

Methodology for Bioprocess Analysis: Mass Balances, Yields and Stoichiometries

Farges Bérangère, Poughon Laurent,
Pons Agnès and Dussap Claude-Gilles
*Clermont Université, Université Blaise Pascal,
Laboratoire de Génie Chimique et Biochimique,
Clermont-Ferrand
France*

1. Introduction

The stoichiometry of a chemical reaction provides basic information about the nature and the quantities of chemical species consumed and produced. It also intrinsically contains all the information on transformation yields. Such information is useful and necessary for the design of any biotechnological process. In the case of microbiological reactions that support microbial growth, this information deals with the carbon and energy sources consumed, the terminal electron acceptor utilized, other metabolic products formed, as well as the quantity of the biomass produced.

In the first part, general mass balances principles/methodology for the stoichiometric analysis of a bioprocess will be presented. These methods will lead to stoichiometric coefficients estimation including statistical analysis and data reconciliation in case of redundant information. Redundant information means more information than the minimum required to calculate all the conversion yields with a suitable approach of mass balances; this concept of minimum information required is presented (degree of freedom or number of unknowns of the system); conversely over-determined systems, in the case of experimental data in excess, are associated to a statistical treatment.

In the second part, the previous stoichiometry principles will be applied to two practical examples. The first examined case is the continuous anaerobic cultures of *Fibrobacter succinogenes*. This strictly anaerobic bacterium was grown in continuous culture in a bioreactor at different dilution rates (0.02 to 0.092 h^{-1}) on a fully synthetic culture medium with glucose as carbon source. Robustness of the experimental information is checked by C and N balances estimations. A detailed overall stoichiometry analysis of the process for each dilution rate examined, including all substrates and products of the culture, is proposed. The mass balances involved in stoichiometric equations were solved using data reconciliation and linear algebra methods in order to take into account errors measurements.

In the last part, a second practical case,i.e. batch aerobic cultures of *Saccharomyces cerevisiae*, is presented. In this example, the bioprocess is analysed using different methodologies: (i) a simple mass balance with a minimal set of experimental data, (ii) a mass balance with a large set of experimental data including error measurement and (iii) a mass balance with experimental data obtained with 3 repetitions of the batch culture.

2. Main principles and methods of biochemistry stoichiometry

The quantitative description of a microbial growth and product formation has maturated considerably during the past few decades due on one part to major improvements in the controlled technical equipments and on the other part to important theoretical progress thanks to the application of elemental mass balancing methods.

The mass balance of a fermentation has become more and more recognized as a valuable tool for analytical data validation, for detection of measurement errors and/or unnoticed products (Wang and Stephanopoulos, 1983) for estimation of variables for which no direct analytical methods are available (Humphrey, 1974), and for improving the accuracy and reliability of fermentation parameter estimation (Solomon *et al.*, 1982, 1984). The mass balancing theory principles were developed in the late seventies by Minkevich, Erickson, Roels and others (Minkevich and Eroshin, 1973; Erickson *et al.*, 1978; Minkevich, 1983; Roels, 1980, 1983). The theory uses the formalism of linear algebra to express the relationships between measurable (macroscopic) flows. Practical applications are mostly in the field of numerical procedures to solve a system for unknown flows or to calculate maximum likelihood estimators in case of over-determined systems. Thus, it is now recognized that biological reactions stoichiometry is mandatory for analysing biological processes.

2.1 Mass-balance equations

The universal principle (Lavoisier principle) that matter cannot be created or destroyed (unless there is a nuclear reaction) holds in biochemical systems. In any closed system the total mass of every element, C, N, O, H, P, etc, is constant over time.

Mass balance of a compound

As a first step in analyzing a biochemical reaction system, the system, its boundary and the surroundings must be defined. A physical entity, such as a cell or a bioreactor, is often defined as a system, and material and energy balance is performed on it. In other cases the balance is done on a set of reactions that is a representative subset of the reaction network in the cell. Material balance can be performed on either a compound (a chemical specie) or an element (Nielsen *et al*, 2003). For a chemical species i, the material balance in a system can be written as:

Accumulation of i = rate of inputs of i - rate of outputs of i + net rate of production/consumption of i from all reaction.

or

$$\frac{d(i)}{dt} = E_{(i)} - S_{(i)} + \sum_{k=1}^{n} R_{k(i)} \tag{1}$$

with $R_{k(i)}$ being the rate of consumption/production of i in the kth reaction.

Elemental Mass balance

Typically, chemical reactions are written as a single or a system of stoichiometric equations into which elements should be conserved. For a given element, such as C, it can shift from one compound to another due to chemical reaction, but the total amount is conserved. For the system, it is written:

rate of accumulation of elements = rate of input of element - rate of output of element

or

$$\frac{d(element)}{dt} = E_{(element)} - S_{(element)} \quad (2)$$

As a consequence, at steady state, the net rate of accumulation being zero, the net production/consumption of all elements is zero in the system. Moreover, for each reaction, the net balance for all elements must also be equal to 0. This can be written for the different elements as a linear system of equations, a special set of equation being representative of a particular stoichiometric equation:

$$\sum_{i,1}^{n} \alpha_{k,i} [C]_i = 0 \quad (3)$$

$$\sum_{i,1}^{n} \alpha_{k,i} [H]_i = 0$$

where $\alpha_{k,i}$ is the relational coefficient of compound *i* in the reaction k and $[X]_i$ the composition in element [X] in the compound *i*.

Usually one reaction is represented by stoichiometric reaction. With respect of the elemental balance the general expression is:

$$\alpha_1 [C_a H_b O_c N_d]_1 + \alpha_2 [C_a H_b O_c N_d]_2 + \ldots. \longrightarrow \alpha_5 [C_a H_b O_c N_d]_5 + \ldots\ldots. \quad (4)$$

In the previous equation, the stoichiometric coefficients (α) have opposite sign for reactants and products. By convention the products are given positive stoichiometric coefficients, while substrates stoichiometric coefficients are negative.

Multiple stoichiometries

When multiple reactions occur in a system, an overall stoichiometric equation can be written as a linear combination of the stoichiometric equations. This is possible if, and only if, the ratios between the rates of all reactions remain at constant values whatever the external conditions. This means that if all the rates remain proportional, the total set of reactions can be replaced by one single stoichiometric equation. This resulting stoichiometric equation is established by summation of the different stoichiometric coefficients of substrates and products with suitable proportionality constants calculated from the ratios between the rates. When dealing with biochemical systems stoichiometric equations are used for describing reactions in biochemical pathways, as well as for depicting complex systems such as the conversion of nutrients into cells or organisms. Considering that biochemical pathways are proceeding at constant ratios between the biochemical rates (due to metabolic regulation and enzymatic control), the formulation of traditional chemical reactions and biochemical reactions are virtually identical.

Conversely, when within a set of reactions the ratio between the reactions rates do not remain constant, the resulting stoichiometry may vary with the external conditions, *i.e.* the substrates/products concentrations, time, development phases...etc.. This leads to a variable stoichiometry, *i.e.* variable conversion yields. An instantaneous stoichiometry may be calculated as previously as a rates-weighted sum of the different stoichiometric equations leading to account for instantaneous conversion yields. But, in any case, the balance equations for the compounds must be written by using the reaction rates of all equations separately. This is easily understandable by considering the previous Equation 1, noticing that the instantaneous stoichiometry and the instantaneous overall reaction rate that are established from the set of elementary equations cannot be used directly without considering a second-order term for accounting of yields variations.

Pseudo- stoichiometry

When using stoichiometric equations for non-chemically defined compounds, the elemental composition of which being non-completely defined, such as macro-compounds (proteins, biomass), transaction will only consider C, H, O, N, and P in most cases. The other elements participate only in a small fraction of all biochemical reactions and only slightly contributeto the biomass. Therefore, stoichiometric equations can be written for reactions that occur inside a biological system, such as a cell whether they are enzyme, catalysed or not; stoichiometric equation are also used for characterising cell growth and compounds production inside a reactor. Whatever the case, the material balance involves input and output flows and the reaction rates in the system. In the case of a pseudo-stoichiometry it must be kept in mind that the elemental composition accuracy of macro-compounds is limited by experimental measurements errors (generally not exceeding 10^{-3} relative error), generating a systematic inaccuracy in balance equations.

2.2 Method for stoichiometric coefficients estimation and statistical analysis

2.2.1 Mathematical description of the equation system

Considering the following stoichiometric equation, involving n compounds and c elements:

$$\alpha_1[CHON]_1 + \alpha_2[CHON]_2 + ... \longrightarrow \alpha_5[CHON]_3 + ... \quad (5)$$

The elemental balances imply a system of c equations (here c = 4: C, H, O and N) and n unknown stoichiometric coefficients α_i:

$$\text{C} \quad \sum_{i=1}^{n} \alpha_i [C]_i = 0$$

$$\text{H} \quad \sum_{i=1}^{n} \alpha_i [H]_i = 0 \quad (6)$$

$$\text{O} \quad \sum_{i=1}^{n} \alpha_i [O]_i = 0$$

$$\text{N} \quad \sum_{i=1}^{n} \alpha_i [N]_i = 0$$

In order to know if the system can be solved by linear algebra, it is necessary to analyse its **degree of freedom d** at first. Normally the previous equations are linearly independent. The kernel matrix dimension is n - c.

In all cases, one unknown coefficient (α) is fixed. This leads to:

$$d = n - c - 1 \tag{7}$$

In order to solve the system, it is necessary to provide d more independent information resulting from experimental yields determination and/or theoretical assumptions. Three cases are thus possible:

1. The minimum of experiments or theoretical independent information for solving the system is available; that is to say that d experiments or theoretical independent information are available; thus, the resolution of the system can be realised "by hand" thanks to a substitution method.
2. More information than d is available; the system must be solved with the use of a reconciliation method as well as the use of statistical results.
3. With not enough information, the system cannot be solved.

2.2.2 Mathematical method for data reconciliation

Let the resulting linear system of constraints be written as follows:

$$S\alpha = K \tag{8}$$

α (n) is the aforementioned column vector of stoichiometric coefficients (n rows, negative for the substrates, positive for the products). **S** (p, n) contains the elemental formula of all compounds (4 rows for 4 elements) and additional constraints (additional rows) such as the stoichiometric coefficient choice, that is fixed to 1, and eventually other constraints equations between the coefficients. Therefore, p is the total number of equations. **K** (p) is the known column vector of resulting constraints, for example 0 for corresponding conservation equations, 1 for the fixed stoichiometric coefficient and 0 for the linear constraints equation between the coefficients (Urrieta-Saltijeral *et al*, 2001).

If a detailed analysis of a process leads to consider a set of n compounds, an overall stoichiometric equation with (n-1) unknown coefficients is established, knowing that one coefficient is arbitrarily fixed to a value of 1. To determine these (n-1) stoichiometric coefficients, experimental data are needed, and it is necessary to keep in mind that calculations must be performed by meeting the constraint of Lavoisier principle of elements conservation.

Let us introduce experimental data in a column vector $\hat{\mathbf{Y}}_{\mathbf{exp}}$ (m) of m mass yields, all calculated with the same compound as reference, glucose for example. Let us consider $\boldsymbol{\alpha}$ (n) the column vector of the stoichiometric coefficients, with the relevant value for the reference compound, again glucose for example, being set to 1. Finally, $\mathbf{Y_r}$ (m) is the column vector of the yields values obtained after data reconciliation. The following matricial expression is written:

$$A\,\alpha = Y_r \tag{9}$$

A (m, n) is the matrix enabling to build the mass yields values knowing the stoichiometric coefficients.

The element conservation balances are written once the elemental formula of all compounds are known. This is a constraint for the identification, as well as the need that one stoichiometric coefficient is fixed to 1.

The complete linear system for the stoichiometric coefficients calculation is obtained by concatenation of the previous expressions, leading to:

$$M\,\alpha = H \tag{10}$$

where **M** is a (m + p, n) matrix composed of matrix **A** and **S**, and **H** is a (m + p) column vector formed by concatenation of $\mathbf{Y_r}$ (m) and **K** (p). Similarly, $\hat{\mathbf{H}}_{\mathbf{exp}}$ (m+p) is the column vector formed by concatenation of $\hat{\mathbf{Y}}_{\mathbf{exp}}$ (m,) and **K** (p). A weighted diagonal matrix **W** (m + p, m +p) is also be filled with the inverse of experimental variances for the n experimental data and with 1 for the constraint relationships. **W** enables to account for the difference in experimental errors of the measurement yields. The system **M α = H** can be solved by direct inversion of the matrix **M**, if matrix rank and (m + p) are equal to α (determined system). In such case:

$$\alpha = M^{-1}\,H \tag{11}$$

In the case of redundant information (more independent rows than columns, *i.e.* (m + p) > α), a data reconciliation method must be used to solve the constrained and over-determined system. We propose to use a Lagrange method for solving this problem of optimisation, with the assumption that errors measurements (*i.e* variances) follow a Gaussian law (Himmelblau, 1970). The method is developed as follows.

The variable to be minimised is the least square estimate (Φ) given by:

$$\Phi = (\hat{H}_{exp}\ \text{-}H)^t\ (W)\ (\hat{H} - H) \tag{12}$$

i.e.

$$\Phi = (\hat{H}_{exp}\ \text{-}M\ \alpha)^t\ (W)\ (\hat{H}_{exp} - M\ \alpha) \tag{13}$$

Φ is a dimensionless number if **W** is used.

In this study the experimental values are known, and both the confidence interval (i_y) and the variance (σ_y) of the model are given:

$$\begin{aligned} y &= \hat{y} \pm i_y \\ \Delta_y &= 2\, i_y \\ \Delta_y &= 2\, t_{1-\alpha/2}\, \sigma_y \\ \sigma_y &= i_y / t_{1-\alpha/2} \end{aligned} \tag{14}$$

If the number of points for the estimation is sufficiently large, $t_{0,975} \approx 2$ ($\alpha = 0.05$), and the interval is a confidence interval of 95%. The weights for all measured yields are given by:

$$W_{yj} = \frac{1}{\sigma_{y_j}^2} = \frac{4}{i_{y_j}^2} \tag{15}$$

Estimation of the vector α components can be directly obtained through matrix calculus from the previous equation. However, a direct inversion does not guarantee that the obtained set of stoichiometric coefficients (vector α) will obey the Lavoisier principle (elements conservation). The originality of the proposed method is to add as constraints the first element conservation equations. The constraints to fulfil are given as previously by:

$$S\alpha = K \tag{16}$$

Calculation of components of vector α is therefore obtained by the classical method of Lagrange multipliers. The Lagrangian function to be minimized is:

$$L = \Phi - \Lambda\,(S\,\alpha - K) \tag{17}$$

where **Λ** is the unknown row vector (p) of the Lagrange multipliers.

The p Lagrange multipliers and the n stoichiometric coefficients are obtained by solving the (p + n) system of equations formed by:

$$\begin{aligned} \frac{\partial L}{\partial \alpha} &= 0 \quad (\alpha \text{ equations}) \\ S\,\alpha &= K \quad (\text{p equations}) \end{aligned} \tag{18}$$

$$\frac{\partial L}{\partial \alpha} = 0$$

is a matrix derivation which leads to the n following equations :

$$\frac{\partial L}{\partial \alpha} = -2\, M^t\, W\, (\hat{H}_{exp} - M\,\alpha) - S^t\, \Lambda^t = 0 \tag{19}$$

This leads to:

$$2\,(M^t\, W\, M)\,\alpha = 2\, M^t\, W\, \hat{H}_{exp} + S^t\, \Lambda^t \tag{20}$$

then:

$$\alpha = (M^t\ W\ M)^{-1}\ M^t\ W\ \hat{H}_{exp} + 1/2\ (M^t\ W\ M)^{-1}\ S^t\ \Lambda^t \quad (21)$$

and:

$$S\ (M^t\ W\ M)^{-1}\ M^t\ W\ \hat{H}_{exp} + 1/2\ S\ (M^t W\ M)^{-1}\ S^t\ \Lambda^t = K \quad (22)$$

considering that:

$$\Lambda^t = 2\ [\ S\ (M^t\ W\ M)^{-1}\ S^t]^{-1}\ [K - S\ (M^t W\ M)^{-1}\ M^t\ W\ \hat{H}_{exp}\ ] \quad (23)$$

if we denote $\psi = M^t\ W\ M$, **α** is given by:

$$\alpha = \psi^{-1}\ M^t\ W\ \hat{H}_{exp} + \psi^{-1}\ S^t\ [S\ \psi^{-1}\ S^t]^{-1}\ [K - S\ \psi^{-1}\ M^t\ W\ \hat{H}_{exp}\ ] \quad (24)$$

Summarizing and combining computed matrices, the calculation leads to:

$$\psi = M^t\ W\ M \quad (25)$$

$$\Omega = M^t\ W\ \hat{H}_{exp} \quad (26)$$

The solution is given by:

$$\alpha = \psi^{-1}\ [\ \Omega + S^t\ (S\ \psi^{-1}\ St)^{-1}\ (K - S\ \psi^{-1}\ \Omega)] \quad (27)$$

The standard deviations of the calculated coefficients are estimated by diagonal elements of matrices of covariances:

$$\mathrm{Covar}\ (\ \hat{\alpha}\ ) = (M^t\ W\ M)^{-1} = \Psi^{-1} \quad (28)$$

(if W is known from variances)

$$\mathrm{Covar}\ (\ \hat{\alpha}\ ) = (M^t\ M)\ \frac{\Phi}{n + p - \alpha} \quad (29)$$

(if W is not known)

Covariance on estimates of the model is:

$$\mathrm{Covar}(\hat{H}_{exp}\ ) = M\ \mathrm{Covar}\ (\hat{\alpha})\ M^t \quad (30)$$

This set matrix equations determines the stoichiometric coefficients (vector α), the covariance vector of the estimated coefficients and the covariance of the model prediction. The constraint of elements conservation is intrinsically fulfilled, which is a prerequisite of any robust modeling including mass balance.

3. First application: Stoichiometric analysis of *Fibrobacter succinogenes* growth

3.1 Introduction

Fibrobacter succinogenes is one of the main fibrolytic bacteria in the bovine rumen (Hungate, 1950). It's a strictly anaerobic bacterium with enzymatic equipment well adapted to the degradation of vegetable fibers and plants, especially when these are highly branches and lignified. The degradation steps lead to the production of cellobiose and glucose that are further metabolized by the bacterium. The fermentative metabolism of this bacterium has been studied and leads to the production of succinate, acetate and formate. *Fibrobacter succinogenes* is also able to store intracellular glycogen, even in cells of young cultures (Gaudet *et al*, 1992) and it can produce and release oligosaccharides (Nouaille *et al*, 2005).

However, there is little information on the global stoichiometric description of this metabolism. Such quantitative information is necessary for further understanding the growth of *Fibrobacter succinogenes,* for example through a global stoichiometric approach prior to metabolic flux modelling.

The aim of this work was to establish the overall stoichiometry of the*Fibrobacter succinogenes* S85 growth, cultivated in a standardized continuous anaerobic culture process on a fully synthetic culture medium with glucose as carbon source for different dilution rates (Guiavarch *et al,* 2010). Linear algebra and data reconciliation methods previously developed were applied to solve the overdetermined system obtained from the large number of collected experimental data.

3.2 Culture conditions

The strain used was *Fibrobacter succinogenes* S85 (ATCC 19169), and was grown anaerobically under 100% CO_2 in a synthetic medium with glucose as carbon source. The reactor was a B.BRAUN culture unit (Biostat ED, B.BRAUN Germany). The working volume was 5 L and the stirring speed 100 rpm. Temperature was controlled at 39°C and the pH was maintained at 6.3 by automatic addition of Na_2CO_3 (70 g.L^{-1}). The culture vessel was fed with fresh medium completed with various glucose concentrations (from 8.2 to 19.1 g.L^{-1}) at three volumetric flow rates (99, 255 and 464 mL.h^{-1}) corresponding to three dilution rates (D = 0.02, 0.051 and 0.092 h^{-1}). Culture vessel and all tanks were interconnected by a gas system and the pressure was maintained at 0.2 bars above atmospheric pressure. The whole gas system was continuously flushed with 5 sccm of sterile oxygen-free CO_2 during the culture to preserve anaerobic conditions. This flow rate was controlled using a mass flow controller (0-5 sccm, Tylan), while the gas flow at the exit of the reactor was measured with a mass flow meter (0-20 sccm, Brooks).

Samples were taken at regular time intervals during the experiment. Microscopic observations showed that the culture was always axenic. For each sample, the absorbance was measured at 600 nm. HPLC apparatus was used to determine glucose and organic acids concentrations (Agilent 1100 series fitted with two Phenomenex Rezex ROA columns, 7.8 mm diameter and 300 mm length).

Culture supernatants were obtained after centrifugation of an aliquot (10 000*g*, 5 min), and used to perform the colorimetric assays of ammonium ions, proteins and total carbohydrates. Soluble carbohydrates production was calculated by difference between total carbohydrates and glucose concentrations.

The pellets resulting from centrifugation step were dried in an oven at 100°C for 24 h to obtain biomass dry weight. A typical correlation OD-cell dry weight was established from data collected during the exponential growth phase of a batch experiment carried out in the same culture conditions as:

$$\text{cell dry weight} = 0.482\ (\pm\ 0.034)\ OD_{600\ nm} \qquad (31)$$

where the cell dry weight is expressed in $g.L^{-1}$ (correlation coefficient 0.989).

At steady-state, one sample was centrifuged (10 000*g*, 15 min, 5°C), washed with 0.9% NaCl and dried under vacuum at 65°C (48 h) to determine an average biomass formula (CHONSP) by elemental analysis.

Gas at the exit of the bubble column was analyzed by gas chromatography (Hewlett Packard 5890 series II, fitted with a Thermal Conductivity Detector). Two 1.5 m length, 1/8" diameter stainless steel columns (Porapak Q and 5 Å molecular sieves) connected with a 6-port commutation valve were used.

3.3 Experimental data: Biomass formulae and element recoveries

The average molar biomass formulae established after elemental analysis during steady-state are presented in Table 1.

Dilution rate D	Average biomass formula				
(h^{-1})	C	H	O	N	S
0.020	3.688	6.760	2.665	0.247	0.010
0.051	3.656	6.821	2.791	0.255	0.009
0.092	3.799	6.981	2.545	0.380	0.008

Table 1. Average biomass formulae for different dilution rates.

The biomass formula changed weakly with the dilution rate, the most important modification concerning the nitrogen mass fraction that increases with the dilution rate. This modification could be explained by the variation in glycogen to protein ratio that has been evidenced when the growth rate is increased.

To calculate C-recovery, consumptions of sodium carbonate and glucose were both taken into account as carbon sources as well as production of biomass, soluble proteins, succinate, acetate, formate, and soluble carbohydrates. As reported in Table 2, C-balance was between 97 and 101%. Data considered in N-recovery were the nitrogen source consumption (ion ammonium), the nitrogen content in cell dry weight and the soluble proteins measured in the culture supernatant. At low dilution rate (0.02 h^{-1}), N-balance was satisfactory with a value of 98% but at high dilution rates (0.051 and 0.092h^{-1}), N-balances were low with respectively 62 and 82%.

N-recovery was dilution rate dependent and thus growth rate dependent. This dependence has already been shown in *Fibrobacter succinogenes* by Wells and Russell (1996). Growing cultures of *Fibrobacter succinogenes* were reported to assimilate more ammonia than could be accounted for cellular protein, RNA, or DNA, and released large amounts of non ammonia nitrogen that were not identified and quantified.

Dilution rate D (h^{-1})	C recovery (%)	N recovery (%)	Redox potential (mV)	Dissolved CO_2 partial pressure (mbar)
0.02	101	98	-358	1167
0.051	98	62	-347	1191
0.092	97	82	-345	1193

Table 2. C and N element recoveries, redox potential and dissolved CO_2 partial pressure for different dilution rates.

All these results showed a rather good consistency of the experimental results obtained during the course of the culture, indicating that the data reconciliation technique can be valuably applied.

3.4 Stoichiometric equation analysis and data reconciliation

The following detailed stoichiometric equation was proposed to describe the culture (Guiavarch *et al*, 2008). The chemical dissociation imposed by the pH value (6.3) was taken into account in the elementary formulae of the organic acids. Nevertheless, it could be assumed that, in the range of pH supported by this bacterium (from 6.0 to 7.0), the relevant formulae remained rather identical. The stoichiometric equation included 13 compounds and therefore 12 stoichiometric coefficients had to be determined, the coefficient for glucose being, as already pointed out, set to 1:

$$\begin{aligned} C_6H_{12}O_6 + \alpha_1\ (NH_4)_2SO_4 + \alpha_2\ Na_2CO_3 \rightarrow\ & \alpha_3\ C_{3.69}H_{6.76}O_{2.66}N_{0.25}S_{0.010}\ \text{(biomass, see table 1)} \\ & + \alpha_4\ C_4H_{4.1864}O_4Na_{1.8136}\ \text{(sodium succinate)} \\ & + \alpha_5\ C_2H_3O_2Na\ \text{(sodium acetate)} \\ & + \alpha_6\ CHO_2Na\ \text{(sodium formate)} \\ & + \alpha_7\ C_6H_{10}O_5\ \text{(carbohydrates)} \\ & + \alpha_8\ C_{4.43}H_{7.09}O_{1.29}N_{1.27}S_{0.042}\ \text{(proteins)} \\ & + \alpha_9\ H_2O + \alpha_{10}\ NaHCO_3 \\ & + \alpha_{11}\ CO_2 + \alpha_{12}\ Na_2SO_4 \end{aligned} \tag{32}$$

At least 12 theoretical and/or experimental data were necessary. On-line and off-line parameters measured during the culture provided nine experimental mass yields ($\hat{Y}_{exp}$) related to ammonium sulfate, sodium carbonate, biomass, succinate, acetate, formate, carbohydrates, carbon dioxide and protein, each value being weighted by a standard deviation associated to the measured value (Table 3). For these data, a A (9, 13) matrix and $\hat{Y}_{exp}$ (9) column vector could be built with molar mass of compounds and nine experimental mass yields. Elemental balances on C, H, O, N, S and Na provided 6 linear equations of constraints. Coefficient of glucose was here again fixed to 1, allowing to build a S (7, 13) matrix filled with chemical formulae of compounds and coefficient of glucose, and a K (7) column vector filled with 0 for conservation equations and 1 for fixed stoichiometric coefficient.

The resulting system of 16 linear equations was made of 9 relationships obtained from experimental measurements and 7 constraints relationships resulting from elemental balances (C, H, O, N, S, Na) and glucose coefficient fixed to 1. It was over-determined since there were only 12 unknown coefficients to calculate. The advantage of data reconciliation was to allow the use of all available information to reduce inaccurate data due to experimental errors. Reconciled molar yields (Y_r) were thus estimated from the calculated stoichiometric coefficients.

At first , this linear system composed of 9 weighted relations from experimental measurements and 7 constraints from elemental balances was used to reconcile molar yields obtained at three different dilution rates (Table 3).

Dilution rate D (h^{-1})	Substrat and Product	$\hat{Y}_{exp}$ mass	Y_{exp} molar	Standard deviation of $Y_{exp\ molar}$	Y_r	Standard deviation of Y_r	Confidence interval after data reconciliation	Y_r/Y_{exp}
0.02	$(NH_4)_2SO_4$	-0.044	-0.060	0.008	-0.071	0.004	0.008	1.19
	Na_2CO_3	-0.603	-1.024	0.038	-1.025	0.019	0.038	1.00
	Biomass	0.207	0.387	0.047	0.343	0.024	0.048	0.89
	Succinate	0.553	0.630	0.030	0.630	0.015	0.030	1.00
	Acetate	0.147	0.322	0.028	0.322	0.014	0.028	1.00
	Formate	0.004	0.108	0.012	0.108	0.006	0.012	1.00
	Carbohydrates	0.237	0.235	0.139	0.260	0.067	0.134	1.11
	CO_2	0.000	0.000	0.939	0.389	0.423	0.846	-
	Proteins	0.026	0.048	0.004	0.047	0.002	0.004	0.97
0.051	$(NH_4)_2SO_4$	-0.140	-0.191	0.017	-0.124	0.009	0.018	0.65
	Na_2CO_3	-0.553	-0.939	0.048	-0.940	0.024	0.048	1.00
	Biomass	0.448	0.814	0.041	0.844	0.020	0.040	1.04
	Succinate	0.502	0.572	0.017	0.569	0.009	0.018	0.99
	Acetate	0.141	0.310	0.021	0.308	0.010	0.020	0.99
	Formate	0.055	0.147	0.014	0.146	0.007	0.014	1.00
	Carbohydrates	0.157	0.173	0.131	0.000	0.063	0.126	-
	CO_2	0.007	0.027	1.297	0.537	0.541	1.082	20.0
	Proteins	0.014	0.025	0.003	0.026	0.001	0.002	1.03
0.092	$(NH_4)_2SO_4$	-0.165	-0.225	0.018	-0.159	0.009	0.018	0.71
	Na_2CO_3	-0.589	-0.999	0.027	-1.000	0.024	0.048	1.00
	Biomass	0.496	0.906	0.038	0.751	0.020	0.040	0.83
	Succinate	0.562	0.641	0.018	0.606	0.009	0.018	0.95
	Acetate	0.168	0.369	0.036	0.340	0.010	0.020	0.92
	Formate	0.058	0.152	0.005	0.149	0.007	0.014	0.98
	Carbohydrates	0.038	0.042	0.347	0.000	0.063	0.126	-
	CO_2	0.055	0.227	1.144	0.670	0.494	0.988	2.95
	Proteins	0.014	0.026	0.005	0.025	0.003	0.006	0.98

Table 3. Experimental mass yields values ($\hat{Y}_{exp\ mass}$) (g substrate or product. (g glucose)$^{-1}$) and comparative values of experimental ($Y_{exp\ molar}$) and reconciled (Y_r) average molar yields (mol substrate or product. (mol glucose)$^{-1}$) with the associated variances for different dilution rates.

At a dilution rate of $0.02 h^{-1}$, reconciled molar yields of acid production and sodium carbonate consumption were equal to experimental yields (Table 3). Biomass and protein yields were slightly decreased which led to an increase of ammonium sulfate yield from -0.060 (σ = 0.008) to -0.071 (σ = 0.004). These variations were of the same order of magnitude than the standard deviation. There was also a slight increase in soluble carbohydrates yield from 0.234 (σ = 0.139) to 0.260 (σ = 0.067) at this dilution rate ($0.02 h^{-1}$) although the standard deviation associated to this value was high. So, this linear system was sufficient to obtain satisfactory results at a dilution rate of $0.02 h^{-1}$.

At the other dilution rates of 0.051 and $0.092 h^{-1}$, this linear system did not give satisfactory results for the soluble carbohydrates yield since a negative value was calculated. This result would lead to consider that, under these conditions, soluble carbohydrates were a substrate. This idea could not be considered as realistic since glucose was the sole carbon source in the fresh medium. It was thus necessary to modify the linear system by adding a new constraint on soluble carbohydrates for dilution rates of 0.051 and $0.092 h^{-1}$. This supplementary constraint was to fix the coefficient of soluble carbohydrates to zero.

The new system also resulted in a new over-determined linear system of equations, then made of 8 relationships from experimental measurements, 6 constrained equations from elemental balances (C, H, O, N, S, Na) and 2 reference coefficients (glucose set to 1 and carbohydrate set to 0). $\mathbf{A}(8, 13)$ was the matrix of known constant coefficients and $\hat{\mathbf{Y}}_{exp}(8)$ was the column vector of experimental yields. These data allowed to build a matrix $\mathbf{S}(8, 13)$ filled with chemical formulae of compounds, and a $\mathbf{K}(8)$ column vector.

3.5 Discussion

The average reconciled yields and the relevant variances were calculated from this second linear system using data reconciliation. Experimental and reconciled values were compared in Table 3.

This modified linear system gave rather satisfactory results for dilution rates of 0.051 and $0.092 h^{-1}$ with very close experimental and identified yield values. Particularly Y_r/Y_{exp} ratios were often close to 1 except for carbohydrates that had been set to zero by the supplementary constraint. The same major reconciliations were observed on carbon dioxide and ammonium sulfate yields. The discrepancy between Y_r and Y_{exp} on ammonium sulfate was explained by N-balances that were not satisfactorily assessed at these dilution rates. Y_r took into account only ammonium sulfate used for cellular growth and protein production. During continuous culture, no significant carbon dioxide gas production or consumption had been measured and there was an important standard deviation on these measurements. Carbon dioxide gas production or consumption was calculated by difference between inlet and outlet gas. The whole gas system was flushed with a regular gas flow of 5 sccm of carbon dioxide minimum to preserve correct anaerobic conditions during the continuous culture. However, effluent and medium tank volumes were about 10 times higher than the reactor volume and were not regulated in temperature. Therefore, carbon dioxide solubility was permanently modified by ambient temperature variations that consequently led to unreliable carbon dioxide flow rate at the exit of the culture vessel. As carbon dioxide yield, carbohydrates yield was obtained indirectly by difference between total carbohydrates and glucose concentrations.

These results showed that the stoichiometric equation was dilution rate dependent. When the dilution rate increased from 0.020 to 0.092h^{-1}, biomass and ammonium sulfate yields significantly increased as well. The biomass yield was improved from 0.343 (σ = 0.024) to 0.751 (σ = 0.020) mol biomass (mol glucose)$^{-1}$ (from 0.183 to 0.412 g biomass (g glucose)$^{-1}$). An important result was to notice that no significant variations were observed on succinate, acetate, formate and sodium carbonate yields. In the range of the studied dilution rates, the rates of succinate, acetate, and formate production were proportional to the rate of glucose consumed into the system. This tended to demonstrate that the metabolism of *Fibrobacter succinogenes* was not limited by the production of these acids which were directly linked to energy metabolism.

These results showed that assays used to track products of fermentation, consumption of nitrogen and carbon source were efficient as well as analysis of the biomass. This information was reliable to establish a stoichiometric equation for each dilution rate. It should also be pointed out that soluble carbohydrates production should be measured using a more specific technique. This information must be accurately available to go further in the analysis of *Fibrobacter succinogenes* growth by the use of a metabolic flux model.

4. Application 2: Stoichiometry for an aerated batch culture of *Saccharomyces cerevisiae*

In this second example of application, stoichiometric equations were established using experimental data obtained for the growth of a strain of *Saccharomyces cerevisiae* in an aerated and controlled bioreactor. The method of data reconciliation to establish the stoichiometry is applied here considering 3 approaches for exploiting the experimental results:

1. analysis of a single batch experiment with the minimal experimental data required for the stoichiometry (i.e. simple mass balance approach)
2. analysis of a single batch experiment and use of all experimental data for establishing the stoichiometry, including the experimental uncertainty (i.e. variance) estimation of the experimental results.
3. analysis of several batch experiments (repeatability of experiments) for establishing the stoichiometry, including the statistical analysis of the repetition.

4.1 Batch culture of *Saccharomyces cerevisiae*

4.1.1 Culture conditions, monitoring and analysis

A strain of *Saccharomyces cerevisiae* ATCC 7754 is grown in a controlled 6 liters bioreactor (Biostat A. B-Braun, Germany). *Sc. cerevisiae* is a facultative anaerobic microorganism and can metabolise glucose into ethanol (fermentative metabolism) or/and into CO_2 (oxidative metabolism). It is also a glucose sensitive microorganism, as for glucose concentration above 0.1 g.L^{-1}, the "Crabtree effect" can be observed. The Crabtree effect reflects the respiratory chain saturation, which is the main path for regenerating reduced co-factors, and thus even in an aerated system the alternate route to ethanol is used to regenerating the co-factors.

The bioreactor is operated during 8 hours in liquid batch conditions (4.4 L liquid volume), air flow rate (1.5 NL.min^{-1}) and perfectly mixed (6 blades stirrer at 500rpm). The dissolved oxygen is monitored (Ingold probe 34-100-3003), and temperature and pH are controlled (respectively at 30°C and pH 5). Bioreactor data (pH, PO2, temperature, stirring rate) are acquired by the digital control unit of the reactor (Micro DCU 300 – B.BRAUN, Germany) as well as the online analysis of the gas output O_2 and CO_2 molar fractions ($y_{O_2}^{out}$ $y_{CO_2}^{out}$) which are measured by an Oxymat 5E (Siemens) and an infrared CO_2 analyser (Schlumberger), respectively.

The growth medium is taken from Kristiansen (1994) (glucose 50 g.L^{-1}, yeast extract 6 g.L^{-1}, KH_2PO_4 5 g.L^{-1}, $(NH_4)_2SO^4$ 2 g.L^{-1}). Organic acids and ethanol products are measured by HPLC (ionic exclusion column Shodex SH1011, 300 x 7.8 mm). Glucose is measured by the 3,5 dinitrosalicylic acid (DNS) method of Summer and Howell (1935). Amino Acids concentrations (yeast extract content) are measured as a leucine equivalent by a colorimetric method after reaction with ninhydrin (Ruhemann's purple read at 570 nm). Ammonium ions (NH_4^+) are measured by the colorimetric method of Patton and Crouch (1977). The biomass growth is followed by optical density at 550 nm and dry mass measurements.

4.1.2 Analysis of a batch culture: Results and theoretical stoichiometry

The main substrates and products identified and expected during the growth of *Sc. cerevisiae* are reported in table 4. It can be noticed that the previously detailed analyses allows quantifying all these compounds during the batch culture. The culture is performed during 8 hours with an initial glucose concentration of about 50 g.L^{-1}, which leads to a growth with a glucose saturated metabolism of *Sc. cerevisiae* (Crabtree effect), *i.e.* a mixed oxidative/fermentative metabolism with ethanol production. It is also considered that the produced metabolites are primary metabolites, which in turns means that all metabolic rates, including biomass synthesis and metabolites production, remain proportional. This justifies that a single stoichiometry approach is applied.

Theoretically, the mass balance on the culture can be expressed with the following stoichiometric equation:

$$\alpha_1\, glucose + \alpha_2\, O_2 + \alpha_3\, NH_3 + \alpha_4\, Amino.Acid$$

$$\rightarrow \alpha_5\, biomass + \alpha_6\, CO_2 + \alpha_7\, ethanol + \alpha_8\, glycerol + \alpha_9\, acetoin + \alpha_{10}\, H_2O \qquad (33)$$

Considering the 4 elements (C H O N) balance and that one of the stoichiometric coefficients is arbitrary fixed to 1, the degree of freedom d = n - c - 1 = 10 – 4 - 1 is equal to 5. This means that a minimal set of 5 independent additional information are required to calculate the 10 stoichiometric coefficients. We will obtain these data from the experimental yields calculated from the various experimental data acquired.

All compounds, except water, can be experimentally measured during the culture. An example of the results obtained for the experiment 1 (Exp 1) is reported in table 5 and figure 1. CO_2 production and O_2 consumption have been computed from the integration of the instantaneous CO_2 and O_2 respiration rates (r_{CO2}, r_{O2}) acquired from the online gas balance measurements. The respiratory quotient (RQ = r_{CO2} / r_{O2}) is also computed and its value above 1 is an indicator of the growth fermentative metabolism.

Compound	Formula (CHON)	Molar mass (g.mol-1)	% Carbon content	% N content
Biomasse	$C_6H_{1.62}O_{0.52}N_{0.15}P_{0.01}$	24.35	49.28	8.6
Glucose	$C_6H_{12}O_6$	180	40	0
AA	$CH_{2.24}O_{0.48}N_{0.24}$	25.28	47.47	13.3
N-NH3	N	14	0	100
Ethanol	C_2H_6O	46	52.17	0
Glycerol	$C_3H_8O_3$	92	39.13	0
Acetoine	$C_4H_8O_2$	88	54.55	0
CO2	CO_2	44	27.27	0
O2	O_2	32	0	0

Table 4. Compounds involved in the batch culture of *Sc. cerevisiae* and their characteristics. The biomass composition was obtained from elemental analysis of dry sample. The amino acids composition was obtained from average content of amino acids in yeast extract.

Time (h)	Biomass (g.L-1)	Glucose (g.L-1)	Amino. Ac.(g.L-1)	$N\text{-}NH_3$ (g.L-1)	Ethanol (g.L-1)	Glycerol (g.L-1)	Acetoin (g.L-1)	CO_2 (g.L-1)	O_2 (g.L-1)	RQ
0.1	0.82	42.88	1.808	0.4226	0.854	0	0.16	0.294	0.049	-
1.1	0.847	42.59	1.936	0.426	0.869	0.045	0.167	0.908	0.118	5.4
2.02	1.033	43.90	1.816	0.4111	1.352	0.06	0.224	2.011	0.212	7.1
3.01	1.486	41.71	1.599	0.394	1.886	0.088	0.242	2.855	0.267	10.2
3.5	1.925	37.65	1.513	0.3931	2.37	0.097	0.269	3.930	0.330	11.7
4	2.235	37.21	1.332	0.3652	3.498	0.115	0.367	5.207	0.404	12.7
4.5	2.61	34.12	1.264	0.3462	2.92	0.11	0.303	6.748	0.498	12.4
5	3.13	31.91	1.095	0.3102	5.015	0.204	0.41	8.588	0.617	11.5
5.51	3.875	27.78	0.544	0.2571	7.46	0.288	0.467	10.766	0.758	11.1
6	4.425	25.93	0.508	0.2129	7.814	0.305	0.426	13.361	0.916	11.4
6.5	5.515	18.90	0.541	0.1363	10.91	0.41	0.491	16.395	1.091	12.2
7.01	6.205	12.85	0.3131	0.0607	11.79	0.51	0.3	0.294	0.049	12.8

Table 5. Results obtained for the growth of *Sc. cerevisiae* - Experiment 1.

A first treatment of the results obtained for the batch culture consists in the calculation of the experimental yields. Considering all products as primary metabolites, the ratios between all production or consumption rates are constant (*i.e* constant yields). Consequently the yield between a compound A and a compound B ($Y_{A/B}$) is calculated by a linear regression (figure 2) using the concentrations obtained in batch:

$$A(t)= \hat{Y}_{A/B}\, B(t) + cst\,,$$

$$A(t)= \hat{Y}_{A/B}\, B(t), \text{ (when initial values are 0: } A(0)=B(0)=0). \qquad (34)$$

The regression line slope is the yield, and calculation of the estimation variance gives the standard deviation. A complete statistical analysis leads to examine the reliability of the linearity assumption between the concentrations of A and B (constant yield and stoichiometry).

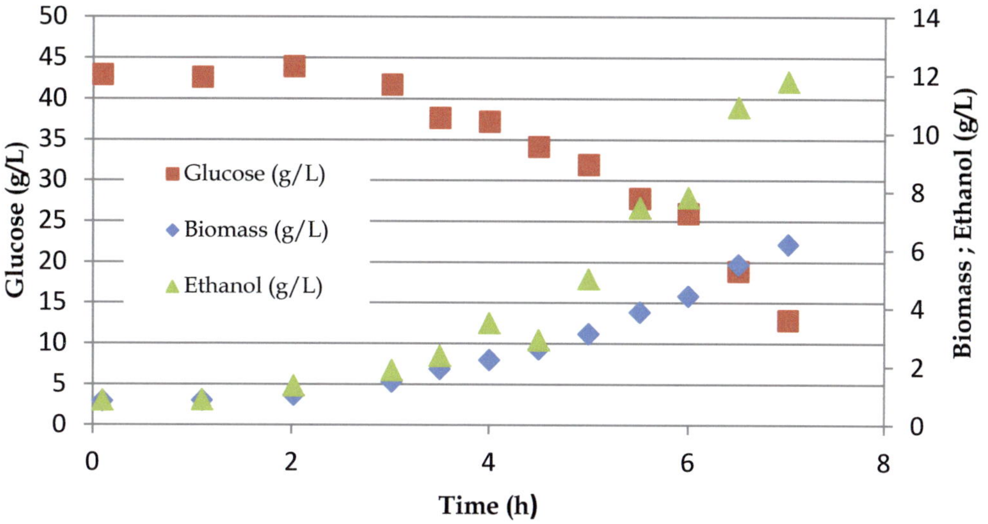

Fig. 1. Glucose consumption, biomass and ethanol production measured for the growth of *Sc. cerevisiae* - Experiment 1.

Some yields calculated for the experiment 1 are reported in table 6 with their standard deviation and correlation coefficient. It is possible to take the minimum of 5 relations required to solve the stoichiometric equation from these results. Besides, the C and N balance can be evaluated, being 0.91 and 0.78 (using $Y_{X/?}$ yields), respectively. These experimental balances may be an indicator of the success for solving the stoichiometric equation, as the theory implies that balances are equal to 1.

	Mass yield (g.g-1)	Standard deviation	correlation coefficient	
$Y_{x/glu}$	-0.1806	+/- 3.4%	0.988	
$Y_{AA/glu}$	0.0374	+/- 5.8%	0.965	*
$Y_{N\text{-}NH3/glu}$	0.0096	+/- 2.5%	0.993	*
$Y_{eth/glu}$	-0.3798	+/- 5.6%	0.970	
$Y_{gly/glu}$	-0.0156	+/- 5.7%	0.969	
$Y_{acet/glu}$	-0.0076	+/- 34.2%	0.461	
$Y_{CO2/glu}$	-0.5245	+/- 3.4%	0.990	
$Y_{O2/glu}$	-0.0332	+/- 4.2%	0.984	
$Y_{x/AA}$	-3.0418	+/- 8.1%	0.939	
$Y_{x/N\text{-}NH3}$	-14.9807	+/- 4.8%	0.977	
$Y_{x/Eth}$	0.5498	+/- 4.2%	0.981	*
$Y_{x/gly}$	13.6788	+/- 5.1%	0.973	*
$Y_{x/acet}$	9.2216	+/- 11.8%	0.866	*
$Y_{x/CO2}$	0.4193	+/- 4.8%	0.977	*
$Y_{x/O2}$	6.0254	+/- 2.5%	0.994	*

Table 6. Yields calculated for Exp. 1. * means that a linear regression without intercept was used.

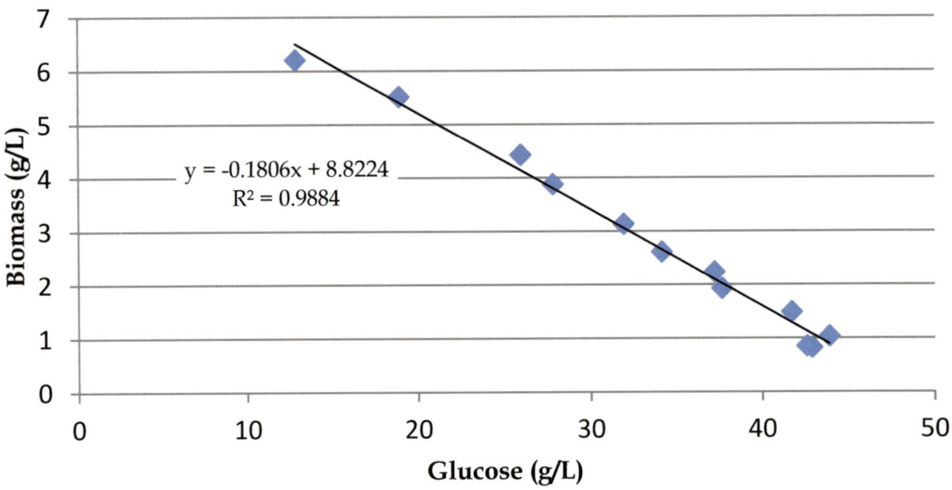

Fig. 2. Graphical representation of the linear regression Biomass(t)= $\hat{Y}_{X/Glucose}$ Glucose(t) + constant.

4.2 Stoichiometry for a minimal set of experimental data (simple elemental balance approach)

If it is chosen to solve the system using the minimal set of 5 experimental data (d=5) and without using reconciliation methods, it is crucial to use strictly independent relations. In the case of the Exp. 1, for instance, it is impossible to select simultaneously the biomass coefficient to 1 and to use the yields $Y_{x/N\text{-}NH3}$ and $Y_{x/AA}$. The 3 information are linked through the N balance (biomass, Amino Acid and NH_3 are the 3 compounds involved in the N-balance) in such a way that only two independent information are really introduced.

The most simple way to solve the stoichiometric equation with the list of yields presented in table 6 is to choose fixing the biomass coefficient $\alpha_5$to 1, considering 4 independent results within the list of the yield $Y_{x/?}$.

Taking for example $Y_{x/Eth}$, we can write :

$$Y_{X/Eth} = \frac{Mass\ Biomass}{Mass\ Ethanol} = \frac{\alpha_5}{\alpha_7} \cdot \frac{Molar\ mass\ biomass}{Molar\ mass\ Ethanol}$$

$$\alpha_7 = \frac{\alpha_5}{Y_{X/Eth}} \cdot \frac{Molar\ mass\ biomass}{Molar\ mass\ Ethanol} = \frac{1}{Y_{X/Eth}} \frac{24.35}{46} = 0.9628 \quad (35)$$

Thus, the ethanol stoichiometric coefficient is experimentally fixed and can be used as a relation to set up one of the system degree of freedom..

In the same way, taking the 3 other yields $Y_{x/AA}$, $Y_{x/gly}$ and $Y_{x/O2}$, the following stoichiometry can be established :

$$0.7492\ glucose + 0.1263\ O_2 + 0.074\ NH_3 + 0.3167\ Amino.Acid \rightarrow 1\ biomass + \\ +1.1305\ CO_2 + 0.9228\ ethanol + 0.0193\ glycerol + 0.1745\ acetoin + 0.7491\ H_2O \quad (36)$$

By taking other experimental data, a different stoichiometric equation is obtained. For example using the experimental yields $Y_{x/CO2}$ instead of $Y_{x/Eth}$ (it can be noticed in table 6 that the two yields were calculated with quite the same accuracy), the stoichiometric equation becomes:

$$0.7492\,glucose + 0.1263\,O_2 + 0.074\,NH_3 + 0.3167\,Amino.Acid \rightarrow 1\,biomass + \\ +1.1305\,CO_2 + 1.1928\,ethanol + 0.0193\,glycerol + 0.0121\,acetoin + 0.4651\,H_2O \quad (37)$$

In this last expression of the stoichiometry, the coefficient for ethanol is 20% higher and the one of acetoin is hundred times lower than in the previous one. This illustrates the influence of the experimental date choice used to establish the stoichiometric equation, as with the minimal set of information necessary to solve the system, all the weight of the constraint for the C H O N conservation remaining on the coefficients that are not given experimentally.

4.3 Stoichiometry using the full set of experimental data

It was previously outlined that even if using only the required experimental data to fulfil the degree of freedom is the easiest methodology, this approach is very sensitive to the experimental data choice and to their accuracy. A way to solve this problem is to use all the available experimental information, with an accuracy evaluation of these data. Such an approach requires the reconciliation method presented in 2.2.2.

With the 8 experimental yields Yx/? of table 6 (and their standard deviation), and by fixing the biomass coefficient $\alpha_5$to 1, a system of 13 equations is built for computing the 10 stoichiometric coefficients of the reaction.

If the variance of $Y_{x/?}$ is computed as:

$$\sigma_Y = (std\ deviation\,\% \,*\, Y_{X/?})^2 \quad (38)$$

the variance of 1/ $Y_{x/Eth}$ can be estimated to be :

$$\sigma_{1/Y} = \frac{1}{(Y_{X/?})^4} . \sigma_Y \quad (39)$$

Thus, assuming a variance of 0 for the fixed reference stoichiometric coefficient (the one of the biomass), the variance of each stoichiometric coefficient used as a new experimental relation (as detail previously for α_7) can be calculated as

$$\sigma_{\alpha ?} = \frac{Molar\ mass\ biomass}{Molar\ mass\ ?} . \sigma_{1/y} \quad (40)$$

The system is computed using the Matlab® (or Octave®) script presented in figure 3.

The resulting stoichiometric equation coefficients are determined, and their confidence interval is calculated (table 7).

The results are consistent with those computed with the previous classical approach. It is noticed that the main uncertainties concern the compounds that have the highest experimental uncertainty (i.e. acetoin and amino acid). This is one of the reconciliation method objectives: to have a high weight on the data that have been obtained with a high accuracy. The standard deviation for the coefficients is lower than the experimental ones but remains in the same order of magnitude.

$$0.7128\,glucose + 0.1267\,O\_2 + 0.0980\,NH\_3 + 0.2166 Amino.Acid \rightarrow 1\,biomass + 1.2019\,CO\_2 + 1.0557\,ethanol + 0.0193\,glycerol + 0.0306\,acetoin + 0.5358\,H\_2\,O$$

Compound	Stoichiometric coefficient	Standard deviation
Biomass	1.0000	0.0000
Glucose	-0.7128	+/- 0.0145 (2.03%)
AA	-0.2166	+/- 0.0172 (7.94%)
N-NH3	-0.0980	+/- 0.0041 (4.18%)
Ethanol	1.0557	+/- 0.0287 (2.72%)
Glycerol	0.0193	+/- 0.0010 (5.18%)
Acetoin	0.0306	+/- 0.0036 (11.76%)
CO2	1.2019	+/- 0.0286 (2.38%)
O2	-0.1267	+/- 0.0032 (2.53%)
H2O	0.5358	+/- 0.0096 (1.79%)

Table 7. Stoichiometric equation with reconciliation with all the experimental data "Yx/?" obtained during a batch culture.

4.4 Stoichiometry using several repetition of the batch growth of *Sc. cerevisiae* in bioreactor

It is generally recommended that an experiment is repeated several times in order to check its reproducibility and thus to confirm the results obtained. There are several ways for using the data obtained from the replication of the experiment:

1. By analyzing the results of each experiment independently and comparing the final results. For this purpose, it is necessary to express the results of each experiment (as presented in table 5) into yields (as presented in table 6) and to compute the resulting stoichiometric equations by either simple mass balance or data reconciliation method. In such an approach the reproducibility is checked by comparing the equations obtained for each experiment.
2. By analyzing the results of each experiment independently, but instead of computing one stoichiometric equation for each experiment, the yields calculated are used as a set of information to compute a single average stoichiometry for the repeated experiments. The reproducibility is tested either by comparing the results with the experimental yields or by analyzing the standard deviation computed for the stoichiometric coefficients.
3. By compiling all the results of the experiments as a single set of data and calculating a single average yield from all experiments. The stoichiometric equation should then be computed using a reconciliation data method and the reproducibility is tested with the standard deviation computed for the stoichiometric coefficients.

4.4.1 Experimental yields of 3 repetition of the batch growth of *Sc. cerevisiae*

The results obtained for 3 repetitions of the batch growth of *Sc. cerevisiae* are reported in table 8. The experimental carbon and nitrogen conservation balances reported in the table are calculated using the Yx/? yields (the balance can be different if calculated using the other yields). In experiment 2, the redundant information gives bad results in terms of conservation of elements. This is due to the large standard deviation calculated for the yields. It can also be observed that within the 3 repetitions there is about 20% of variation in the mass yields calculated.

	Experiment 1 *C balance = 0.92* *N balance = 0.78*			*Experiment 2* *C balance = 0.75* *N balance = 0.71*			*Experiment 3* *C balance = 0.72 *** *N balance = 0.89*		
	Yield ($g.g^{-1}$)	Standard deviation	r^2	Yield ($g.g^{-1}$)	Standard deviation	r^2	Yield ($g.g^{-1}$)	Standard deviation	r^2
$Y_{x/glu}$	**-0.1806**	+/- 3.4%	0.988	**-0.1775**	+/-10.8%	0.887	**-0.1495**	+/-3.9%	0.983
$Y_{AA/glu}$	**0.0374***	+/- 5.8%	0.965	**0.0532 ***	+/-3.8%	0.983	**0.0266 ***	+/-6.1%	0.957
$Y_{N\text{-}NH3/glu}$	**0.0096***	+/- 2.5%	0.993	**0.0104 ***	+/-3.3%	0.987	**0.0079 ***	+/-3.3%	0.987
$Y_{eth/glu}$	**-0.3798**	+/- 5.6%	0.970	**-0.3039**	+/-11.2%	0.878	**-0.3047**	+/-4.5%	0.978
$Y_{gly/glu}$	**-0.0156**	+/- 5.7%	0.969	**-0.0222**	+/-11.3%	0.876	-	-	-
$Y_{acet/glu}$	**-0.0076**	+/- 34.2%	0.461	**-0.0130**	+/-14.7%	0.807	-	-	-
$Y_{CO2/glu}$	**-0.5245**	+/- 3.4%	0.990	**-0.4288**	+/-12.1%	0.873	**-0.4065**	+/-2.8%	0.992
$Y_{O2/glu}$	**-0.0332**	+/- 4.2%	0.984	**-0.0410**	+/-11.3%	0.888	**-0.0388**	+/-4.0%	0.984
$Y_{x/AA}$	**-3.0418**	+/- 8.1%	0.939	**-2.4486**	+/-7.5%	0.942	**-4.0251**	+/-6.4%	0.957
$Y_{x/N\text{-}NH3}$	**-14.9807***	+/- 4.8%	0.977	**-15.0498 ***	+/-7.1%	0.948	**-15.6974***	+/-9.2%	0.916
$Y_{x/Eth}$	**0.5498***	+/- 4.2%	0.981	**0.6869 ***	+/-3.8%	0.983	**0.5732 ***	+/-4.2%	0.979
$Y_{x/gly}$	**13.6788***	+/- 5.1%	0.973	**10.4657 ***	+/-7.8%	0.932	-	-	-
$Y_{x/acet}$	**9.2216***	+/- 11.8%	0.866	**10.6540 ***	+/-6.0%	0.959	-	-	-
$Y_{x/CO2}$	**0.4193***	+/- 4.8%	0.977	**0.5549 ***	+/-7.1%	0.947	**0.4441**	+/-4.6%	0.978
$Y_{x/O2}$	**6.0254***	+/- 2.5%	0.994	**5.4944 ***	+/-5.3%	0.970	**4.7570**	+/-5.7%	0.965

Table 8. Yields calculated for 3 repetitions of the batch growth of *Sc. cerevisiae*. . * means that a linear regression without intercept was used. ** balance is obtained without glycerol and acetoin. r^2 is the correlation coefficient of the linear regression used to calculate the yield.

4.4.2 Stoichiometric equation and comparison with experiments

With the 22 experimental yields Yx/? of table 8 (and their standard deviation), and by fixing the biomass coefficient $\alpha_5$to 1, a system of 29 equations is built for computing the 10 stoichiometric coefficients of the reaction. The system is highly over determined and information given is redundant. The solution is computed using the same script (figure 3), by changing the file experimental matrix and imposing the element conservation equations.

The stoichiometric equation computed is reported in table 9. The result obtained remains closed to the one obtained in table 7. It can also be observed that the standard deviations of all coefficients are significantly lower than the results presented in the table 8. In fact, repetitions of the experiment coupled with the over-determined system have increased the computation robustness (on a statistical point of view). Obviously, the stoichiometry remains theoretical and is an average of 3 experiments, but it is representative of the batch growth of *Sc. cerevisiae* and it can be also considered as reproducible for any growth of the strain in the same condition.

$$0.6613\ glucose + 0.1322\ O\_2 + 0.0946\ NH\_3 + 0.2310 Amino.Acid \rightarrow 1\ biomass + 1.109\ CO\_2 + 0.9595\ ethanol + 0.0207\ glycerol + 0.0272\ acetoin + 0.5292\ H\_2\ O$$

Compound	Stoichiometric coefficient	Standard deviation	Ratio table 7 / table 9
Biomass	1.0000	0.0000	100%
Glucose	-0.6613	+/- 0.0083 (1.26%)	92.8%
AA	-0.2310	+/- 0.0098 (4.24%)	106.6%
N-NH3	-0.0946	+/- 0.0024 (2.54%)	96.5%
Ethanol	0.9595	+/- 0.0163 (1.70%)	90.9%
Glycerol	0.0207	+/- 0.0009 (4.35%)	107.3%
Acetoin	0.0272	+/- 0.0015 (5.51%)	88.9%
CO2	1.1090	+/- 0.0164 (1.48%)	92.3%
O2	-0.1322	+/- 0.0028 (2.12%)	104.3%
H2O	0.5292	+/- 0.0053 (1.00%)	98.8%

Table 9. Stoichiometric equation with reconciliation with all the experimental data "Yx/?" obtained with the 3 repetitions of the same batch culture.

	Mass yield ($g.g^{-1}$)	*Standard deviation*
$Y_{x/glu}$	-0.2046	-0.55%
$Y_{x/AA}$	-4.1697	-0.23%
$Y_{x/N\text{-}NH3}$	-18.3857	-0.02%
$Y_{x/Eth}$	0.5517	1.56%
$Y_{x/gly}$	12.7862	0.00%
$Y_{x/acet}$	10.1730	0.00%
$Y_{x/CO2}$	0.4990	1.82%
$Y_{x/O2}$	-5.7560	-0.04%

Table 10. Theoretical yields computed with reconciliation with all the experimental data "Yx/?" obtained with the 3 repetitions of the same batch culture.

One of the main feature of these computation remains in the fact that the computed coefficients satisfy elements conservation; this provides the robustness of the stoichiometric model; on the other hand, it must also be kept in mind that the model, even robust, intrinsically assumes *(i)* that all substrates and products have really been identified and taken in the stoichiometry and *(ii)* that all yields remain constant during the observation time (culture duration) taken for estimation of experimental yields. This is certainly the main difficulty here, both for the estimation of experimental yields from linear regression and for imposing a single stoichiometry model that summarizes three different experiments obtained in batch cultures. Any experimental deviation from the assumption of constant yields creates a lack of adequacy of the model that results in an increase of the variance of the model.

Nevertheless, it can be concluded that the results obtained, within their confidence intervals (table 10), fairly represent the experimental data obtained from the 3 different experiments, knowing that it is not clear if a more complex model (with more coefficients to identify) would be justified by the available degree of experimental information.

```
%==========================================================================================
% Programm for Stoichiometry resolution by data reconciliation and statistical approach.
% AUTHOR : L. POUGHON
%==========================================================================================
% [1] ---> Problem definition <-----------------------------------------------------------
clear all; % clear all previous variables of the workspace
%.....Compounds list. The compounds are ordered from 1 to N
name={'Biomass','Glucose','Amino.Acid.','NH3','Ethanol','Glycerol','Acetoine','CO2','O2','H2O'};
%.....S1 = Compounds composition matrix (CHONSP balance).
S1=[1     6    1     0    2   3   4  1  0 0
           1.62  12   2.24  3    6   8   5  0  0 2
           0.52  6    0.48  0    1   3   2  2  2 1
           0.15  0    0.24  1    0   0   0  0  0 0];
K1=[0 ; 0 ; 0 ; 0];
%....S2 =. Theoreticals relations (typicaly one of the coefficients of the stoichiometry is fixed
S2=[1 0 0 0 0 0 0 0 0 0];
K2=1;
%....A =.Experimentals relations. IF There is No variance then write variance_exp=[]
A =[0      1       0       0       0       0        0        0       0       0
           0       0       1       0       0       0        0        0       0       0
           0       0       0       1       0       0        0        0       0       0
           0       0       0       0       1       0        0        0       0       0
           0       0       0       0       0       1        0        0       0       0
           0       0       0       0       0       0        1        0       0       0
           0       0       0       0       0       0        0        1       0       0
           0       0       0       0       0       0        0        0       1       0];
Y =[-0.7492 ; -0.3167 ;-0.1161 ; 0.9628 ; 0.0193 ; 0.03 ; 1.3199 ; -0.1263];
variance_exp=[  0.0257^2 ; 0.0256^2 ;  0.0056^2 ; 0.0406^2 ; 0.0010^2 ; 0.0036^2 ; 0.0640^2 ;
0.0032^2];
% [2] ---> Solving problem <--------------------------------------------------------------
%.... Be care for errors (matrix must be homogenous in size)
M=[S1 ; S2 ; A]; R=[K1 ; K2 ; Y];
S=[S1 ; S2 ] ;K=[K1 ; K2] ;
%... matrix for weight
if isempty(variance_exp)
   w=eye(size(A));
else
    w=diag(1./[1e-10*ones(size(K,1),1) ; [variance_exp] ] );
end
%.... Solving the problem
if (size(M,2)==size(M,1) )
   %-- the system is determined (no reconciliations)
   coefficients=M\R;
   covar_coeff=zeros(size(coefficients));
   covar_Acc=zeros(size(R));
   w=zeros(size(R)); % for simplifying the result display
elseif (size(M,2)<size(M,1))
   %-- the system is over determined : reconciliation by lagrangian approach
   V=inv([M]' * w * [M] );
   G=[M]' * w* [R];
   H=inv([ S ] * V * [ S ]' );
   coefficients=V * (G + [S]' * H * ( K - S * V * G ) );
   covar_coeff= [ [R-M*coefficients]' * w * [R-M*coefficients] ] * V ./ ( size(M,1)-size(M,2));
   covar_Acc=[M]*covar_coeff * [M]';
else
   %-- the system cannot be solved.
   disp('System under determined : cannot be solved') ;  return
end
% [3] ---> Display Solution of the problem (coefficients and accumulation vector)<---------------
for i=1:size(coefficients,1)
    display=sprintf('%10s\t   :  %10.4f\t   +/-   %10.4f'   ,char(name(i)),   coefficients(i)    ,
sqrt(covar_coeff(i,i))); disp(display);
end
Acc=M*coefficients;
disp(' ') ; disp('Accumulation vector')
for i=1:size(Acc,1)
    display=sprintf('line[%2d] : %7.4f\t +/- %7.4f  (theoretical = %7.4f +/- %7.4f)' ,i, Acc(i) ,
sqrt(covar_Acc(i,i)),R(i),sqrt(1./w(i,i)) ); disp(display);
end
```

Fig. 3. Octave/Matlab script used to compute stoichiometric coefficients with the data reconciliation method.

5. Conclusion

Elements conservation laws are a prerequisite to evaluate a solid mass balance model in fermentation technology. As in Chemistry, the perfect vehicle for accounting for elements conservation is the stoichiometric equation. Application of this representation to biochemical systems (and particularly to microbial growth processes) presents some difficulties. The first one is linked to the fact that macromolecules and biomass constituents have seldom a well-determined elemental composition. This is a source of inaccuracy and variability. However general observation of biomass composition clearly shows that it is seldom highly variable (except in the case a product is accumulated into the cells in high quantities). The second obstacle is related to the fact that a single stoichiometry representation intrinsically assumes that the yields are constant. This is certainly a good assumption for continuous processes where biomass metabolism is confined in a constant environment. This is more inaccurate in the case of batch cultures.

Provided a complete statistical analysis is performed, including the calculation of both the coefficients and the model variances, the single stoichiometry approach can be applied for characterizing bioreactions.

We have presented here a data reconciliation technique coupled with the constraint of elements conservation. The main interest of this approach is that the coefficients are obtained with a flexible method applicable with linear algebra techniques, the result being "stoichiometrically" valid.

This technique has been applied to two cases. In the first case, results on the continuous culture of the rumen anaerobic bacteria *Fibrobacter succinogenes* lead to characterize the culture by a stoichiometric equation, slightly depending on the dilution rate. In the second case, batch experiments for the culture of *Saccharomyces cerevisiae* clearly indicate that a single stoichiometry approach is less accurate than for continuous cultures. Nevertheless, a stoichiometric equation has been obtained and realistic mean square deviations have been calculated for the coefficients. The technique has been applied to lump the experimental information from three independent experiments. This shows that this first-order stoichiometric model, including elements balance conservation, is certainly a valuable characterization of the biomass growth and of primary metabolites production. It must also be kept in mind that more complex models would involve more coefficients finally resulting in inaccurate predictions without creating more robustness.

6. References

Erickson, L.E., Minkevich, I.G. & Eroshin, V.K. (1978) Application of mass and energy balance regularities in fermentation. *Biotechnology and Bioengineering*, Vol.20, No.10, pp. 1595-1621.

Gaudet, G., Forano, E., Dauphin, G. & Delort, A.M. (1992). Futile cycle of glycogen in *Fibrobacter succinogenes* as shown by in situ ^{1}H NMR and ^{13}C NMR investigations. *European Journal of Biochemistry*, Vol.107, pp. 155-162.

Guiavarch, E., Pons, A., Creuly, C. & Dussap, C.G. (2008). Application of a data reconciliation method to the stoichiometric analysis of *Fibrobacter succinogenes* growth. *Applied Biochemistry and Biotechnology*, Vol.151, pp.201-210.

Guiavarch, E., Pons, A., Christophe, C., Creuly, C. & Dussap, C.G. (2010). Analysis of a continuous culture of *Fibrobacter succinogenes* S85 on a standardized glucose medium. *Bioprocess and Biosystems Engineering*, Vol.33, pp.417-425.

Himmelblau, D.M. (1970). *Process analysis by statistical methods*, John Wiley Ed, New-York.

Humphrey, A.E. (1974) Current developments in fermentation. *Chemical Engineering*. Vol.81, No.26, pp. 98-112

Hungate, R.E. (1950). The anaerobic mesophilic cellulolytic bacteria. *Bacteriological Review*, Vol.14, No.1, pp.1-49.

Kristiansen B. (1994). Integrated desugn of a fermentation plant. The production of baker's yeast. VCH (Ed.) Weinheim.

Minkevich, I.G. (1983) Mass-energy balance for microbial product synthesis—biochemical and cultural aspects. *Biotechnology and Bioengineering*, Vol.25, No.5, pp. 1267-1293.

Minkevich, I.G. & Eroshin, V.K., (1973) Folio Microbiol, Vol. 18, pp. 376-385.

Nielsen, J., Villadsen, J. & Liden, G. (2003) Bioreaction Engineering Principles, 2nd Ed, Kluwer, Dordrecht.

Nouaille, R., Matulova, M., Delort, A.M. & Forano, E. (2005). Oligosaccharide synthesis in *Fibrobacter succinogenes* S85 and its modulation by the substrate. *FEBS Journal*, Vol. 272, pp.2416-2427.

Patton, C.J., & Crouch, S.R. (1977). Spectrophotometric and kinetics investigation of the Berthelot reaction for the determination of ammonia: *Analytical Chemistry*, Vol.49, pp. 464-469.

Roels, J.A. (1980) Application of macroscopic principles to microbial metabolism. *Biotechnology and Bioengineering*, Vol. 22, No.12, pp.2457-2514.

Roels, J.A. (1983) Energetics and kinetics in Biotechnology, Elsevier Biomedical Press, 117, Amsterdam

Solomon, B.O., Erickson, L.E., Hess, J.E. & Yang, S.S. (1982) Maximum likelihood estimation of growth yields. *Biotechnology and Bioengineering*, Vol. 24, pp.633-649.

Solomon, B.O., Oner, M.D., Erickson, L.E. & Yang, S.S. (1984) Estimation of parameters where dependent observations are related by equality constraints. *AIChE Journal*, Vol.30, pp. 747-757

Summer, J.B. & Howell, S.F. (1935). A method for determination of saccharase activity. *Journal of Biochemical Chemistry*., Vol.108, pp. 51-54.

Urrieta-Saltijeral, J.M., Dussap, C.G., Pons, A., Creuly, C. & Gros, J.B. (2001). Metabolic flux modeling as a tool to analyse the behavior of a genetically modified strain of *Saccharomyces cerevisiae*. *Engineering and Manufacturing for Biotechnology*, pp.143-156.

Wang, N.S. & Stephanopoulos, G. (1983) Application of macroscopic balances to the identification of gross measurement errors. *Biotechnology and Bioengineering*, Vol.25, pp. 2177-2208.

Wells, J.E. & Russel, J.B. (1996). The effect of growth and starvation on the lysis of the ruminal cellulolytic bacterium *Fibrobacter succinogenes*. *Applied and Environmental Microbiology*, Vol. 62, No.4, pp.1342-1346.

13

Distribution Diagrams and Graphical Methods to Determine or to Use the Stoichiometric Coefficients of Acid-Base and Complexation Reactions

Alberto Rojas-Hernández[1], Norma Rodríguez-Laguna[1], María Teresa Ramírez-Silva[1] and Rosario Moya-Hernández[2]
[1]*Depto. de Química, Área de Química Analítica, Universidad Autónoma Metropolitana-Iztapalapa,*
[2]*Facultad de Estudios Superiores-Cuautitlán, Lab. 10, UIM, Universidad Nacional Autónoma de México, Mexico*

1. Introduction

Graphical methods to study the behaviour of systems showing different chemical equilibrium are known and very used in several fields of Chemistry (particularly in Bioinorganic, Medicinal and Pharmaceutical Chemistry) in order to establish the chemical species that are related with drugs behaviour in different systems. Among these methods, the most commonly used are the distribution diagrams (Högfeldt, 1979), the titration curves (Asuero & Michałowski, 2011) and the molar ratio and continuous variations methods (Hartley et al., 1980).

In the present work we have selected two molecules used extensively like drugs. In order to exemplify some novelties related with distribution diagrams and titration curves for acid-base systems we have selected the case of oxine (HOX, 8-hydroxiquinoline) that has been used as antiseptic and disinfectant. On the other hand, we have selected the complexation interaction between Fe(III) and tenoxicam (Tenox) to show other novelties related with more complicated distribution diagrams and molar ratio and continuous variations methods, because tenoxicam has been extensively used as non-steroidal anti-inflammatory drug that may be complexed with several metal ions. The chemical developed formulae of these compounds are presented in Scheme 1.

2. Distribution diagrams for acid-base and complexation systems

Graphic representations of chemical systems have found wide application because a simple look at them allows for solve specific problems and have a panorama, qualitative and quantitative, for different problems and phenomena. Moreover, some of these representations also permit to graphically solve the stated problem with a predetermined error (Vicente-Pérez, 1985). Distribution diagrams of species are some of the most used graphic representations since the second half of 20th century; nevertheless, there have been some novelties on the field in the last decade (e.g. Moya-Hernández et al., 2002a, 2002b).

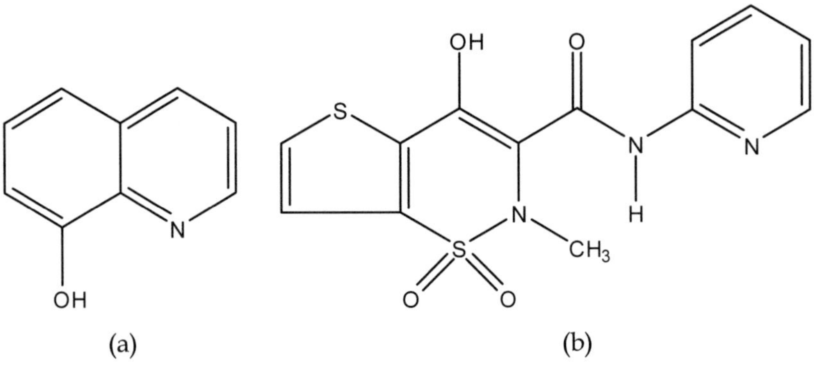

Scheme 1. Developed formulae of a) oxine (HOX) and b) tenoxicam (Tenox).

2.1 Typical representations of distribution diagrams

In this section some typical representations will be quickly reviewed to introduce the newest representations given in section 2.2.

2.1.1 Acid-base systems

In Chemistry the study of polyprotic systems, whose global formation equilibrium are represented in Eq. 1, is of crucial importance, because many substances, drugs among them, follow this Brϕnsted acid-base behaviour.

$$L^{a-} + jH^{+} \rightleftarrows LH_j^{j-a} \text{ with } \beta_j = \frac{[LH_j^{j-a}]}{[L^{a-}][H^{+}]^{j}} \tag{1}$$

The typical way to define the molar fractions to describe the species distribution of the component L in this system with respect to the proton (H^{+}) is given in Eq. 2, as well as its factorization in the substance amount balance equation of this component in the system - using the set of Eq. 1 (Rojas-Hernández, 1995).

$$f_j = \frac{[LH_j^{j-a}]}{[L]_T} = \frac{\beta_j[H^{+}]^{j}}{1+\sum_{j=1}^{n}\beta_j[H^{+}]^{j}} \tag{2}$$

where $[L]_T$ is L total concentration in the system.

An example of distribution diagram is given in Fig. 1a, showing the case of oxine hydrochloride (H_2OXCl, 8-hydroxiquinolinol = HOX).

Fig. 1b represents the function known as Average Proton Number ($\overline{n}$), introduced and developed by Niels and Jannik Bjerrum (Hartley et al., 1980). Eq. 3 shows the definition and factorization of $\overline{n}$ as a function of pH (taking into account the sets of Eq. 1 and 2) for aqueous solutions.

$$\overline{n} = \frac{[H^+]_T - [H^+]}{[L]_T} = \frac{\sum_{j=1}^{n} j\beta_j [H^+]^j}{1 + \sum_{j=1}^{n} \beta_j [H^+]^j} = \sum_{j=1}^{n} jf_j \tag{3}$$

$[H^+]_T$ is the protons total concentration in the system, which requires the balance of proton equation. In aqueous solutions, this equation needs the autoprotolysis constant and special considerations.

The chemical information given in the curves of Fig. 1 is the same, as expected from Eq. 2 and 3. In fact, the Average Proton Number is the set of statistical means of the subjacent distributions resumed by the distribution diagram of Fig. 1, as it will be explained in the section 2.2.

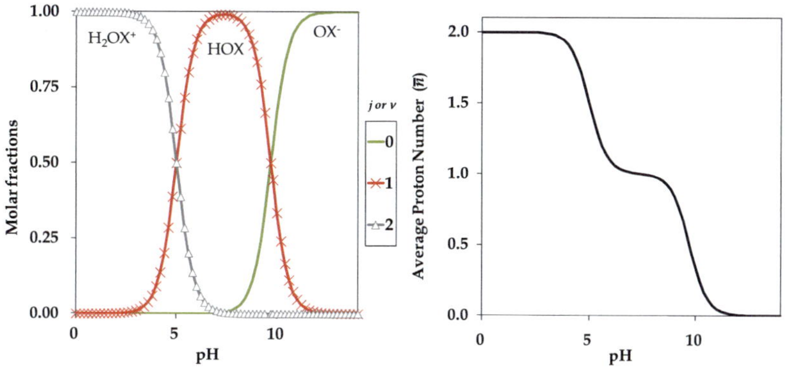

(a) (b)

Fig. 1. Typical graphic representations of the oxine hydrochloride (H_2OXCl) in water as a function of pH. j (or ν) represents the proton stoichiometric coefficient for each species. a) Distribution diagram. b) Average proton number. Data were taken from Ringbom (1963): $pK_{a1} = 5.0$, $pK_{a2} = 9.7$.

2.1.2 Complexation systems

Even though the knowledge of Brϕnsted acid-base behaviour is important, the interaction of substances with metal ions is remarkable as well (e.g., the interaction of drugs with metal ions may potentiate or suppress its pharmacological activity or toxicity).

The formation of several coordination compounds, or complexes, between a metal ion (M) and a ligand (L) can be described by the global formation equilibrium represented in Eq. 4.

$$iM + jL \rightleftarrows M_iL_j \text{ with } \beta_{ij} = \frac{[M_iL_j]}{[M]^i [L]^j} \tag{4}$$

where $i \in \{1, 2, ..., m\}$ and $j \in \{(0, 1, ..., n[i]\}$

In Eq. 4, the charge of the species has been omitted for notation simplicity. When $i = 1$ the complexes are called mononuclear, but when $i \geq 2$ the corresponding complexes are called polynuclear. The formation of polynuclear complexes on a given system is thermodynamically favoured when the total concentration of M ($[M]_T$) is high and placed over the mononuclear wall (Ringbom, 1963).

In complexation chemistry, several distributions have to be considered. In general, it is preferred to study the way the component L is distributing on M species, but studying how the component M is distributing on L species may be interesting as well. In both cases there are two possible descriptions, depending on what is considered between the amount or the concentrations of the species. When polynuclear compexes are formed in the system all the distribution diagrams representing the formation of the species depends on $[M]_T$ and $[L]_T$.

Distributions of L in M

The M substance amount fractions are defined by Eq. 5.

$$^{L/M}f_{10} = \frac{[M]}{[M]_T} = \frac{1}{1+\sum_{i=1}^{m}\left(\sum_{j=0}^{n[i]} i\beta_{ij}[M]^{(i-1)}[L]^j\right)} \quad \text{and} \quad ^{L/M}f_{ij} = \frac{i[M_iL_j]}{[M]_T} = {}^{L/M}f_{10}\left(i\beta_{ij}[M]^{(i-1)}[L]^j\right) \tag{5}$$

where $i \in \{1, 2, ..., m\}$ and $j \in \{0, 1, ..., n[i]\}$

When polynuclear M species are not forming in a given system ($i = 1$), this distribution only depends on $[L]_T$, but when polynuclear species appear, the substance amount fractions depend on $[L]_T$ and $[M]_T$; furthermore in this last case the simple sum of the concentrations of M species (Σ_M) is lower than $[M]_T$, in agreement with Eq. 6.

$$\Sigma_M = \sum_{i=1}^{m}\left(\sum_{j=0}^{n[i]}[M_iL_j]\right) < \sum_{i=1}^{m}\left(\sum_{j=0}^{n[i]} i[M_iL_j]\right) = [M]_T \tag{6}$$

In this particular case, M concentration fractions can be defined by Eq. 7.

$$^{L/M}\varphi_{10} = \frac{[M]}{\Sigma_M} = \frac{1}{1+\sum_{i=1}^{m}\left(\sum_{j=0}^{n[i]} \beta_{ij}[M]^{(i-1)}[L]^j\right)} \quad \text{and} \quad ^{L/M}\varphi_{ij} = \frac{[M_iL_j]}{\Sigma_M} = {}^{L/M}\varphi_{10}\left(\beta_{ij}[M]^{(i-1)}[L]^j\right) \tag{7}$$

where $i \in \{1, 2, ..., m\}$ and $j \in \{0, 1, ..., n[i]\}$

The substance amount and concentration fractions of M species are related by means of Eq. 8.

$$^{L/M}\varphi_{ij} = {}^{L/M}f_{ij}\frac{[M]_T}{\Sigma_M} \tag{8}$$

Distributions of M in L

Following the same approach, several distributions of *L* species may be defined. Then, the L substance amount fractions are defined in Eq. 9, while the L concentration fractions are described in Eq. 10.

$$^{M/L}f_{01} = \frac{[L]}{[L]_T} = \frac{1}{1+\sum_{j=1}^{n}\left(\sum_{i=0}^{m[j]} j\beta_{ij}[M]^i[L]^{(j-1)}\right)}$$
$$\text{and} \quad ^{M/L}f_{ij} = \frac{j[M_iL_j]}{[L]_T} = {}^{M/L}f_{01}(j\beta_{ij}[M]^i[L]^{(j-1)}) \tag{9}$$

where $i \in \{0, 1, ..., m[j]\}$ and $j \in \{1, 2, ..., n\}$

$$^{M/L}\varphi_{01} = \frac{[L]}{[L]_T} = \frac{1}{1+\sum_{j=1}^{n}\left(\sum_{i=0}^{m[j]} j\beta_{ij}[M]^i[L]^{(j-1)}\right)}$$
$$\text{and} \quad ^{M/L}\varphi_{ij} = \frac{j[M_iL_j]}{[L]_T} = {}^{M/L}\varphi_{01}(j\beta_{ij}[M]^i[L]^{(j-1)}) \tag{10}$$

where $i \in \{0, 1, ..., m[j]\}$ and $j \in \{1, 2, ..., n\}$

The substance amount and concentration fractions of *L* species are related by means of Eq. 11.

$$^{M/L}\varphi_{ij} = {}^{M/L}f_{ij}\frac{[L]_T}{\Sigma_L} \tag{11}$$

because the following inequality is always confirmed.

$$\Sigma_L = \sum_{j=1}^{n}\left(\sum_{i=0}^{m[j]}[M_iL_j]\right) < \sum_{j=1}^{n}\left(\sum_{i=0}^{m[j]} j[M_iL_j]\right) = [L]_T \tag{12}$$

Distribution diagrams for the Fe(III)-tenoxicam system in acetone

In order to exemplify the typical distributions diagrams of *M* and *L* species, Fig. 2 is reported for the Fe(III) - tenoxicam (Tenox) system in acetone from previously reported data by Moya-Hernández et al. (2009). The equilibrium constants of this reference have been collected in Table 1.

Species	***i***	***j***	**logβ_{ij}**
Fe_2Tenox	2	1	9.04 ± 0.03
Fe_2Tenox_2	2	2	14.75 ± 0.06
Fe_2Tenox_3	2	3	18.45 ± 0.07

Table 1. Global formation constants of Fe(III)-tenoxicam species in acetone (Moya-Hernández et al., 2009).

The distribution diagrams that represent the substance amount fractions, calculated from global formation constants given in Table 1, have been constructed with the aid of program MEDUSA (Puigdomenech, 2010). The distribution diagrams that represent the concentration fractions have been obtained by means of Excel (*Microsoft®*) worksheets applying Eq. 8 and 11. Some of the typical distribution diagrams are shown in Fig. 2 and 3.

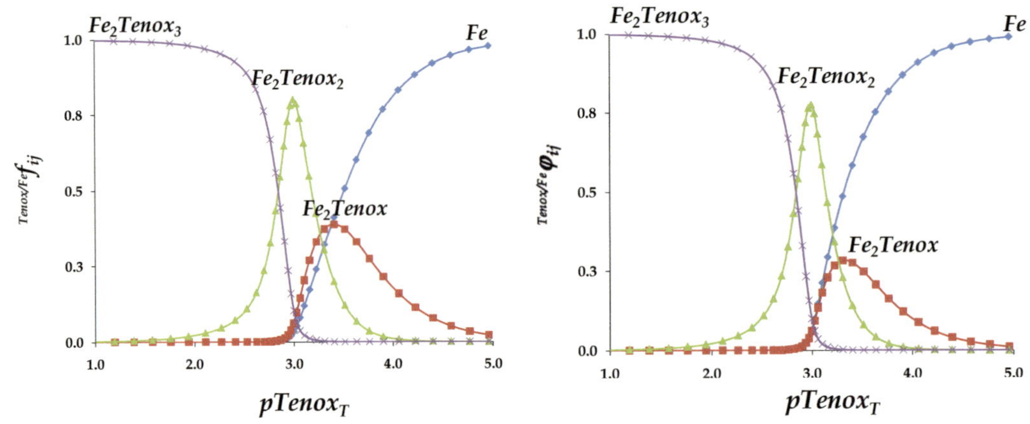

(a) (b)

Fig. 2. Typical graphic representations of the Fe(III)-tenoxicam system in acetone as a function of p$Tenox_T$. $[Fe(III)]_T = 1\times10^{-3}$ M and p$Tenox_T$ = -log$[Tenox]_T$. a) Distribution diagram of substance amount of Fe(III) species taking into account the quantity of Fe(III) in each species. b) Distribution diagram of concentration of Fe(III) species taking in account which Fe(III) species is more concentrated in the system.

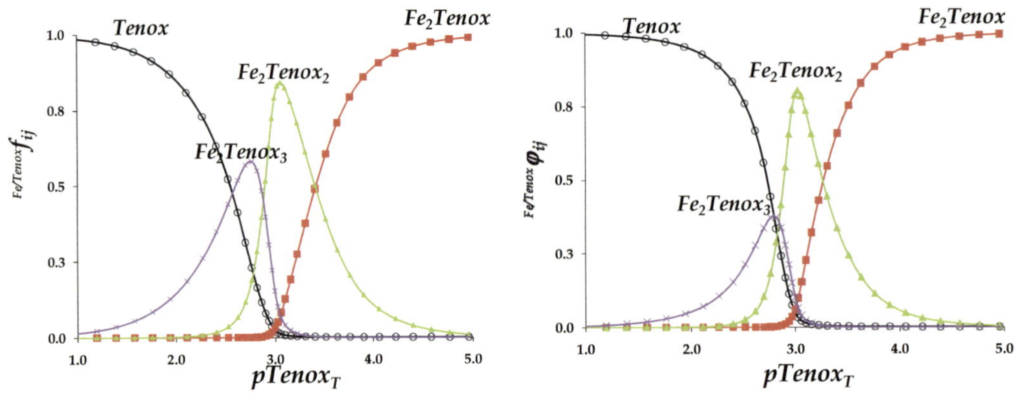

(a) (b)

Fig. 3. Typical graphic representations of the Fe(III)-tenoxicam system in acetone as a function of p$Tenox_T$. $[Fe(III)]_T = 1\times10^{-3}$ M and p$Tenox_T$ = -log$[Tenox]_T$. a) Distribution diagram of substance amount of Tenoxicam species, taking in account the quantity of tenoxicam in each species. b) Distribution diagram of concentration of tenoxicam species, taking in account which tenoxicam species is more concentrated in the system.

The independent variable of these figures, in all cases, has been selected to be the p*Tenox*$_T$, in order to compare directly the shape of each fraction in Fig. 2 and 3. Nevertheless this axis could represent another variable (like $p\Sigma_M$, $p\Sigma_L$, p*L*, p*M*, etc.)

It is noteworthy than distribution of substance amount and concentration are similar for the same component, even though slightly differences can be shown comparing Fig. 2a and 2b, or Fig. 3a or 3b; some of their differences are crucial and related with the physical-chemical meaning of each distribution.

A distributions of Fe(III) and tenoxicam species comparison allows for the conclusion that they are very different, obviously representing distributions of two different components in the system.

2.2 Distribution diagrams as a function of stoichiometric coefficients

The sentence "distribution diagram" could have an implicit idea concerning possible statistical distributions subjacent to the graphic representations given in Fig. 1, 2 and 3. This idea was first explored by Moya-Hernández et al. (2002a) for the case of Brφnsted acid-base systems. In the next subsection (2.2.1) the conclusions of this work will be applied to the case of oxine species as a function of pH while in the other subsection (2.2.2) this treatment will be generalized to the case of complex systems of the M-L kind, where polynuclear species are forming.

2.2.1 Distribution diagrams of one discrete variable (the proton stoichiometric coefficient for an acid-base system species)

If an aqueous solution of oxine at a certain concentration has a known pH value, the distribution of the oxine species will be fixed, as it is shown in Fig. 1a. Then a 3D graph could represent all the distributions of oxine species for each pH value. The set of distributions of oxine species is represented in Fig. 4 as well as one of them, at pH = 5.0.

In agreement with Mathematical Statistics (Kreyszig, 1970; Reichl, 1980), the meaning of each distribution of discrete variable is defined by Eq. 13.

$$\bar{\nu} = \sum_{j=0}^{n} j f_j \tag{13}$$

Furthermore, each of these statistical distributions has a variance. The variance of each distribution of discrete variable is defined by Eq. 14.

$$s_{\nu}^2 = \sum_{j=0}^{n} (j - \bar{\nu})^2 f_j \tag{14}$$

The equality of Eq. 3 and 13 demonstrate that the set of means of the oxine species distributions is the one given in Fig. 1b. In this way, the mean of the distribution offers the value in which the proton number is centered, as an average, at each pH value.

The set of variances of these distributions is related with an intrinsic buffer capacity (Moya-Hernández et al., 2002a). A graphic representation of the oxine set of variances as a function of pH is given in Fig. 5. When the variance has a value near to zero one species is present in the system with a fraction near 1; when the variance reaches a maximum, two or more species are present in the system with comparable fraction values. In the case of oxine system the maxima of the variance function are reached for pH values equal to pK_{a1} and pK_{a2}, because $pK_{a2} >> pK_{a1}$.

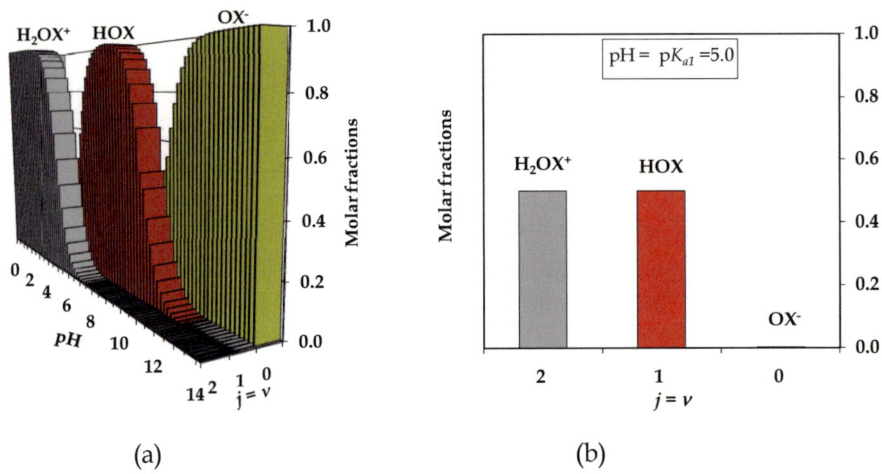

Fig. 4. Statistical distributions of oxine species. a) Set of distributions of the stoichiometric coefficient of protons as the discrete variable. b) Specific distribution diagram at pH = 5.0.

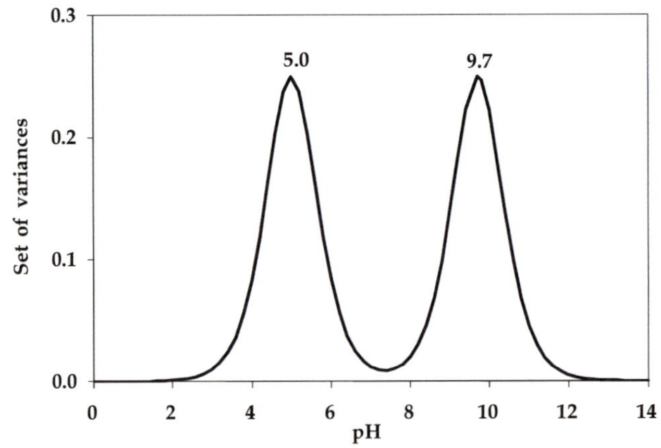

Fig. 5. Set of variances of the distributions of discrete variable of oxine as a function of pH. The maxima of these function are placed in the pK_a values.

2.2.2 Distribution diagrams of two discrete variables (the M and L components stoichiometric coefficients for complexation systems)

It can be demonstrated that the distribution diagrams as those of Fig. 2 and 3 for *M-L* complexation systems represent sets of distributions of two discrete variables,where these variables are the M and L stoichiometric coefficients.

Examples of substance amount and concentration distributions of tenoxicam in Fe(III), for only one of the systems represented in Fig. 2 are shown in Fig. 6.

In this case, each one of the statistical distributions that can be defined has two means, two variances and one covariance (Reichl, 1980).

Just as a mere example, the definition of the two means of the substance amount distribution of Tenoxicam in Fe(III) is given in Eq. 15, while the definition of the two variances and the covariance for the same distribution is given in Eq. 16.

$$\begin{aligned} {}^{L/M}_{f}\overline{\nu}_M &= \sum_{i=1}^{m}\sum_{j=0}^{n[i]}[i({}^{L/M}f_{ij})] \\ {}^{L/M}_{f}\overline{\nu}_L &= \sum_{j=0}^{n}\sum_{i=1}^{m[j]}[j({}^{L/M}f_{ij})] \end{aligned} \tag{15}$$

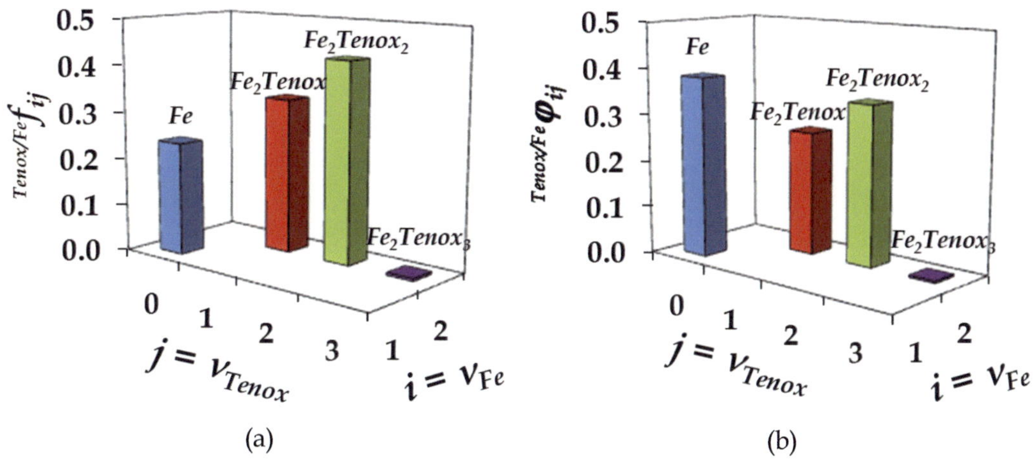

Fig. 6. Statistical distributions of tenoxicam in Fe(III) species in acetone. $[Fe(III)]_T = 1\times10^{-3}$M and $[Tenox]_T = 6\times10^{-4}$M. a) Substance amount fractions of Fe(III) species. b) Concentration fractions of Fe(III) species.

The set of means and variances for the distributions of two discrete variables of Tenoxicam in Fe(III), represented typically in Fig. 2a like a "distribution diagram", are shown in Fig. 7.

The interpretation of each of the two means is to be the stoichiometric coefficient average for the corresponding component. The two variances grow when two or more species are forming: higher variance increases the number of species with different stoichiometric coefficient of the corresponding component.

The possible consequences of this statistical view should be studied exhaustively, but this kind of study would be beyond the objectives of the present work. The distribution diagrams applications to determine or to use stoichiometric coefficients are developed in the following sections.

$$
\begin{aligned}
{}^{L/M}_{\ f}S_{M,L} &= \sum_{i=1}^{m}\sum_{j=0}^{n[i]}\{[i-({}^{L/M}_{\ f}\bar{\nu}_M)]^2({}^{L/M}f_{M_iL_j})\} \\
{}^{L/M}_{\ f}S_{M,L} &= \sum_{j=0}^{n}\sum_{i=1}^{m[j]}\{[j-({}^{L/M}_{\ f}\bar{\nu}_L)]^2({}^{L/M}f_{ij})\} \qquad (16) \\
{}^{L/M}_{\ f}S_{M,L} &= \sum_{i=1}^{m}\sum_{j=0}^{n[i]}[(i-{}^{L/M}_{\ f}\bar{\nu}_M)(j-{}^{L/M}_{\ f}\bar{\nu}_L)({}^{L/M}f_{M_iL_j})]
\end{aligned}
$$

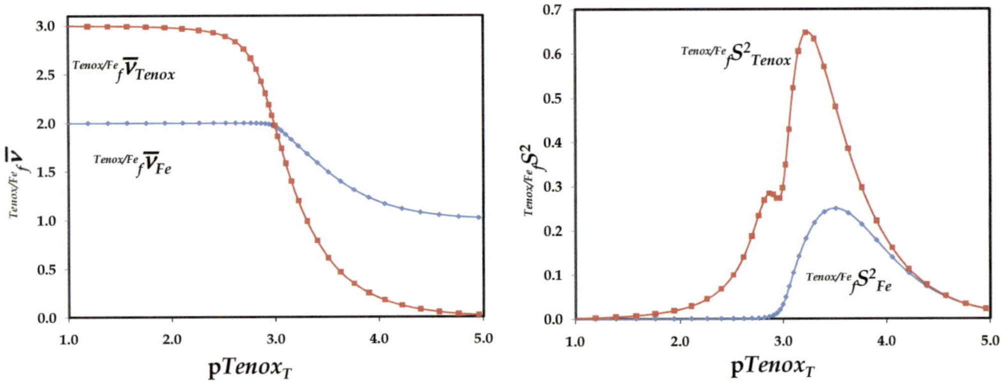

(a) (b)

Fig. 7. Statistical parameters for the substance amount distributions of Tenoxicam in Fe(III) in acetone corresponding to Fig. 2a. a) Set of the two means of the distribution. b) Set of the two variances of the distribution.

3. Acid-base titration curves for polyprotic systems

This section deals with titration curves, pH = f(volume of strong acid or base), of polyacid and polybase systems by means of a description given by a thermodynamic model. This allows for the theoretical building of this kind of curves as well as their first derivative and the buffer capacity curves as a function of pH. The model is deducted from electroneutrality equation relating the global formation equilibrium and molar fractions of the distribution diagram of the system. Some previous works concerning this mater can be found in literature, by Fleck, 1967; Högfeldt, 1979; King & Kester, 1990; Efstathiou, 2000; Rojas-Hernández & Ramírez-Silva, 2002; Tarapčík & Beinrohr, 2003; Asuero, 2007; Gutz, 2010; Asuero & Michałowski, 2011.

3.1 Titration curves, pH = f(added volume of strong acid or base), of a mixture of species in the same polyprotic system

A system formed by a mixture of V_{oj} volumes of solutions of H_jL^{j-a} species, with concentrations C_{oj}, giving a total initial volume $V_o = \Sigma V_{oj}$, has been considered. The H_jL^{j-a} species form part of the same polyprotic system ($H_nL^{(n-a)+}/H_{(n-1)}L^{(n-a-1)+}/.../H_aL/.../HL^{(a-1)-}/L^{a-}/H^+$). Each charged species has associated a contra-cation or a contra-anion (M^{z+} or X^{z-}) that do not have acid-base properties, depending if $(j-a)$ is negative or positive.

3.1.1 Titrations with a strong base: *MOH*

If the mixture described at the beginning of section 3.1 is titrated with a strong base *MOH*, of C_b concentration, it is possible to write the electroneutrality equation, for each added volume of *MOH* (V_b), in the form:

$$[M^+]+\frac{\sum_{j=0}^{a-1}(a-j)\{V_{oj}C_{oj}\}}{V_o+V_b}+\sum_{j=a+1}^{n}(j-a)[LH_j^{j-a}]+[H^+]=\frac{\sum_{j=a+1}^{n}(j-a)\{V_{oj}C_{oj}\}}{V_o+V_b}+\sum_{j=0}^{a-1}(a-j)[LH_j^{j-a}]+[OH^-] \tag{17}$$

where $[M^+] = V_bC_b/(V_o + V_b)$, the second term in the first member of Eq. 17, represents the contra-cations charge associated to the anions of the polyprotic system for $j \in \{0, 1, ..., a\text{-}1\}$, while the first term in the second member represents the contra-anions charge associated to the cations of the polyprotic system for $j \in \{a+1, a+2, ..., n\}$.

Introducing Eq. 1 and 2 in Eq. 17 and algebraically rearranging it, it is possible to arrive to Eq. 18.

$$V_b=\frac{\sum_{j=0}^{n}\{(j-a)(V_{oj}C_{oj})\}-\left[\sum_{j=0}^{n}(V_{oj}C_{oj})\right]\left[\sum_{j=0}^{n}\{(j-a)f_j\}\right]-V_o\left(\left[H^+\right]-\frac{K_w}{\left[H^+\right]}\right)}{C_b+\left[H^+\right]-\frac{K_w}{[H^+]}} \tag{18}$$

3.1.2 Titrations with a strong acid: *HX*

If the mixture described at the beginning of the section 3.1 is titrated with a strong acid *HX*, of C_a concentration, it is possible to write the electroneutrality equation, for each added volume of *HX* (V_a), in the form:

$$\frac{\sum_{j=0}^{a-1}(a-j)\{V_{oj}C_{oj}\}}{V_o+V_b}+\sum_{j=a+1}^{n}(j-a)[LH_j^{j-a}]+[H^+]=\frac{\sum_{j=a+1}^{n}(j-a)\{V_{oj}C_{oj}\}}{V_o+V_b}+\sum_{j=0}^{a-1}(a-j)[LH_j^{j-a}]+[OH^-]+[X^-] \tag{19}$$

where $[X^-] = V_aC_a/(V_o + V_a)$. Introducing Eq. 1 and 2 conveniently in Eq. 19 and algebraically rearranging it, it is possible to arrive to Eq. 20.

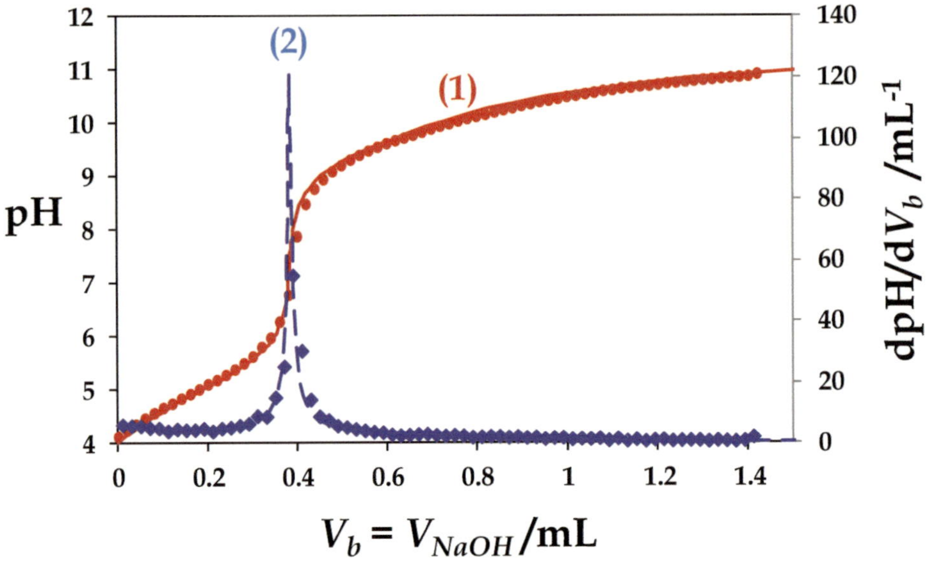

(a)

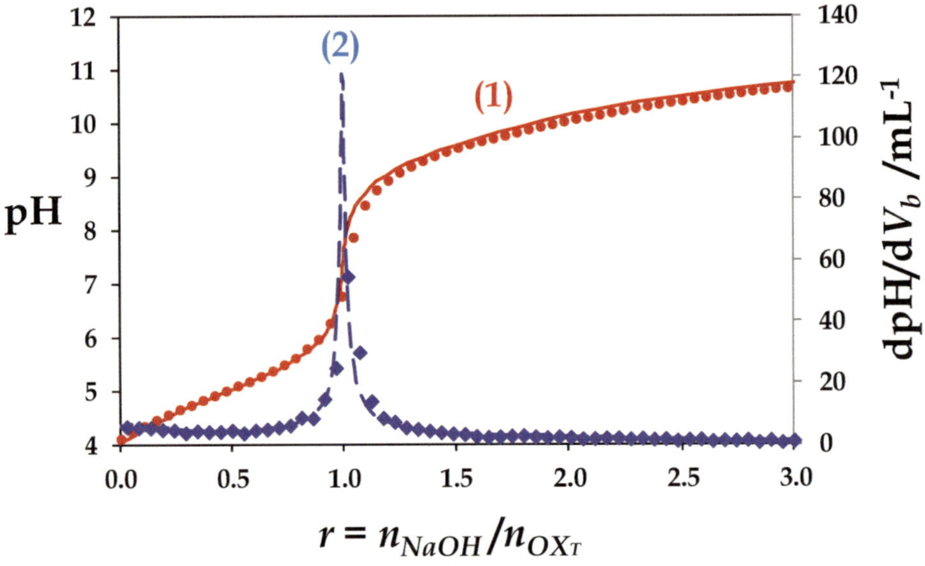

(b)

Fig. 8. Titration curve of 50 mL of aqueous solution of H_2OXCl with an aqueous solution of NaOH 0.1315 M. The values used to obtain the fitting shown are the following: $pK_{a1} = 5.0$, $pK_{a2} = 9.7$, $pK_w = 13.7$, $[H_2OXCl]_{\text{initial}} = 0.00101$ M.
1) The circles represent the experimental points of the pH = $f(V_b)$ curve and the solid line is the fitted curve obtained with Eq. 18. 2) The rhombuses represent the experimental points of the $(dpH/dV_b) = g(V_b)$ curve and the dashed line is the fitted curve obtained with Eq. 22.
a) Curves as a function of added volume of the titrand. b) Curves as a function of molar ratio (r) of the titrand.

Practically all the simulators, available nowadays, to predict acid-base titration curves, using strong base or acid as titrand agent, are based on Eq. 18 and 20. They are analytical expressions to calculate exactly the added volume of strong base or acid, given a set of pH values. In the following subsections this feature will be used to obtain important applications of these equations.

$$V_a = \frac{-\sum_{j=0}^{n}\{(j-a)(V_{oj}C_{oj})\} + \left[\sum_{j=0}^{n}(V_{oj}C_{oj})\right]\left[\sum_{j=0}^{n}\{(j-a)f_j\}\right] + V_o\left(\left[H^+\right] - \frac{K_w}{\left[H^+\right]}\right)}{C_b - \left[H^+\right] + \frac{K_w}{[H^+]}} \quad (20)$$

3.1.3 Titration of aqueous solution of oxine hydrochloride (*H_2OXCl*) with *NaOH*

In order to compare the predicted results with the experimental ones, 50 mL of an aqueous solution 0.001M H_2OXCl where titrated with a solution of NaOH 0.1315 M at 25°C.

The comparison of the experimental titration curve with the fitted curve through the model given by Eq. 18 is shown in Fig. 8a.

As it is shown in curves 1 of Fig. 8, the observed fitting for the titration curve is good. In the case of Fig. 8b, the molar ratio (r) is defined as the ratio of the added titrand (NaOH), with respect to the analyte (OX_T). The solution pH has a great change near 1, meaning that the quantitative reaction consumes 1 mol of H_2OX^+ for each added mol of OH^-. In other words, the stoichiometric coefficients of these reagents are 1 and 1 for the reaction that permits the quantification of oxine with the hydroxide ion:

$$H_2OX^+ + OH^- \rightleftharpoons HOX + H_2O \quad (21)$$

3.2 The first derivative of the titration curve: dpH/dV

The first derivative method of an acid-base titration curve is well known to determine the equivalence point volumes in order to accomplish quantitative chemical analysis.

Nevertheless, being Eq. 18 and 20 functions of only one variable (the pH), it is possible to obtain the analytical expressions of their first derivatives and their reciprocal functions, to arrive to the exact algebraic expressions of the titration first derivatives curves. These expressions are given in Eq. 22 and 23.

$$\frac{dpH}{dV_b} = \frac{C_b + 10^{-pH} - 10^{pH-pK_w}}{-2.303\left[\sum_{j=0}^{n}(V_{oj}C_{oj})\right]\left[\sum_{j=0}^{n}\left\{jf_j\sum_{i=0}^{n}[(i-j)f_i]\right\}\right] + 2.303(V_o + V_b)\left[10^{-pH} + 10^{pH-pK_w}\right]} \quad (22)$$

$$-\frac{dpH}{dV_a} = \frac{C_a - 10^{-pH} + 10^{pH-pK_w}}{-2.303\left[\sum_{j=0}^{n}(V_{oj}C_{oj})\right]\left[\sum_{j=0}^{n}\left\{jf_j\sum_{i=0}^{n}[(i-j)f_i]\right\}\right] + 2.303(V_o + V_a)\left[10^{-pH} + 10^{pH-pK_w}\right]} \quad (23)$$

3.2.1 Titration first derivative curve of an oxine hydrochloride (*H_2OXCl*) aqueous solution with *NaOH*

The curves 2 in Fig. 8 compare the titration experimental first derivative, described at the beginning of subsection 3.1.3, with the curves obtained by Eq. 22.

The experimental first derivative was obtained approximately as the ratio of finite differences of measured pH values and volumes during titration, using the average of volumes, or molar ratios, for each interval.

As it can be seen, the fitting attained is quite good and the maximum observed in Fig. 8a and 8b is sharp. In the first case, this maximum signals the volume position of the first equivalence point, while in the second case it indicates the ratio of the titrand stoichiometric coefficients with respect to the analyte for the quantitative reaction.

The first derivative is usually better than the pH curve to experimentally determine the volumes of the equivalence points (Fig. 8a) and the titration reactions (titrand/analyte) ratio of stoichometric coefficients (Fig. 8b) when these are quantitative.

In the case of the *HOX* reaction with OH^-, the second titration reaction, is not quantitative because its corresponding equilibrium constant is not high enough for a 0.001 M analyte initial concentration. For this reason there are no visible changes in the second equivalence point volume in curves 1 or 2 in Fig. 8a, nor in Fig. 8b for $r = 2$.

3.3 The buffer capacity (β) of a polyprotic system

In many chemical and biological processes it is essential that the medium pH be kept within certain limits, which is possible through the use of buffer solutions. They possess a specific buffer capacity and are used to maintain constant the pH with a very small uncertainty.

In the chemical literature, there are two ways to define a buffer capacity (β): one is defined in terms of concentration of strong acid or base added to the system, in order to simplify the mathematical treatment, as firstly proposed by Van Slyke (1922), and then used by others, as Urbansky & Schock (2000) or Segurado (2003). The other way to define the buffer capacity is in terms of the amount of strong acid or base added to the system, as King and Kester did (1990), as well as Skoog et al. (2005); they also derive equations with the concentration, but considering explicitly 1L of solution.

3.3.1 A buffer capacity with dilution effect (β_{dil})

According to the definition given by King & Kester (1990) it is possible to apply the derivative of the added amount of strong base or acid with respect to the pH, and then obtaining mathematical expressions for the buffer capacity as function of pH, by considering the dilution effect, i.e. $\beta_{dil} = f(pH)$. In the present work, this implies to take Eq. 22 and 23 reciprocals and multiply them by C_b or C_a, respectively.

The typical way to represent a buffer capacity curve, consists in plotting it as a function of pH, even though it may be represented as a function of the titrand volume or the molar ratio titrand/analyte.

$$\beta_{\text{dil}_b} = \frac{dV_bC_b}{dpH} = \frac{2.303C_b}{C_b + (10^{-pH} - 10^{pH-pK_w})}$$
$$\left\{\left[\sum_{j=0}^{n}(V_{oj}C_{oj})\right]\left[-\sum_{j=0}^{n}\left(jf_j\sum_{i=0}^{n}[(i-j)f_i]\right)\right] + (V_o+V_b)\left[10^{-pH} + 10^{pH-pK_w}\right]\right\} \tag{24}$$

$$\beta_{\text{dil}_a} = -\frac{dV_aC_a}{dpH} = \frac{2.303C_a}{C_a - (10^{-pH} - 10^{pH-pK_w})}$$
$$\left\{\left[\sum_{j=0}^{n}(V_{oj}C_{oj})\right]\left[-\sum_{j=0}^{n}\left(jf_j\sum_{i=0}^{n}[(i-j)f_i]\right)\right] + (V_o+V_a)\left[10^{-pH} + 10^{pH-pK_w}\right]\right\} \tag{25}$$

As Moya-Hernández et al. (2002b) have demonstrated, Eq. 14 is equal to the double sum between brackets in Eq. 24 and 25. For this reason, the set of variances is related with the intrinsic buffer capacity of a polyprotic system.

$$s_{\bar{v}}^2 = \sum_{j=0}^{n}(j-\bar{v})^2 f_j = \left[-\sum_{j=0}^{n}\left(jf_j\sum_{i=0}^{n}[(i-j)f_i]\right)\right] = \textit{intrinsic buffer capacity} \tag{26}$$

It is noteworthy that the intrinsic buffer capacity, i.e. the set of variances of the proton stoichiometric coefficient distributions for this kind of systems, is a function that only depends on the molar fractions and the stoichiometric coefficients.

The second term between keys in Eq. 24 and 25 is due to the acid and basic particles of the amphiprotic solvent (H^+ and OH^- in the case of water). (See Segurado (2003), Urbansky & Schock (2000).)

3.3.2 Buffer capacity with dilution of aqueous solution of oxine hydrochloride (H_2OXCl) with *NaOH*

Fig. 9 shows the comparison of experimental buffer capacity, with effect of dilution, and the curve obtained by Eq. 24 and 25 for the titrations of the system defined at the beginning of subsection 3.1.3.

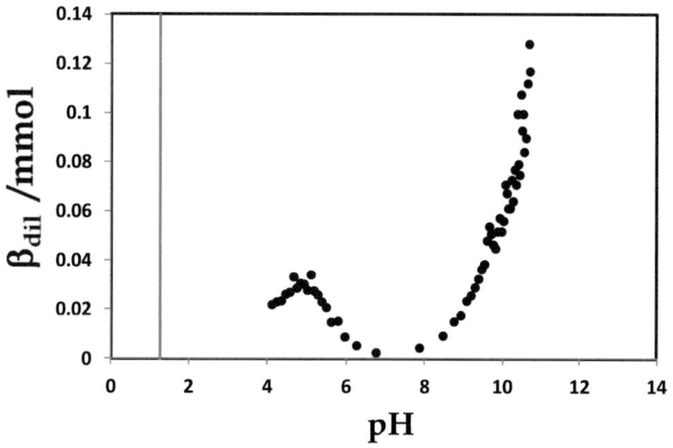

Fig. 9. Comparison of experimental (markers) and calculated (solid line) buffer capacity with effect of dilution.

The experimental β_{dil} has been determined approximately by taking the ratio of the titrand concentration and the first derivative experimentally obtained as explained in subsection 3.2.1.

As it can be seen in Fig. 9, there is a good agreement between the theoretical and the experimental data. The expected maximum of the curve at pH = pK_{a2} = 9.7 (see Fig. 5) is lost due to the effect of the hydroxide ion over the pair HOX/OX^- by the low concentration of oxine in the system (0.001 M).

4. Molar ratio and continuous variations methods for complexation systems

For complexation reactions the two traditional methods to determine the stoichiometry of formation reactions and formation equilibrium constants are the molar ratio and the continuous variations methods (this last also known as Job's method). (See Hartley et al., 1980.)

Nevertheless, the explanation of these methods has not always been given in a clear way, and this is particularly evident for equilibrium considering the formation of polynuclear species. Furthermore, these treatments are disappearing from modern text books. For this reason, the aim of this part of the chapter is to describe a way to deduct the equations and the curves that appear in some Inorganic and Analytical Chemistry books.

4.1 Tables of Variation of Substance Amount (TVSA)

Professor Gaston Charlot (1969), in France, has used a teaching tool to explain the advance degree in the formation of acid-base, complexation and redox reactions. It has been called by him the Table of Variation of Substance Amount. In the following subsections this tool will be applied to the systems equilibrium states using the molar ratio and continuous variations methods.

For a system where only one reaction takes place, quantitatively:

$$aM + bL \rightleftarrows M_aL_b \quad \text{with} \quad \beta_{ab} = \frac{[M_aL_b]}{[M]^a[L]^b} >> 1 \tag{27}$$

4.1.1 Table of Variation of Substance Amount for the molar ratio method

In the molar ratio method several amounts of one of the reagents, i. e. L, is added to another reagent, i. e. M, and typically the dilution of the solutions is controlled in volumetric flasks of the same capacity V_T in order to measure a response R that is directly proportional to the reaction product, M_aL_b, through the equation:

$$R = k_{M_aL_b}[M_aL_b] = k_{M_aL_b}(n_{M_aL_b} / V_T) \tag{28}$$

This experiment is described in Table 2 for a quantitative reaction.

If all the amounts in the first column of Table 2 are divided by the M quantity (n_M), and the amounts in the other columns are divided by V_T and multiplied by the corresponding response factor, Table 3 will be obtained.

	$a\,M$	+ $b\,L$	⇆ M_aL_b
Initial	n_M	n_L	
$n_L < \frac{b}{a} n_M$	$n_M - (a/b)n_L$	$b\epsilon \approx 0$	$(1/b)n_L$
$\frac{b}{a} n_M = {}_{SC}n_L$	$a\epsilon \approx 0$	$b\epsilon \approx 0$	$(1/a)n_M$
$\frac{b}{a} n_M < n_L$	$a\epsilon \approx 0$	$n_L - (b/a)n_M$	$(1/a)n_M$

Table 2. TVSA for molar ratio method. n_M is a constant for all the systems, n_L is variable, all systems are in solution in thermodynamic equilibrium and the total volume is the same and equal to V_T. ${}_{SC}n_L$ represents the amount of L for the stoichiometric condition.

The functions deducted for molar ratio method and presented in Table 3, with the given restrictions, lead to represent their behaviour in Fig. 10 assuming Eq. 28 and giving R in arbitrary units.

	$a\,M$	+ $b\,L$	⇆ M_aL_b
Initial	n_M	n_L	
$r_L < \frac{b}{a}$	$k_M(n_M - (a/b)n_L)/V_T$	$b\epsilon \approx 0$	$k_{MaLb}(1/b)r_L(n_M)/V_T$
${}_{SC}r_L = \frac{b}{a}$	$a\epsilon \approx 0$	$b\epsilon \approx 0$	$k_{MaLb}(1/a)n_M/V_T$
$\frac{b}{a} < r_L$	$a\epsilon \approx 0$	$k_L(n_L - (b/a)n_M)/V_T$	$k_{MaLb}(1/a)n_M/V_T$

Table 3. TVSA for molar ratio method expressed in terms of molar ratio of L (r_L) and response (R) of the system. ${}_{SC}r_L$ represents the amount of L for the stoichiometric condition. For this study it has been assumed that $k_M = k_L = 0$.

It should be noticed in Fig. 10 that the intersection between the two formed straight lines indicates the molar ratio corresponding to stoichiometric conditions; in other words, this value is equal to the L stoichiometric coefficient ratio divided by the M stoichiometric coefficient : ${}_{SC}r_L = b/a$.

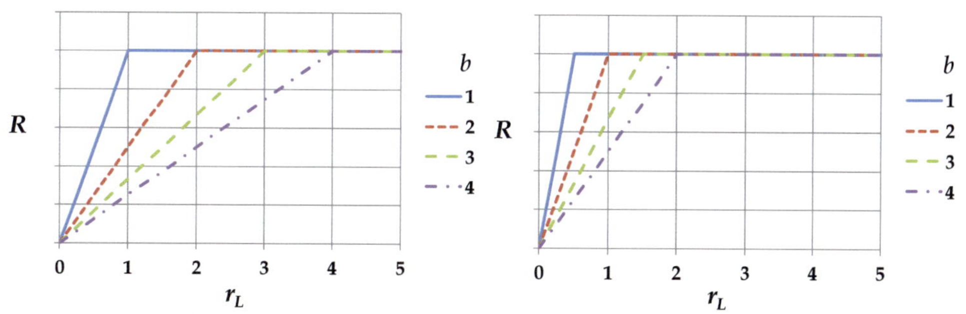

(a) (b)

Fig. 10. Curves *Response* = R= f(r_L) for experiments of molar ratio method. a) a = 1 for the formation of species of the ML_b kind. b) a = 2 for the formation of species of the M_2L_b kind.

If some of the assumptions formulated in this work are avoided there will be some deviations of the curves shown in Fig. 10. As an example, if more species linearly contribute to the response, the parameters of the straight lines change, but their intersection still indicates the molar ratio of the stoichiometric conditions. If the formation reaction in Eq. 27 is not quantitative there will be some deviations of the linearity near the stoichiometric conditions. Finally, if there are more species forming in the system at the same time, in principle, there will be more straight lines in the molar ratio curve, one for each species appearing in the system (if all the reactions are quantitative, if all the contributions to the response are linear and the response factors are different enough).

4.1.2 Tables of Variation of Substance Amount for the continuous variations method

In the continuous variations method several amounts of the reagents, L and M, are mixed in such a way that the total amount of both reagents is constant: $n_M + n_L = n_T =$ constant. Typically, the solutions dilution is controlled in volumetric flasks of the same capacity V_T in order to measure a response R that is directly proportional to the reaction product, M_aL_b, through Eq. 28. This experiment is described in Table 4 for a quantitative reaction.

Generally, in this method the equilibrium conditions are expressed in terms of the molar fraction of one of the components, x_L or x_M. So the ${}_{SC}x_L$ (the component L molar fraction at stoichiometric conditions) can be deducted, as it is shown in Eq. 29.

$$\frac{b}{a} = \frac{{}_{SC}n_L}{n_T - {}_{SC}n_L} \Rightarrow \frac{b}{a}(n_T - {}_{SC}n_L) = {}_{SC}n_L$$
$$\Rightarrow {}_{SC}x_L = \frac{b}{a}(1 - {}_{SC}x_L) \Rightarrow {}_{SC}x_L = \frac{\frac{b}{a}}{1+\frac{b}{a}} \tag{29}$$
$$\therefore {}_{SC}x_L = \frac{b}{a+b}$$

$n_M + n_L = n_T$	$a\,M$	+	$b\,L$	⇆	M_aL_b
Initial	$n_T - n_L$		n_L		
$n_L < {}_{SC}n_L$	$n_T - n_L - (a/b)n_L$		$b\epsilon \approx 0$		$(1/b)n_L$
$n_L = {}_{SC}n_L$	$a\epsilon \approx 0$		$b\epsilon \approx 0$		$(1/b)({}_{SC}n_L)$
${}_{SC}n_L < n_L$	$a\epsilon \approx 0$		$n_L - (b/a)(n_T - n_L)$		$(1/a)(n_T - n_L)$

Table 4. TVSA for continuous variations method. n_T is a constant for all the systems, n_M and n_L are variable, all systems are in solution in thermodynamic equilibrium and the total volume is the same and equal to V_T. ${}_{SC}n_L$ represents the amount of substance of L for the stoichiometric condition.

If all the amounts in the first column of Table 4 are divided by n_T, while the amounts in the other columns are divided by V_T and multiplied by the corresponding response factor, Table 5 will be obtained.

The functions deducted for continuous variations method and presented in Table 5, with the given restrictions, lead to represent their behaviour in Fig. 11 assuming Eq. 28 and giving R in arbitrary units.

$x_M+x_L=1$	$a\,M$	+	$b\,L$	$\leftrightarrows$	M_aL_b
Initial	$n_T - n_L$		n_L		
$0 \le x_L \le \frac{b}{a+b}$	$k_M(n_T-((b-a)/b)n_L)/V_T$		$b\epsilon \approx 0$		$(k_{MaLb}/b)x_L n_T/V_T$
$\frac{b}{a+b} = {}_{SC}x_L$	$a\epsilon \approx 0$		$b\epsilon \approx 0$		$(k_{MaLb}/(a+b))n_T/V_T$
$\frac{b}{a+b} \le x_L \le 1$	$a\epsilon \approx 0$		$k_L(n_L-(b/a)(n_T-n_L))/V_T$		$(k_{MaLb}/a)(1-x_L)n_T/V_T$

Table 5. TVSA for continuous variations method expressed in terms of L molar fraction (x_L) and response (R) of the system. ${}_{SC}x_L$ represents the amount of L substance for the stoichiometric condition. For this study it has been assumed that $k_M = k_L = 0$.

It should be remarked in Fig. 11 that the intersection between the two formed straight lines indicates the molar fraction corresponding to stoichiometric conditions; in other words, this molar fraction is equal to the following relationship: ${}_{SC}x_L = b/(a+b)$.

Moreover, in this method, as it has been discussed for the molar ratio method, if some of the assumptions formulated in this work are avoided there will be some deviations of the curves shown in Fig. 11. As an example, if more species contribute to the response, the parameters of the straight line change, but their intersection still indicates the molar fraction of the stiochiometric conditions. If the formation reaction in Eq. 27 is not quantitative, there will be some deviations of the linearity near the stoichiometric conditions. Finally, if there are more species forming in the system at the same time, in principle, there will be more straight lines in the molar ratio curve, one for each species appearing in the system (if all the reactions are quantitative, if all the contributions to the response are linear and the response factors are different enough).

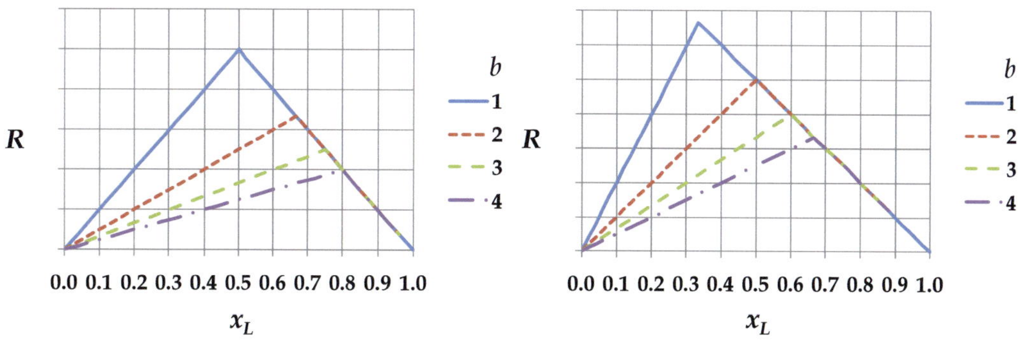

(a) (b)

Fig. 11. Curves *Response* = R= f(x_L) for experiments of continuous variations method. a) $a = 1$ for the formation of species of the ML_b kind. b) $a = 2$ for the formation of species of the M_2L_b kind.

4.1.3 Some remarks for the use of Tables of Variation of Substance Amount

The TVSA are a very powerful tool to understand the composition of thermodynamic equilibrium states when chemical reactions are involved. In the subsections 4.1.1 and 4.1.2 the dependent and independent variables are those typically selected. Nevertheless other selections could be used if the description and interpretation of chemical behaviour require it. Then, in the molar ratio method the representation of the curves could be done as a function of metal ion ratio (r_M), while for the continuous variations method the molar fraction of metal ion (x_M) could be used.

Furthermore, the TVSA could be used for the treatment of several complexes forming in the system at the same time.

In this work we have presented only the curves that may help interpreting the system that will be treated in the following section.

4.2 Application of the methods to determine the stoichiometry and equilibrium constants: The case of Fe(III)-tenoxicam system in acetone

A spectroscopic study in the visible region of electromagnetic spectrum was undertaken to determine the complexes formed as well as their formation constants for the Fe(III)-tenoxicam system in acetone, due to the red colour observed when both reagents are mixed. The solutions preparation and the details of the spectra acquisition have been given elsewhere (Moya-Hernández et al., 2009).

The absorption spectra obtained in this study are presented in Fig. 12, for molar ratio and continuous variations methods.

In order to be near the fulfilment of the conditions selected in section 4.1, (e.g. absorption only due to the complexes formed) a wavelength of 520 nm was selected to represent the typical curves of molar ratio and continuous variations, which are shown in Figure 13.

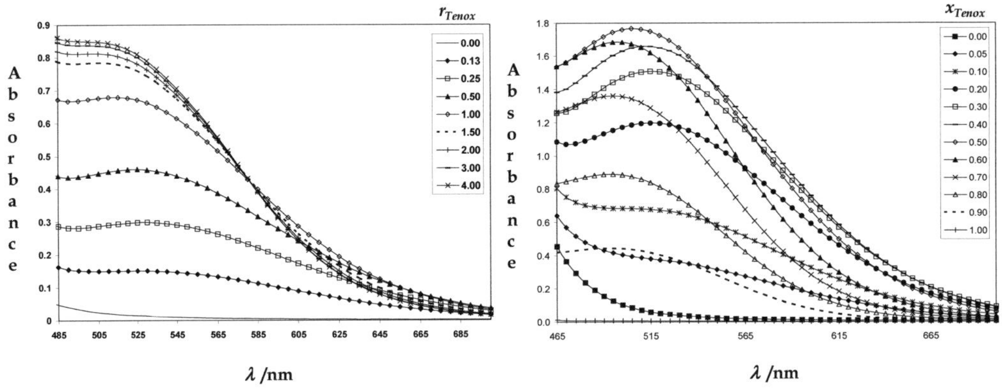

(a) (b)

Fig. 12. Absorption spectra in the visible region for the Fe(III)-tenoxicam system in acetone. [Fe(III)] = 0.001M or [Fe(III)] + [Tenox] = 0.001M. a) Molar ratio method. b) Continuous variations method.

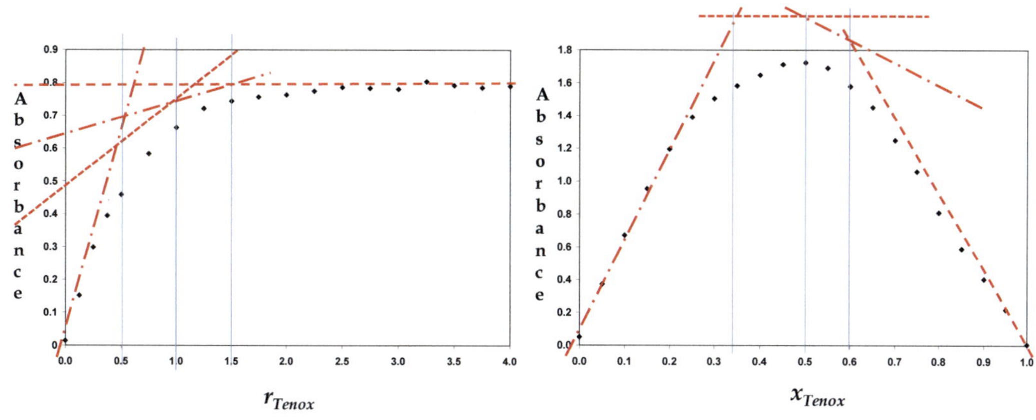

(a) (b)

Fig. 13. Spectral behaviour, at 520 nm, of the Fe(III)-tenoxicam system in acetone where different complexes are forming. [Fe(III)] = 0.001M or [Fe(III)] + [Tenox] = 0.001M. a) Molar ratio method. b) Continuous variations method. The dashed lines and the thin vertical lines only have been added to help follow the discussion given in the text.

The shape of the curves presented in Fig. 13 demonstrates the formation of polynuclear species in the system, both methods clearly showing an abrupt change of slope before the molar ratio or molar fraction corresponding to 1:1 stoichiometry ($r_{Tenox} < 1$ and $x_{Tenox} < 0.5$), as it can be concluded form Fig. 10b and 11b. The other changes in slope support the possibility of the formation of several complexes; in other words, two straight lines are not enough to explain the shape of the curves. The thin vertical lines indicate the position of the molar ratio or the molar fraction that fulfil the stoichiometric conditions of the Fe(III)-tenoxicam complexes (Fe_2Tenox, Fe_2Tenox_2 and Fe_2Tenox_3) obtained in the treatment of spectrophotometric data (Moya-Hernández et al., 2009 and Table 1).

In order to better describe the physical-chemical behaviour observed in the molar ratio method, the distribution diagrams of discrete variable of tenoxicam in Fe(III) (for the concentration of Fe(III) species) for the thin vertical lines shown in Fig. 13a, are presented in Fig. 14.

As it can be seen in Fig. 14, the predominant complex in the system corresponds to the molar ratio of each system, with other Fe(III) species been important as well. This is the reason why the experimental points are placed outside straight (dashed) lines in Fig. 13a.

Although some of these distribution diagrams of discrete variable could be represented for the continuous variations method, Fig. 13b may be the best graphic representation could be a distribution that consider Fe(III) and tenoxicam species at the same time, being the sum of substance amount of Fe(III) and tenoxicam ($n_{Fe} + n_{Tenox} = n_T$ = constant) the biggest restriction of this method. A look of this kind of distributions have been previously developed (Moya-Hernández, 2003).

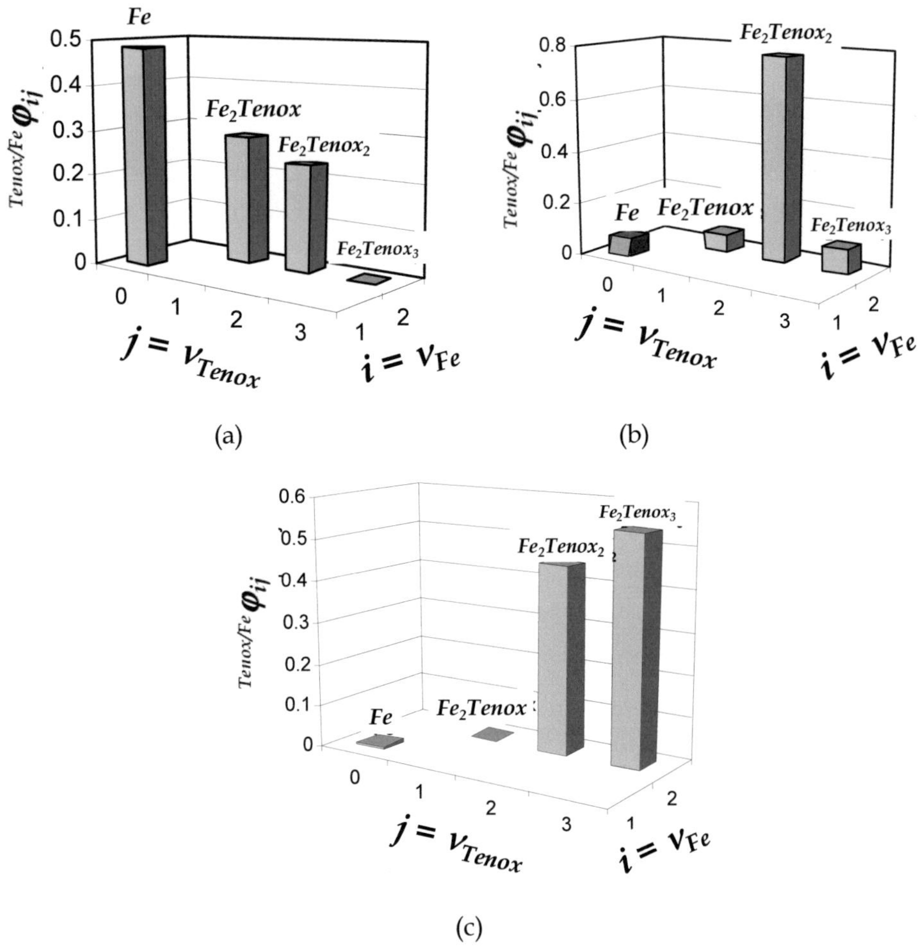

Fig. 14. Distribution diagrams of concentration of tenoxicam in Fe(III), for Fe(III) species, of some of the systems related with Fig. 13a. a) $r_{Tenox} = 0.5$. b) $r_{Tenox} = 1.0$. c) $r_{Tenox} = 1.5$.

5. Conclusion

In this work, some novelties related with the distribution diagrams, understood as statistical distributions of discrete variables, have been presented. We have extended this vision for two component systems. Moreover, the fractions of the distribution diagrams have been used to develop analytical equations to calculate exactly pH-metric titration curves as well as their first derivatives and a buffer capacity with effect of dilution. Finally the molar ratio and continuous variations methods have been reviewed, according to Charlot's methods, and explained with the discrete variables statistical distributions for complexation systems.

6. Acknowledgments

NR-L wants to acknowledge CONACyT for the stipend to follow PhD studies. MTR-S, RM-H and AR-H are in debt with SNI by the stipend and recognition like National Researchers.

MTR-S and AR-H acknowledge PROMEP for partial financial support, through Cuerpo Académico de Química Analítica (CA-UAMI-33), to develop this study.

RM-H and AR-H acknowledge αlfa Program of the EC and UNAM (through the 201855(B_1), PAPIIT-IN222011and PACIVE GC-11 projects) for partial financial support.

AR-H acknowledge Dr. Julio Arturo Soto-Guerrero, from 3M company, for helpful comments.

7. References

Asuero, A. G. Buffer Capacity of a Polyprotic Acid: First Derivative of the Buffer Capacity and pK_a Values of Single and Overlapping Equilibria. *Critical Reviews in Analytical Chemistry*, Vol.37, (July 2007), pp. 269-301.

Asuero, A. G. & Michałowski, T. Comprehensive Formulation of Titration Curves for Complex Acid-Base Systems and Its Analytical Implications. *Critical Reviews in Analytical Chemistry*, Vol.41, (May 2011), pp. 151-187.

Charlot, G. (1969). Cours de Chimie Analytique Générale, Vol.1. Solutions Aqueuses et Non Aqueuses, Masson, Paris, France

Efstathiou, C. E. (2000). Acid-base titration curves, Applet, Department of Chemistry, University of Athens, Greece, Available from http://www.chem.uoa.gr/Applets/AppletTitration/Appl_Titration2.html

Fleck, G. M. (1967). *Equilibrios en Disolución,* Alhambra, Madrid, Spain

Gutz, I. G. R. (September 2011). Simulator: CurTiPot. Version 3.5.4, MS Excel. Institute of Chemistry, University of Sao Paulo, Brazil. Available from http://www2.iq.usp.br/docente/gutz/Curtipot_.html

Hartley, F. R., Burgess, C. & Alcock R. M. (1980). *Solution Equilibria,* Ellis Horwood, Chichester, UK

Högfeldt, E. (1979). Chapter 15, In: *Treatise on Analytical Chemistry,* Kolthoff, I. M., Elving, P. J. Part 1, Vol.2, Section D, Interscience, ISBN: 978-047-1055-10-5, New York, USA

King, D. W.; Kester, D. R. (1990). A General Approach for Calculating Polyprotic Acid Speciation and Buffer Capacity. *Journal of Chemical Education,* Vol.67, No. 11, pp. 932-933.

Kreyszig, E. (1970). *Introductory Mathematical Statistics: Principles and Methods,* Wiley, New York, USA

Moya-Hernández, R.; Rueda-Jackson, J. C.; Ramírez-Silva, M. T.; Vázquez-Coutiño, G. A.; Havel, J. & Rojas-Hernández, A. (2002a). Statistical Study of Distribution Diagrams for Two-component Systems: Relationships of Means and Variances of the Discrete Variable Distributions with Average Ligand Number and Intrinsic Buffer Capacity. *Journal of Chemical Education,* Vol.79, No.3, (March 2002), pp. 389-392.

Moya-Hernández, R.; Rueda-Jackson, J. C.; Ramírez-Silva, M. T.; Vázquez-Coutiño, G. A.; Havel, J. & Rojas-Hernández, A. (2002b). Statistical Study of Distribution Diagrams for Two-component Systems: Relationships of Means and Variances of the Discrete Variable Distributions with Average Ligand Number and Intrinsic Buffer Capacity. *Journal of Chemical Education,* Vol.79, No.3, (March 2002), pp. 389-392. Supplemental Material for Journal of Chemical Education On Line, Available form http://jchemed.chem.wisc.edu/Journal/Issues/2002/Mar/PlusSub/JCESupp/supp389.html

Moya-Hernández, R. (2003). Estudio de Especiación Química de los Fármacos Antiinflamatorios Tenoxicam y Piroxicam con Cationes Metálicos de Interés Biológico, Ph. D. Thesis, Universidad Autónoma Metropolitana, Unidad Iztapalapa, México, D. F., Mexico.

Moya-Hernández, R., Gómez-Balderas R., Mederos A., Domínguez S., Ramírez-Silva M. T. & Rojas-Hernández A. (2009). *Journal of Coordination Chemistry*, Vol.62, No.1, pp. 40-51.

Puigdomenech, I. (May 2011). Make Equilibrium Diagrams Using Sophisticated Algorithms (MEDUSA), Available from http//www.kemi.kth.se/medusa

Reichl, L. E. (1980). A *Modern Course in Statistical Physics*, University of Texas Press, Austin, USA

Ringbom, A. (1963). *Complexation in Analytical Chemistry*, Wiley, New York, USA

Rojas-Hernández, A.; Ramírez, M. T.; González, I. & Ibanez, J. G. Predominance-Zone Diagrams in Solution Chemistry. Dismutation Processes in Two-Component Systems (M-L). *Journal of Chemical Education*, Vol.72, No.12, (December 1995), pp. 1099-1105

Rojas-Hernández, A. & Ramírez-Silva M. T. (2002). Modelo Termodinámico General para Curvas de Valoración Ácido-Base de Mezclas de Sistemas Poliácidos o Polibásicos (Sin Polinucleación) Con Ácido o Base Fuertes, In: *Química Inorgánica en la UAM-Iztapalapa 2002*, López-Goerne, T. M. & Rojas-Hernández, A. Vol. 1. pp. 133-158, ISBN: 970-31-0149-6, México, D. F., Mexico

Segurado, M. A. P. (2003). Extreme Values in Chemistry: Buffer capacity. *Chemical Educator*, Vol.8, pp. 22-27

Skoog, D. A. West, D. M., Holler, F. J. & Crouch, S. R. (2004). Fundamentals of Analytical Chemistry, 8th Ed., Brooks/Cole, Thompson Learning, Belmont, USA

Tarapčík, P., & Beinrohr, E. (2003). Implementation of a Universal Algorithm for pH Calculation into Spreadsheet and its Use in Teaching in Analytical Chemistry, Bratislava, Eslovaquia, Available from http://jchemed.chem.wisc.edu/JCEDLib/WebWare/collection/open/JCEWWOR012/

Urbansky, E. & Schock, M. R. (2000). Understanding, Deriving, and Computing Buffer Capacity. *Journal of Chemical Education*, Vol.77, pp. 1640-1644

Van Slyke, D. D. (1922). On the Measurement of Buffer Values and on the Relationship of Buffer Values to the Dissociation Constant of the Buffer and the Concentration and Reaction of the Buffer Solution. *Journal of Biological Chemistry*, Vol. 52, pp. 525-570

Vicente-Pérez, S. (1985). *Química de las Disoluciones. Diagramas y Cálculos Gráficos.* Alhambra. Madrid, Spain

14

Limiting Reactants in Chemical Analysis: Influences of Metals and Ligands on Calibration Curves and Formation Constants for Selected Iron-Ligand Chelates

Mark T. Stauffer, William E. Weller,
Kimberly R. Kubas and Kelly A. Casoni
University of Pittsburgh at Greensburg, Greensburg, Pennsylvania
USA

1. Introduction

1.1 The limiting reactant concept in chemical analysis

The concept of the limiting reactant in chemical reactions is one of the fundamental concepts learned by all students enrolled in introductory courses in chemistry at the high school and early undergraduate levels. Practicing chemists, and just about every technical professional involved in at least some aspect of chemistry, use the concepts of stoichiometry, and particularly the limiting reactant concept, in the workplace daily. In the practice of analytical chemistry, one makes use of an analytical method that relies upon a chemical reaction of an *analyte* (i.e., a chemical species present in a sample to be analyzed, for which concentration and other information is to be sought) with a suitable analytical reagent to generate a desired product, which yields a signal due to a change in a physical property (e.g., color, temperature, current, conductivity, etc.) of the product that is quantifiable and can be related to analyte concentration. The balanced chemical equation for the reaction must also be known. In a chemical analysis, the analyte is deliberately made the limiting reactant, with the analytical reagent added in excess, to ensure that **all** of the analyte reacts to yield the product and its signal, which in turn are proportional to the analyte concentration. The stoichiometric ratios among the analyte, analytical reagent, and product must be established for the analytical determination to yield reliable results.

Analytical chemistry makes use of chemical reactions that reach equilibrium. The Law of Mass Action (Baird, 1999) describes the relatively fixed ratio of product to reactant concentrations at the equilibrium state. For a generic chemical reaction described by a balanced equation, the Law of Mass Action is described in Equation 1:

$$aA\ (aq) + bB\ (aq) \rightleftharpoons cC\ (aq) + dD\ (aq) \qquad K = \frac{[C]^c[D]^d}{[A]^a[B]^b} \qquad (1)$$

In Equation 1, the uppercase and lowercase letters represent the reactants and products and their stoichiometric coefficients, respectively, the square brackets represent mole/L concentrations of the species at equilibrium, and K is the *equilibrium constant*, which is the numerical value of the product-to-reactant concentration ratio. The magnitude of the equilibrium constant K indicates the extent of conversion of reactants to products upon attainment of equilibrium. As K values are generally either greater than or less than unity, a K value of 10^{16} is considered very large and characteristic of a reaction that goes essentially to completion (i.e., the equilibrium favors the products). Conversely, $K = 10^{-5}$ represents a reaction in which there is partial formation of products and most of the reactants still intact (i.e., the equilibrium favors the reactants) (Brown et al., 2006). Metal-ion chelation reactions have values of K that are generally much greater than unity, indicating that such reactions proceed spontaneously, without energy assistance from outside (Harris, 2010)

Complexation of a metal ion M^{n+} with a coordinating ligand L, both in aqueous solution, proceeds sequentially in a manner analogous to that described by Equations 2-4:

$$M^{n+}\ (aq) + L\ (aq) \rightleftharpoons ML^{n+}\ (aq) \qquad K_{f1} = \frac{[ML^{n+}]}{[M^{n+}][L]} \tag{2}$$

$$ML^{n+}\ (aq) + L\ (aq) \rightleftharpoons ML_2^{n+}\ (aq) \qquad K_{f2} = \frac{[ML_2^{n+}]}{[ML^{n+}][L]} \tag{3}$$

$$ML_2^{n+}\ (aq) + L\ (aq) \rightleftharpoons ML_3^{n+}\ (aq) \qquad K_{f3} = \frac{[ML_3^{n+}]}{[ML_2^{n+}][L]} \tag{4}$$

Each step in the overall complexation process reaches equilibrium and thus has an associated equilibrium constant, K_f, the *formation* or *stability* constant, the magnitude of which denotes the strength or tightness of binding of M^{n+} by L (Butler, 1998). The stepwise coordination sequence described by Equations 2-4 may be described as well in terms of summary, or *overall*, formation constants, described by Equations 5–7, and denoted by the lowercase Greek β_x, in which x is the number of individual complex-forming reaction steps that contribute to the overall complexation reaction (Butler, 1998):

$$M^{n+}\ (aq) + L\ (aq) \rightleftharpoons ML^{n+}\ (aq) \qquad \beta_1 = \frac{[ML^{n+}]}{[M^{n+}][L]} \tag{5}$$

$$M^{n+}\ (aq) + 2\,L\ (aq) \rightleftharpoons ML_2^{n+}\ (aq) \qquad \beta_2 = \frac{[ML_2^{n+}]}{[M^{n+}][L]^2} \tag{6}$$

$$M^{n+}\ (aq) + 3\,L\ (aq) \rightleftharpoons ML_3^{n+}\ (aq) \qquad \beta_3 = \frac{[ML_3^{n+}]}{[M^{n+}][L]^3} \tag{7}$$

Ligands that are weak acids can undergo dissociation of their acidic hydrogens during metal-ion complexation, in a manner similar to that shown in Equations 8 and 9 for the diprotic weak acid Tiron (1,2-dihydroxybenzene-3,5-disulfonic acid disodium salt, Na_2H_2L) (Cheng et al., 1992):

$$H_2L^{2-}\ (aq) \rightleftharpoons H^+(aq) + HL^-\ (aq) \qquad K_{a1} = \frac{[H^+][HL^-]}{[H_2L^{2-}]} \tag{8}$$

$$HL^-\ (aq) \rightleftharpoons H^+(aq) + L^{2-}\ (aq) \qquad K_{a2} = \frac{[H^+][L^{2-}]}{[HL^-]} \tag{9}$$

The deprotonation steps occur sequentially, with each step possessing its own *acid dissociation* or *acid ionization* constant, K_a. K_a values are less than unity; the smaller the magnitude of K_a, the more difficult the acidic hydrogen is to ionize. Weak bases, on the other hand, can directly chelate a metal ion such as Fe^{2+}, and can also undergo protonation at low pH.

1.2 Spectrophotometric determinations of metal ions

One of the most established and widely used analytical methods employed by analytical chemists and many other technical professionals, for determination of a plethora of analytes in a wide variety of samples, is ultraviolet-visible spectrophotometry, also known as UV-visible spectrophotometry, UV-vis, spectrophotometry, or colorimetry. As this topic alone is immense in scope, and most readers are perhaps already familiar with spectrophotometry, the reader is referred to any number of references on this subject (Thomas, 1996; Skoog et al., 2007; Kellner, 1998). Most metal ions such as iron are weakly absorbing species that can be made very strongly absorbing via complexation of iron ions with an appropriate complexing agent, which is usually selective for a particular valence of iron (i.e., Fe^{2+} or Fe^{3+}) (McBryde, 1964; Stookey, 1970).

As with any analytical method, UV-visible spectrophotometry requires prior knowledge, e.g,, the stoichiometric ratio of metal ion to ligand, of the chemical reaction that occurs between the metal ion and its chelating ligand, equilibrium information such as formation constants, and the useful concentration range for determination of the metal analyte. Knowledge of the stoichiometry of the metal-ion complexation required for the spectrophotometric determination of a given metal ion guides the analyst in proper selection of the amount of ligand to use to ensure complete coordination of the metal ion analyte.

As this chapter will focus on the stoichiometric aspects of the spectrophotometric determination of iron (as Fe^{2+}) using the clinical iron-marking chelators Ferene S and Ferrozine, one needs to know about Beer's Law (Thomas, 1996; Skoog et al., 2007; Kellner, 1998; Harris, 2010), which is perhaps most familiar as

$$A = \varepsilon bC \tag{10}$$

The *molar* absorptivity (ε, in L mole^{-1} cm^{-1}), is a function of the wavelength used for absorbance measurements and the nature of the analyte (Harris, 2010); thus, it is actually a measure of the light-absorbing ability of the analyte in its absorbing form. The term b is the path length of the cuvet or sample container used for absorbance measurements. For the most sensitive results, the wavelength of maximum absorption (λ_{max}) should be used in a spectrophotometric analysis, to yield the maximum absorptivity possible.

1.3 Stoichiometry of metal ion chelates

Perhaps the best known and most widely used spectrophotometric method for studying metal-ion complex stoichiometry is the *method of continuous variations* (Harvey & Manning, 1950). Also known as the *Job method* (Job, 1928), it is best suited for metal-ion complex systems in which only one complex predominates. Additionally, the chelate in question must follow Beer's Law.

The Job method involves mixing aliquots of metal-ion (M) and ligand (L) solutions, with dilution to constant volume, to obtain solutions with a constant total concentration of metal ion (C_M) plus ligand (C_L), or $C_M + C_L$ = constant. A series of solutions of the chelate are prepared, with the ratios of M and L varied but the total concentration of each solution kept constant, as depicted in Figure 1. The absorbance of each solution in the series is measured at the maximum absorbing wavelength of the chelate (λ_{max}), followed by generation of a plot of corrected absorbance as a function of the mole fraction of L (X_L) in each solution. The maximum corrected absorbance in the continuous variations plot corresponds to the stoichiometric ratio M:L, which gives the chelate formula. The corrected absorbance is calculated according to Equation 11 (Harris, 2010):

$$A_{corr} = A_{meas} - A_M(1 - X_L) - A_L(X_L) \tag{11}$$

In Equation 11, A_{meas} is the measured absorbance of the solution, and A_M and A_L are the absorbances of the all-metal-ion and all-ligand solutions, respectively. X_L is simply the ratio of the moles of L to the total moles of (M + L), or X_L = moles L / total moles of M + L. The value of X_L at the apex of the Job plot represents the stoichiometry of the complex, e.g., when $X_L = 0.5$, the complex has a 1:1 M:L ratio.

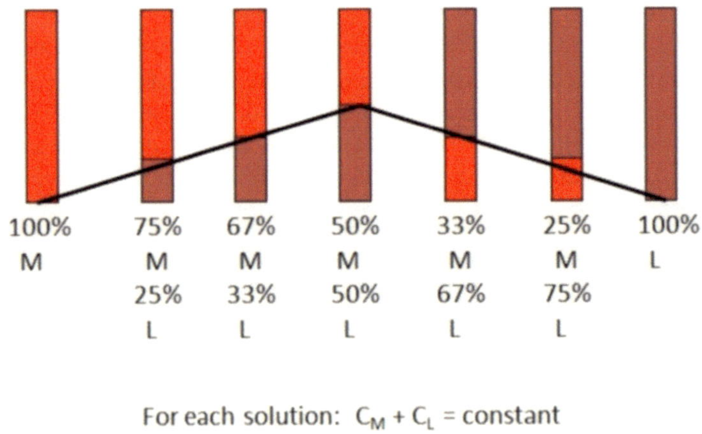

Fig. 1. Preparation of solutions of metal ion M and ligand L for a continuous variation experiment.

If equimolar solutions of M and L are used, calculation of X_L is then based on the volumes of stock M and stock L used in each solution. Again, the reader is referred to the published literature regarding the method of continuous variations (Harvey& Manning, 1950; Job, 1928; Harris, 2010; Vosburgh & Cooper, 1941; Foley & Anderson, 1948).

1.4 Formation constants of metal ion chelates

Formation constants for metal-ion complexes provide quantitative information on the extent of coordination of a metal ion M by a ligand L. Bjerrum and coworkers (Bjerrum, 1941; Bjerrum & Nielsen, 1948) have contributed immensely to the development and implementation of potentiometric and spectrophotometric techniques for determination of formation constants of a huge number of metal-ion complexes. Other analytical methods, e.g., NMR, have been employed for formation constant determinations (Irwin et al., 1996). In this chapter, the focus will be on the pH-based potentiometric and spectrophotometric methods for determination of the overall formation constant β_3 for the Ferene S and Ferrozine chelates of iron(II).

The Bjerrum pH-spectrophotometric method (Billo, 2001) utilizes low values of pH to promote only partial complexation and thus permits calculation of equilibrium concentrations of the chelate, free metal ion, and free ligand, and subsequently, the overall formation constant. The procedure involves preparation of a series of solutions, all of the same volume and containing the same concentrations of metal ion and ligand, but at different low values of pH. The absorbance of each solution is measured at the wavelength of maximum absorption (λ_{max}) for the chelate (ML_n), and the chelate concentration in each solution is calculated from Beer's Law:

$$[ML_n] = \frac{A_{ML_n}}{\varepsilon_{ML_n} b} \quad (12)$$

From here, the equilibrium concentrations of free M ([M]) and free L in all its forms at the selected pH ([L′]) are calculated according to Equations 13 and 14:

$$[M] = C_M - [ML_n] \quad (13)$$

$$[L'] = C_{L'} - n[ML_n] \quad (14)$$

From the K_a of the ligand and the pH (to yield $[H^+]$), the concentration of free ligand in its unprotonated form ([L]) is calculated from the fraction of free L to free L′ in solution (i.e., $\alpha_L = [L]/[L']$). For a monoprotic weak acid or a weak monobase, α_L is described by Equation 15.

$$\alpha_L = \frac{K_a}{K_a + [H^+]} \quad (15)$$

The concentration of free L is then calculated by Equation 16:

$$[L] = \alpha_L [L'] \quad (16)$$

Having now obtained [M], [L], and $[ML_n]$, one can calculate the overall formation constant, β_n, for the complexation reaction

$$M\,(aq) + n\,L\,(aq) \rightleftharpoons ML_n\,(aq) \quad (17)$$

by use of its β_n expression:

$$\beta_n = \frac{[ML_n]}{[M][L]^n} \quad (18)$$

The Bjerrum pH-potentiometric method makes use of a pH titration of a solution containing known concentrations of metal ion M, ligand L, and an acid. If the ligand is a weak acid, then no additional acid is necessary. If the ligand is a weak base, then either a stoichiometric amount of strong acid (e.g., HCl) is added, or the conjugate acid of the weak base ligand is used. Details on the procedures used in this type of formation constant determination are obtainable from the published literature (Rossotti & Rossotti, 1961; Martell & Motekaitis,

1992). The calculations involved in obtaining formation constants (usually stepwise formation constants, or K_f values) for the complex ML_n are extensive and involved. The reader is referred to appropriate texts on the pH-potentiometric method and its variations (Rossotti & Rossotti, 1961; Martell & Motekaitis, 1992).

1.5 The ligands Ferene S and Ferrozine in the spectrophotometric determination of iron, and their role as iron markers in clinical analysis

Two organic molecules that are known chelating agents for iron in its divalent state, Ferene S and Ferrozine, have been selected by the authors for a study of the effects of the iron-to-ligand ratio on the linearity of calibration curves produced for the spectrophotometric determination of iron by these two chelators, and on the determination of formation constants for the iron chelates of the two ligands.

Ferene S (3-(2-pyridyl)-5,6-difurylsulfonic acid-1,2,4-triazine disodium salt, Figure 2a) and Ferrozine (3-(2-pyridyl)-5,6-bis(4-phenylsulfonic acid)-1,2,4-triazine disodium salt, Figure 2b) are members of a class of pyridyl- and triazine-containing molecules referred to as "ferroins" due to their renowned capacity to bind with iron in its divalent oxidation state (Fe^{2+}) (Almog et al., 1996). Other members of this class of well-known iron(II) chelators include 1,10-phenanthroline, 2,2′-bipyridine, and 2,4,6-tripyridyl-1,3,5-triazine (TPTZ). Both Ferene S and Ferrozine are structurally analogous except for the different groups attached to the 5- and 6- positions on the triazine ring. The iron(II) chelates of both ligands possess high molar absorptivities – 3.55×10^4 L mole^{-1} cm^{-1} (λ_{max} = 593 nm) for Fe(II)-Ferene S (Higgins, 1981), and 2.79×10^4 L mole^{-1} cm^{-1} (λ_{max} = 562 nm) for Fe(II)-Ferrozine (Stookey, 1970) – making the two ligands ideal for sub-µg-per-mL iron determinations, particularly Ferene S. The UV-vis spectra of the Fe(II) chelates of Ferene S and Ferrozine are shown in Figure 3. Neither Ferene S nor Ferrozine absorbs in the visible region. Both compounds are sulfonated derivatives of their parent ferroins, making both molecules water-soluble and thus desirable for analytical applications involving quantitation of iron in aqueous media, and they are commercially available from major chemicals suppliers.

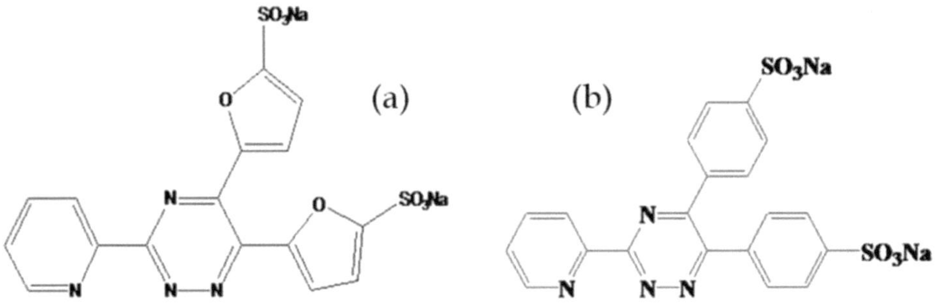

Fig. 2. The iron(II)-chelating ferroin-type ligands (a) Ferene S and (b) Ferrozine.

Ferene S and Ferrozine are strong, effective, and highly selective chelators for iron as the divalent cation Fe^{2+}. Both molecules, particularly Ferene S, are well known iron markers in clinical determinations of iron in blood cells, serum, and a host of biological and biomedical sample types. The first account of the use of Ferene S as an iron(II) chelating agent for determination of iron in serum was published in 1981 (Higgins, 1981), followed by papers on the analytical utility of Ferene S (Artiss et al., 1981) and its unsulfonated analogue, Ferene Triazine (Smith et al., 1984), for determination of serum iron. More recent papers (Camberlein et al., 2010) indicate that Ferene S is still widely used in biological iron determinations. A paper describing application of flow-injection spectrophotometry to the determination of aluminum and iron in potable and treated waters, using Ferene S for determination of iron, shows an environmental application of Ferene S (Benson & Worsfold, 1993). There is also a paper describing the pedagogical use of a number of ferroin ligands, Ferene S and Ferrozine among them, for teaching Beer's Law in analytical chemistry (Stauffer, 2007).

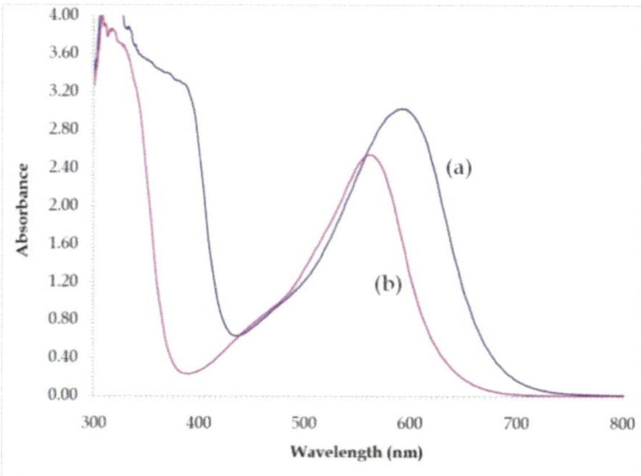

Fig. 3. The UV-visible spectra of (a) $Fe(Ferene\ S)_3^{2+}$, 1.00×10^{-4} mol L^{-1}, and (b) $Fe(Ferrozine)_3^{2+}$, 1.00×10^{-4} mol L^{-1}.

Ferrozine has experienced extensive application inside and outside the realm of biological/biomedical analysis. Ferrozine was introduced in 1970 as a potential Fe(II) chelator, and was first used extensively for determinations of iron in serum (Carter, 1971). Other applications over the years have included hemoglobin (Riemer et al., 2004), wine (Argyri et al., 2006), plants (Yamamoto et al., 2010), foods (Alexandropoulou et al., 2006), natural waters (Viollier et al., 2000), and a host of other sample types. Ferrozine is a trade name of the Hach Chemical Company and was originally applied to iron determinations in water (Stookey, 1970).

1.6 Purpose and aims of this chapter

The purpose of this chapter is to present and emphasize the role of the metal ion as the limiting reactant in spectrophotometric determinations of metal ion analytes. For our studies of this topic, the ligands Ferene S and Ferrozine were chosen for their ability to chelate divalent iron ions (Fe(II)) strongly and selectively as well as their prevalent use as iron markers in clinical analysis. In this chapter, the effect of the concentration ratio of Fe(II) to ligand on the Beer's Law behavior of calibration curves for the determination of iron will be presented and discussed. Along with considerations of Fe(II):ligand ratio effects on calibration curves, the stoichiometries of the Ferene S and Ferrozine chelates of Fe(II) will be examined in light of the results obtained from the calibration curve study. This chapter will explore our attempts to determine formation constants for the Fe(II)-Ferene S and Fe(II)-

Ferrozine chelates by spectrophotometry and potentiometry, and to gain insights into the binding of Fe(II) by each of the two ligands. The chapter will conclude with presentation and discussion of an application of Ferene S to the spectrophotometric determination of iron outside the realm of clinical analysis, e.g., in abandoned mine drainage (AMD) and other natural waters.

2. Experimental section

2.1 Equipment, reagents, solutions

2.1.1 Equipment and reagents

Spectral measurements were made with a Hitachi Model U-3010 scanning double-beam UV-visible spectrophotometer (Hitachi High Technologies America, San Diego, CA, USA) and 1.00-cm quartz cuvets (Fisher Scientific, Inc., Pittsburgh, PA, USA), a battery-operated WPA Colourwave 7500B eight-filter colorimeter and 1.00-cm plastic cuvets (Biochrom, Ltd., Cambridge, UK), and a Vernier SpectroVis diode-array spectrophotometer plus battery-operated LabQuest microprocessor with software (for operation of the SpectroVis spectrophotometer), and 1.00-cm plastic cuvets (Vernier Software & Technology, Beaverton, OR, USA). A Perkin-Elmer AAnalyst 100 flame atomic absorption spectrophotometer with air-acetylene flame, 10-cm single-slot burner head, and Lumina iron hollow cathode lamp Model No. N3050126 (Perkin-Elmer Corporation, Norwalk, CT, USA), was used for verification of total iron concentration in some field determinations of iron. Adjustments of pH for optimum color formation of the Fe^{2+}-Ferene S and Fe^{2+}-Ferrozine chelate solutions, and for carrying out pH titrations of ligand and chelate solutions, were made with an Oakton pHTestr 30 handheld combination electrode pH meter with built-in temperature probe (Fisher Scientific, Inc.). Temperature control for the spectrophotometric and potentiometric formation constant experiments was achieved using an Isotemp Model 2340 programmable constant temperature water bath (Fisher Scientific, Inc.).

Ferene S (3-(2-pyridyl)-5,6-difurylsulfonic acid-1,2,4-triazine disodium salt) and Ferrozine (3-(2-pyridyl)-5,6-bis(4-phenylsulfonic acid)-1,2,4-triazine disodium salt) were purchased from GFS Chemicals, Inc. (Powell, OH, USA) and Sigma-Aldrich (St. Louis, MO, USA) and used without further purification. Other reagents include hydroquinone ($C_4H_6O_2$, reducing agent for Fe^{3+}), sodium acetate trihydrate ($NaC_2H_3O_2 \cdot 3H_2O$, pH buffering agent), iron(II) ammonium sulfate hexahydrate ($Fe(NH_4)_2(SO_4)_2 \cdot 6H_2O$), potassium hydrogen phthalate ($KHC_8H_4O_4$), concentrated hydrochloric acid (12 mole HCl L^{-1}), sodium hydroxide (NaOH), 1000 mg Fe L^{-1} stock standard solution, and NIST-traceable pH 5.00 buffer solution (Fisher Scientific, Inc.).

2.1.2 Solution preparation

Aqueous solutions of hydroquinone were prepared at 2-3% (w/v) concentration. Aqueous solutions of sodium acetate were prepared at 2.0 mole $NaC_2H_3O_2$ L^{-1} concentration. Dilute (1 mole L^{-1}) solutions of HCl and NaOH were prepared from reagent grade concentrated HCl and NaOH pellets, respectively. Solutions of the water-soluble Ferene S and Ferrozine were easily prepared. Aqueous stock solutions of Ferene S and Ferrozine were prepared at concentrations between 5.00 x 10^{-3} to 5.00 x 10^{-2} mole ligand L^{-1}. Standard aqueous Fe stock solutions (1000 mg Fe L^{-1} or 1.79 x 10^{-2} mole Fe L^{-1}, Fisher Scientific, Inc.) were used to prepare aqueous Fe working standard solutions (100 mg Fe L^{-1} or 1.79 x 10^{-3} mole Fe L^{-1}), according to established procedures (McBride, 1980). Calibration standards ranging from 0.05 - 10 mg Fe L^{-1} (or approximately 10^{-6} - 10^{-4} mole Fe L^{-1}) were prepared from the working standard. The 1 mole L^{-1} NaOH titrant solution for the pH titrations of the ligands and their Fe(II) chelates was standardized against potassium hydrogen phthalate.

2.2 Experimental procedures

2.2.1 Calibration curve study for Fe(II)-Ferene S and Fe(II)-Ferrozine chelates

A series of six sets of calibration solutions, each containing at least one reagent blank and ten Fe-containing calibration solutions (2.00 x10^{-6}, 4.00 x10^{-6}, 6.00 x10^{-6}, 8.00 x10^{-6}, 1.00 x10^{-5}, 2.00 x10^{-5}, 4.00 x10^{-5}, 6.00 x10^{-5}, 8.00 x10^{-5}, 1.00 x10^{-4} mole Fe L^{-1}), were prepared according to a series of steps common to the colorimetric determination of iron by ferroin ligands (McBride, 1980). These steps are: (1) pipetting an appropriate aliquot of Fe working standard into a small (30-60 mL) cup, beaker, or equivalent containing a small (5-10 mL) amount of distilled or deionized water; (2) pipetting fixed aliquots of ligand (1.00 mL of Ferene S or Ferrozine) solution, Fe(III) reducing agent (hydroquinone, 1.00 mL) solution, and buffering (sodium acetate, 2.00 mL) solution; (3) pH adjustment of the analysis solution to pH 5.0 ± 0.05 for optimum color formation (for both Ferene S and Ferrozine chelates of Fe(II)); (4) quantitative transfer of the analysis solution to a small (e.g., 25-mL) volumetric flask and dilution to volume, followed by spectrophotometric determination of iron, with absorbance measurements at 591, 593, and 595 nm (vs. H_2O) for the Fe(II)-Ferene S chelate, and 560, 562, and 564 nm (vs. H_2O) for the Fe(II)-ferrozine chelate. For each set of calibration solutions, the ligand concentration was based on the highest Fe concentration in the set (i.e., 1.00 x 10^{-4} mole Fe L^{-1}), increased from one set to the next, and kept constant throughout each calibration solutions set. The ratio of Fe to ligand for each calibration set is given in Table 1.

Calibration Solution Set Number	Highest Fe Concentration in Set (mole Fe L^{-1})	Concentration of Ligand Used in Set (mole ligand L^{-1})	Ratio of Fe to Ligand
1	1.00 x 10^{-4}	5.00 x 10^{-5}	1 : 0.5
2	1.00 x 10^{-4}	1.00 x 10^{-4}	1 : 1
3	1.00 x 10^{-4}	2.00 x 10^{-4}	1 : 2
4	1.00 x 10^{-4}	5.00 x 10^{-4}	1 : 5
5	1.00 x 10^{-4}	1.00 x 10^{-3}	1 : 10
6	1.00 x 10^{-4}	2.00 x 10^{-3}	1 : 20

Table 1. Ratios of Fe:ligand used in the calibration curve experiments involving the Ferene S and Ferrozine chelates of Fe(II). The ratio is based upon the highest Fe concentration in the set and the ligand concentration (which is kept constant in all the solutions in the set).

For each calibration set, an absorbance-concentration plot was generated, and the Beer's Law region was subjected to linear regression to obtain the calibration slope and the molar absorptivity (ε_λ). The absorbance data used were those measured at 593 nm (vs. H_2O) for the Fe(II)-Ferene S chelate, and at 562 nm (vs. H_2O) for the Fe(II)-Ferrozine chelate.

Absorption spectra of Ferene S and Ferrozine, and their Fe(II) chelates, were measured from 300-800 nm (vs. H_2O) using the Hitachi U-3010 spectrophotometer.

2.2.2 Stoichiometries of Fe(II)-Ferene S and Fe(II)-Ferrozine chelates

The method of continuous variations was employed for determination of the stoichiometries of the two Fe(II) chelates. For each chelate, three series of solutions, of total concentrations (Fe(II) + ligand) of 5.00-6.00 x 10^{-5}, 1.00 x 10^{-4}, and 2.50 x 10^{-4} mol L^{-1} and containing from 11 to 15 solutions each, were prepared according to the common steps outlined in section 2.2.1 and analyzed for Fe. In each series, the moles of Fe and ligand were varied in accordance with the method of continuous variations while keeping the total moles of all solutions in the series constant. The measured absorbances (at 593 nm vs. H_2O for Fe(II)-Ferene S and 562 nm vs. H_2O for Fe(II)-Ferrozine) were corrected as recommended by the Job method, and the mole fraction of ligand (X_L) calculated for each solution in the series. The corrected absorbances were plotted as a function of X_L, and the Fe:ligand ratio for the chelates determined from the apex of each plot (Stauffer, 2007).

2.2.3 Determination of K_a for conjugate acids of Ferene S and Ferrozine

The determination of acid dissociation constants (K_a) for Ferene S and Ferrozine was performed by manual pH titration. For each ligand, a 50.00-mL titration solution containing 0.01 mole ligand L^{-1} and 0.10 mole KCl L^{-1} to maintain constant ionic strength was prepared and transferred to a beaker, which was placed in a constant-temperature water bath at 20°C and allowed to stand for several minutes before the titration began. Titration of Ferrozine was carried out using the monosodium salt; titration of Ferene S was performed in the presence of a mole equivalent of HCl (per mole of Ferene S) added to the titration solution before dilution to volume. The titration solution was stirred manually (glass stirring rod) for at least 5 seconds after addition of each increment of standard NaOH, followed by measurement of the solution pH (no stirring) with a calibrated Oakton pHTestr 30 handheld pH meter, with combination glass electrode. The titration was carried out from the initial solution pH (usually pH 2.0-3.0) to pH 11.5-12.0. Between 60-100 data points were collected for each titration. The pK_a of each ligand was determined graphically (Harris, 2010).

2.2.4 Determination of formation constants for Fe(II)-Ferene S and Fe(II)-Ferrozine chelates

Both spectrophotometric and potentiometric methods (Billo, 2001; Martell & Motekaitis, 1992; Rossotti & Rossotti, 1961) were employed for the determination of the overall formation constant (β_3) for the Fe(II)-Ferene S and Fe(II)-Ferrozine chelates.

For the spectrophotometric experiments, a series of solutions containing known, fixed concentrations of Fe(II) and ligand were prepared according to the common protocol given in section 2.2.1, except that no sodium acetate solution was added, and the pH of the solutions in the series ranged from 1.20 to 2.80 via adjustment with dilute HCl and NaOH. The solutions were placed in a constant-temperature bath at 20°C for 30-60 minutes prior to measuring the absorbance of each solution (593 nm vs. H_2O for Fe(II)-Ferene S and 562 nm vs. H_2O for Fe(II)-Ferrozine). For the Fe(II)-Ferene S chelate, four series of 5-11 solutions, ranging in pH from 1.20-2.80, and with each solution containing 2.00 x 10^{-5} mole Fe(II) L^{-1}, were prepared and analyzed for Fe in the manner just described. The Fe(II):Ferene S concentration ratios in the four series were 1:1, 1:4, 1:5, and 1:10, respectively. For the Fe(II)-Ferrozine chelate, two series made up of 7-11 solutions with the same Fe(II) concentration in each solution, the same pH ranges, and with 1:1, 1:4, 1:5, and 1:10 Fe(II):Ferrozine ratios, were prepared and analyzed for Fe in the aforementioned manner.

For the potentiometric experiments, 50.00-mL titration solutions containing 1:1, 1:2, 1:3, and 1:4 ratios of Fe(II):Ferene S, in which the Fe(II) concentration was 5 x 10^{-3} mol L^{-1} and which were prepared in a manner analogous to that described in section 2.2.3, were titrated with standard 1 mole NaOH L^{-1} titrant solution and measured for pH in the same manner as described in section 2.2.3. In the titrations involving Ferene S, one mole equivalent of HCl was added for every mole of Ferene S in the titration mixture. For the titrations involving Ferrozine, Fe(II):ligand ratios of 1:2 and 1:4 were used, and the Fe(II) concentration was kept at 1.88 x 10^{-4} mol L^{-1} in both experiments.

2.2.5 Applications of Ferene S to the determination of iron in natural waters

Samples of abandoned mine drainage (AMD) and other types of natural waters were analyzed for total Fe (as Fe(II)) by the spectrophotometric Ferene S method, according to the common protocol described earlier in section 2.2.1. Water samples that contained suspended solids or coarser debris were filtered by established procedures (Stauffer, 2007; Stauffer et al., 2007). If necessary, samples were digested by traditional wet ashing or microwave digestion (Eperesi et al., 2010); the digestion step was, in the bulk of determinations, unnecessary.

AMD samples that were investigated for Fe(II)/Fe(III) speciation were analyzed for Fe, as Fe(II) and Fe(III), by the spectrophotometric Ferene S method, in a somewhat different manner. Between 50-200 μL of water sample were used for this determination, along with 80.0 μL of 0.01-0.05 mole Ferene S L^{-1} solution and 80.0 μL of 2-3% (w/v) hydroquinone solution. An aliquot of pH 5.00 buffer solution (KHP/NaOH), ranging from 1640-1790 μL, was selected to bring the total volume of the analysis solution to 2000 μL (2.000 mL). The color-forming reaction was carried out in a 1.00-cm plastic cuvet, with calibrated adjustable-volume micropipettors used for transfer of solution and sample aliquots to the cuvet. Absorbance measurements were made at 590 nm (vs. H_2O) with a WPA Colourwave 7500B colorimeter, or at 593 nm (vs. H_2O) with a Vernier SpectroVis diode-array spectrophotometer, operated in kinetics mode. Once the desired sample volume was selected, the appropriate volume of pH 5.00 buffer solution was added first, followed by the Ferene S solution aliquot and then the sample aliquot. At this point, the solution volume in the cuvet was 1.920 mL. Upon addition of the sample to the cuvet, with brief (2-3 seconds) stirring, absorbance measurements were initiated and recorded at a predetermined time interval throughout the course of the determination. When the absorbance began to plateau after an initial increase, hydroquinone solution was added to the cuvet (with brief stirring) to reduce Fe(III) to Fe(II). Depending on the amount of Fe(III) present in the sample, an additional absorbance increase occurred, with subsequent leveling of absorbance to a fairly constant value. All recorded absorbances were corrected to a total volume of 2.000 mL for the Fe determination, with an average corrected absorbance ($A_{corr,1}$) calculated from the first plateau (due to Fe(II)) and one ($A_{corr,2}$) calculated from the second plateau (due to total Fe).

Blanks and calibration standards were analyzed for Fe in the same manner. The calibration factor obtained was expressed in terms of the total Fe concentration in the standard as Fe(II). The concentrations of Fe(II) and total Fe were determined from $A_{corr,1}$ and $A_{corr,2}$, respectively. The concentration of Fe(III) was determined by the difference between the total Fe and Fe(II) concentrations.

2.3 Data manipulations

Data and results from the calibration curve, stoichiometry, formation constant, and Ferene S application studies were processed using Microsoft® Excel™.

3. Results and discussion

3.1 Study of calibration curves for iron(II) chelates of Ferene S and Ferrozine

The effect of varying Fe:ligand ratios on the Beer's Law behavior of calibration curves for colorimetric determination of Fe using Ferene S and Ferrozine is depicted by Figures 4a and 4b, respectively. For each Fe(II) complex, six sets of calibration solutions, composed of one blank and ten Fe standard solutions (2.00×10^{-6} to 1.00×10^{-4} mol Fe^{2+} L^{-1} concentrations) were prepared, and their absorbances measured, according to the common protocols outlined in section 2.2.1. The stated ratio of Fe(II) to ligand is the ratio of the concentration of the highest Fe(II) standard in the series (1.00×10^{-4} mol Fe^{2+} L^{-1}, for all six calibration sets) to the concentration of ligand used for the particular set (refer to Table 1). From Figures 4a and 4b, the Beer's Law region for each calibration set is readily apparent. For both iron(II) chelates, the trends are almost identical, with the calibration set possessing the lowest ligand concentration exhibiting a shortened Beer's Law range in concentration to 1.00×10^{-5} mol Fe^{2+} L^{-1}, and the set with the highest ligand concentration exhibiting linearity of absorbance with Fe(II) concentration nearly throughout the entire Fe(II) concentration range used for our studies. It becomes apparent that for equimolar concentrations of Fe(II) and ligand, the ligand, and not the analyte iron, becomes the limiting reactant at higher iron concentrations in the calibration scheme.

The calibration results shown in Figures 4a and 4b for Fe(II)-Ferene S and Fe(II)-Ferrozine, respectively, are based on absorbance measurements at 593 nm for the Ferene S chelate and at 562 nm for the Ferrozine chelate. Calibration slopes (Table 2) are the product of molar absorptivity and cuvet path length (1.00 cm), and ranged from 3.12×10^4 to 3.34×10^4 L (mol Fe^{2+})$^{-1}$ for Fe(II)-Ferene S, and from 2.54×10^4 to 2.64×10^4 L (mol Fe^{2+})$^{-1}$ for Fe(II)-Ferrozine. The R^2 and standard error of the estimate were greater than 0.999 and less than 0.009, respectively, indicating excellent linearity of the Beer's Law regions for each calibration set. The lower limit of the Beer's Law concentration range (Table 2) for each set is an estimated limit of detection (LOD), or minimum Fe concentration detectable by the colorimetric method, and is calculated by Equation 19 (Miller & Miller, 1993):

$$LOD = 3s_{blk}/m_{calib} \tag{19}$$

where s_{blk} is the standard deviation of the blank (i.e., the standard deviation of the y intercept of the Beer's Law curve), m_{calib} is the calibration slope, and the factor of 3 corresponds to the 99% confidence level (Miller & Miller, 1993).

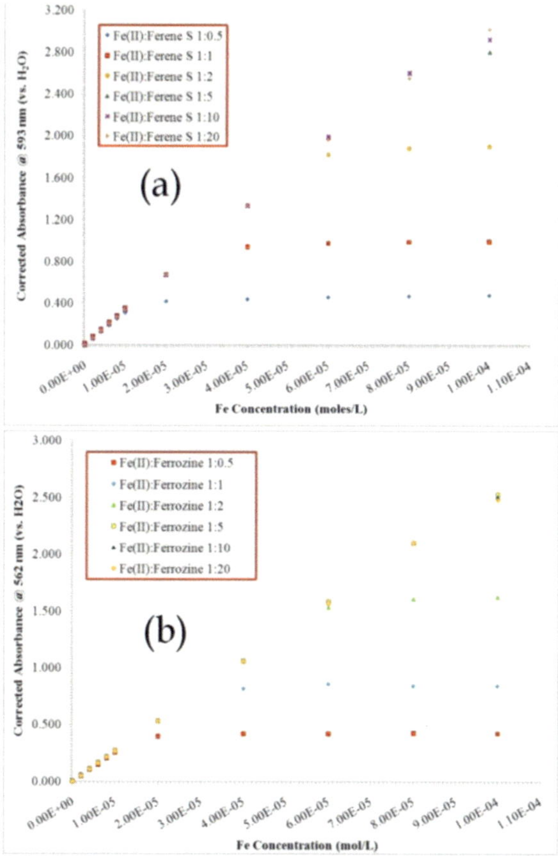

Fig. 4. Calibration curves for spectrophotometric determination of Fe(II) using (a) Ferene S and (b) Ferrozine at varying ratios of Fe(II) to ligand.

Fe(II):Ligand Ratio	Calibration Slope Fe(II)-Ferene S (L (mol Fe)$^{-1}$)	Beer's Law Conc. Range (mol Fe L^{-1})	Calibration Slope Fe(II)-Ferrozine (L (mol Fe)$^{-1}$)	Beer's Law Conc. Range (mol Fe L^{-1})
1 : 0.5	3.12×10^4	2.57×10^{-7} – 1.00×10^{-5}	2.54×10^4	2.21×10^{-7} – 1.00×10^{-5}
1 : 1	3.30×10^4	1.29×10^{-7} – 2.00×10^{-5}	2.59×10^4	1.94×10^{-7} – 2.00×10^{-5}
1 : 2	3.34×10^4	1.29×10^{-7} – 4.00×10^{-5}	2.63×10^4	1.97×10^{-7} – 4.00×10^{-5}
1 : 5	3.32×10^4	1.63×10^{-7} – 6.00×10^{-5}	2.64×10^4	1.60×10^{-7} – 6.00×10^{-5}
1 : 10	3.31×10^4	1.10×10^{-7} – 6.00×10^{-5}	2.63×10^4	2.40×10^{-7} – 8.00×10^{-5}
1 : 20	$3. 28 \times 10^4$	3.86×10^{-7} – 6.00×10^{-5}	2.62×10^4	2.52×10^{-7} – 8.00×10^{-5}

Table 2. Calibration slopes (L (mol Fe)$^{-1}$) and corresponding Beer's Law concentration ranges (mol Fe L^{-1}) for the calibration plots for Fe(II)-Ferene S (Figure 4a) and Fe(II)-Ferrozine (Figure 4b).

3.2 Stoichiometries of the iron(II) chelates of Ferene S and Ferrozine by the method of continuous variations

The stoichiometries of the iron(II) chelates of Ferene S and Ferrozine were investigated by the method of continuous variations (a.k.a. Job method) according to the procedure described in section 2.2.2, and are illustrated by the Job plots of Figures 5a and 5b for Fe(II)-Ferene S and Fe(II)-Ferrozine, respectively. For all six Job plots, the Fe(II):ligand ratio corresponding to the apex of each plot is 1:3 ($X_L = 0.75$) and is readily apparent from the shape of each plot. Thus, the stoichiometry of Fe(II)-Ferene S and Fe(II)-Ferrozine is 1:3 for each chelate, indicating compositional formulae of Fe(Ferene S)$_3^{2+}$ and Fe(Ferrozine)$_3^{2+}$. The 1:3 stoichiometry found in our studies agrees with published findings for the Ferrozine chelate (Gibbs, 1976) and those for the unsulfonated analogue of Ferene S (Smith et al., 1984).

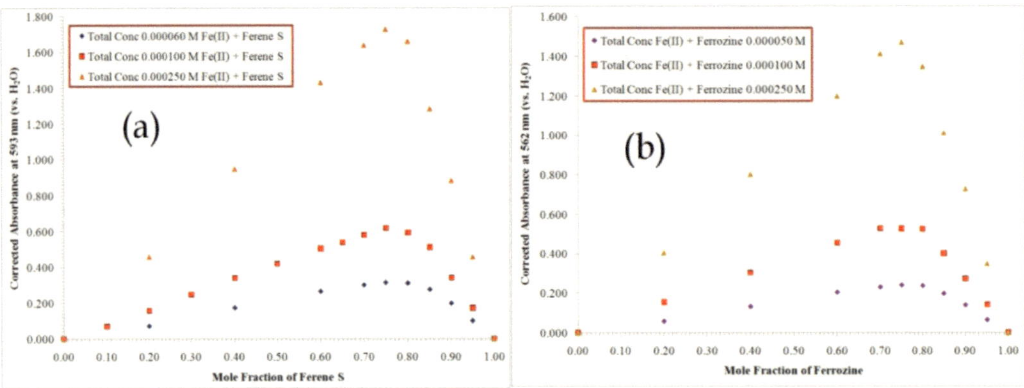

Fig. 5. Continuous variation plots for (a) Fe(Ferene S)$_3^{2+}$ and (b) Fe(Ferrozine)$_3^{2+}$, at three different total concentrations of Fe(II) + ligand (in mol L^{-1}).

The degree of sharpness at the apex of a continuous variations plot gives a qualitative estimate of the tightness of binding of the metal ion by the ligand in a complex, and can also be used for determination of an overall formation constant for the complex if there is sufficient rounding at the apex (Harris, 2010). The lower-concentration Job plots shown in Figures 5a and 5b appear quite rounded at their apices relative to the highest-concentration Job plots. Upon closer inspection of each Job plot individually, it was found that the lower-concentration plots are much sharper than expected; the roundedness observed in Figures 5a and 5b may simply be a result of plotting together three continuous variations plots of differing total concentrations. Yet, in the Job plots of Figures 5a and 5b, there is slight rounding at the apex evident in all of them, which may be characteristic of the chelates themselves or due to the concentrations of Fe(II) and ligand employed in these experiments. Nonetheless, the sharp apices of the continuous variation plots of Figures 5a and 5b indicate strong coordination of Fe^{2+} by Ferene S and Ferrozine. The results obtained for Fe(Ferene S)$_3^{2+}$ and Fe(Ferrozine)$_3^{2+}$ appear to be typical of stoichiometric Fe(II):ligand ratios for other ferroins, e.g. 1,10-phenanthroline and 2,2′-bipyridine (Stauffer, 2007 and references cited therein).

3.3 Determination of formation constants for the chelates of Ferene S and Ferrozine with iron(II)

Prior to determination of formation constants for the Fe(II) chelates of Ferene S and Ferrozine, determination of the pK_a of each ligand was carried out by pH titration, according to the procedure described in section 2.2.3, followed by graphical analysis of the generated titration curves to obtain the pK_a of each ligand from the midpoint of the buffer region (Harris, 2010). The pK_a values of Ferene S and Ferrozine were found to be 3.13 and 3.21, respectively. Our experimental pK_a for Ferrozine is in fairly good agreement with the published value (Thompsen & Mottola, 1984). Attempts to locate a published pK_a for Ferene S were unsuccessful; the experimental pK_a for Ferene S appears to be a reasonable one, in view of the structural similarities between Ferene S and Ferrozine.

Potentiometric determination of formation constants for $Fe(Ferene\ S)_3^{2+}$ and $Fe(Ferrozine)_3^{2+}$ proved exceedingly difficult; thus, values of the overall formation constants (β_3) of both chelates were determined spectrophotometrically, as described in sections 1.4 and 2.2.4. The $\log_{10}\beta_3$ values ranged from 16.30 to 16.82 (mean = 16.45 ± 0.25, %RSD = 1.5) for $Fe(Ferene\ S)_3^{2+}$, and from 17.24 to 18.01 (mean = 17.46 ± 0.37, %RSD = 2.1) for $Fe(Ferrozine)_3^{2+}$. The average $\log_{10}\beta_3$ results indicate that β_3 is not affected by changes in ligand concentration, as predicted by LeChatelier's Principle. The results also indicate that Ferrozine chelates Fe(II) more tightly than Ferene S. The experimental $\log_{10}\beta_3$ obtained for Ferrozine differs from a published value (Thompsen & Mottola, 1984) by about 2 units; the difference is most likely due to any number of experimental factors, such as temperature control, instrument problems, or differences in the methods for determination of $\log_{10}\beta_3$. Attempts to find a published value for comparison with our experimental $\log_{10}\beta_3$ for $Fe(Ferene\ S)_3^{2+}$ were unsuccessful. Again, the structural similarities between Ferene S and Ferrozine suggest that the overall formation constant for $Fe(Ferene\ S)_3^{2+}$ may be reasonable.

Figures 6a and 6b are the absorbance-pH curves ("formation curves") associated with the spectrophotometric determination of β_3 for $Fe(Ferene\ S)_3^{2+}$ and $Fe(Ferrozine)_3^{2+}$ and, as such, illustrate the formation of the two chelates at low pH, at which partial complexation is expected to occur due to competition between Fe^{2+} and H^+ for the binding site on the ligand. For $Fe(Ferene\ S)_3^{2+}$ and $Fe(Ferrozine)_3^{2+}$, a predicted absorbance for complete chelation was calculated using Beer's Law and a cuvet path length of 1.00 cm and a Fe(II) concentration of 2.00×10^{-5} mol L^{-1}. This absorbance is indicated in Figures 6a and 6b by a dashed line. The results provided by Figures 6a and 6b suggest that while β_3 does not appreciably change due to increasing ligand concentration, the extent of complexation does. This trend is observed for both $Fe(Ferene\ S)_3^{2+}$ and $Fe(Ferrozine)_3^{2+}$, and even more so for $Fe(Ferrozine)_3^{2+}$, as its formation curves at higher Ferrozine concentrations are closer together near the predicted absorbance for complete chelation than are the formation curves for $Fe(Ferene\ S)_3^{2+}$. The 1:10 Fe(II):Ferrozine formation curve in particular shows that, as pH increases beyond a value of 2.00, Fe(II) is essentially completely chelated by Ferrozine. A similar trend is observed for the 1:10 Fe(II):Ferene S formation curve. For both chelates, the 1:1 Fe(II):ligand formation curves are expected to give much lower absorbances, as the ligand now becomes the limiting reactant and only partial complexation occurs. It was noted that, even for the 1:1 Fe(II):ligand experiments, the indigo color of $Fe(Ferene\ S)_3^{2+}$ and the magenta color of $Fe(Ferrozine)_3^{2+}$ are readily formed and apparent. This suggests tight binding of Fe(II) by the ligands and a tendency to preferentially form $Fe(Ferene\ S)_3^{2+}$ and

Fe(Ferrozine)$_3^{2+}$, even at low pH. Additionally, a data point each in the 1:1 and 1:10 Fe(II):Ferrozine formation curves in Figure 6b is anomalous and is outside the trend exhibited by the other data points in the curve. This may be due to a pipetting error for either the stock Fe^{2+} or Ferrozine solutions.

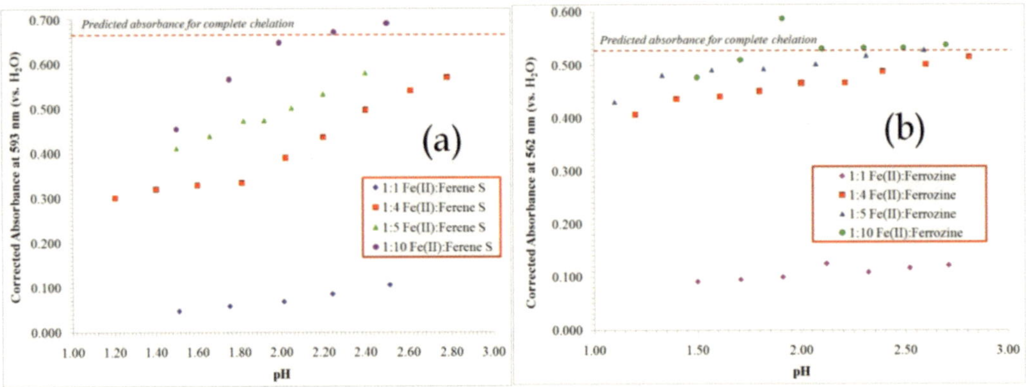

Fig. 6. Absorbance-pH formation curves for the spectrophotometric determination of the overall formation constant β_3 for (a) Fe(Ferene S)$_3^{2+}$ and (b) Fe(Ferrozine)$_3^{2+}$ at varying Fe(II):ligand ratios.

Even though the potentiometric determination of formation constants was unsuccessful, the pH titrations of Fe(Ferene S)$_3^{2+}$ and Fe(Ferrozine)$_3^{2+}$ at different ratios of Fe(II) to ligand, performed as described in section 2.2.4, yielded useful information toward understanding the complexation of Fe(II) by Ferene S and Ferrozine. Figures 7a and 7b depict the pH-vs.-titrant volume curves generated by titration of the chelates with standard 1 mol NaOH L^{-1} titrant, at Fe(II):ligand ratios of 1:1 through 1:4 for Fe(Ferene S)$_3^{2+}$, and ratios of 1:2 and 1:4 for Fe(Ferrozine)$_3^{2+}$. At the lower ratios of Fe(II) to ligand, a slight stepwise curve was obtained for Fe(Ferene S)$_3^{2+}$, and a curve with a large single equivalence point inflection, similar to that for a strong acid-strong base titration, was observed for Fe(Ferrozine)$_3^{2+}$.

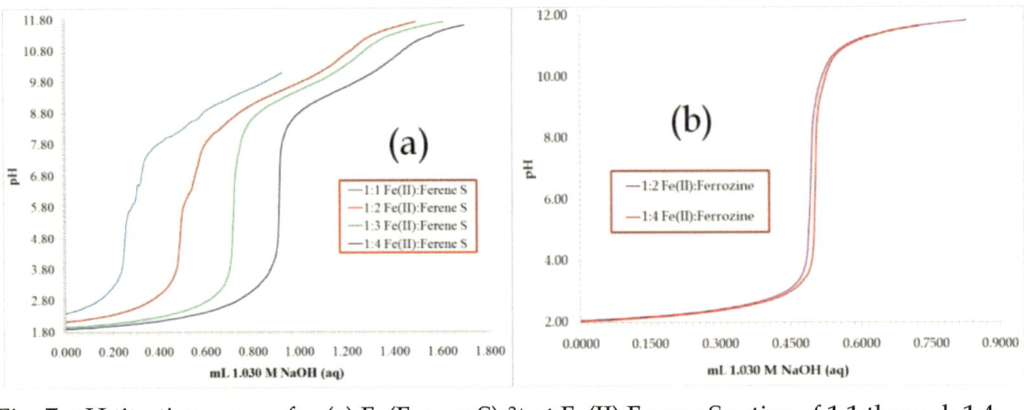

Fig. 7. pH titration curves for (a) Fe(Ferene S)$_3^{2+}$ at Fe(II):Ferene S ratios of 1:1 through 1:4, and (b) Fe(Ferrozine)$_3^{2+}$ at Fe(II):Ferrozine ratios of 1:2 and 1:4.

For the higher Fe(II):ligand ratios, titration curves resembling those for strong acid-strong base neutralizations were obtained for Fe(Ferene S)$_3^{2+}$ and Fe(Ferrozine)$_3^{2+}$. These results suggest that Fe(II) is coordinated strongly by Ferene S and Ferrozine, and support the results obtained by the pH-spectrophotometric method.

3.4 Application of Ferene S to iron determinations in natural waters

The results presented in this section will focus on the application of Ferene S to the spectrophotometric determination of total iron, and speciation of Fe^{2+} and Fe^{3+}, in abandoned mine drainage (AMD) and other types of natural waters.

Table 3 gives results for determination of total iron in water from Pigeon Creek (Washington County, Pennsylvania, USA) during March and October 2007. The iron concentrations (± their standard deviations) given are averages of triplicate and quadruplicate determinations, and are reported as mol Fe L^{-1} and mg Fe L^{-1}. Relative precision of replicates ranged from 2.2-10.2 percent, which is fairly good for these low part-per-million Fe levels. Calibration slopes given in Table 3 are in the range expected for Fe(Ferene S)$_3^{2+}$, with R^2 values approaching unity, indicating excellent linearity of the Fe calibration range (7.16×10^{-7} - 6.00×10^{-5} mol Fe L^{-1}, or 0.04 - 3.35 mg Fe L^{-1}) used in these determinations. The estimated limit of detection (LOD) was calculated to be 7.2×10^{-7} mol Fe L^{-1} (0.04 mg Fe L^{-1}), using the standard deviation of the y intercept obtained from linear regression of the calibration data via the LINEST function in Microsoft® Excel™ (Billo, 2001) and Equation 19 (section 3.1).

Sample	Avg. Fe Conc. ± Std. Dev. (mol Fe L^{-1})	Avg. Fe Conc. ± Std. Dev. (mg Fe L^{-1})	Calibration Slope (L (mol Fe)$^{-1}$)	Calibration Slope (L (mg Fe)$^{-1}$)
PIGEON-02-10172007	$(2.67 \pm 0.06) \times 10^{-5}$ (n = 3)	1.49 ± 0.03 (n = 3)	3.24×10^4 (R^2 = 0.9995)	0.581 (R^2 = 0.9995)
PIGEON-07-03202007	$(1.17 \pm 0.12) \times 10^{-5}$ (n = 4)	0.65 ± 0.06 (n = 4)	3.38×10^4 (R^2 = 0.9995)	0.605 (R^2 = 0.9995)
PIGEON-05-03202007	$(3.17 \pm 0.07) \times 10^{-5}$ (n = 4)	1.77 ± 0.04 (n = 4)	3.38×10^4 (R^2 = 0.9995)	0.605 (R^2 = 0.9995)
PIGEON-00-03202007	$(2.80 \pm 0.16) \times 10^{-5}$ (n = 4)	1.56 ± 0.09 (n = 4)	3.38×10^4 (R^2 = 0.9995)	0.605 (R^2 = 0.9995)

Table 3. Results from determination of total iron in water from Pigeon Creek (Washington County, PA, USA) in 2007, using the colorimetric Ferene S method.

A precision study of the spectrophotometric Ferene S method for determination of iron in AMD was conducted by the authors on runoff water collected near an abandoned coal mine in the vicinity of Coal Bluff in Washington County, PA in October 2006. The mean total Fe concentration in this AMD sample was found to be 13.9 ± 0.09 mg Fe L^{-1} (n = 8 replicates), with a 95% confidence interval of ± 0.07 mg Fe L^{-1}, suggesting good accuracy. A separate accuracy study for the Ferene S method was conducted in January 2007 in our laboratory on a series of water samples prepared in our laboratory and spiked with standard Fe solution to yield concentrations of 5.00 mg Fe L^{-1} in each sample. The samples were analyzed for total iron (as Fe^{2+}) by the common protocols outlined in section 2.2.1, with determination of the percent recovery of iron in each sample. Iron recoveries for the spiked water samples ranged from 100.6 - 101.4 percent, indicating essentially complete recovery of Fe and good accuracy. Additionally, our group has compared total Fe results for samples determined by the spectrophotometric Ferene S method to total Fe for the same samples determined by flame atomic absorption spectrophotometry (FAAS). Table 4 lists average Fe concentrations (in mg Fe L^{-1}) found in water from clean and AMD-contaminated portions of Gillespie Run (Allegheny County, PA, USA), determined by the colorimetric Ferene S method and by FAAS. The results from Table 4 indicate good agreement between the spectrophotometric Ferene S and FAAS methods.

Sample ID	UV-Vis/Ferene S Avg. µg Fe mL^{-1} in original sample	FAAS Avg. µg Fe mL^{-1} in original sample
Gillespie Site 1 09052008	13.1	13.8
Gillespie Site 2 09052008	33.1	34.9
Gillespie Site 4-1-09182008	29.5	27.5
Gillespie Site 4-2-09182008	27.3	26.4
Gillespie Site 3-1-10172008	$<0.08_5$	<0.3
Gillespie Site 3-2-10172008	$<0.08_5$	<0.3

Table 4. Comparison of the colorimetric Ferene S method with flame atomic absorption spectrophotometry (FAAS) for determination of total iron in abandoned mine drainage (AMD).

Current work in our laboratory involves, among other things, the use of the spectrophotometric Ferene S method for speciation of iron (i.e., Fe^{2+}, Fe^{3+}, and total Fe) in runoff from abandoned mines and other natural waters. The experimental approach used in these studies is given in section 2.2.5. In the speciation experiments, a spectrophotometer or colorimeter with absorbance-versus-time measurement capability is used to monitor formation of $Fe(Ferene\ S)_3^{2+}$ due to Fe^{2+} present in the sample. Upon chelation of Fe^{2+} initially present in the sample, the absorbance reaches a temporary plateau, at which time a reducing agent, e.g., hydroquinone, is added to reduce any Fe^{3+} present to Fe^{2+}. Depending on the concentration of Fe^{3+}, the absorbance at 590 nm (or 593 nm) increases accordingly until it reaches a maximum value and levels off, allowing for subsequent determination of total iron, and then Fe^{3+}, in the sample. Figure 8a shows results from initial experiments that addressed the amount of hydroquinone reducing agent to add to achieve rapid, successful reduction of Fe(III) to Fe(II). For these investigations, 1120.0 µL of a 3.04 x 10^{-5} mol Fe^{3+} L^{-1} solution was pipetted into a 3.00-mL capacity, 1.00-cm path length plastic cuvet containing 800.0 µL of pH 5.00 KHP/NaOH buffer solution and 80.0 µL of 9.76 x 10^{-3} mol Ferene S L^{-1} chelating solution. A kinetic absorbance-time run at 590 nm, using a WPA Colourwave CO7500 B colorimeter, was initiated upon addition of the sample. At t = 240 s, 20.0 µL of 2% aqueous hydroquinone was pipetted into the cuvet (with brief mixing), followed by a significant increase and eventual leveling of the absorbance at 590 nm, indicating reduction of Fe^{3+} to Fe^{2+}. This process required approximately 9 minutes, using 20.0 µL of 2%

hydroquinone. A second experiment, using 80.0 μL of 2% aqueous hydroquinone reducing agent and performed under the same conditions as before, required 3-5 minutes to achieve complete reduction of Fe^{3+} to Fe^{2+}. All absorbances in both experiments were adjusted to the total solution volume in the cuvet after addition of hydroquinone. Sine wave-like fluctuations of the absorbance at the plateaus of both absorbance-time curves are attributed to insufficient mixing after addition of hydroquinone. Conversion of Fe^{3+} to Fe^{2+}, expressed as the percent ratio of the concentration of Fe^{3+} initially present and the Fe^{2+} concentration determined at the end of the kinetic run (via the average absorbance at 590 nm at the plateau and Beer's Law), was found to be 103 and 107%, respectively, for the two experiments. Though the conversions are rather high, they do suggest essentially complete reduction of Fe^{3+} to Fe^{2+}.

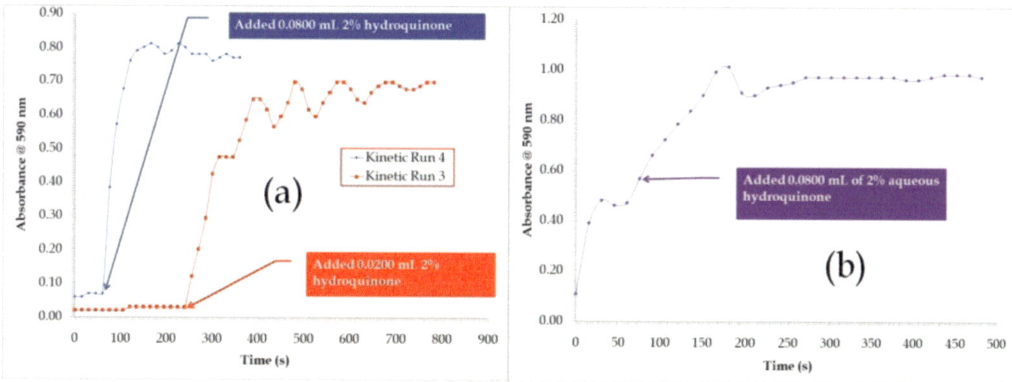

Fig. 8. Determination of (a) the amount of hydroquinone reducing agent to add for conversion of 3.04×10^{-5} mol Fe^{3+} L^{-1} solution to Fe^{2+}, and (b) the speciation of a synthetic sample containing 2.95×10^{-5} mol Fe^{2+} L^{-1} and 1.52×10^{-5} mol Fe^{3+} L^{-1}.

Further recovery experiments were conducted, involving speciation of iron in synthetic samples containing known concentrations of Fe(III) and Fe(II) and analyzed for Fe^{2+} by the procedures described in section 2.2.5. The purpose of these experiments was to check the iron recovery and efficiency of reduction of Fe^{3+} to Fe^{2+}. Table 5 gives the added and found Fe^{2+}, Fe^{3+}, and total Fe concentrations (in mol Fe L^{-1}) for three such recovery experiments, and Figure 8b illustrates the absorbance-time curve obtained for one of these recovery runs. The recoveries obtained for the forms of Fe in the samples are generally good, despite the high recoveries of 110.8 and 105.9%, and the rather low recovery of 84.3%. The recoveries suggest that complete Fe recoveries, and Fe(II)/Fe(III) speciation, are possible with this method. In Figure 8b, there is a very small leveling point prior to addition of hydroquinone, at which point apparent reduction of Fe^{3+} to Fe^{2+} was occurring, possibly promoted by Ferene S. Our group plans to further investigate this tendency.

Average Fe(II) and Fe(III) results from the speciation of Fe^{2+} and Fe^{3+} in AMD samples collected from a mine runoff tributary of Gillespie Run, and analyzed for Fe by the procedure given in section 2.2.5, were found to be 33.7 ± 0.5 mg Fe^{2+} L^{-1} and 0.6 ± 0.2 mg Fe^{3+} L^{-1} for one sample, and 35.5 ± 1.0 mg Fe^{2+} L^{-1} and 0.7 ± 0.2 mg Fe^{3+} L^{-1} for a different sample. These results suggest that the form of iron in AMD is mainly Fe^{2+}, with a very small Fe^{3+} concentration present. Calibration slopes associated with these determinations ranged from

3.50 x 10^4 to 3.60 x 10^4 L (mol Fe)$^{-1}$, with excellent Beer's Law behavior (R^2 ranged from 0.9993 to 1.000, and standard error of the estimate ranged from 0.0030 to 0.017) over the 1.00 x 10^{-6} – 3.94 x 10^{-5}mol Fe L^{-1} (0.05 – 2.20 mg Fe L^{-1}) concentration range.

Experiment	1	2	3
Fe^{2+} Added (mol L^{-1})	2.95 x 10^{-5}	1.88 x 10^{-5}	1.88 x 10^{-5}
Fe^{2+} Found (mol L^{-1})	2.85 x 10^{-5}	2.08 x 10^{-5}	1.77 x 10^{-5}
% Recovery Fe^{2+}	96.9	110.8	94.3
Fe^{3+} Added (mol L^{-1})	1.52 x 10^{-5}	1.79 x 10^{-5}	1.79 x 10^{-5}
Fe^{3+} Found (mol L^{-1})	1.56 x 10^{-5}	1.51 x 10^{-5}	1.90 x 10^{-5}
% Recovery Fe^{3+}	103.0	84.5	105.9
Total Fe Added (mol L^{-1})	4.47 x 10^{-5}	3.67 x 10^{-5}	3.67 x 10^{-5}
Total Fe Found (mol L^{-1})	4.43 x 10^{-5}	3.60 x 10^{-5}	3.67 x 10^{-5}
% Recovery Total Fe	99.3	98.0	100.0

Table 5. Recovery of Fe^{2+}, Fe^{3+}, and total Fe from synthetic water samples spiked with known concentrations of each form of Fe, using the colorimetric Ferene S method for speciation of iron.

3.5 Discussion

The results obtained from our studies of the effect of metal ion to ligand on the Beer's Law behavior of calibration data (Figures 3a and 3b) support our initial hypothesis that insufficient ligand stunts the range of linearity of absorbance with analyte concentration due to the ligand becoming the limiting reactant rather than the Fe(II) analyte. There is also an instrumental limit on Beer's Law: the ability of the spectrophotometer to detect changes in transmittance (usually very small at high concentrations) with respect to large changes in analyte concentration (Skoog et al., 2007; Stauffer, 2007), usually associated with the high-concentration end of the calibration curve. Advances in spectrophotometer design over the past few decades have enabled more sophisticated instruments to extend Beer's Law linearity into the 2.0 – 3.0 absorbance unit region, which is unattainable with low-end photometers and simple colorimeters. Regardless, the limiting reactant concept must be kept in mind when performing spectrophotometric determinations of any analyte.

The results of our formation constant studies indicated that coordination of Fe^{2+} by Ferene S and Ferrozine is strong, based on the average $\log_{10}\beta_3$ of 16.45 ± 0.25 and 17.46 ± 0.37 for Fe(Ferene $S)_3^{2+}$ and $Fe(Ferrozine)_3^{2+}$, respectively. As the formation constants for each chelate are means of quadruplicate determinations, their standard deviations suggest that LeChatelier's Principle is essentially followed. What does change, however, is the extent of chelation at low pH with changes in the ligand concentration used, which further emphasizes the importance of maintaining the analyte Fe^{2+} as the limiting reactant. Previous unpublished studies by our group regarding optimum formation of Fe(Ferene $S)_3^{2+}$ as a function of pH indicated that the range for optimum chelation was pH 3 – 7. For

$Fe(Ferrozine)_3^{2+}$, the published pH range for optimum chelation is pH 3 - 9 (Gibbs, 1976; McBride, 1980). The tendency of both ligands to readily chelate Fe^{2+} even at low pH values was suggested by qualitative observations of formation of the indigo and magenta colors of $Fe(Ferene\ S)_3^{2+}$ and $Fe(Ferrozine)_3^{2+}$, respectively, further suggesting that the 1:3 chelates are formed preferentially, though incompletely, even at low pH. The pH titration curves for $Fe(Ferene\ S)_3^{2+}$ and $Fe(Ferrozine)_3^{2+}$ at varying Fe(II):ligand ratios (Figures 7a and 7b) provide some support for this hypothesis, as do the absorbance-pH formation curves (Figures 6a and 6b) from the pH-spectrophotometric formation constant experiments. The absorbance-pH formation curves show that for a typical Fe(II):ligand ratio, e.g., 1:4, that can be used in colorimetric determinations of iron using either of these ligands, that a significant absorbance (ca. 0.3 - 0.4) is obtained even at pH values as low as 1.20 (Figures 6a and 6b), which signifies extensive chelate formation at such low pH. The pH titration curves for $Fe(Ferene\ S)_3^{2+}$ and $Fe(Ferrozine)_3^{2+}$ at the 1:4 Fe^{2+}:ligand ratio resemble strong acid-strong base titration curves, suggesting that competition between Fe^{2+} and H^+ for the coordination site on the ligand occurs overwhelmingly in favor of Fe^{2+}, leaving H^+ to be titrated by standard base. The indigo and magenta colors of $Fe(Ferene\ S)_3^{2+}$ and $Fe(Ferrozine)_3^{2+}$, respectively, were already intense at the start of the titrations, even for the low Fe(II):ligand ratios and added acid.

The application our group selected was the spectrophotometric determination of iron in natural waters, using a ligand that would yield lower detection limits for iron, particularly in consideration of the US Environmental Protection Agency (USEPA) mandated limit of 0.3 mg Fe L^{-1} for water (Heakin, 2000). The idea of using Ferene S was appealing due to the high molar absorptivity (published value of 3.55×10^4 L mol^{-1} cm^{-1}) (Higgins, 1981). The results given in Figures 8a and 8b, and Tables 3 - 5, suggest that the colorimetric Ferene S method is suitable for accurate and precise determinations of iron in natural waters, and that speciation of Fe^{2+} and Fe^{3+} in abandoned mine drainage is feasible with Ferene S. The portability of the Ferene S method has also made it useful in our attempts to determine iron in runoff from old coal mines on-site, in a "real-time" manner. The method has been microscaled so that solution mixing and absorbance measurements can be performed in the same 1-cm cuvet. The Ferene S reagent is not prohibitively expensive, is available from major chemicals suppliers, and is water-soluble. Portable, battery-operated clorimeters and spectrophotometers are inexpensive, low-maintenance, and yield reliable absorbance and transmittance measurements.

4. Conclusions, future directions

In this chapter, the concept of the limiting reactant in analytical chemistry was examined through studying the effects of the metal ion to ligand ratio on calibration curves, determinations of stoichiometries, and determination of formation constants for the iron(II) chelates of Ferene S and Ferrozine, two well known chelating agents for the spectrophotometric determination of iron in serum and other biomedical samples. The results of our studies for both chelates show that using insufficient ligand for spectrophotometric determination of iron produces premature deviations from Beer's Law that are not instrumental but due to the ligand becoming the limiting reactant. The results further indicate that the formation constant of each chelate is relatively unaffected by changes in ligand concentration, but that the extent of complexation is influenced by increasing the concentration of ligand used. The results of our studies for the two chelates also indicate good agreement of molar absorptivities and stoichiometries with published values, and some disagreement with the published formation constant for $Fe(Ferrozine)_3^{2+}$ due most likely to experimental differences in the methods employed. Finally, an application of Ferene S to the colorimetric determination of total and speciated (Fe^{2+}, Fe^{3+}) iron in natural waters was presented and discussed.

Future plans for this research include continuation of efforts toward further development, implementation, and refinement of the field-portable colorimetric determination and speciation of iron in natural waters using Ferene S. Work on using Ferene S for spectrophotometric quantitation of iron in sample types other than natural waters continues in our laboratory. Additionally, other ferroin ligands besides the two examined in this chapter will be investigated for use in colorimetric quantitation of iron in various sample types. Finally, ferroin ligands and other types of iron(II) and even iron(III) complexing agents will be explored for pedagogical use in effective teaching of the limiting reactant concept in analytical chemistry courses.

5. Acknowledgements

The authors gratefully acknowledge the moral and financial support of the University of Pittsburgh at Greensburg in this endeavor. The generous support of the McKenna Foundation, the Fisher Fund of the Pittsburgh Foundation, the Society for Analytical Chemists of Pittsburgh (SACP), and the Spectroscopy Society of Pittsburgh (SSP) is gratefully acknowledged for making this research possible. MTS thanks his wife, Resa, for her moral support and patience during this work, his colleagues in the Chemistry Department at Pitt-Greensburg for their support and input, his former and current research students as well as the many students who enrolled in his analytical chemistry and instrumental analysis courses over the past several years for their contributions to this research, and to Mrs. Cynthia Genard for helping with administrative functions during the last few weeks of manuscript preparation.

6. References

Alexandropoulos, I.; Komaitis, M. & Kapsokefalou, M. (2006). Effects of iron, ascorbate, meat, and casein on the antioxidant capacity of green tea under conditions of in vitro digestion. *Food Chemistry*, Vol. 94, No. 3, (February 2006), pp. 359-365, ISSN 0308-8146

Almog, J.; Hirshfeld, A.; Glattstein, B.; Sterling, J. & Goren, Z. (1996). Chromogenic reagents for iron(II): studies in the 1,2,4-triazine series. *Analytica Chimica Acta*, Vol. 22, pp. 203-208, ISSN 0003-2670

Argyri, K.; Komaitis, M. & Kapsokefalou, M. (2006). Iron decreases the antioxidant capacity of red wine under conditions of in vitro digestion. *Food Chemistry*, Vol. 96, No. 2, (May 2006), pp. 281-289, ISSN 0308-8146

Artiss, J. D.; Vinogradov, S. & Zak, B. (1981). Spectrophotometric study of several sensitive reagents for serum iron. *Clinical Biochemistry*, Vol. 14, No. 6, (December 1981), pp. 311-315, ISSN 0009-9120

Baird, J. K. (1999). A Generalized Statement of the Law of Mass Action. *Journal of Chemical Education*, Vol. 76, No. 8, (August 1999), pp. 1146-1150, ISSN 0021-9584

Benson, R. L. & Worsfold, P. J. (1993). A flow-injection approach to the continuous monitoring of residual coagulants (aluminium and iron) in potable and treated waters. *Science of the Total Environment*, Vol. 135, No. 1-3, (August 1993), pp. 17-25, ISSN 0048-9697

Billo, E. J. (2001). *Excel® for Chemists: A Comprehensive Guide,* 2nd edition, Wiley-VCH, ISBN 0-471-39462-9, New York, New York, USA

Bjerrum, J. (1941). *Metal Ammine Formation in Aqueous Solution*, P. Haase & Son, OL 15056032M, Copenhagen, Denmark

Bjerrum, J. & Nielsen, E. J. (1948). Metal Ammine Formation in Aqueous Solution. VI. Stability and Light Absorption of Copper Ethylenediamine Ions. *Acta Chemica Scandinavica*, Vol. 2, pp. 297-318, ISSN 0001-5393

Brown, T. L.; LeMay, H. E. & Bursten, B. E. (2006). *Chemistry: The Central Science*, 10th edition, Pearson Education, Inc., ISBN 0-13-146489-2, Upper Saddle River, New Jersey, USA

Butler, J. N. (1998). *Ionic Equilibrium: Solubility and pH Calculations*, John Wiley & Sons, ISBN 0-471-58526-2, New York, New York, USA

Camberlein, E.; Abgueguen, E.; Fatih, N.; Cannone-Hergaux, F.; Leroyer, P.; Turlin, B.; Ropert, M.; Brissot, P. & Loreal, O. (2010). Hepcidin induction limits mobilisation of splenic iron in a mouse model of secondary iron overload. *Biochimica et Biophysica Acta – Molecular Basis of Disease*, Vol. 1802, No. 3, (March 2010), pp. 339-346, ISSN 0925-4439

Carter, P. (1971). Spectrophotometric Determination of Serum Iron at the Submicrogram Level with a New Reagent (Ferrozine). *Analytical Biochemistry*, Vol. 40, pp. 450-458, ISSN 0003-2697

Cheng, K. L.; Ueno, K. & Imamura, T. (1992). *Handbook of Organic Analytical Reagents*, 2nd edition, CRC Press, ISBN 9780849342875, Boca Raton, Florida, USA

Eperesi, C. A.; Nelson, D. E. & Stauffer, M. T. (2010). Preliminary Investigations of Correlations Between Total Mercury in Tuna and Quality Control, and Mercury Recoveries using Microwave Digestion. *Spectroscopy Letters*, Vol. 43, No. 7, (November-December 2010), pp. 597-601, ISSN 0038-7010

Foley, R. T. & Anderson, R. C. (1948). Spectrophotometric Studies on Complex Formation with Sulfosalicylic Acid. *Journal of the American Chemical Society*, Vol. 70, No. 3, (March 1948), pp. 1195-1197, ISSN 0002-7863

Gibbs, C. R. (1976). Characterization and Application of FerroZine Iron Reagent as a Ferrous Iron Indicator. *Analytical Chemistry*, Vol. 48, No. 8, (July 1976), pp. 1197-1201, ISSN 0003-2700

Harris, D. C. (2010). *Quantitative Chemical Analysis*, 8th edition, W. H. Freeman & Co., ISBN 978-1-4292-1815-3, New York, New York, USA

Harvey, Jr., A. E. & Manning, D. L. (1950). Spectrophotometric Methods of Establishing Empirical Formulas of Colored Complexes in Solution. *Journal of the American Chemical Society*, Vol. 72, No. 10, (October 1950), pp. 4488-4493, ISSN 0002-7863

Higgins, T. (1981). Novel Chromogen for Serum Iron Determinations. *Clinical Chemistry*, Vol. 27, No. 9, pp. 1619-1620, ISSN 0009-9147

Irwin, A. E.; DeRamos, C. M. & Stout, B. E. (1996). Solution and Solid State ^{13}C NMR Studies of Alginic Acid Binding with Alkaline Earth, Lanthanide, and Yttrium Metal Ions. *Humic and Fulvic Acids*, Chapter 15, *ACS Symposium Series*, Vol. 651, (November 14, 1996), pp. 244-258, ISSN 0097-6156

Job, P. (1928). Formation and Stability of Inorganic Complexes in Solution. *Annales de Chimie et du Physique*, Vol. 9, pp. 113-163, ISSN 0365-1444

Kellner, R. A. (1998). UV-Vis Spectrophotometry, Emission and Luminescence, In: *Analytical Chemistry*, Kellner, R. A.; Mermet, J.-M.; Otto, M. & Widmer, H. M., Eds., pp. 527-540, Wiley-VCH, ISBN 3-527-28610-1, Weinheim, Germany

Martell, A. E. & Motekaitis, R. J. (1992). *Determination and Use of Stability Constants*, John Wiley & Sons, ISBN 978-0-471-18817-9, New York, New York, USA

McBride, L. (1980). *The Iron Reagents*, 3rd edition, G. Frederick Smith Chemical Co., Columbus, Ohio, USA

McBryde, W. A. E. (1964). A Spectrophotometric Reexamination of the Spectra and Stabilities of the Iron(III)-Tiron Complexes. *Canadian Journal of Chemistry*, Vol. 42, No. 8, (August 1964), pp. 1917-1927, ISSN 0008-4042

Miller, J. C. & Miller, J. N. (1993). *Statistics for Analytical Chemistry*, 3rd edition, Ellis Horwood Limited, ISBN 0-13-030990-7, Chichester, West Sussex, United Kingdom

Riemer, J.; Hoepken, H. H.; Czerwinska, H.; Robinson, S. R. & Dringen, R. (2004). Colorimetric ferrozine-based assay for the quantitation of iron in cultured cells. *Analytical Biochemistry*, Vol. 331, No. 2, (August 2004), pp. 370-375, ISSN 0003-2697

Rossotti, F. C. & Rossotti, H. (1961). *The Determination of Stability Constants*, McGraw-Hill, New York, New York, USA

Skoog, D. A.; Holler, F. J. & Crouch, S. R. (2007). *Principles of Instrumental Analysis*, 6th edition, Cengage Learning, ISBN 9780495012016, Florence, Kentucky, USA

Smith, F. E.; Herbert, J.; Gaudin, J.; Hennessy, D. J & Reid, G. R. (1984). Serum Iron Determination Using Ferene Triazine. *Clinical Biochemistry*, Vol. 17, (October 1984), pp. 306-310, ISSN 0009-9120

Stauffer, M. T. (2007). Undergraduate Analytical Chemistry: To Use and Evaluate Organic Chelators for Spectrophotometric Determination of Iron. *Spectroscopy Letters*, Vol. 40, No. 3, (May-June 2007), pp. 439-452, ISSN 0038-7010

Stauffer, M. T.; Hunter, L. J. & Troncone, S. K. (2007). Determination of Iron in Abandoned Mine Drainage by UV-Vis Spectrophotometry and Flame Atomic Absorption Spectrophotometry. *Spectroscopy Letters*, Vol. 40, No. 3, (May-June 2007), pp. 429-437, ISSN 0038-7010

Stookey, L. L. (1970). Ferrozine – A New Spectrophotometric Reagent for Iron. *Analytical Chemistry*, Vol. 42, No. 7, (June 1970), pp. 779-781, ISSN 0003-2700

Thomas, M. (1996). *Ultraviolet and Visible Spectroscopy*, 2nd edition, John Wiley & Sons, Ltd., ISBN 0-471-96743-2, West Sussex, England, United Kingdom

Thompsen, J. C. & Mottola, H. A. (1984). Kinetics of the Complexation of Iron(II) with Ferrozine. *Analytical Chemistry*, Vol. 56, No. 4, (April 1984), pp. 755-757, ISSN 0003-2700

Viollier, E.; Inglett, P. W.; Hunter, K.; Roychoudhury, A. N. & Van Cappellen, P. (2000). The ferrozine method revisited: Fe(II)/Fe(III) determination in natural waters. *Applied Geochemistry*, Vol. 15, No. 6, (July 2000), pp. 785-790, ISSN 0883-2927

Vosburgh, W. C. & Cooper, G. R. (1941). Complex Ions I. The Identification of Complex Ions in Solution by Spectrophotometric Measurements. *Journal of the American Chemical Society*, Vol. 63, No. 2, (February 1941), pp. 437-442, ISSN 0002-7863

Yamamoto, M.; Nishida, A.; Otsuka, K.; Komai, T. & Fukushima, M. (2010). Evaluation of the binding of iron(II) to humic substances derived from a compost sample by a colorimetric method using ferrozine. *Bioresource Technology*, Vol. 101, No. 12, (June 2010), pp. 4456-4460, ISSN 0960-8524

Part 6

Biomedicine and Environment: The Future is Now?

15

Recent New Characterizations on the Giant Extracellular Hemoglobin of *Glossoscolex paulistus* and Some Other Giant Hemoglobins from Different Worms

Marcel Tabak[1], Francisco A.O. Carvalho[1], José W.P. Carvalho[1], Jose F.R. Bachega[2] and Patrícia S. Santiago[1,3]
[1]*Instituto de Química de São Carlos, Universidade de São Paulo, São Carlos, SP,*
[2]*Instituto de Física de São Carlos, Universidade de São Paulo, São Carlos, SP,*
[3]*Campus Experimental de Registro, UNESP, SP,*
Brazil

1. Introduction

Giant extracellular hemoglobins, also known as erythrocruorins, have been investigated as a model of extreme complexity in oxygen-binding heme proteins [1,2]. They are characterized by a very high molecular mass (*MM*) of several megadalton (MDa), and their oligomeric structure together with the crowded and protected heme environment are two of the main factors responsible for the high redox stability [3,4]. Superoxide dimustase (SOD)-like intrinsic activity, observed for hemoglobins of *Lumbricus terrestris* (HbLt) and of *Arenicola marina* (HbAm), is another important factor [5,6]. These hemoglobins present a highly cooperative oxygen binding and a peculiar behavior associated to their oligomeric dissociation into smaller subunits and possible rearrangement back into the native oligomeric structure [7,8].

Moreover, a strong motivation to study these giant hemoglobins is related to their potential use in medicine as blood substitutes. Studies have been performed in the past for HbLt [9], and are presently underway to test and validate the use of HbAm in this direction [6,10]. They seem to be very promising due to the lack of undesirable immunological reactions in tests with animals, explained by the absence of cell membranes as occurs with human hemoglobin in red blood cells [6,10]. Besides, the resistance to oxidation of extracellular hemoglobins, as noticed by their redox stability, is also an advantage as compared to the use of human hemoglobin in this medical application.

The giant extracellular hemoglobin of *Glossoscolex paulistus* (HbGp) is similar to several homologous proteins described in the literature [11-14]. These extracellular hemoglobins are constituted by a large number of globin-like subunits containing heme groups with *MM* in the range 15–19 kDa. These globin subunits form monomers of 16 kDa (***d***) and disulphide bound hetero-trimers of 51-52 kDa (***abc***), linked by non-heme structures (24–32 kDa), named linkers (***L***) [12,13]. Recent partial characterization of *MM* of HbGp by matrix assisted laser desorption time-of-flight mass spectrometry (MALDI-TOF-MS) confirmed the similarity of its subunits to those of homologous proteins of this class, mentioned above, especially HbLt [15]. This characteristic multi-subunit content confers to the whole protein a double-layered hexagonal oligomeric structure. A common model for the quaternary structure, so-called "bracelet model", has been employed to explain the assembly of this class of proteins into their oligomeric structure.

It is worth of notice that HbGp belongs to the same class of hemoglobins as HbLt, which is one of the most studied hemoglobins in this group. Despite the fact that HbLt has been extensively studied over the past 20 years, the issue of its true *MM* is still not fully understood. HbLt was one of the proteins studied by Theodore Svedberg and collaborators in 1933 [16], and later work by Daniel et al. has argued that the *MM* of HbLt could vary between 3.6 and 4.4 MDa [17]. They propose a model for the whole protein, consisting of twelve equal structures involving a dodecamer, $(abcd)_3$, and three linkers L_3, together with twelve tetramers (*abcd*), in such a way that the protomer corresponding to the 1/12 of the whole oligomer is given by $(abcd)_3L_3(abcd)$, or alternatively, $(abcd)_4L_3$ [17,18]. On the other hand, Vinogradov et al. [19] have proposed a model for HbLt, where 1/12 of the whole molecule is given by $(abcd)_3\ L_3$, so that the difference between the two models is the presence of twelve additional tetramers in the former occupying the central part of the hexagonal bilayer.

Royer et al. describing the crystal structure of HbLt [11,20] has suggested that the Vinogradov model is very consistent with the crystal structure. Besides, very recent preliminary work on the crystal structure of HbGp [21] has also suggested a strong similarity between HbGp and HbLt, both belonging to class 1, where the two hexagonal layers forming the bilayer are rotated to 16 degree one relative to another. It is worthy of mention, that another extracellular hemoglobin from a sea worm, HbAm, has also been investigated by Zal et al. [22,23]. In this case the structure belongs to class 2, where the two hexagonal layers are exactly eclipsed one relative to the other, as demonstrated in recent crystallographic studies at low resolution [24]. Besides, the assembly of the protomer corresponding to 1/12 of the whole HbAm oligomer is different: a dodecamer formed by two monomeric units a_1 and a_2 together with a trimer (*T*) gives $(a_1)_3(a_2)_6T$ associated to an average of 3.5 linkers resulting in a structure of $[(a_1)_3(a_2)_6T]L_{3.5}$ [23,25]. This arrangement implies a different number of globin and linker chains for HbAm. In this assembly the contacts between the subunits are quite different as compared to those in HbLt. Moreover, quite recently, the primary sequence of a fourth linker chain for HbLt has been reported, $\boldsymbol{L_4}$ [1]. The unanswered question remains as an open issue regarding the role of four linker chains in a structure that, apparently, only needs three of them. Another interesting question, relevant to the understanding of the overall oligomeric subunit stoichiometry, is the existence of several isoforms for some of the globin chains. This has also been elusive in the description of the crystal structure of the whole assembly at atomic resolution. So, the precise characterization of the several globin and linker subunits that constitute the native extracellular hemoglobins still remains a matter for further research.

In conclusion, this review chapter addresses the issue of the molecular masses of HbGp subunits, as monitored by sodium dodecyl sulfate polyacrylamide gel electrophoresis (SDS-PAGE) and MALDI-TOF-MS, and their hydrodynamic properties, as monitored by analytical ultracentrifugation (AUC). Also new data from other three giant hemoglobins are added, to compare the differences and similarities between these systems: namely hemoglobins of *Rhinodrilus alatus*, *Eisenia andrei* and *Perionyx excavatus*. The focus of this study is the characterization of the different subunits that constitute each protein, aiming to assess in detail the nature of the subunit interactions that maintain the whole extraordinary oligomeric structure. These three new hemoglobins belong to different worm species that have been classified and studied previously only in relation to their biological effects upon the soil condition in their living habitat. Comparing the composition and structures of their subunits could be interesting also in relation to the understanding of the evolutionary changes evolved as a function of their different living environments. Finally, recent results concerning the subunits composition and architecture of HbAm, in connection with its possible medical application as a blood substitute, are described.

1.1 Some new extracellular hemoglobins from different worms

The giant extracellular hemoglobins found in the Annelids, are characterized by high molecular mass and by an overall hexagonal symmetry [23]. Hemoglobin provides a fascinating example of molecular evolution. In this work four types of extracellular hemoglobins from different earthworms were studied.

These species of worms have very specific habitat and are found and live only in some restricted regions. It is not possible to produce some of these earthworm species in large amounts and captivity. *Glossoscolex paulistus* is a worm of the Glossoscolecidae family, very common and endemic in the cities of Piracicaba and Rio Claro, in state of São Paulo, Brazil [26]. The more common use of these earthworms is in the fishing, as baits. However, the extracellular hemoglobin of *Glossoscolex paulistus*, HbGp, has now been studied for more than twenty years, focusing its physical-chemical and structural properties, by several research groups in Brazil [27,28].

Rhinodrilus alatus is a species endemic and prevalent in sites in the regions of Sete Lagoas and Paraopeba, in the state of Minas Gerais, Brazil [29]. This species was considered to be threatened of extinction, due to its extensive use to achieve natural fertilizer as well as for bait in fishing. This species was well characterized and its anatomy is known [30], especially regarding the circulatory system. *Rhinodrilus alatus* is a giant earthworm, of 56 to 63 cm of length and 11 to 12 mm of diameter [30]. In the period of drought, between April and September, the earthworms of this species enter into spontaneous dormancy, in a camera protected by mucus. *Rhinodrilus alatus* belongs to the same family as the *Glossoscolex paulistus* worm. Differently from HbGp, the extracellular hemoglobin of *Rhinodrilus alatus*, HbRa, is not known from the structural point of view.

Perionyx excavatus is a worm of the family Megascolecidae and genus Perionyx. *Perionyx excavatus* is an earthworm found commonly over a large area of tropical Asia although it has been transported to Europe and North America [31]. This is an endemic species which lives in organic wastes and high moisture contents, and adequate amounts of suitable organic material are required for populations to become fully established and for them to process organic wastes efficiently [32].

Perionyx excavatus had been shown to have efficient biological potential for conversion of organic wastes into high-value useful plant growth media [32]. Differently from the other two species, the *Perionyx excavatus* is produced in earthworm culture and its marketing is allowed around the world. For this reason, it is often used in the process of vermicomposting, which is a mesophilic process associated to ingestion, digestion, and absorption of organic waste carried out by earthworms followed by excretion of castings through the worm's metabolic system [32].

Another extracellular hemoglobin that is discussed in this work is collected from the annelid *Eisenia andrei*, HbEa. This is an earthworm of the family Lumbricidae and is known as the red California worm. This earthworm is between 5 to 10 cm in length and 4 to 8 mm in diameter, and it is the most used species in the world for decomposition of organic material [33]. The easy adaptation and reproduction of this species partly justify the *Eisenia andrei* large use around the world.

Some interesting studies suggest that earthworms can be used as biological indicators of soil contamination. Vampré et al. [34] showed that soil contamination by hexachlorobenzene (HCB) can be identified by analysis of soil and earthworm tissue extracts [34]. The earthworm has an important role in the equilibrium of the soil nutrients distribution, in particular, the increase of soil stability, infiltration rates, besides playing an important role in the phosphorus (P) and nitrogen (N) cycles [35]. In this context, interesting work has been developed by Brown et al. regarding the worms population of the state of Paraná, Brazil, aiming to evaluate the soil characteristics of this region [36].

1.2 Extracellular worm hemoglobins as potential blood substitutes

Giant extracellular hemoglobins are easily purified to a homogeneous product avoiding expensive synthetic steps. Besides, it is a product easy to store, the auto-oxidation is quite a slow process and it is less likely to cause immunogenic responses since cell membranes are not present and HbAm, for instance, is not glycosilated [27]. Preliminary experiments have been performed many years ago with the naturally polymerized HbLt. Mice and rats undergoing exchange transfusion with HbLt revealed no apparent behavioral and physical changes [9]. A report on the potential use of HbAm, showing that its structural and functional properties are consistent with the requirements for blood substitutes, has been published recently [6]. These properties should prevent kidney damage, reduce vasoconstrictor effect and oxygen radical formation, often associated with the administration of dissolved mammalian Hb.

Structural analyses of HbAm under simulated human physiological conditions *in vitro* revealed its dissociation into high molecular weight and functional subunits, while *in vivo* experiments performed on mice revealed no apparent behavioral or physiopathological changes and absence of allergic response [6]. Recent effort has also been devoted to express some of the globin chains of HbAm considering the possibility of producing larger amounts of material aiming at reconstituting a recombinant hexagonal bilayer hemoglobin (HBL-Hb) by genetic engineering in order to provide a new oxygen carrier for therapeutic applications [10]. Considering the similarity of HbGp and HbLt with HbAm it is possible to conclude that all of them could be potentially useful for blood substitutes. Therefore, our studies aiming to obtain a deeper understanding of the structural and physical-chemical properties of HbGp and the new giant hemoglobins presented in this report can be quite relevant to a better evaluation of their potential biomedical applications.

2. Experimental methods

In the present work, a review is presented of recent work performed in our laboratory, focusing on the molecular mass *MM* of HbGp, based on electrophoresis, AUC, and MALDI-TOF-MS [3,15]. SDS-PAGE electrophoresis is an extremely useful technique, especially to monitor the subunits contents present in different fractions of the protein obtained from gel exclusion chromatography [26]. Though this technique is not as precise as direct mass spectrometry, it is able to provide informations about the mass characteristic and migration properties of these subunits under the effect of an applied electric field at the same time.

X-Ray crystallography is a powerful structural technique, providing models of complex protein structures with atomic resolution [21].

3. Results

3.1 Equilibrium of HbGp species obtained from alkaline dissociation at pH 10

Our recent *MM* determination performed on two HbGp samples, at pH 7.0, one in the reduced oxy- form, and the other in the oxidized cyanomet- form, have given values of 3.6 ± 0.1 MDa and 3.7 ± 0.1 MDa, respectively [3]. This value is in excellent agreement with the prediction of the *MM* for the whole molecule, based on the Vinogradov model, and our previous MALDI-TOF-MS analysis [15]: a tetramer *abcd* of 52.1+16.4 = 68.5 kDa is observed, and assuming further an average *MM* for the linkers of 28 kDa, plus 144 heme groups (~0.6 kDa each), a total *MM* of 12×[68.5×3+28×3]+144×0.6 = 3560 kDa is expected for HbGp.

Very recent ultracentrifugation studies regarding the HbGp subunits, obtained from alkaline dissociation at pH 10, provided further information on subunits masses, underlining the difficulties in separating, by simple SEC experiments, the linker chains from the trimer globin subunits due to their similar hydrodynamic properties [37]. In this study, analysis of the equilibrium dissociation of HbGp, at pH 10.0, has shown that the whole protein is constituted by several species. For oxy-HbGp, at pH 10.0, no contribution from un-dissociated whole protein is observed, suggesting that the reduced form is completely dissociated under this alkaline condition. However, for cyanomet-HbGp, 17 % of the protein remains in the native un-dissociated form, implying a higher oligomeric stability of the oxidized cyanomet- form [37]. Results are shown in Tables 1 and 2 and can be summarized as follows: 1) AUC experiments for the monomer *d* alone indicated that this species is quite pure. However, equilibrium is observed involving monomers and dimers of monomers. The dimer contribution is relatively low, around 10%, similar to that observed in previous experiments by MALDI–TOF-MS, increasing at higher protein concentrations. 2) Analysis of oxy-HbGp solution, at pH 10.0, showed the existence of four species in equilibrium, assigned to the following subunits: monomer *d*, dimers of monomers d_2, trimers *abc* and a fourth species associated to the tetramer *abcd*. The second species (dimers of monomers, d_2) revealed a significant intensity increase as compared to the pure monomer. This increase in intensity is, possibly, due to a superposition of the contribution from some linker chains, having masses near to the dimers of monomers d_2 one, around 32 kDa. Linker chains are characterized by mass values *MM* in the range of 24-32 kDa, and are, probably, detected as a single peak, corresponding to the peak of the dimers of monomers. The third species, trimers *abc*, is not observed for samples containing the reducing agent, β-mercaptoethanol, since the disulfide bonds are disrupted with the formation of the monomeric species that compose the trimers, monomers *a, b* and *c,* consistent also with the increase in the contribution of the monomeric fraction, observed for this sample (Tables 1 and 2). Calculations of the sedimentation coefficients for the HbLt subunits based on the reported crystal structure [11,20] gave additional useful informations for the interpretation of the obtained AUC data for HbGp: first of all, according to these estimates, the linker chains could appear together either with the monomeric globin chains or with the dimeric globins. Besides, the presence of linker chains associated to globin tetramers would not alter in significant ways the value of s for the pure globin tetramer.

Samples	pH	Observed species[a] $s^0_{20,w}$ 1	2	3	4	5
Monomer	7.0	2.05 ± 0.05	2.81± 0.03	-	5.7 ± 0.1	
	10.0	1.86 ±0.06	2.9 ± 0.5	-	4.6 ± 0.9	
Oxy-HbGp	10.0	1.7 ± 0.1	2.67 ± 0.03	4.12±0.06	6.2 ± 0.2	
Oxy-HbGp[1]	10.0	1.64 ± 0.06	2.67 ± 0.02	-	4.6 ± 0.2	
Cyanomet-HbGp	10.0	2.0 ± 0.1	3.06 ± 0.09	3.98 ±0.02	6.6 ± 0.2	58.3 ± 0.5

Oxy-HbGp[1] -HbGp in the presence of 2-mercaptoethanol. All data obtained at 236 nm. [a]Observed species 1, 2, 3, 4 and 5 correspond to pure monomer *d*, dimer of monomers d_2, trimer *(abc)*, tetramer (*abcd*) and tetramer of monomers d_4 and un-dissociated cyanomet-HbGp, respectively.

Table 1. Sedimentation coefficients for the pure monomer ***d***, and for HbGp, dissociated in alkaline medium, under the indicated conditions.

Samples	pH	Observed species[a] % (Area) 1	2	3	4	5
Monomer	7.0	84 ± 8	14 ± 8	-	2 ± 1	-
	10.0	89 ± 4	8 ± 4	-	3 ± 1	-
Oxy-HbGp	10.0	24 ± 8	29 ± 10	38 ± 3	9 ± 6	-
Oxy-HbGp[1]	10.0	47 ± 4	38 ± 3	-	15 ± 3	-
Cyanomet-HbGp	10.0	20 ± 4	20 ± 7	40 ± 3	3 ± 1	17 ± 2

Oxy-HbGp[1] – HbGp in the presence of 2-mercaptoethanol. All data obtained at 236 nm. [a]The species are the same described in Table 1.

Table 2. Percentage contributions of different species observed in the equilibrium of HbGp, dissociated at alkaline medium, pH 10.0, and of monomer *d*, shown in Table 1.

As mentioned above, for oxy-HbGp no contribution from un-dissociated protein was observed, implying that the reduced form is fully dissociated at pH 10.0. However, for cyanomet-HbGp, around 17 % of un-dissociated protein remains in its native oligomeric form, consistent with a greater oligomeric stability for this oxidized form, in alkaline medium (Tables 1 and 2). Finally, equilibrium sedimentation data allowed an estimate of the masses *MM* for the four globin chains, monomers *a*, *b*, *c* and *d*. Due to the small difference of masses for monomers *b* and *d* they appear as a single unresolved peak in AUC and MALDI-TOF-MS [15] experiments.

3.2 Initial characterization of the new extracellular hemoglobins from different worms

In this section new data are presented regarding both electrophoretic and MALDI-TOF-MS measurements of HbGp subunits. Four linker chains are observed for this species by SDS-PAGE, but with quite different concentrations that preclude their detection in the mass spectra experiments. Moreover, multiple chains were detected for the monomeric *c* chain obtained by reduction of the trimer *abc*, as for the isoforms of monomeric subunit *d*, reported earlier [15]. Together with the studies on HbGp, we have recently started to look at three different hemoglobins obtained from different worms, namely HbRa, HbPe, and HbEa. Some preliminary results based on SDS-PAGE, AUC, and MALDI-TOF-MS studies are here reported for the first time, showing a great similarity, but not identity, among the subunit composition and masses for these extracellular hemoglobins as compared to HbGp.

3.2.1 SDS-PAGE electrophoresis data

In Figs.1A and 1B SDS-PAGE gels are shown for the extracellular hemoglobins of HbGp, HbRa, HbPe and HbEa, in the absence and the presence of 2-mercaptoethanol, respectively. The slot (S) corresponds to the standard masses used for calibration. The four hemoglobins in the present study showed a similar, but not identical, band pattern with mass values around 52 ± 2 kDa, associated to the trimer subunit, and also very similar masses for the monomer *d*, around 12 kDa (Fig.1A). The slots II and III correspond to HbGp. The slots IV and V, corresponding to HbRa, showed some differences as compared to HbGp: apparently two bands were observed in the trimer position, while the four linker subunits with different intensities were shifted as compared to HbGp bands. Furthermore, two linkers showed masses similar to those of HbGp and the other two smaller ones. The HbPe bands, shown in slots VI and VII, presented three linker chains, one of them with a higher mass as compared to HbGp and HbRa (mass value around 37 ± 2 kDa). For the HbEa bands presented in slots from VIII to X, also three linker chains were observed, two of them with masses very close to those of HbRa and the third one with a greater one (around 49 kDa).

In Fig.1B a SDS-PAGE gel image is shown for the four different hemoglobins, in the presence of the 2-mercaptoethanol. The absence of the band corresponding to the trimer around 52 kDa (see Fig.1A) was observed, as a result of the disulfide bond reduction into the three corresponding monomeric subunits. The linker pattern for HbGp and HbRa were essentially maintained upon addition of the reducing agent (slots II-III and IV-V, respectively). In the slots IV and V it was noticed that the monomeric subunits ***a*, *b*** and ***c*** for HbRa were similar to those for HbGp. HbRa had two of these monomers with mass values very close, basically unresolved as a single broad band. HbPe, shown in slots VI and VII, presented one of the trimer monomeric subunits heavier than that for HbGp and HbRa.

However, the other two reduced monomeric subunits from the trimer were very similar, as observed for HbGp and HbRa. The linkers pattern for HbPe changed upon disulfide bonds reduction in the presence of the 2-mercaptoethanol. It is not clear if this was only due to partial denaturation of the protein in the presence of the reducing agent, leading to a change in protein migration.

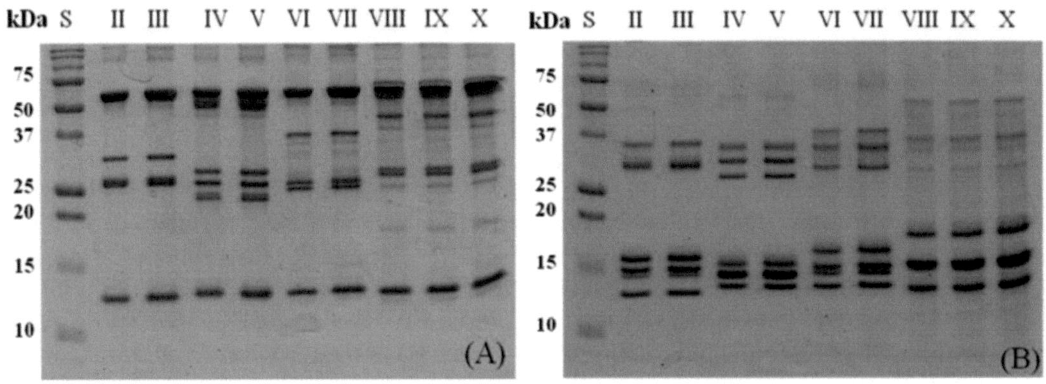

Fig. 1. SDS-PAGE gel electrophoresis for the different extracellular hemoglobins analyzed in this work. The gel concentration was 15% in 25 mmol/L Tris-HCl, 192 mmol/L glycine, pH 8.3, and stained with Comassie Blue R-250. The slot (S) corresponds to the standard masses. (A) Gel electrophoresis in the absence of 2-mercaptoethanol and (B) with the reducing agent. The slots II and III correspond to HbGp, slots IV and V to HbRa, VI and VII to HbPe, and VIII, IX and X to HbEa.

Based on SDS-PAGE, HbEa is the hemoglobin that presents subunits with the highest mass values. All the monomeric subunits obtained from the trimer are heavier as compared to the other hemoglobins studied in this work. Its monomeric subunits have mass values in the range from 12.5 to 18.5 kDa (Fig. 1B). It is also observed one of the linkers with *MM* of 47 ± 2 kDa. These heavier subunits should confer a higher value of *MM* to the whole HbEa as compared to HbGp, HbRa and HbPe. Although, some heavier chains are observed in HbPe and HbEa, it seems that no stoichiometry change occurs for the whole oligomer as compared to HbRa, since the same number of subunits is observed when the disulfide bonds are reduced: namely, four globin monomers and four linkers are detected. This implies that the hemoglobins HbRa, HbPe and HbEa should have a stoichiometry for the whole protein of $[(abcd)_3L_3]_{12}$. Nevertheless, for HbGp only two linker chains are observed in the SDS-PAGE, but, probably, each observed band contains two linkers superposed or, alternatively, the amounts of two of the linkers are too low to be observed in the gel.

Interestingly, some differences observed in the migration for the monomeric subunits ***d*** for all the studied hemoglobins, in the presence of the reducing agent 2-mercaptoethanol, can be associated to the higher unfolding of these subunits, due to the reduction of all disulfide bonds in the hemoglobins. For this reason, when the subunits undergo partial unfolding, their migration through the SDS-PAGE gel becomes more difficult. Being SDS-PAGE electrophoresis alone rather limited, more detailed characterization of the subunits for these hemoglobins by mass spectrometry was performed.

3.2.2 MALDI-TOF-MS data

Fig.2 shows the MALDI-TOF-MS spectrum of a solution of hemoglobin of *Rhinodrilus alatus*, at pH 7.0, using sinapinic acid as matrix in positive ion mode. Fig. 2A shows the peaks obtained for the monomer *d* subunit, the trimer (*abc*) and the linker chains. In agreement with previous studies of hemoglobin of *Glossoscolex paulistus* [15], Fig. 2A shows an intense peak centered around 16.3 kDa, corresponding to the monomer *d*, which is consistent with its relatively easy ionization. Fig.2B shows the expanded region from 15,500 to 18,200 Da, corresponding to the single protonation of the monomer *d*. The contribution of two more intense isoforms, d_1 and d_2, and another less intense isoform d_3 is evident in Fig.2B.

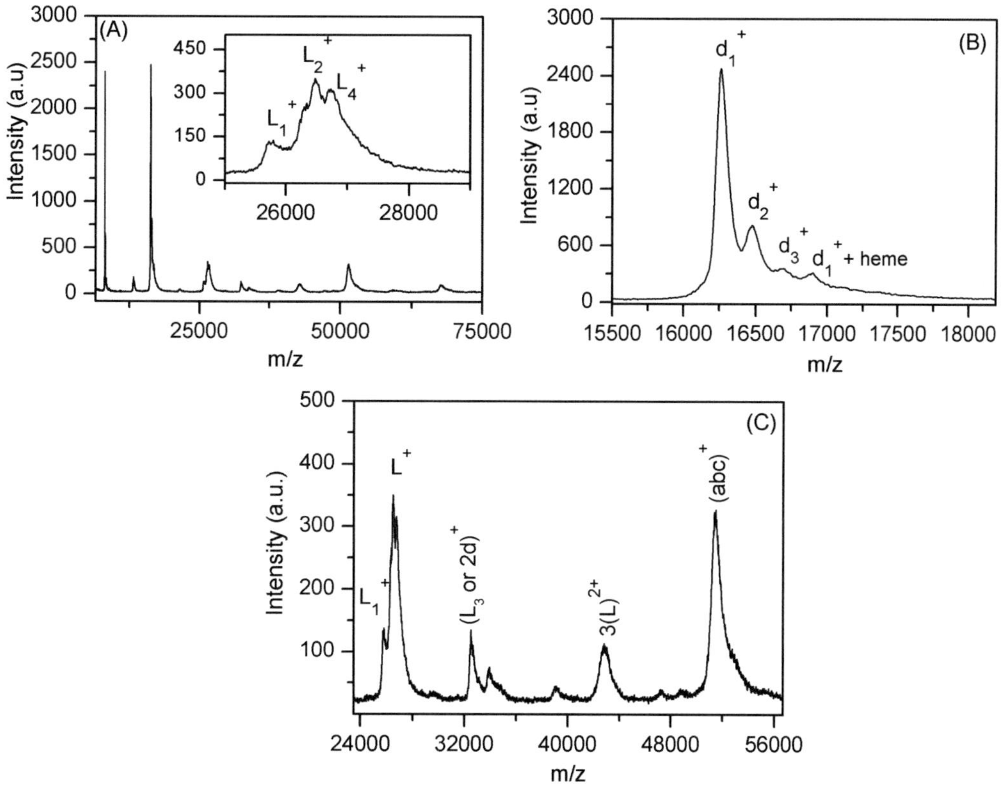

Fig. 2. (A) MALDI-TOF-MS spectrum of *Rhinodrilus alatus* hemoglobin, HbRa, at pH 7.0. The insert shows the expanded ordinate, corresponding to the intensity in arbitrary units, highlighting the linkers peaks; (B) the expanded region for the mono-protonated monomer d^+ from 15,500 to 18,300 Da; (C) the expanded region for the mono-protonated trimer abc^+ and linkers from 24,000 to 56,000 Da.

Moreover, a small contribution around 16,900 ± 30 Da can be associated to d_1 + heme, which is not observed for the other isoforms. In Fig. 2C the expanded region from 24,000 to 56,100 Da is displayed, corresponding to the single protonation of the linker chains *L* and trimer subunits (*abc*). The spectrum clearly shows the existence of three linker chains L_1, L_2 and L_4, with 25,770, 26,540 and 26,740 Da, respectively. The remaining linker chain, L_3, at 32,515 Da, can be superposed with the dimers of monomer *2d*. Finally, an intense contribution at 51,470 Da is observed, associated to the trimer $(abc)^+$, while the less intense species at 67,690 Da is due to the contribution of the tetramer $(abcd)^+$ (Table 3).

Our results for HbRa suggest that the molecular masses of its subunits are very similar to those for HbGp, but the presence of two isoforms for the trimer subunit, as noticed for HbGp [15], is not observed in this hemoglobin. This might indicate that the monomers *a*, *b* and *c* do not have isoforms.

In Table 3, the results of analysis of MALDI-TOF-MS data for hemoglobin of *Eisenia andrei* are shown. In Fig. 3A the peaks obtained for the mono- and di-protonated monomer *d* subunit are significantly more intense as compared to the trimer (*abc*) and the linker chains ones. The molecular mass of the monomer *d* subunit is very similar to those for the HbGp and HbRa hemoglobins, but the peak corresponding to d_1 bound to the heme is not observed. In Fig.3B the three linker chains L_1, L_2 and L_4, with masses of 25,110, 26,470 and 27,445 Da, respectively, and another linker L_3 with a more intense peak at 32,775 Da, are shown. Two additional contributions at 53,270 ± 80 and 69,590 ± 100 Da are also shown in Fig. 3C, which can be assigned to the trimer (*abc*) and tetramer (*abcd*), respectively. Differently from the HbRa and HbGp, the hemoglobin of *Eisenia andrei* has only one predominant monomeric isoform d_1 with molecular mass at 16,344 ± 24 Da. The remaining monomeric isoforms have low intensities.

Mass of the extracellular hemoglobins in (Da)				
Subunits	HbGp	HbRa	HbEa	HbPe
d_1	16,370	16,272 ± 16	16,344 ± 24	16,220 ± 19
d_2	16,415 ± 10	16,490 ± 20	16,495 ± 12	16,438 ± 20
d_3	16,650 ± 40	16,710 ± 25	16,560	16,656 ± 25
d_4	16,850 ± 40	-	16,790	-
$d_1 + heme$		16,900 ± 30		16,844 ± 20
L_1	25,780 ± 30	25,770	25,110	25,670
L_2	26,750 ± 80	26,540	26,470	27,145
L_4	-	26,740	27,445	-
L_3 *or2d**	32,870	32,515	32,775	32,410
T_1 *(abc)*	51,200	51,470	53,270 ± 80	51,240
T_2 *(abc)*	51,985	-	-	-
abcd	68,400	67,690	69,590 ± 100	67,620

*The value of mass corresponds very closely to the dimer of the monomer isoform d_2

Table 3. Molecular masses in (Da) of extracellular hemoglobin subunits, obtained from MALDI-TOF-MS, and for different worms.

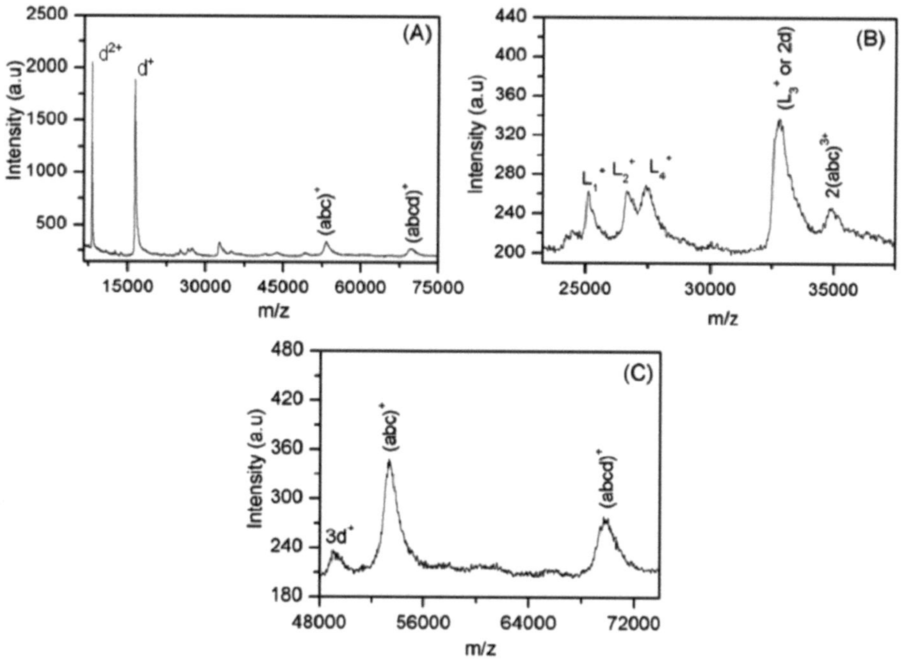

Fig. 3. MALDI-TOF-MS spectrum of *Eisenia andrei* hemoglobin, HbEa. (A) at pH 7.0, full mass range. (B) Corresponds to the intensity in arbitrary units, highlighting the linkers and triple-protonated dimer of trimer; (C) the expanded region for the mono-protonated trimer abc^+ and tetramer $abcd^+$ from 48,000 to 75,000 Da.

Our results indicate that the HbEa presents two significant differences when compared with the HbGp: one of the monomeric chains *a*, *b* or *c*, that constitute the trimer *abc*, has a molecular mass higher than the corresponding HbGp one, due to the mass difference of 2 kDa observed in the trimer of the HbEa (Table 3). The second is the presence of one additional linker chain (L_4) in the oligomeric structure of HbEa.

The data for hemoglobin of *Perionyx excavatus* are shown in Table 3. In this case the molecular mass of monomer *d* is analogous to that observed for the other hemoglobins. Moreover, it was noticed that a small proportion of the monomer *d* remained associated to heme with a mass of 16,844 ± 20 Da. In general, the subunits of the HbPe are very similar to those of HbGp, since no significant differences in the molecular masses are observed. Very recent studies of HbGp, in the presence of 2-mercaptoethanol [38], have shown that the monomer ***c*** chain presents also four isoforms with *MM* in the range of 17.3-17.6 kDa. This is, probably, why the trimer ***T*** is also characterized by two isoforms (Table 3). Further experiments in the future, in the presence of 2-mercaptoethanol will be necessary to elucidate more clearly the masses differences of the globin subunits forming the trimer *abc*, especially regarding the new hemoglobins.

3.2.3 AUC data

All AUC experiments were performed in 100 mmol/L Tris-HCl containing 50 mmol/L NaCl, at pH 7.0 or 5.0, and at 20 °C. The protein concentrations were in the range 100 to 300 μg/mL, and the speed rotor was 20,000 rpm. The SEDFIT software was used in the analysis of sedimentation velocity (SV) data. The V_{bar} parameter used in the fits was the standard value of 0.733 mL/g and f/f_0 was allowed to float being a regularization parameter.

Fig.4 shows sedimentation coefficient distributions c(S), at 200 μg/mL, for the four extracellular hemoglobins. Our results indicate that three of the four hemoglobins present a good homogeneity with a single species in solution. However, for the extracellular hemoglobin of *Eisenia andrei* two different populations are observed, the first one around 10 S can be associated to the dodecamer subunits while the other species at 64 S corresponds to the whole protein. Although these proteins are quite stable in these conditions [3], the observed dissociation is, probably, due to the purification process used for this hemoglobin.

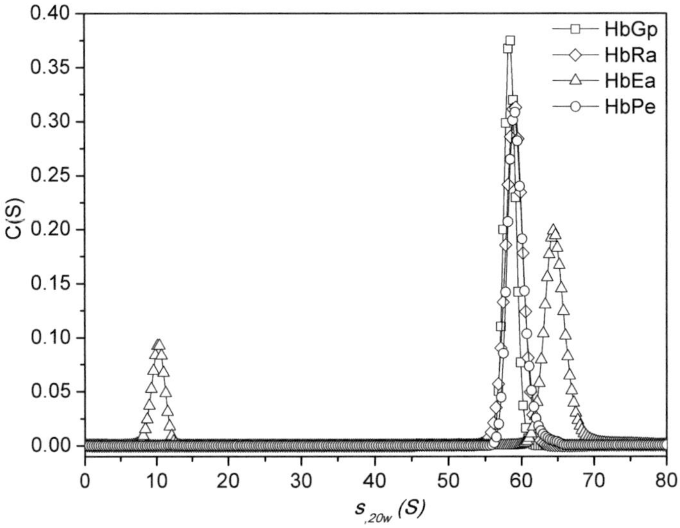

Fig. 4. Continuous sedimentation coefficient distribution of extracellular hemoglobins. The c(S) fittings for hemoglobins, at a concentration of 200 μg/mL, in 100 mmol/L Tris–HCl containing 50 mmol/L NaCl, are shown. The $s_{,20w}$ for each fitted curve was determined as the maximum of the peaks of c(S) curves. Absorbance was monitored at 415 nm.

The work of Krebs et al [39] on the properties of the dodecamer subunit, $(abcd)_3$, of HbLt showed that the dodecamer obtained from urea dissociation of the whole protein consisted of an equilibrium of three species with sedimentation coefficients of 8.5 - 9.4 S, 3.6 - 4.4 S and 1.9 S. According to our AUC data for HbGp, the dodecamer is associated to the 8.5 - 9.4 S species. The other two species correspond to trimers and monomers, in order of decreasing *s*, implying that urea dissociation in HbLt [39] produces an equilibrium of three species.

The *s* values were corrected to standard conditions (water and 20 °C), and the $s^0_{20,w}$ values, corresponding to $s_{20,w}$ at 0 mg/mL protein, were obtained by linear regression extrapolation. The $s^0_{20,w}$, values for the oxy-HbGp at pH 5.0 and 7.0 were 58.6 ± 0.4 and 58.1 ± 0.4 S, respectively, as shown in Table 4. These results suggest that HbGp is very stable in both pH values, and does not undergo oligomeric dissociation at pH 5.0. For the other two hemoglobins, HbRa (*Rhinodrilus alatus*) and HbPe (*Perionyx excavatus*), similar results were observed as for HbGp [3], with $s^0_{20,w}$ around of 59 S. The mass values are very similar, within the experimental error, with the exception of HbEa that has a higher mass (Table 4).

Hemoglobins	$s^0_{20,w}(S)$	*MM* by c(*M*) **(kDa)**
Glossoscolex paulistus (HbGp)[1]	58.6 ± 0.4	3600 ± 80
Glossoscolex paulistus (HbGp)[2]	58.1 ± 0.4	3500 ± 100
Rhinodrilus alatus (HbRa)	59.1 ± 0.1	3500 ± 70
Eisenia andrei (HbEa)	64.6 ± 0.4	3850 ± 50
Perionyx excavatus (HbPe)	58.9 ± 0.2	3500 ± 50

[1]HbGp at pH 5.0. [2]HbGp at pH 7.0.

Table 4. AUC hydrodynamic data analysis, for extracellular hemoglobins from different worms, at 20.0 ± 0.1 °C and pH 7.0.

In Fig.5 the c(M) distributions are shown for the four types of studied extracellular hemoglobins, at a protein concentration of 300 µg/mL. It is noticed that HbEa has a higher *MM* than the other three hemoglobins one (Table 4). This 330 kDa difference can be attributed to two factors: 1) the difference of the subunits masses constituting the oligomeric structure, and 2) a different subunit stoichiometry for the HbEa oligomer. Thus, the inclusion of another linker chain in the structure of HbEa, giving a model like $[(abcd)_3L_4]_{12}$, could contribute with a 326 kDa increase in the total mass of the molecule, consistent with the results observed for HbEa in the c(M) values. This fourth linker chain would have an average mass of 326/12 =27 kDa.

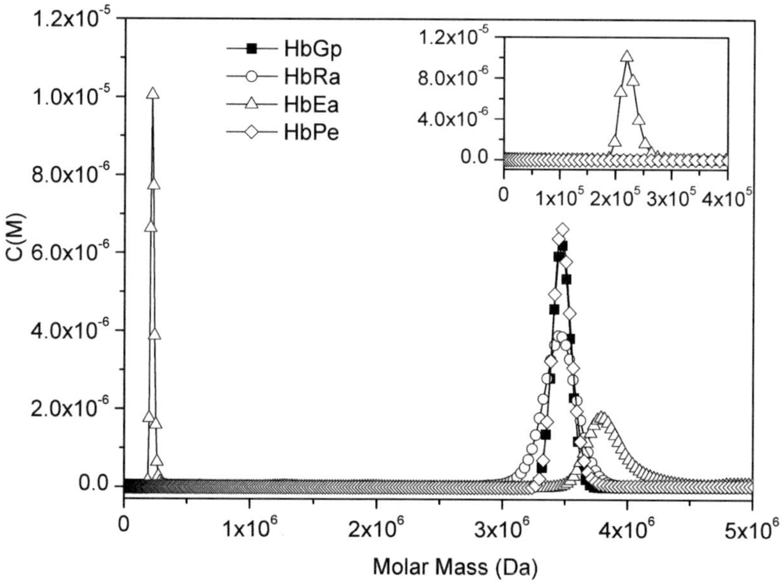

Fig. 5. Continuous molecular mass distribution of extracellular hemoglobins. The c(M) fittings for hemoglobins, at a concentration of 300 µg/mL, in 100 mmol/L Tris-HCl containing 50 mmol/L NaCl are shown. The insert shows the enhanced plot in the *MM* range from 0 to 400 kDa. The *MM* for each fitted curve was determined as the maximum of the peaks of c(M) curves. Absorbance was monitored at 415 nm.

In the c(M) distribution curve for the hemoglobin of *Eisenia andrei* an additional species of 210 kDa is observed, which is assigned to the dodecamer $(abcd)_3$. This mass value is in agreement with the literature reports of 205 kDa [19]. Moreover, the peak at 3.8 MDa corresponding to the whole native protein is broadened, which is, probably, due to a superposition of two contributions: from species lacking the dodecamer and from the whole protein.

The *MM* of three of the hemoglobins shown in Table 4 is around 3.6 MDa, indicating that these proteins have the same stoichiometry and subunits with quite similar mass. Moreover, these *MM* values strongly suggest that the Vinogradov's model $[(abcd)_3L_3]_{12}$ [19] is adequate for the hemoglobins of *Glossoscolex paulistus*, HbGp, *Rhinodrilus alatus*, HbRa, and *Perionyx excavatus*, HbPe. However, our results indicate that for the hemoglobin of *Eisenia andrei* this model is not appropriate, since a significant mass difference is observed corresponding to 12 additional linker chains (with an average mass of 27 kDa).

3.3 Structural model and stoichiometry

The first crystallization experiments with giant hemoglobins are dated from 1840, when crystals from HbLt were obtained. Indeed, HbLt was the first protein crystallized ever [40]. Nevertheless, it took more than one hundred and sixty years to obtain a complete crystallographic structure [20]. The crystal structure of HbLt, at 3.5 Å of resolution, elucidated how the hierarchical levels of an erythrocruorin is made, and represented a fundamental step to better understand these structures. Recently, our group, reported the preliminary structure of HbGp, at 3.15 Å of resolution [21]. The HbGp and HbLt share an estimated identity for the monomer subunit *d* of 54 % [41], with the HbGp structure showing the same hierarchical levels as HbLt (Fig. 6), and the same global association, into type 1. It was the second time that an entire type 1 erythrocrurin has been reported. As in HbLt, the electron density map of the HbGp reveals important details, such as the conserved calcium biding sites, inter/intra chains disulfide bonds and heme group positions. Very recently, crystals from the giant hemoglobins from HbEa, and HbPe were also obtained in our group and the preliminary structure for HbEa has been solved, with a resolution of 4.7 Å, which is enough to conclude that, like HbGp and HbLt, HbEa also belongs to type 1 array. Further experiments are needed to improve the resolution and find evidences on the electron density map where HbEa shows an accumulation of mass [42].

Another very recent relevant advance in the structural analysis was the characterization of the isolated subunit *d* from HbGp. In the biological unit, subunits type *d* form an interface with subunits type *a*, involving the heme groups from both chains, and at the same time an interface with two other subunits *d*, forming a trimeric array, as shown in Fig. 6. We showed that once isolated, the subunit *d* shows, as a first level of aggregation, a dimer *d-d*, with an interface involving heme groups, similar to the one observed between *a-d* in the biological unit (where *a* and *d* shares 27% of identity). In the next level, the crystal lattice shows a stable dimer of dimers *d-d.* This tetrameric array is unrelated with the hetero tetramer (*abcd*) in the biological unit [43]. The existence of these oligomeric structures has also been confirmed by AUC, which shows that the pure monomer *d* solution contains also three species, monomer, dimer and tetramer, and increasing the protein concentration the contribution of the monomeric species reduces from 90 to 80 % [44]. On the other hand, the trimer formed by the subunits *d* in the biological unit has not been observed for the isolated subunit *d*, which leads us to conclude that such an arrangement is a consequence of associations between subunits *d* and *a* in the whole oligomer.

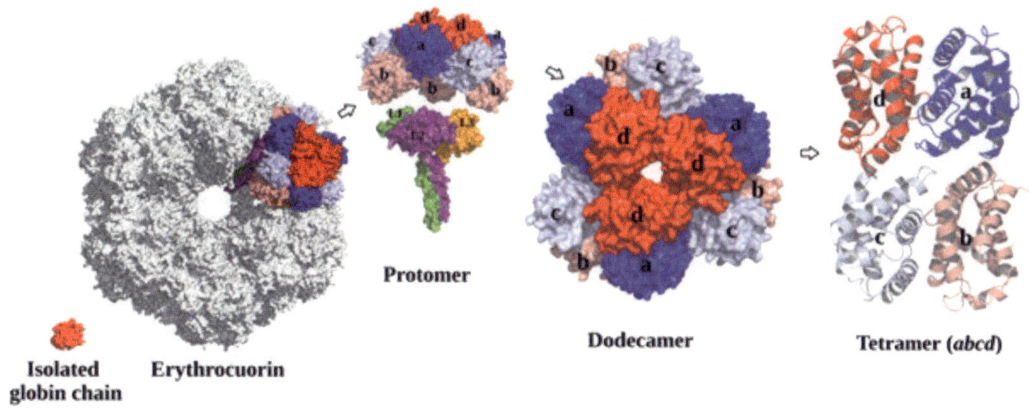

Fig. 6. Schematic representation of the hierarchy in the oligomeric assembly of HbGp into the native structure as obtained from crystallographic data analysis. The whole HbGp structure is composed by twelve protomers, each of them containing a dodecameric structure of globins and three linker subunits, $(abcd)_3L_3$. The dodecameric structure is composed by four types of globin chains: *a*, *b*, *c* and *d*. The four globin chains are associated as a hetero-tetramer (where *a*, *b*, and *c* form a trimer, linked by disulfide bonds).

4. Conclusions

In order to evaluate the potential usefulness of such a giant protein such as HbGp for biomedical applications, a detailed knowledge of its constituent subunits is very relevant. In the present review chapter, recent results for HbGp were described, based on the use of SDS-PAGE, MALDI-TOF-MS and AUC. Preliminary characterization of three new extracellular hemoglobins of different worm species was also described for the first time. The electrophoresis analysis of these hemoglobins shows that they have a subunits structure very similar to that described for HbGp. Moreover, our present results based on AUC data show that two of the new hemoglobins have a total *MM* similar to that of HbGp, namely 3.6 MDa, while the fourth one has a higher *MM* of 3.8 MDa. It appears clear from our data that the globin chains are a total of four with a trimer of 52 - 53 kDa and a monomer of 16 kDa as a common feature for all these hemoglobins. The highest *MM* hemoglobin, HbEa, has heavier linker chains as well as one of the globin monomers. MALDI-TOF-MS analysis for HbGp showed that the monomer *c* presents four isoforms and that the trimer, *abc*, is characterized by two isoforms, T_1 and T_2. In the final part of this review some crystal structures are also reported, which might be helpful in understanding the oligomeric structure of this class of proteins. Our present studies for HbGp are consistent with literature reports on several other extracellular hemoglobins, such as the HbLt and HbAm. Future more detailed characterization of the new hemoglobins will be important to assess all the subunit masses to model their oligomeric structure. We believe our results represent a nice contribution and an important and necessary step in the complete characterization of HbGp oligomeric structure.

5. Acknowledgments

Thanks are due to the Brazilian agencies FAPESP, CNPq, and CAPES for partial financial support. P.S. Santiago is grateful to FAPESP and CNPq for postdoctoral grants. F. A. O. Carvalho is the recipient of a PhD. grant from FAPESP (2009/17261-6). J. W. P. Carvalho is the recipient of a PhD. grant from FAPESP (2010/09719-0). M. Tabak is grateful to CNPq for a research grant. Thanks are also due to Mr. Ézer Biazin for efficient support in the sample preparations and size exclusion chromatography experiments. The authors are indebted to Prof. Paolo di Mascio from Instituto de Química, Universidade de São Paulo, São Paulo, for making available the MALDI-TOF-MS instrumentation and to Mrs. Izaura N. Toma for excellent technical support in the experiments. The authors are greatful to Prof. Richard Garrat and Mr. Fernando Maluf, from the Instituto de Física de São Carlos, University of São Paulo, São Carlos, Brazil, respectively, for constant interest on the crystal structure analysis and support with purification of HbEa and HbPe. Thanks are also due to Mr. Afrânio Augusto Guimarães, from Minhobox (www.minhobox.com.br) for making available *Eisenia andrei* and *Peryonix excavatus* worms.

6. References

[1] Vinogradov, S.N. (2004). The stoichiometry of the four linker subunits of *Lumbricus terrestris* hemoglobin suggests an asymmetric distribution. *Micron,* Vol.35, No. 1-2, (January-February 2004), pp. 127-129, ISSN 0968-4328.

[2] Weber, R.E; Vinogradov, S.N. (2001). Nonvertebrate hemoglobins: functions and molecular adaptations. *Physiological Reviews,* Vol. 81 No. 2, (April 2001), pp. 569–628, ISSN 0031-9333.

[3] Carvalho, F.A.O; Santiago, P.S; Borges, J.C; Tabak, M. (2008). On the molecular mass of the extracellular hemoglobin of *Glossoscolex paulistus*: Analytical ultracentrifugation reexamination. *Analytical Biochemistry,* Vol. 385, No. 2, (February 2009), pp. 257-263, ISSN 0003-2697.

[4] Ohtsuki, M; Crewe, A.V. (1983). Evidence for a central substructure in a Lumbricus terrestris hemoglobin obtained with stem low-dose and digital processing techniques. *Journal of ultrastructure Research.* Vol. 83, No. 3, (1983), pp. 312–318, ISSN 0022-5320.

[5] Weber, R.E; Fago, A. (2004). Functional adaptation and its molecular basis in vertebrate hemoglobins, neuroglobins and cytoglobins *Respiratory Physiology & Neurobiology*. Vol. 144, No.2-3, (December 2004), pp. 141–159, ISSN 1569-9048.

[6] Rousselot, M; Delpy, E; La Rochelle, C.D; Lagente, V; Pirow, R; Rees, J; Hagege, A; Le Guen, D; Hourdez, S; Zal, F. (2006). Arenicola marina extracellular hemoglobin: a new promising blood substitute. *Biotechnology Journal*. Vol. 1, No.3, (March, 2006), pp. 333-345, ISSN 1860-7314.

[7] Zhu, H; Ownby, D.W; Riggs, C.K; Nolasco, N.J; Stoops, J. K; Riggs, A. F. (1996). Assembly of the gigantic hemoglobin of the earthworm *Lumbricus terrestris* - Roles of subunit equilibria, non-globin linker chains, and valence of the heme iron. *Journal of Biological Chemistry*. Vol. 271, No. 47, (June, 1996), pp. 30007-30021, ISSN 0021-9258.

[8] Fushitani, K; Riggs. A. F. (1991). The extracellular hemoglobin of the earthworm *Lumbricus terrestris*-oxygenation properties of isolated chains, trimer, and re-associated products. *Journal of Biological Chemistry*. Vol. 266, No. 16, (June, 1991), pp. 10275-10281, ISSN 0021-9258.

[9] Hirsch, R.E; Jelicks, L.A; Wittenberg, B.A; Kaul, D.K; Shear, H.L; Harrington. J.P. (1997). A first evaluation of the natural high molecular weight polymeric *Lumbricus terrestris* hemoglobin as an oxygen carrier. *Artificial Cells Blood Substitutes and Immobilization Biotchnoplogy*. Vol. 25, No. 5, (1997) 429–444, ISSN 1073-1199.

[10] Harnois, T; Rousselot, M; Rogniaux, H; Zal, F. (2009). High-level Production of Recombinant Arenicola Marina Globin Chains in Escherichia Coli: A New Generation of Blood Substitute. *Artificial Cells Blood Substitutes and Immobilization Biotchnoplogy*. Vol. 37, No. 3, (2009), pp. 106-116, ISSN 1073-1199.

[11] Royer, W.E; Sharma, H; Strand, K; Knapp, J.E; Bhyravbhatla, B. (2006). *Lumbricus* Erythrocruorin at 3.5 Å Resolution: Architecture of a Megadalton Respiratory Complex. *Structure*. Vol. 14, No. 7, (May, 2006), pp. 1167–1177, ISSN 0969-2126.

[12] Martin, P.D; Kuchumov, A; Green, B.R; Oliver, R.W.A; Braswell, E.H; Wall, J.S; Vinogradov, S.N. (1996). Mass spectrometric composition and molecular mass of Lumbricus terrestris hemoglobin: A refined model of its quaternary structure. *Journal of Molecular Biology*. Vol. 255, No.1, (January,1996), pp. 154–169, ISSN 0022-2836.

[13] Viana, E; Silva, C.H.T.P; Tabak, M; Imasato, H; and Garrat, R.C. (1998). A molecular model for the d chain of the giant haemoglobin from *Lumbricus terrestris* and its implications for subunit assembly. *Biochimical et Biophysical Acta-Protein Structure and Molecular Enzymology*. Vol. 1383, No.1, (March, 1998), pp. 130–142, ISSN 0167-4838.

[14] Ownby, D.W.; Zhu, H.; Schneider, K.; Beavis, R.C.; Chait, B.T.; Riggs, A.F. (1993). The extracellular hemoglobin of the earthworm Lumbricus terrestris-determination of subunit stoichiometry. *Journal of Biological Chemistry*. Vol. 268, No. 18, (June, 1993), pp. 13539–13547, ISSN 0021-9258.

[15] Oliveira, M.S; Moreira, L.M; Tabak, M. (2007). Partial characterization of giant extracellular hemoglobin of *Glossoscolex paulistus*: A MALDI-TOF-MS study. *International Journal of Biological Macromolecules*. Vol. 40, No. 5, (April 2007), pp. 429-436, ISSN 0141-8130.

[16] Svedberg, T; Inga-Britta, E. (1933). The molecular weight of erythrocruorin. *Journal of the American Chemical Society*. Vol. 55, No. 7, (May-August, 1933), pp. 2834-2841, ISSN 0002-7863.

[17] Daniel, E.; Lustig, A.; David, M.M.; Tsfadia. Y. On the molecular mass of *Lumbricus* erythrocruorin. *Micron*, Vol. 35, No.1-2, (2004), pp. 131-132, ISSN 0968-4328.

[18] Daniel, E; Lustig, A; David, M.M; Tsfadia, Y. (2003). Towards a resolution of the long-standing controversy regarding the molecular mass of extracellular erythrocruorin of the earthworm *Lumbricus terrestris*. *Biochimica et Biophysica Acta- Protein and Proteomics*. Vol. 1649, No. 1, (June 2003), pp. 1–15, ISSN 1570-9639.

[19] Vinogradov, S.N; Lugo, S; Mainwaring, M.G; Kapp, O.H; Crewe, A.V. (1986). Bracelet Protein: A Quaternary Structure Proposed for the Giant Extracellular Hemoglobin of *Lumbricus terrestris*. *Proceeding of the Academy of Sciences of the United States of America.* Vol. 83, No. 21, (November 1986), pp. 8034-8038, ISSN 0027-8424.

[20] Royer, W.E; Strand, K; Van Heel. M; Hendrickson, W.A. (2000). Structural hierarchy in erythrocruorin, the giant respiratory assemblage of annelids. *Proceedings of the National Academy of Science of the United States of America.* Vol. 97, No.13, (June, 2000) 7107–7111, ISSN 0027-8424.

[21] Bachega, J.F.R; Bleicher, L; Horjales, E.R; Santiago, P.S; Garratt, R.C; Tabak M. (2011). Crystallization and preliminary structural analysis of the giant haemoglobin from *Glossoscolex paulistus* at 3.2 angstrom. *Journal of Synchrotron Radiation,* Vol. 18, (January 2011), pp. 24-28, ISSN 0909-0495.

[22] Zal, F; Green, B.N; Martineau, P; Lallier, FH; Toulmond, A; Vinogradov, S.N; Childress, J.J. (2000). Polypeptide chain composition diversity of hexagonal-bilayer haemoglobins within a single family of annelids, the Alvinellidae. *European Journal of Biochemistry.* Vol. 267, No. 16, (August 2000), pp. 5227-5236, ISSN 0014-2956.

[23] Zal, F; Green, N; Lallier, F.H; Vinogradov S.N; Toulmond, A. (1997). Quaternary structure of the extracellular haemoglobin of the lugworm *Arenicola marina*: a multi-angle-laser-light-scattering and electrospray-ionisation-mass-spectrometry analysis. *European Journal of Biochemistry,* Vol. 243, No. 1-2, (January 1997), pp. 85–92, ISSN 0014-2956.

[24] Royer, W.E, Omartian, M.N, Knapp, J.E. (2007). Low resolution structure of*Arenicola* erythrocruorin: Influence of coiled coils on the architecture of a megadalton respiratory protein. *Journal of Molecular Biology,* Vol. 365, No. 1, (January 2007), pp. 226–236, ISSN 0022-2836.

[25] Rousselot, M; Le Guen, D; Chabasse, C; Zal, F. (2006). Novel dissociation mechanism of a polychaetous annelid extracellular haemoglobin. *FEBS Journal,* Vol. 273, No. 7 (April 2006), pp. 1582-1596, ISSN 1742-464X.

[26] Santiago, P.S; Moura, F; Moreira, L.M; Domingues, M.M; Santos, N.C; Tabak, M. (2008). Dynamic light scattering and optical absorption spectroscopy study of pH and temperature stabilities of the extracellular hemoglobin of *Glossoscolex paulistus. Biophysical Journal,* Vol. 94, No. 6, (March 2008), pp. 2228-2240, ISSN 0006-3495.

[27] Agustinho, S.C.M; Tinto, M.H; Imasato, H; Tominaga, T.T; Perussi, J.R; Tabak, M. (1996). Spectroscopic studies of the met form of the extracellular hemoglobin from *Glossoscolex paulistus. Biochimica et Biophysica Acta (BBA) - Protein Structure and Molecular Enzymology,* Vol. 1298, No. 2, (December 1996), pp. 148-158, ISSN 0167-4838.

[28] Bispo, J.A.C; Santos, J.L.R; Landini, G.F; Goncalves, J.M; Bonafe, C.F.S. (2007). PH dependence of the dissociation of multimeric hemoglobin probed by high hydrostatic pressure. *Biophysical Chemistry,* Vol. 125, No. 2-3, (February 2007), pp. 341-349, ISSN 0301-4622.

[29] Righi, G. (1971). Sobre a família Glossoscolecidae (Oligochaeta) no Brasil. *Arquivos de Zoologia S. Paulo 20*, Vol. 29, pp. 1-95, ISSN 0066-7870 (in Portuguese).

[30] Righi, G. (1972). Bionomic Considerations Upon Glossoscolecidae (Oligochaeta). *Pedobiologia*, Vol. 12, No. 4, pp. 254-260, ISSN 0031-4056.

[31] Maboeta, M.S; Reinecke, A.J; Reinecke, S.A. (1999). Effects of Low Levels of Lead on Growth and Reproduction of the Asian Earthworm *Perionyx excavatus* (Oligochaeta). *Ecotoxicology and Environmental Safety*, Vol. 44, No. 3, (November 1999), pp. 236-240, ISSN 0147-6513.

[32] Edwards, C.A, Dominguez, J, Neuhauser, E.F. (1998). Growth and reproduction of Perionyx excavatus (Perr.) (Megascolecidae) as factors in organic waste management. *Biology and Fertility of Soils*. Vol. 27, No. 2, (June 1998), pp.155–161, ISSN 0178-2762.

[33] Buch, A.C. (2010). *Pontoscolex Corethrurus* (Müller, 1857) e *Eisenia Andrei*, Bouché 1972, Como Bioindicadoras De Solos Contaminados por Agrotóxicos. Universidade Federal do Paraná, Curitiba-Brazil (in Portuguese).

[34] Vampré, T.M; Fuccillo, R; de Andréa, M.M. (2010). Oligoqueta *Eisenia Andrei* Como Bioindicador De Contaminação De Solo Por Hexaclorobenzeno(1). *Revista Brasileira de Ciência do Solo*, Vol. 34, No. 1, pp. 59-66, ISSN 0100-0683

[35] Cortez, J; Billes, G; Bouché, M.B. (2000). Effect of climate, soil type and earthworm activity on nitrogen transfer from a nitrogen-15-labelled decomposing material under field conditions. *Biology and Fertility of Soils*, Vol. 30, No. 4, (January 2000), pp. 318–327, ISSN 0178-2762.

[36] Sautter, K.D; Brown, G.G; James, S.W; Pasini, A; Nunes, D.H; Benito, N.P. (2006). Present knowledge on earthworm biodiversity in the State of Paraná, Brazil. *European Journal of Soil Biology*, Vol. 42, No. 42, (August 2006), pp. S296-S300, ISSN 1164-5563.

[37] Carvalho, F.A.O; Santiago, P.S; Borges, J.C; Tabak, M. (2011). Molecular masses and sedimentation coefficients of extracellular hemoglobin of *Glossoscolex paulistus*: Alkaline oligomeric dissociation. *International Journal of Biological Macromolecules*, Vol. 48, No. 1, (January 2011), pp. 183-193, ISSN 0141-8130.

[38] Carvalho, F.A.O; Carvalho, J.W.P; Santiago, P.S; Tabak, M. (2011). Further characterization of the subunits of the giant extracellular hemoglobin of *Glossoscolex paulistus* (HbGp) by SDS-PAGE electrophoresis and MALDI-TOF-MS. *Process Biochemistry*, Vol.46 (August 2011), pp. 2144-2151.

[39] Krebs, A; Kuchumov, A.R; Sharma, P.K; Braswell, E.H; Zipper, P; Weber, R.E; Chottard, G; Vinogradov, S.N. (1996). *Journal of Biological Chemistry*, Vol. 271, No. 31, (August 1996), pp. 18695-18704, ISSN 0021-9258

[40] McPherson, A. (1999) *Crystallization of Biological Macromolecules*. Cold Spring Harbor Lab. Press, Plain view, NY.

[41] Cabral, B.C; Imasato, H; Rosa, JC; Laure, H.J; da Silva, C.H; Tabak, M; Garratt, R.C; Greene, L.J. (2002). Fluorescence properties of tryptophan residues in the monomeric *d*-chain of *Glossoscolex paulistus* hemoglobin: an interpretation based on a comparative molecular model. *Biophysical Chemistry*, Vol. 97, No. 2-3, (June 2002), pp. 139-157, ISSN 0301-4622

[42] Bachega, J.F.R et al, work in progress.

[43] Bachega JFR, Horjales ER, Tabak M, Garratt RC. (2011). Preliminary Crystallographic Structure of Subunit D from the Giant Hemoglobin of *Glossoscolex paulistus. XL Reunião Anualda Sociedade Brasileira de Bioquímica e Biologia Molecular - SBBq*. No. M-54, pp. 76

[44] Bachega, J.F.R et al., manuscript in preparation.

16

Biological Stoichiometry: The Elements at the Heart of Biological Interactions

Mehdi Cherif
McGill University, Department of Biology,
Montreal, Quebec
Canada

1. Introduction

All organisms in their complexities of shapes, structures and functions use the same building blocks, elements, assembled and cemented together by energy. But only a subset of the elements available on Earth is used by the organisms in their biomass (Figure 1). Furthermore, the elements most commonly used by living beings (e.g., H, C, N, O, P, S, Na, K, Ca, Fe) are essential components of all organisms biomass. This reveals on one hand the common origin of all species and on the other hand the very specific requirements of the various life processes, to which only a subset of the elements are adapted (see Fraústo da Silva & Williams 2001 for a thorough discussion of the adequacy of elements to their biological functions).

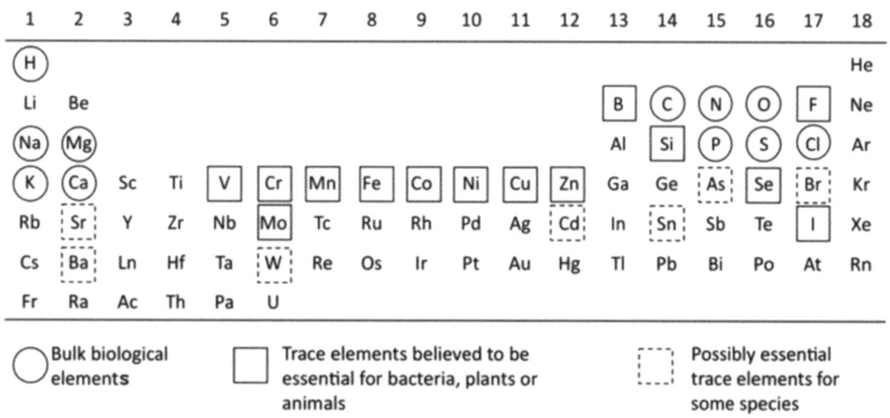

Fig. 1. The distribution of elements essential for life in the periodic table (from Fraústo da Silva & Williams 2001).

Organisms need to get their elements from the environment. To do so, they engage in a variety of interactions with their physical environment and with the other species surrounding them. This fundamental need for elements and energy is thus the fulcrum of many ecological interactions. Furthermore, the sum of all element and energy consumption rates in an ecosystem represents a major driver of the biogeochemical cycles of elements. On geological timescales, organism-driven cycling of elements has effected great changes at a biosphere level, which fed back on life itself (Lovelock & Margulis 1974; Mcelroy 1983).

One would thus expect that the elemental nutrition of organisms would have been an early concern of ecologists and biogeochemists. Oddly enough, this was not the case, despite the fact that, very early on, Alfred James Lotka, a founding figure of ecology, called the attention of ecologists towards the crucial role of elements in shaping what he called the "drama of life", i.e., the sum of all ecological interactions (Lotka 1925). His call has been mostly ignored during the following six decades. Instead, ecologists focused almost exclusively on energy fluxes between organisms. Apart from some specialized fields of ecology, and until recently, most ecological approaches ignored the potential role of elements in shaping ecological interactions, emphasizing instead the importance of energy acquisition. The reasons are many, some conceptual, others practical. Energy in ecosystems is generally fixed from light in newly-formed organic matter by photosynthetic plants (hence the term primary producers used to describe photosynthetic organisms). It is then transmitted to those organisms that consume plant production, herbivores and decomposers. Energy then moves up the food web, thanks to predators eating other consumers. Once organic matter is consumed, the energy is either used for growth, excreted in molecules that cannot be used by plants, or dissipated as heat. Hence, there is no recycling of energy back to plants. The fate of all energy entering ecosystems through plants is either to be rapidly degraded into heat or buried into organic matter recalcitrant to decomposition. Energy flow within ecosystems is thus relatively simple. Consequently, its study led to straightforward, successful theories and concepts, such as Eltonian pyramids (Elton 1927), ecological efficiencies and food webs (Lindeman 1942).

On the other hand, the nutrients flow in ecosystems is a cycle. For a given element, autotrophic organisms are those that incorporate in their biomass the element in its mineral form from the environment. Generally, they are also primary producers, but many heterotrophic microorganisms show this ability, too. Mineral elements in ecosystems come partly from external outputs, but the bulk comes from the decomposition of carcasses and wastes from the organisms themselves. On very long timescales, because the Earth is virtually a closed system, most available elements should cycle at least once through living organisms, short of those spurted from the depths of the planet by volcanoes. This cycling adds a level of complexity that can hardly translate into simple, general laws, as is the case for energy (Loreau 2010). Faced with this complexity, few theoreticians attempted to look for generalities about the flows of matter in food webs and ecosystems, despite Lotka's (1925) longstanding call (DeAngelis 1992).

Admittedly, there have been some fields in which approaches based on elemental composition were applied. Moreover, there have been some sporadic attempts at taking into account the repercussions of the organisms elemental composition on their interactions or on the availability of nutrients in ecosystems. The next section is dedicated to a presentation of these fields that considered the role of elements in biology, but did not serve in their time as stepping stones towards a comprehensive theory of the role of elements in biological interactions. The field of ecology had to wait until the early nineties for such a theory, called "Ecological Stoichiometry", to emerge. It is a recent, exciting theory, presented in the third section, which tackles the role of elements in ecological interactions with a novel and promising approach. It views organisms as a single molecule, made of a combination of the various essential elements (C, N, P, Fe...). Accordingly, it treats ecological interactions as chemical reactions, during which elements are exchanged between a consumer, its resource and the environment. It generally assumes that the organisms stoichiometry is constant, i.e., that their elemental composition is homeostatic. But this assumption is not essential to the theory. More essential is the mass conservation principle, which constrains the ecologists to track the fate of all the important elements exchanged in an ecological interaction.

This theory has led to major advances in our understanding of ecological interactions across biological scales. Among them, there are: the realization that the growth of higher, complex organisms can be limited by the availability of one specific element in their food (Urabe & Watanabe 1992); the uncovering of indirect effects from plants on their supply of mineral nutrients through herbivores, because of mismatches between their elemental compositions (Sterner 1990); the exposure of a causal relationship between the elemental compositions of organisms and their growth rates (Elser *et al.* 2003a). Surprising insights from the theory also extend to other fields of biology, such as reproductive biology (Bertram *et al.* 2006), human cancer (Elser *et al.* 2007), evolution (Souza *et al.* 2008) and genomics (Acquisti *et al.* 2009). The earliest contributions of ecological stoichiometry to biology are covered in the 4th section. The latest contributions are covered in the 5th section. These advances led to the coinage of a new term, "Biological Stoichiometry". This term is meant to emphasize the potential of the theory to link processes across all the scales of biology, from molecules to the biosphere. The last section of this chapter will briefly evaluate how far the theory has gone in this unifying endeavour and what are the challenges ahead of biological stoichiometry, before it can claim to realistically portray some of the important interrelations between molecular and ecosystemic processes.

2. The long road to ecological stoichiometry

Justus von Liebig was probably the first influential scientist to apply chemistry to study plant and animal physiologies in a systematic way. It is probably his vision, that there was no distinction between chemical reactions within and outside organisms, that led him to investigate the elemental compositions of organisms and the effects of this composition on biotic processes such as plant growth and decomposition (Playfair & Liebig 1843).

He came to realize that plant nutrition could be entirely satisfied by inorganic compounds, as long as they contained all the elements that made up plant biomass. Liebig's law of the minimum (Figure 2) emerged from this work and has become a central law of ecology. This law was the first example of an application of the principle of conservation of matter to the biological realm, albeit restricted to plants. For society at large, Liebig's work led to the invention and large-scale application of inorganic fertilizers, in other words, what was later known as the "Green Revolution".

Liebig's work on plant mineral nutrition started a long tradition of research on plant growth limitation by elements. It also oriented researchers towards the pursuit of the original source of mineral nutrients in soils. Quickly, it was understood that microbes (bacteria and fungi) were the main providers of mineral nutrients to plants through their decomposition of organic matter in soils. This organic matter itself originates from dead parts of plants (shed leaves, fallen twigs and trunks, dead roots...) or from animal waste.

To a lesser degree, Liebig's work also attracted attention to the role of animals as resuppliers of elements to plants. Overall, it helped entrench a prevalent view of ecosystems where plants are at the centre, bringing inorganic nutrients into the world of organic matter, and consumers are dissipators of energy and resuppliers of inorganic nutrients to plants, with decomposers taking the largest stack. The abiotic components of ecosystems considered are mainly those that affect mineral uptake by plants and the decomposition of organic matter into minerals (e.g., atmospheric deposition of minerals, leaching, temperature, light conditions…). This model came to reinforce the energy-based food chain model formalized by Lindeman (1942). The effect of elements on the growth and reproduction of animals and microbes was seldom considered, although Liebig himself invoked the possibility that the availability of elements in an animal's diet could limit its growth (Playfair & Liebig 1843). Elements were not yet seen as a factor able to affect the food webs structure and dynamics.

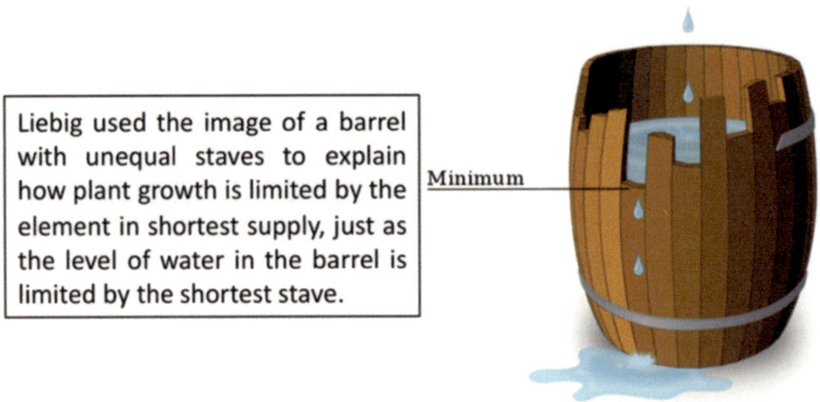

Fig. 2. Liebig's Law of the Minimum and the barrel analogy.

Later developments, however, made it harder to ignore the importance of the elemental needs of some consumers, both for their growth and for their recycling of nutrients. For example, it was known since a long time that microbial decomposers could, in some circumstances, take up inorganic elements instead of mineralize them (Waksman 1917). This uptake of mineral nutrients by heterotrophic microbes was called immobilization. It was quickly understood that the main controlling factor for microbial decomposition or immobilization of nutrients was the mineral content of the microbial biomass in relation to the content of organic matter (Figure 3).

The ecological consequences of the microbial decomposers making up shortages of essential elements in their resource by tapping into the stocks of inorganic nutrients were worked out later on (Bratbak & Thingstad 1985; Harte & Kinzig 1993; Daufresne & Loreau 2001a; Cherif & Loreau 2007). Nutrient-limited primary producers tend to generate carbon-rich organic matter, promoting microbial immobilization. This leads to a paradox, with nutrient-limited plants driving themselves towards stronger nutrient limitation by promoting immobilization. How, then, do limiting nutrients cycle back to plants and support continuous primary productivity if they are locked into the biomass of microbial decomposers? The solution to this paradox was found when food web studies in both aquatic and terrestrial ecosystems established that most bacterial production is generally consumed by heterotrophic predators also called microbivores (mainly protists, such as amoebae, ciliates and flagellates and, in soils, nematodes). The elements locked in the biomass of the ingested microbial decomposers are then mineralized as catabolic by-products, or because microbivores themselves fall prey to other predators higher up the food web, closing what was called the "microbial loop" (Caron 1994; Clarholm 1994; figure 4).

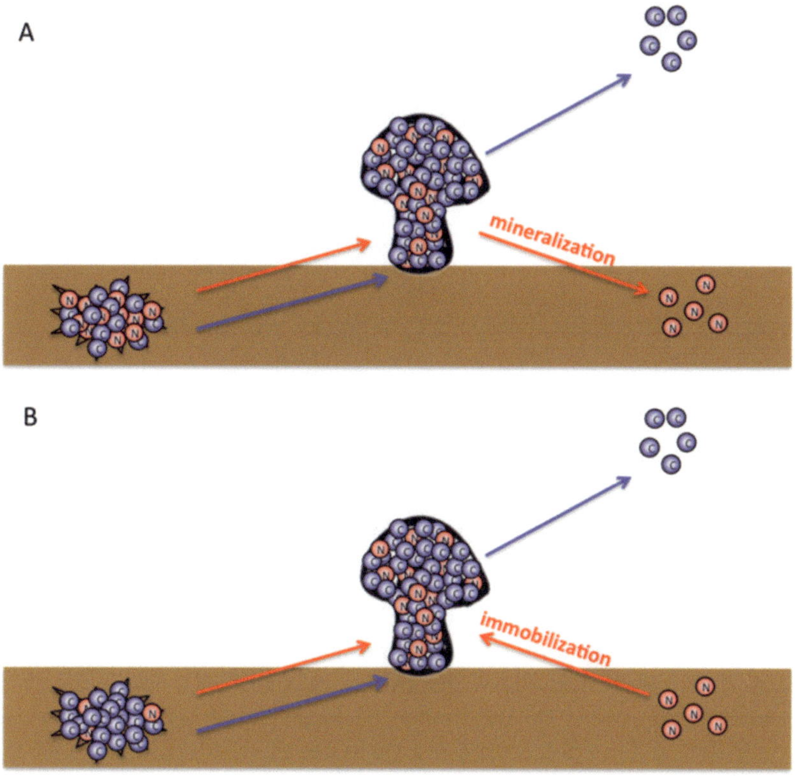

Fig. 3. Mineralization (A) and immobilization (B) of mineral nitrogen by a microbial decomposer, depending on whether organic matter is too rich or too poor in nitrogen, respectively, in comparison to the decomposer nitrogen requirement.

Following the breakthrough of the microbial loop concept, a change in the paradigm of decomposition occurred. Now, the whole detrital food web, not only microbial decomposers, was seen as contributing to the mineralization of the elements essential to plant growth. In this new model, the elemental composition of microbial decomposers plays a central role. On one hand, it determines the extent of immobilization occurring. On the other hand, it also affects the excretion of elements by microbivores, since elements in excess of microbivores needs are excreted (Nakano 1994). Unfortunately, this increasing awareness of the roles of the elemental compositions of microbes, organic matter and microbivores within the communities of researchers interested in soils, did not spread to other fields of ecology, at least until the emergence of the ecological stoichiometry theory.

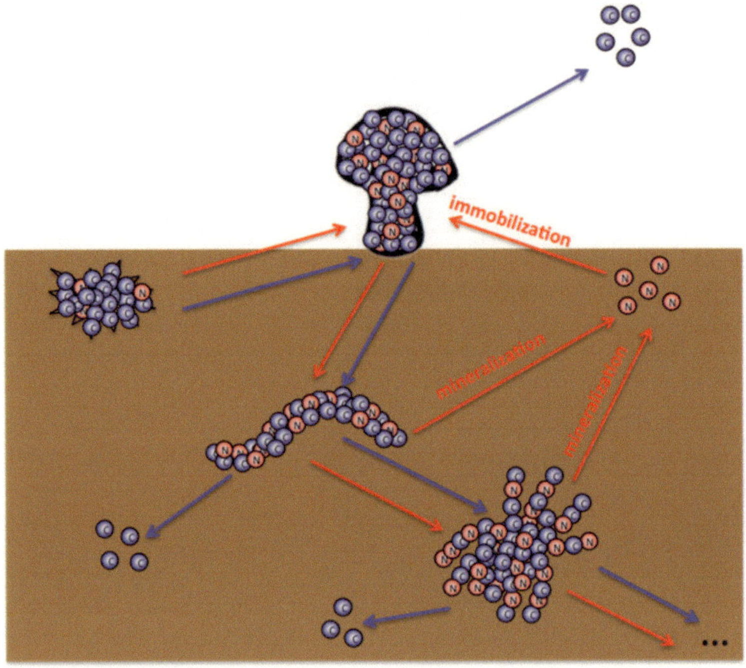

Fig. 4. The microbial loop in soils. Microbial decomposers (fungi and bacteria) immobilize the inorganic elements (here N). They are consumed by microbivores (here nematodes) who release the immobilized N as a by-product of catabolism and are consumed by other consumers (here mites).

The closest to an early stoichiometric thinking, anterior to the ecological stoichiometry theory, appeared in oceanography, a discipline interested into patterns at a larger spatial scale than most other disciplines, but which turned its attention towards the phytoplankton, among the smallest organisms on the planet. Biomass elemental composition was part of oceanographic thinking since at least the 40s, thanks to the work of Alfred Clarence Redfield (1934). Redfield compared the contents of carbon, nitrogen and phosphorus in the phytoplankton of open ocean areas to dissolved nutrient concentrations in surface water and regenerated in the deep ocean (Table 1). The similarity between these ratios led him to state that the plankton chemical composition determined, on geological time, the chemical composition of the ocean (Redfield 1958).

	P	*N*	*C*
Analyses of plankton	1	16	106
Changes in sea water	1	15	105
Available in sea water	1	15	1000

Table 1. Atomic ratios of elements in components of the oceanic biochemical cycle (Adapted from Redfield 1958)

Furthermore, Redfield proposed that the phytoplankton balanced its consumption of nitrogen relative to phosphorus by fixing the atmospheric nitrogen when P was in excess, so that their ratio became equal to that of their chemical composition (the now famous N:P Redfield ratio equal to 16). This is equivalent to assuming that it was the phosphorus that, on geological timescales, limited the growth of phytoplankton, while nitrogen was simply adjusted by the biological activity of the nitrogen-fixing phytoplankton (Redfield 1958).

This stoichiometric model of the oceanic biogeochemical cycle has prompted work on the elemental stoichiometry of recycling in oceans (e.g., Berner). Moreover, it encouraged much speculation on the genesis and maintenance of the ocean and the atmosphere chemical properties (Walker 1974; Griffith *et al.* 1977; Lovelock & Watson 1982). Curiously, this did not lead to any serious attempt to generalize these results to other ecosystems, other elements beyond nitrogen, phosphorus and carbon, or the roles of other trophic levels beyond the phytoplankton.

On the other hand, the assertion that phosphorus should be the element limiting the growth of phytoplankton contradicted accumulated empirical evidence showing that the oceanic phytoplankton was primarily limited by nitrogen (Smith 1984). This contradiction spurred several decades of studies on the growth and chemical composition of phytoplankton grown in the presence of several potentially limiting factors, especially nitrogen and phosphorus (Droop 1974; Rhee 1978; Goldman *et al.* 1979; Tett *et al.* 1985). These experiments showed that both the chemical composition and type of growth-limiting element vary among phytoplankton species. Although constant at the scale of ocean basins, the Redfield ratio is thus probably the result of several processes rather than a fixed property of the phytoplankton (Falkowski 2000; Geider & La Roche 2002; Klausmeier *et al.* 2004).

The accumulation of knowledge on the diversity of elemental requirements, limitations and chemical compositions among phytoplankton species led to believe that it was possible to explain the "paradox of the plankton" proposed by George Evelyn Hutchinson (1961). Hutchinson wondered how the phytoplankton could harbour so many species (in the order of several tens) in the relatively homogeneous environment of surface waters, despite the low number of resources shared by these species. This seemed to contradict the principle of competitive exclusion, which predicts that there cannot be more species than limiting resources at equilibrium (Hardin 1960).

Based on earlier work (Macarthur & Levins 1964; Rapport 1971; Leon & Tumpson 1975), David Tilman developed a theory that could predict the outcome of resource competition between several species of phytoplankton according to their elemental requirements, their chemical compositions and external supplies of elements in the ecosystem (Tilman 1980). Later, expanding his theory to integrate spatiotemporal fluctuations in external supplies, he demonstrated that these variations allowed the coexistence of more species than resources (Tilman *et al.* 1982). He thus provided what he considered as a definitive response to Hutchinson's "paradox of the plankton". Furthermore, seeking to explain possible sources of variation in the supplies of elements, he advanced the hypothesis that "If some nutrients (e.g., phosphorus) are regenerated more rapidly than others, zooplankton may significantly affect phytoplankton community structure by changing nutrient supply rates and ratios" (Tilman *et al.* 1982). Only a few steps remained until the ecological stoichiometry theory.

3. Ecological stoichiometry: An attempt at a systematic approach

In 1988, Elser and colleagues observed a correlation between the type of element limiting the growth of the phytoplankton and the species composition of the zooplankton community of experimental lakes in Michigan (Elser *et al.* 1988). When the zooplankton community was dominated by copepods, the phytoplankton was limited by nitrogen, whereas it was limited by phosphorus when dominated by cladocerans such as Daphnia. They already knew that the zooplankton recycled nitrogen and phosphorus with different efficiencies (Lehman 1984). They could not explain, though, the different effects of copepods and cladocerans, especially since many differences between the two types of zooplankton could intervene: copepods are mainly small and select the species they consume, while cladocerans are generally larger (up to several millimetres) and consume very effectively all the species captured in their filters. An explanation was soon offered by R. W. Sterner (1990) when he showed theoretically that zooplankton species with different chemical compositions should recycle elements with different efficiencies, provided that their chemical composition is kept constant over time. Andersen and Hessen (1991) then found that copepods and cladocerans were widely dissimilar in their chemical composition; copepods are rich in nitrogen while Daphnia are richer in phosphorus. Moreover, they found little variation in their compositions over time, despite variations in the composition of their resources.

All these related observations and hypotheses merged together to give the first fully-stoichiometric description of a trophic interaction: " Herbivore species with a high ratio of N:P in their tissues should resupply nutrients at a relatively low N:P ratio compared to herbivore species with low body N:P" (Sterner *et al.* 1992). The increased availability of the element in excess of the herbivores needs should drive the phytoplankton to a limitation by the same factor that limits the growth of herbivores (N for herbivores with a high ratio of N: P and P for those with a low N: P) (Figure 5).

Surprisingly, the main criticisms of this hypothesis concerned a point that is not essential to the mechanism that underlies it, but derives from subsequent works (Hessen 1992; Urabe & Watanabe 1992). The possibility of a direct limitation of the growth of the zooplankton by mineral elements, either N or P, raised many objections from researchers thinking that resource limitation of growth was possible only by biochemical substances such as amino acids or fatty acids (Brett 1993, Müller-Navarra 1995). Links between growth rate and diet elemental content were seen as simple correlations. Much research was then devoted to prove or disprove the negative effects of nitrogen and phosphorus-deficient phytoplankton on the growth of the zooplankton (Sterner *et al.* 1993; Anderson & Hessen 1995; Urabe *et al.* 1997; Urabe & Sterner 2001).

Regeneration of nitrogen and phosphorus by the zooplankton with a ratio reflecting the difference between its chemical composition and that of its resources is a part of the hypothesis that was largely confirmed afterwards (Sterner & Smith 1993; Urabe 1993; Balseiro *et al.* 1997; Elser & Urabe 1999). On the other hand, the alteration of phytoplankton limitation that is supposed to result from this differential recycling of elements by zooplankton was, if not less studied, rarely highlighted. Some studies showed indeed a strong effect of herbivore chemical composition and recycling on the phytoplankton growth limitation (Carpenter *et al.* 1993; Rothhaupt 1997; MacKay & Elser 1998). Other results did not concur with the predictions from the stoichiometric hypothesis (Moegenburg & Vanni

1991; Urabe 1993). Daufresne and Loreau (2001b) provided an elegant explanation of these discrepancies by showing theoretically that the effect of herbivores on the plants limitation depends not only on their chemical composition, but also on the physiological response of plants to herbivory. Indeed, the decrease in plant biomass caused by herbivory results in increased elemental requirements of plants to compensate for the loss. These additional requirements can vary between elements and between phytoplankton species. The nature of the limiting element promoted by herbivores is determined by the result of these physiological adjustments and the differential recycling of elements by herbivores.

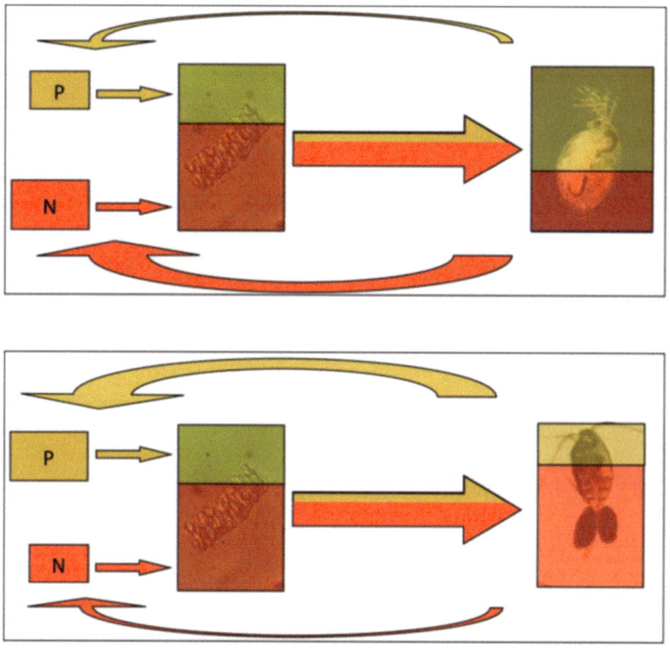

Fig. 5. The stoichiometric hypothesis of consumer-driven elemental limitation of phytoplankton. P-rich Daphnia (upper panel) ingest N in excess from the phytoplankton. Getting rid of this excess, they enrich the environment in N and thus drive the phytoplankton towards P limitation. N-rich copepods (lower panel) drive the phytoplankton towards N limitation by a similar mechanism.

Efforts were also undertaken to broaden the stoichiometric approach beyond the sphere of pelagic freshwater organisms and towards other ecosystems. Several studies have therefore turned to other habitats: marine (Elser & Hassett 1994), arctic (Dobberfuhl & Elser 2000), terrestrial (Elser *et al.* 2000), benthic (Frost *et al.* 2002), arid (Schade *et al.* 2003) and even fossil ecosystems (Elser *et al.* 2006). Other organisms and trophic levels were also investigated: bacteria (Chrzanowski & Kyle 1996; Makino *et al.* 2003), protists (Grover & Chrzanowski 2006), vertebrates (Vanni *et al.* 2002), and insects (Woods *et al.* 2002; Markow *et al.* 2006).

Most of the advances in ecological stoichiometry, from its birth to the early years of this century are well summarized in the book "Ecological stoichiometry: The biology of elements from molecules to the biosphere" published in 2002 by Sterner and Elser. It is worth noting though, that no comprehensive review of the topic has appeared since then.

4. Understanding stoichiometry: The biological bases of the economy of elements in organisms

Different organisms vary widely in their elemental composition. This variation is what makes the study of stoichiometry relevant for developing a better understanding of ecological interactions. On a different level, these elemental differences also lead to questions about the underlying biological causes for these differences. Sterner and Elser's synthetic book (2002) represents the first attempt at an in-depth investigation of the origins of the differences among the elemental stoichiometries of organisms.

A first obvious source of stoichiometric diversity is the various extents to which organisms invest in structural materials that often present distinct stoichiometric signatures. Well-known examples are the investment of molluscs in calcium carbonate shells, which should increase their calcium content, the hydroxyapatite-based bones of vertebrates, the siliceous frustules of diatoms and the carbon-rich, nitrogen-poor woody stems of many terrestrial plants. A precursor to the ecological stoichiometry theory, William A. Reiners (1986) assumed a fixed composition for the protoplasm of all organisms (the cellular components, without any structural material) and assigned all variations in elemental composition to variations in the proportions of different structural material. Since then, it became obvious that protoplasms can differ in their elemental compositions, such that even relatively taxonomically close species can show different stoichiometries (Andersen & Hessen 1991). The basic building blocks of organic matter (amino-acids, lipids, carbohydrates, nucleotides…) and the polymers assembled from them (proteins, nucleotides…) show obvious stoichiometric differences (Figure 6).

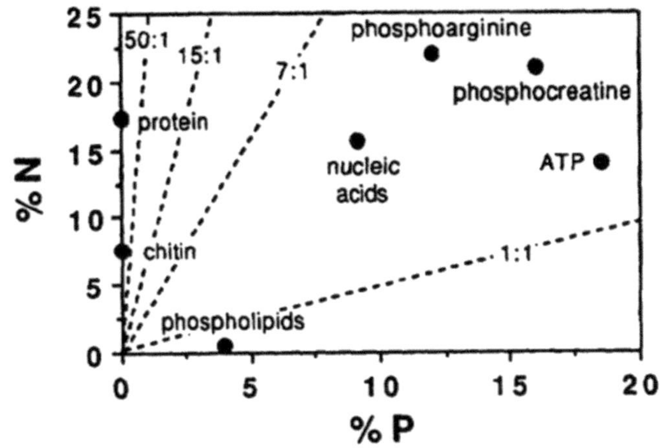

Fig. 6. Nitrogen and phosphorus composition of important biomolecules. Percentage nitrogen and percentage phosphorus are given in terms of weight. Dotted lines depict standard values of atomic (molar) N:P ratios, the most commonly used units reported in ecological stoichiometry studies (reproduced from Elser *et al.* 1996)

Among these biomolecules, proteins and nucleic acids stand out, being very abundant and having contrasting elemental compositions. Proteins are rich in N and nucleic acids are rich in P. It was postulated and then shown that otherwise close organisms that differ in their proportions of proteins and nucleic acids also differ in their N:P ratios (Sterner & Elser 2002). The next step was to look at the distribution of these molecules within cell components and organelles. Through cell fractionation techniques and calculations, it quickly became clear that ribosomal RNA (rRNA) generally represent the major stock of nucleic acids and P within cells (Elser *et al.* 1996). Proteins and associated N atoms are more evenly distributed within cells, although mitochondria emerge as a particularly N-rich organelles (Sterner & Elser 2002). These observations led to one of the first and major unexpected predictions to stem from the ecological stoichiometry theory, namely the "growth rate hypothesis". This hypothesis is simply a causal link made between the observation that rRNA generally represent the major stock of P in cells and organisms on one side, and the observation that the need for ribosomes increases with growth rate on the other side (Elser *et al.* 1996). From there came the hypothesis that there should be a direct relation between the growth rate of organisms and their P content. Since proteins and nucleic acids have similar N contents, replacing one with another should not alter the N content. So, there should be also a direct relation between growth rate and the N:P ratio. The hypothesis was put to test, using data collections and experiments. Many studies showed results that are congruent with the growth rate hypothesis in various taxa (Elser *et al.* 2003a; Karpinets *et al.* 2006). However, it was found to be of limited validity across other taxa, because of species-specific differences in the percentage of P linked to RNA (Matzek & Vitousek 2009). Moreover, maintenance costs for high P levels in biomass can also impair the relation between P content and growth rate (Urabe & Shimizu 2008). Finally, P content was often decoupled from growth rate when organisms were grown under a limiting factor other than P, probably because they can store P that is in excess of their needs (Elser *et al.* 2003a; Matzek & Vitousek 2009).

Curiously, although there is a strong association between mitochondria and cell N content, there was no hypothesis set forth to predict potential relations between cell N content and physiological correlates of mitochondrial cellular density. More generally, the role of N content has been understudied in biological stoichiometry, probably reflecting the fact that: i) N content is less variable than P content ii) P-rich Daphnia are model organisms in many fields of ecology and genetics and iii) P is thought to be the predominant limiting factor in freshwater ecosystems and the main agent of anthropogenic eutrophication.

In summary, there are three main factors that determine the elemental composition of organisms: i) the relative amounts of important biomolecules in cells, such as proteins and RNA; ii) the type and amount of structural material in the organism; and iii) the reserves of elements that are supplied in excess of the organismal requirement. Each of these three factors is related to ecologically relevant life history traits, thus building a bridge between the stoichiometry and the ecology of organisms. For example, P content in P limited organisms, is related to RNA content which itself is a function of growth rate (the Growth Rate Hypothesis). Organisms with more structural material, tending to be larger than related species with fewer structures, show lower specific metabolic rates (Brown *et al.* 2004). Species storing non-limiting resources fare better than similar organisms without storage when the resource becomes limiting, but at the expenses of a higher maximum growth rate (Sommer 1985). Hence, progress in understanding the underlying biological determinants of the organisms stoichiometry is relevant, not only because it advances our knowledge of the physiology of organisms, but also because it sheds light on the ecology of organisms as affected by their stoichiometry. The previous section described how Ecological Stoichiometry opened up the way to link the organisms stoichiometry to the biogeochemical cycles within ecosystems. This section shows how Biological Stoichiometry represents a link from molecules to the ecology of organisms. Since Biological Stoichiometry encompasses Ecological Stoichiometry, then it is a theory that has the potential to link molecules to ecosystems, as claimed by its main proponents in their reference work (Sterner & Elser 2002). Nevertheless, the theory just set the tools (the elemental composition regulation in organisms) and the method (balancing the multi-elemental exchanges between organisms) to reach such integration across the levels of biology, without offering a-priori predictions about how processes at different biological levels articulate. These predictions need to be worked out by mixing stoichiometric reasoning with observations. Such was the case for the Growth Rate Hypothesis, which stemmed from the observations that a majority of P in cells is associated with rRNA, itself associated with growth rate, and concluded that fast-growing organisms should be P-rich and thus more sensitive to P deficiencies in their food. The next section is meant to present some of the most recent advances towards this integrative goal.

5. Recent advances in biological stoichiometry

Following Sterner and Elser's 2002 book, researchers in the field of biological stoichiometry pursued two main directions. On one hand, there was an urge to have a more accurate knowledge of the mechanisms by which organisms regulate their elemental composition, in order to more realistically link their stoichiometric properties to their impacts on the cycles of elements. On the other hand, other researchers carried on with the process of extending the use of the stoichiometric approach to other fields in biology, always with the objective of integrating seemingly separate fields.

Consumers that strive to keep their elemental composition constant, in the face of stoichiometrically imbalanced resources, need to alter their gross growth efficiencies for elements in a controlled way (Figure 7). These gross growth efficiencies, in turn, determine the differential recycling of elements by consumers (Sterner 1990).

How consumers regulate their gross growth efficiencies was, and still is, largely unknown. In the absence of empirical data, in early stoichiometric models, the gross growth efficiency of the element limiting the consumer growth was set to a maximum value, ensuring maximal growth, while the gross growth efficiencies of the other elements were adjusted to yield a constant stoichiometry for the consumer (Figure 7). But theoretically, there is an infinite number of possible alternative strategies (Andersen 1997). Recent experiments also show that net assimilation of the limiting element is not necessarily at its maximal efficiency (DeMott *et al.* 1998) and that non-limiting elements too have impacts on growth (Boersma & Elser 2006; Zehnder & Hunter 2009). Moreover, it was shown that the quantity of resources, besides their stoichiometric compositions, affects the gross growth efficiencies of elements (Anderson & Hessen 2005). Furthermore, models that included a description of the distribution of elements among the various biomolecules in cells have shown that it is not even always possible to set one element as the growth- limiting factor (Anderson *et al.* 2004). It thus became clear that more physiologically grounded models of the use of elements by organisms were needed. Anderson et al's now classical model (2005) strikes a good balance between physiological realism and simplicity, including processes such as biomass turnover, assimilation costs, maintenance costs, and respiration. These endeavours to understand the regulation of organismal stoichiometry by including the metabolism of biomolecules lead to connections between biological stoichiometry and nutritional sciences (Raubenheimer *et al.* 2009).

A

$$G_X = I_X - F_X - R_X$$
$$G_Y = I_Y - F_Y - R_Y$$

C

$$\begin{aligned}\theta_{XY} &= G_X/G_Y \\ &= (GGE_X \times I_X)/(GGE_Y \times I_Y) \\ &= (GGE_X/GGE_Y) \times (I_X/I_Y) \\ &= (GGE_X/GGE_Y) \times \Phi_{XY}\end{aligned}$$

B

$$GGE_X = G_X/I_X$$
$$GGE_Y = G_Y/I_Y$$

D

X is limiting:

$$GGE_X = GGE_{Xmax}$$
$$\begin{aligned}GGE_Y &= GGE_X \times (\Phi_{XY}/\theta_{XY}) \\ &= GGE_{Xmax} \times (\Phi_{XY}/\theta_{XY})\end{aligned}$$

G_X: X newly accumulated in biomass	*GGE_X: gross growth efficiency for X*
I_X: X ingested from resource	*θ_{XY}: consumer's X:Y ratio*
F_X: X egested with fecal matter	*Φ_{XY}: resource X:Y ratio*
R_X: X excreted due to catabolism	

Fig. 7. Relation between the gross growth efficiencies of two unspecified elements (X and Y) as imposed by the constraint of a homeostatic regulation of the stoichiometry of a consumer. A) Mass balance equations for consumption. B) Definition of the gross growth efficiency. C) Stoichiometric constraint imposed on the GGEs for X and Y, as a consequence of the constancy of the X:Y ratio of consumers. D) A simple model that assumes a maximal GGE for the limiting element leads to the GGE of the non-limiting element to be a function of the maximal GGE, and the X:Y ratios of the consumer and its resource (adapted from Sterner 1990).

Physiological adaptation is the short-term response of consumers to imbalanced resources. Analyses at the levels of genomes and transcriptomes, showed that transcriptional changes are among the mechanisms used by consumers to achieve stoichiometric homeostasis. For example, transcriptional changes in the expression of phosphate transporters, activation of alternative metabolic pathways, changes in allocations to roots (for plants), are triggered under P deficiency (Jeyasingh & Weider 2007). Recent studies uncovered long-term evolutionary responses to element deprivations: N-deprived organisms react by substituting N-rich amino-acids by amino-acids with N-poor residues in their expressed proteins or by expressing shorter mRNAs (Grzymski & Dussaq 2011). They also show RNAs with more N-poor nucleotides (Elser *et al.* 2011). As for DNA, since GC and AT pairs have almost the same N content, N limitation seems to have less effect. These advances on the links between elemental limitation and cell polymer composition lead to the coining of a new term: "stoichiogenomics" (Elser *et al.* 2011).

Away from these ventures into the heart of the cellular machinery, other researchers looked for new insights from applying stoichiometric approaches to yet untouched fields. For example, models and experiments had shown that primary producers with a very low nutrient content could drive grazers to extinction and prevent their invasion of a habitat where they are absent (Andersen *et al.* 2004). This barrier to herbivore establishment led to speculations that the lack of grazers before the early Cambrian explosion and their "sudden" appearance afterwards could be linked to a change in the P supply at the scale of the globe (Elser *et al.* 2006). The same authors tested the hypothesis using modern stromatolites, which are very similar to the fossilized Cambrian stromatolites.

Another unexpected fallout from the application of the stoichiometric approach is the uncovering of stoichiometry-related effects on the relation between sexes and on the process of sexual selection. Sexes often differ in their investment in sex-related characters and organs. This difference is likely to be reflected in their elemental needs and use of their resources (Morehouse *et al.* 2010). A well-studied example is the positive correlation found between the phosphorus body content in male crickets and their song performance. Another area in which the stoichiometric approach proved fruitful hits closer to our everyday concerns: our health. An ingenious application of the growth rate hypothesis to cancer, gave rise to the hypothesis that fast-growing cancerous tumours should be richer in P. Thus, they should enter into competition with their neighbouring healthy cells for P and possibly see their growth be P-limited (Elser *et al.* 2007). This hypothesis brought forth by ecologists, that sees tumours as an ecosystem in itself, attracted favourable attention from the medical world (Baudouin-Cornu 2008; Pienta *et al.* 2008) and has potential medical applications ((Elser *et al.* 2003b). Because pathogens share the same requirements for elements as their hosts, they too can be affected by shortages in some key elements, such as iron (Smith 2007). Competition between host cells and pathogens for elements as well as external supplies of elements become an important parameter of the outcome of infections (Hall *et al.* 2009). Hence, the stoichiometry of diseases opens the door for more rational medical treatments through nutrition (Cotter *et al.* 2011).

6. Future needs and challenges ahead

Biological stoichiometry proved to be astonishingly successful in bringing new insights in seemingly disconnected fields of biology, such as molecular evolution, palaeontology and parasitology. But these advances have not yet allowed us to draw a complete picture of the elements role in structuring biological entities from molecules to ecosystems. Huge gaps remain between levels: for example, the stoichiometric theory currently attributes a unique elemental composition to all individuals within one population. But it is known that stoichiometry varies with ontogeny (E.g., Main *et al.* 1997). Hence, the stoichiometry of a population probably differs from the stoichiometry of its individual components and might vary through time, a fact rarely considered (Nakazawa 2011).

Life is complex: different organisms might show different strategies to regulate their elemental composition (Mitra & Flynn 2005, 2007); food webs are diverse, both horizontally (i.e., within the same trophic level) and vertically (i.e., across trophic levels). Predictions that apply to one trophic level may prove erroneous if they neglect other species from the same (Danger *et al.* 2008) or from different trophic levels (Cherif & Loreau 2009). These additional complexities need to be fully incorporated into the theory of Biological Stoichiometry before it really can link molecules to ecosystems. This is obviously a long journey but the road is already drawn on the map!

7. References

Acquisti C., Elser J.J. & Kumar S. (2009). Ecological Nitrogen Limitation Shapes the DNA Composition of Plant Genomes. *Mol Biol Evol*, 26, 953-956.

Andersen T. (1997). *Pelagic nutrient cycles herbivores as sources and sinks*. Springer, Berlin Heidelberg New York.

Andersen T., Elser J.J. & Hessen D.O. (2004). Stoichiometry and population dynamics. *Ecol Lett*, 7, 884-900.

Andersen T. & Hessen D.O. (1991). Carbon, Nitrogen, and Phosphorus-Content of Fresh-Water Zooplankton. *Limnol Oceanogr*, 36, 807-814.

Anderson T.R., Boersma M. & Raubenheimer D. (2004). Stoichiometry: Linking elements to biochemicals. *Ecology*, 85, 1193-1202.

Anderson T.R. & Hessen D.O. (1995). Carbon or Nitrogen Limitation in Marine Copepods. *J Plankton Res*, 17, 317-331.

Anderson T.R. & Hessen D.O. (2005). Threshold elemental ratios for carbon versus phosphorus limitation in Daphnia. *Freshwater Biol*, 50, 2063-2075.

Anderson T.R., Hessen D.O., Elser J.J. & Urabe J. (2005). Metabolic stoichiometry and the fate of excess carbon and nutrients in consumers. *Am Nat*, 165, 1-15.

Balseiro E.G., Modenutti B.E. & Queimalinos C.P. (1997). Nutrient recycling and shifts in N:P ratio by different zooplankton structures in a South Andes lake. *J Plankton Res*, 19, 805-817.

Baudouin-Cornu P. (2008). Stoichiometric, my dear Watson! *M S-Med Sci*, 24, 483-489.

Berner R.A. (1977). Stoichiometric Models for Nutrient Regeneration in Anoxic Sediments. *Limnol Oceanogr*, 22, 781-786.

Bertram S.M., Schade J.D. & Elser J.J. (2006). Signalling and phosphorus: correlations between mate signalling effort and body elemental composition in crickets. *Anim Behav*, 72, 899-907.

Boersma M. & Elser J.J. (2006). Too much of a good thing: On stoichiometrically balanced diets and maximal growth. *Ecology*, 87, 1325-1330.

Bratbak G. & Thingstad T.F. (1985). Phytoplankton-Bacteria Interactions - an Apparent Paradox - Analysis of a Model System with Both Competition and Commensalism. *Mar Ecol-Prog Ser*, 25, 23-30.

Brett M. T. (1993). Possibility of N or P Limitation for Planktonic Cladocerans - an Experimental Test and Nutrient Element Limitation of Zooplankton Production - Comment. Limnol Oceanogr., 38, 1333-1337.

Brown J.H., Gillooly J.F., Allen A.P., Savage V.M. & West G.B. (2004). Toward a metabolic theory of ecology. *Ecology*, 85, 1771-1789.

Caron D.A. (1994). Inorganic Nutrients, Bacteria, and the Microbial Loop. *Microb Ecol*, 28, 295-298.

Carpenter S.R., Morrice J.A., Soranno J.A., Elser J.J., Mackay N.A. & St Amand A. (1993). Dynamics of primary production and nutrients. In: *The trophic cascades in lakes* (eds. Carpenter SR & Kitchell JF). Cambridge University Press Cambridge, UK, pp. 225-251.

Cherif M. & Loreau M. (2007). Stoichiometric constraints on resource use, competitive interactions, and elemental cycling in microbial decomposers. *Am Nat*, 169, 709-724.

Cherif M. & Loreau M. (2009). When microbes and consumers determine the limiting nutrient of autotrophs: a theoretical analysis. *P R Soc B*, 276, 487-497.

Chrzanowski T.H. & Kyle M. (1996). Ratios of carbon, nitrogen and phosphorus in Pseudomonas fluorescens as a model for bacterial element ratios and nutrient regeneration. *Aquat Microb Ecol*, 10, 115-122.

Clarholm M. (1994). The Microbial Loop in Soil. *Beyond the Biomass*, 221-230.

Cotter S.C., Simpson S.J., Raubenheimer D. & Wilson K. (2011). Macronutrient balance mediates trade-offs between immune function and life history traits. *Funct Ecol*, 25, 186-198.

Danger M., Daufresne T., Lucas F., Pissard S. & Lacroix G. (2008). Does Liebig's law of the minimum scale up from species to communities? *Oikos*, 117, 1741-1751.

Daufresne T. & Loreau M. (2001a). Ecological stoichiometry, primary producer-decomposer interactions, and ecosystem persistence. *Ecology*, 82, 3069-3082.

Daufresne T. & Loreau M. (2001b). Plant-herbivore interactions and ecological stoichiometry: when do herbivores determine plant nutrient limitation? *Ecol Lett*, 4, 196-206.

DeAngelis D.L. (1992). *Dynamics of nutrient cycling and food webs*. Chapman & Hall, London New York Tokyo [etc.].

DeMott W.R., Gulati R.D. & Siewertsen K. (1998). Effects of phosphorus-deficient diets on the carbon and phosphorus balance of Daphnia magna. *Limnol Oceanogr*, 43, 1147-1161.

Dobberfuhl D.R. & Elser J.J. (2000). Elemental stoichiometry of lower food web components in arctic and temperate lakes. *J Plankton Res*, 22, 1341-1354.

Droop M.R. (1974). Nutrient Status of Algal Cells in Continuous Culture. *J Mar Biol Assoc Uk*, 54, 825-855.

Elser J.J., Acharya K., Kyle M., Cotner J., Makino W., Markow T., Watts T., Hobbie S., Fagan W., Schade J., Hood J. & Sterner R.W. (2003a). Growth rate-stoichiometry couplings in diverse biota. *Ecol Lett*, 6, 936-943.

Elser J.J., Acquisti C. & Kumar S. (2011). Stoichiogenomics: the evolutionary ecology of macromolecular elemental composition. *Trends Ecol Evol*, 26, 38-44.

Elser J.J., Dobberfuhl D.R., MacKay N.A. & Schampel J.H. (1996). Organism size, life history, and N:P stoichiometry. *Bioscience*, 46, 674-684.

Elser J.J., Elser M.M., Mackay N.A. & Carpenter S.R. (1988). Zooplankton-Mediated Transitions between N-Limited and P-Limited Algal Growth. *Limnol Oceanogr*, 33, 1-14.

Elser J.J., Fagan W.F., Denno R.F., Dobberfuhl D.R., Folarin A., Huberty A., Interlandi S., Kilham S.S., McCauley E., Schulz K.L., Siemann E.H. & Sterner R.W. (2000). Nutritional constraints in terrestrial and freshwater food webs. *Nature*, 408, 578-580.

Elser J.J. & Hassett R.P. (1994). A Stoichiometric Analysis of the Zooplankton-Phytoplankton Interaction in Marine and Fresh-Water Ecosystems. *Nature*, 370, 211-213.

Elser J.J., Kyle M.M., Smith M.S. & Nagy J.D. (2007). Biological Stoichiometry in Human Cancer. *Plos One*, 2, -.

Elser J.J., Nagy J.D. & Kuang Y. (2003b). Biological stoichiometry: An ecological perspective on tumor dynamics. *Bioscience*, 53, 1112-1120.

Elser J.J. & Urabe J. (1999). The stoichiometry of consumer-driven nutrient recycling: Theory, observations, and consequences. *Ecology*, 80, 735-751.

Elser J.J., Watts J., Schampel J.H. & Farmer J. (2006). Early Cambrian food webs on a trophic knife-edge? A hypothesis and preliminary data from a modern stromatolite-based ecosystem. *Ecol Lett*, 9, 292-300.

Elton, C. S. 1927. Animal ecology. London,: Sidgwick & Jackson, ltd.

Falkowski P.G. (2000). Rationalizing elemental ratios in unicellular algae. *J Phycol*, 36, 3-6.

Fraústo da Silva J.J.R. & Williams R.J.P. (2001). *The Biological Chemistry of the Elements: The Inorganic Chemistry of Life*. 2nd Edition edn. Oxford University Press.

Frost P.C., Stelzer R.S., Lamberti G.A. & Elser J.J. (2002). Ecological stoichiometry of trophic interactions in the benthos: understanding the role of C : N : P ratios in lentic and lotic habitats. *J N Am Benthol Soc*, 21, 515-528.

Geider R.J. & La Roche J. (2002). Redfield revisited: variability of C : N : P in marine microalgae and its biochemical basis. *Eur J Phycol*, 37, 1-17.

Goldman J.C., Mccarthy J.J. & Peavey D.G. (1979). Growth-Rate Influence on the Chemical Composition of Phytoplankton in Oceanic Waters. *Nature*, 279, 210-215.

Griffith E.J., Ponnamperuma C. & Gabel N.W. (1977). Phosphorus, a Key to Life on Primitive Earth. *Origins Life Evol B*, 8, 71-85.

Grover J.P. & Chrzanowski T.H. (2006). Stoichiometry and growth kinetics in the "smallest zooplankton" - phagotrophic flagellates. *Arch Hydrobiol*, 167, 467-487.

Grzymski J.J. & Dussaq A.M. (2011). The significance of nitrogen cost minimization in proteomes of marine microorganisms. *ISME J.*

Hall S.R., Knight C.J., Becker C.R., Duffy M.A., Tessier A.J. & Caceres C.E. (2009). Quality matters: resource quality for hosts and the timing of epidemics. *Ecol Lett*, 12, 118-128.

Hardin, G. 1960. Competitive Exclusion Principle. - Science 131: 1292-1297.

Harte J. & Kinzig A.P. (1993). Mutualism and Competition between Plants and Decomposers - Implications for Nutrient Allocation in Ecosystems. *Am Nat*, 141, 829-846.

Hessen D.O. (1992). Nutrient Element Limitation of Zooplankton Production. *Am Nat*, 140, 799-814.

Hutchinson G. E. (1961). The Paradox of the Plankton. Am Nat, 95, 137-145.

Jeyasingh P.D. & Weider L.J. (2007). Fundamental links between genes and elements: evolutionary implications of ecological stoichiometry. *Mol Ecol*, 16, 4649-4661.

Karpinets T.V., Greenwood D.J., Sams C.E. & Ammons J.T. (2006). RNA: protein ratio of the unicellular organism as a characteristic of phosphorous and nitrogen stoichiometry and of the cellular requirement of ribosomes for protein synthesis. *Bmc Biol*, 4.

Klausmeier C.A., Litchman E., Daufresne T. & Levin S.A. (2004). Optimal nitrogen-to-phosphorus stoichiometry of phytoplankton. *Nature*, 429, 171-174.

Lehman J.T. (1984). Grazing, nutrient release, and their impacts on the structure of phytoplankton communities. In: *Trophic interactions within aquatic ecosystems* (eds. Myers DG & Strickler JR). Westview Press Boulder, Colorado, USA, pp. 49-72.

Leon J.A. & Tumpson D.B. (1975). Competition between 2 Species for 2 Complementary or Substitutable Resources. *J Theor Biol*, 50, 185-201.

Lindeman R.L. (1942). The trophic-dynamic aspect of ecology. *Ecology*, 23, 399-418.

Loreau M. (2010). *From Populations to Ecosystems: Theoretical Foundations for a New Ecological Synthesis*. Princeton University Press, Princeton, NJ.

Lotka A.J. (1925). *Elements of Physical Biology*. Williams & Wilkins Company, Baltimore, Md, USA.

Lovelock J.E. & Margulis L. (1974). Atmospheric Homeostasis by and for Biosphere - Gaia Hypothesis. *Tellus*, 26, 2-10.

Lovelock J.E. & Watson A.J. (1982). The Regulation of Carbon-Dioxide and Climate - Gaia or Geochemistry. *Planet Space Sci*, 30, 795-802.

Macarthur R.H. & Levins R. (1964). Competition Habitat Selection + Character Displacement in Patchy Environment. *P Natl Acad Sci USA*, 51, 1207-&.

MacKay N.A. & Elser J.J. (1998). Nutrient recycling by Daphnia reduces N-2 fixation by cyanobacteria. *Limnol Oceanogr*, 43, 347-354.

Main T.M., Dobberfuhl D.R. & Elser J.J. (1997). N : P stoichiometry and ontogeny of crustacean zooplankton: A test of the growth rate hypothesis. *Limnol Oceanogr*, 42, 1474-1478.

Makino W., Cotner J.B., Sterner R.W. & Elser J.J. (2003). Are bacteria more like plants or animals? Growth rate and resource dependence of bacterial C : N : P stoichiometry. *Funct Ecol*, 17, 121-130.

Markow T.A., Watts T., Woods H.A., Hargand S. & Elser J.J. (2006). Biological stoichiometry of growth in Drosophila melanogaster. *J Insect Physiol*, 52, 187-193.

Matzek V. & Vitousek P.M. (2009). N : P stoichiometry and protein : RNA ratios in vascular plants: an evaluation of the growth-rate hypothesis. *Ecol Lett*, 12, 765-771.

Mcelroy M.B. (1983). Atmospheric Composition - Influence of Biology. *Planet Space Sci*, 31, 1065-1074.

Mitra A. & Flynn K.J. (2005). Predator-prey interactions: is 'ecological stoichiometry' sufficient when good food goes bad? *J Plankton Res*, 27, 393-399.

Mitra A. & Flynn K.J. (2007). Importance of interactions between food quality, quantity, and gut transit time on consumer feeding, growth, and trophic dynamics. *Am Nat*, 169, 632-646.

Moegenburg S.M. & Vanni M.J. (1991). Nutrient Regeneration by Zooplankton - Effects on Nutrient Limitation of Phytoplankton in a Eutrophic Lake. *J Plankton Res*, 13, 573-588.

Morehouse N.I., Nakazawa T., Booher C.M., Jeyasingh P.D. & Hall M.D. (2010). Sex in a material world: why the study of sexual reproduction and sex-specific traits should become more nutritionally-explicit. *Oikos*, 119, 766-778.

Müller-Navarra D. (1995). Evidence That a Highly Unsaturated Fatty-Acid Limits Daphnia Growth in Nature. Archiv Fur Hydrobiol, 132, 297-307.

Nakano S. (1994). Carbon - Nitrogen - Phosphorus Ratios and Nutrient Regeneration of a Heterotrophic Flagellate Fed on Bacteria with Different Elemental Ratios. *Arch Hydrobiol*, 129, 257-271.

Nakazawa T. (2011). The ontogenetic stoichiometric bottleneck stabilizes herbivore-autotroph dynamics. *Ecol Res*, 26, 209-216.

Pienta K.J., McGregor N., Axelrod R. & Axelrod D.E. (2008). Ecological Therapy for Cancer: Defining Tumors Using an Ecosystem Paradigm Suggests New Opportunities for Novel Cancer Treatments. *Transl Oncol*, 1, 158-164.

Playfair L., Baron & Liebig J.v. (1843). *Chemistry in its applications to agriculture and physiology, by Justus Liebig,... Edited... by Lyon Playfair,... 3d edition*. printed for Taylor and Walton, London.

Rapport D.J. (1971). Optimization Model of Food Selection. *Am Nat*, 105, 575-&.
Raubenheimer D., Simpson S.J. & Mayntz D. (2009). Nutrition, ecology and nutritional ecology: toward an integrated framework. *Funct Ecol*, 23, 4-16.
Redfield A.C. (1934). *On the proportions of organic derivatives in sea water and their relation to the composition of plankton*. University Press of Liverpool.
Redfield A.C. (1958). The biological control of chemical factors in the environment. *American Scientist*, 46, 205-211.
Reiners W.A. (1986). Complementary Models for Ecosystems. *Am Nat*, 127, 59-73.
Rhee G.Y. (1978). Effects of N-P Atomic Ratios and Nitrate Limitation on Algal Growth, Cell Composition, and Nitrate Uptake. *Limnol Oceanogr*, 23, 10-25.
Rothhaupt K.O. (1997). Grazing and nutrient influences of Daphnia and Eudiaptomus on phytoplankton in laboratory microcosms. *J Plankton Res*, 19, 125-139.
Schade J.D., Kyle M., Hobbie S.E., Fagan W.F. & Elser J.J. (2003). Stoichiometric tracking of soil nutrients by a desert insect herbivore. *Ecol Lett*, 6, 96-101.
Smith S.V. (1984). Phosphorus Versus Nitrogen Limitation in the Marine-Environment. *Limnol Oceanogr*, 29, 1149-1160.
Smith V. (2007). Host resource supplies influence the dynamics and outcome of infectious disease. *Integr Comp Biol*, 47, 310-316.
Sommer U. (1985). Comparison between Steady-State and Non-Steady State Competition - Experiments with Natural Phytoplankton. *Limnol Oceanogr*, 30, 335-346.
Souza V., Eguiarte L.E., Siefert J. & Elser J.J. (2008). Opinion - Microbial endemism: does phosphorus limitation enhance speciation? *Nat Rev Microbiol*, 6, 559-564.
Sterner R.W. (1990). The Ratio of Nitrogen to Phosphorus Resupplied by Herbivores - Zooplankton and the Algal Competitive Arena. *Am Nat*, 136, 209-229.
Sterner R.W. & Elser J.J. (2002). *Ecological stoichiometry : the biology of elements from molecules to the biosphere*. Princeton University Press, Princeton.
Sterner R.W., Elser J.J. & Hessen D.O. (1992). Stoichiometric Relationships among Producers, Consumers and Nutrient Cycling in Pelagic Ecosystems. *Biogeochemistry*, 17, 49-67.
Sterner R.W., Hagemeier D.D. & Smith W.L. (1993). Phytoplankton Nutrient Limitation and Food Quality for Daphnia. *Limnol Oceanogr*, 38, 857-871.
Sterner R.W. & Smith R.F. (1993). Clearance, Ingestion and Release of N and P by Daphnia-Obtusa Feeding on Scenedesmus-Acutus of Varying Quality. *B Mar Sci*, 53, 228-239.
Tett P., Heaney S.I. & Droop M.R. (1985). The Redfield Ratio and Phytoplankton Growth-Rate. *J Mar Biol Assoc Uk*, 65, 487-504.
Tilman D. (1980). Resources - a Graphical-Mechanistic Approach to Competition and Predation. *Am Nat*, 116, 362-393.
Tilman D., Kilham S.S. & Kilham P. (1982). Phytoplankton Community Ecology - the Role of Limiting Nutrients. *Annu Rev Ecol Syst*, 13, 349-372.
Urabe J. (1993). N-Cycling and P-Cycling Coupled by Grazers Activities - Food Quality and Nutrient Release by Zooplankton. *Ecology*, 74, 2337-2350.
Urabe J., Clasen J. & Sterner R.W. (1997). Phosphorus limitation of Daphnia growth: Is it real? *Limnol Oceanogr*, 42, 1436-1443.
Urabe J. & Shimizu Y. (2008). Regulation of phosphorus stoichiometry and growth rate of consumers: theoretical and experimental analyses with Daphnia. *Oecologia*, 155, 21-31.

Urabe J. & Sterner R.W. (2001). Contrasting effects of different types of resource depletion on life-history traits in Daphnia. *Funct Ecol*, 15, 165-174.

Urabe J. & Watanabe Y. (1992). Possibility of N-Limitation or P-Limitation for Planktonic Cladocerans - an Experimental Test. *Limnol Oceanogr*, 37, 244-251.

Vanni M.J., Flecker A.S., Hood J.M. & Headworth J.L. (2002). Stoichiometry of nutrient recycling by vertebrates in a tropical stream: linking species identity and ecosystem processes. *Ecol Lett*, 5, 285-293.

Waksman S.A. (1917). The influence of available carbohydrates upon ammonia accumulation by microorganisms. *J Am Chem Soc*, 39, 1503-1512.

Walker J.C.G. (1974). Stability of Atmospheric Oxygen. *Am J Sci*, 274, 193-214.

Woods H.A., Perkins M.C., Elser J.J. & Harrison J.F. (2002). Absorption and storage of phosphorus by larval Manduca sexta. *J Insect Physiol*, 48, 555-564.

Zehnder C.B. & Hunter M.D. (2009). More is not necessarily better: the impact of limiting and excessive nutrients on herbivore population growth rates. *Ecol Entomol*, 34, 535-543.